Brain Aging and Alzheimer's Disease: Translational and Clinical Research

Brain Aging and Alzheimer's Disease: Translational and Clinical Research

Editor: Nolan Morales

AMERICAN
MEDICAL PUBLISHERS
www.americanmedicalpublishers.com

AMERICAN
MEDICAL PUBLISHERS
www.americanmedicalpublishers.com

Cataloging-in-Publication Data

Brain aging and alzheimer's disease : translational and clinical research / edited by Nolan Morales.
p. cm.
Includes bibliographical references and index.
ISBN 978-1-63927-942-5
1. Brain--Aging. 2. Alzheimer's disease. 3. Central nervous system--Aging.
4. Alzheimer's disease--Pathophysiology. 5. Brain--Aging--Pathophysiology.
6. Alzheimer's disease--Treatment. I. Morales, Nolan.
QP430 .B73 2023
612.82--dc23

American Medical Publishers,
41 Flatbush Avenue,
1st Floor, New York,
NY 11217, USA

ISBN 978-1-63927-942-5 (Hardback)

Contents

Preface

Brain aging refers to the structural, chemical, and functional changes in the brain due to old age. It is a major risk factor for neurodegenerative diseases such as Alzheimer's disease, Parkinson's disease and cerebrovascular disease. Alzheimer's disease is a neurodegenerative disease which results in short term memory loss, mood swings and disorientation. Diagnosis of this medical condition is conducted through diagnostic imaging, medical history and behavioral observations. Imagining techniques such as positron emission tomography (PET) are utilized for extensive imaging of tau tangles and amyloid beta (Aβ) plaques in order to predict the likelihood of Alzheimer's disease. There is no known cure for this disease, therefore clinical and translational research focuses on clinical trials for studying the safety and efficiency of upcoming therapies. This book elucidates the concepts and innovative models around prospective developments with respect to clinical and translational research on brain aging and Alzheimer's disease. The readers would gain knowledge that would broaden their perspective in this area.

This book unites the global concepts and researches in an organized manner for a comprehensive understanding of the subject. It is a ripe text for all researchers, students, scientists or anyone else who is interested in acquiring a better knowledge of this dynamic field.

I extend my sincere thanks to the contributors for such eloquent research chapters. Finally, I thank my family for being a source of support and help.

Editor

1

Early-Life Cognitive Activity is Related to Reduced Neurodegeneration in Alzheimer Signature Regions in Late Life

*Kang Ko[1,2], Min Soo Byun[3], Dahyun Yi[3], Jun Ho Lee[1,4], Chan Hyung Kim[2,5] and Dong Young Lee[1,3,4]**

[1] Department of Neuropsychiatry, Seoul National University Hospital, Seoul, South Korea, [2] Department of Psychiatry, Yonsei University College of Medicine, Seoul, South Korea, [3] Institute of Human Behavioral Medicine, Medical Research Center, Seoul National University, Seoul, South Korea, [4] Department of Psychiatry, Seoul National University College of Medicine, Seoul, South Korea, [5] Institute of Behavioral Science in Medicine, Yonsei University College of Medicine, Seoul, South Korea

***Correspondence:**
Dong Young Lee
selfpsy@snu.ac.kr

†Information of the KBASE Research Group is provided in the online Supplemental Material.

Background: Although increased cognitive activity (CA), both current and past, is known to be associated with a decreased occurrence of Alzheimer's disease (AD) dementia in older adults, the exact neural mechanisms underlying the association between CA during different stages of life and human dementia remain unclear. Therefore, we investigated whether CA during different life stages is associated with cerebral amyloid-beta (Aβ) pathology and AD-related neurodegeneration in non-demented older adults.

Methods: Cross-sectional analyses of data collected between April 2014 and March 2016 from the Korean Brain Aging Study for Early Diagnosis and Prediction of Alzheimer's Disease (KBASE), an ongoing prospective cohort. In total, 321 community-dwelling, non-demented older adults were involved in this study. Cerebral Aβ deposition and Aβ positivity were measured using ^{11}C-Pittsburgh compound B (PiB)-positron emission tomography (PET). AD-signature region cerebral glucose metabolism (AD-CMglu) and AD-signature region neurodegeneration (AD-ND) positivity were measured using ^{18}F-fluorodeoxyglucose (FDG)-PET. In addition, CA in early, mid, and late life was systematically evaluated using a structured questionnaire.

Results: Of the 321 participants, 254 were cognitively normal (CN) and 67 had mild cognitive impairment (MCI). The mean age of participants was 69.6 years old [standard deviation (SD) = 8.0]. Higher early-life CA (CA_{early}) was associated with significantly increased AD-CMglu (B = 0.035, SE = 0.013, P = 0.009) and a decreasing trend of AD-ND positivity (OR = 0.65, 95% CI 0.43–0.98, P = 0.04) but was not associated with Aβ deposition or positivity. We observed no association between midlife CA (CA_{mid}) and any AD-related brain changes. Late-life CA (CA_{late}) showed an association with both global Aβ deposition and AD-CMglu, although it was not statistically significant. Sensitivity analyses controlling for current depression or conducted only for CN individuals revealed similar results.

Conclusion: Our results suggest that CA in early life may be protective against late-life AD-related neurodegeneration, independently of cerebral Aβ pathology.

Keywords: cognitive activity, early life, midlife, late life, Alzheimer's disease, neurodegeneration, amyloid beta deposition, the KBASE study

INTRODUCTION

Increased cognitive activity (CA), both current and past, is known to be associated with reduced cognitive decline (Marquine et al., 2012; Wilson et al., 2012, 2013; Hughes et al., 2015; Arfanakis et al., 2016) and the occurrence of Alzheimer's disease (AD) dementia (Wilson et al., 2002a, 2007; Sattler et al., 2012) in the elderly. However, the exact pathological process underlying this inverse association between CA and AD dementia remains unclear.

To explore the pathological process, several studies investigated the association between the degree of CA and both cerebral amyloid-beta (Aβ) pathology (Landau et al., 2012; Vemuri et al., 2012, 2016, 2017; Wirth et al., 2014; Gidicsin et al., 2015) and neurodegeneration (Valenzuela et al., 2008; Vemuri et al., 2012, 2016, 2017; Gidicsin et al., 2015) using *in vivo* AD neuroimaging biomarkers. The results from these studies are, however, controversial. One possible explanation for this controversy is that the brain has different physiological or pathological properties during different stages of life. The influence of a certain life experience, such as CA, on the brain may vary at different stages of life. Nevertheless, most previous studies exploring the association between CA and AD biomarkers did not take into account different life stages and simply classified all CA into simple categories, mainly current or past (Landau et al., 2012; Vemuri et al., 2012; Gidicsin et al., 2015), or focused only on either midlife CA (CA_{mid}) (Vemuri et al., 2016, 2017) or late-life CA (CA_{late}) (Valenzuela et al., 2008).

Early life (i.e., childhood and early adulthood) is a critical period for brain development characterized by neural plasticity (Chugani et al., 1987; Andersen, 2003; Dekhtyar et al., 2016). Previous studies have shown that early-life CA (CA_{early}) is associated with reduced late-life cognitive decline and progression to cognitive disorders in later life (Wilson et al., 2013, 2015; Dekhtyar et al., 2016), suggesting that CA_{early} is closely related to increases in cognitive reserve (CR). CR refers to functional rather than structural or quantitative aspects of the brain, and may explain why some people are more resilient to cognitive decline than others who present with the same level of pathology (Stern, 2012). In contrast, CA in mid or late life stages is less beneficial to individuals, given that brain plasticity is limited during mid- and late life (Leuner et al., 2007; Kolb and Gibb, 2011).

The accumulation of cerebral Aβ pathology begins 10–20 years prior to AD dementia (Villemagne et al., 2013) and its prevalence in non-demented persons typically increases from mid- to late life (Jansen et al., 2015). Thus, cerebral Aβ pathology is rarely observed in the early-life period. Therefore, it is more reasonable to assume that CA or other brain affecting activities may influence the occurrence of Aβ pathology when they are applied in mid or late life rather than in early life. Some studies have reported an association between CA_{mid} and Aβ deposition (Wirth et al., 2014; Vemuri et al., 2016). In the case of late life, however, about half of the cognitively healthy elderly already have amyloid or neurodegeneration abnormalities and the estimated frequency of normal AD biomarker status decreases continuously with age (Jack et al., 2014). Therefore, the accumulation of amyloid and/or neurodegeneration itself might reduce participation in CA in late life, although a few studies have reported a beneficial effect of congitive training or exercise in late life on brain function as well as cognive performance (Snowball et al., 2013; Shah et al., 2014; Lampit et al., 2015).

We hypothesized that CA during different stages of life is differentially associated with cerebral Aβ pathology and AD-related neurodegeneration in non-demented older adults. More specifically, we formulated three working hypotheses. First, CA_{early} is inversely associated with the degree of AD-related neurodegeneration, including neuronal or synaptic dysfunction in late life. Second, CA_{mid} is inversely associated with cerebral Aβ pathology in late life. Third, CA_{late} is inversely associated with both cerebral Aβ pathology and AD-related neurodegeneration in late life.

To test our hypotheses, we measured cerebral Aβ pathology using ^{11}C-Pittsburgh compound B (PiB)-positron emission tomography (PET) and AD-related neurodegeneration using ^{18}F-fluorodeoxyglucose (FDG)-PET. We selected cerebral glucose metabolism (CMglu) on FDG-PET as a neurodegeneration marker because it is a reliable index of regional neuronal or synaptic function (Sokoloff, 1981; Jueptner and Weiller, 1995), and specific regional hypometabolism in the temporo-parietal cortices is a reliable and sensitive measure of AD-related neurodegeneration, which appears earlier than structural brain changes on magnetic resonance imaging (MRI) (Jack et al., 2014, 2015, 2016). CA in early, mid, and late life was assessed using a structured questionnaire (Wilson et al., 2005, 2007; Barnes et al., 2006). We further investigated the moderating effects of apolipoprotein E ε4 (*APOE4*) on the relationship between CA and AD-related brain changes, as CA is particularly protective in *APOE4* carriers for the risk of dementia onset (Carlson et al., 2008) and Aβ accumulation (Wirth et al., 2014; Vemuri et al., 2016).

MATERIALS AND METHODS

Participants

This study was part of the Korean Brain Aging Study for Early Diagnosis and Prediction of Alzheimer's Disease (KBASE), an ongoing prospective cohort study, which began in 2014 and was designed to identify novel biomarkers for AD and explore various lifetime experiences contributing to AD-related brain changes. The current study included 321 community-dwelling elderly individuals without dementia who were at least 55 years old and enrolled between April 2014 and March 2016.

The study participants consisted of 254 cognitively normal (CN) and 67 subjects with mild cognitive impairment (MCI). All individuals with MCI met the current consensus criteria for amnestic MCI: (1) memory complaints confirmed by an informant; (2) objective memory impairment, (3) preserved global cognitive function; (4) independence in functional activities; and (5) no dementia. All MCI individuals had a global clinical dementia rating (CDR) of 0.5. In terms of Criterion 2, the age-, education-, and gender-adjusted z-scores for at least 1 of the 4 episodic memory tests was less than −1.0. The four memory tests included Word List Memory, Word List Recall, Word List Recognition, and Constructional Recall tests, which are included in the Korean version of the Consortium to Establish a Registry for Alzheimer's Disease (CERAD-K) neuropsychological battery. The CN group consisted of participants with a global CDR of 0 and lack of an MCI or dementia diagnosis. The exclusion criteria were current serious medical, psychiatric, or neurological disorders that may influence mental functioning; the presence of severe communication problems that would hinder the clinical interview or brain imaging process; *in vivo* devices or a mental status that prevented us from performing the brain MRI; absence of a reliable informant; illiteracy; participation in a different clinical trial; and treatment with an investigational product. The Institutional Review Board of the Seoul National University Hospital and Seoul Metropolitan Government-Seoul National University Boramae Medical Center, South Korea, approved this study, and subjects and their legal representatives provided written consent.

Clinical Assessment

All participants received standardized clinical assessments by trained psychiatrists based on the KBASE clinical assessment protocol, which incorporated the CERAD-K (Lee et al., 2002). KBASE neuropsychological assessments incorporating the CERAD-K neuropsychological battery (Lee et al., 2004) were also administered to all participants by trained neuropsychologists. Genomic DNA was extracted from whole blood and apolipoprotein E (*APOE*) genotyping was performed as described previously (Wenham et al., 1991). *APOE4* carrier status was considered positive if the participant had at least one *APOE4* allele.

Assessment of Early-, Mid-, and Late-Life CA

Participant CA was assessed using a 39-item expanded version (Wilson et al., 2005, 2007; Barnes et al., 2006) of a previously reported 25-item autobiographical questionnaire (Wilson et al., 2003; Landau et al., 2012), which was shown to have sufficient internal consistency and temporal stability. Items included relatively common activities with few barriers to participation, such as reading newspapers, magazines, or books; visiting a museum or library; attending a concert, play, or musical; writing letters; and playing games. Individuals completed the questionnaire at a baseline evaluation point. Frequency of participation was rated from 1 (once a year or less) to 5 (daily or approximately daily). There were 9 current (i.e., late life) activities and 30 previous activities including 11 related to childhood (6–12 years of age), 10 related to young adulthood (18 years of age), and 9 related to midlife (40 years of age). Item scores were averaged to yield separate values for each age period. The CA_{early} score was determined by averaging childhood and young adulthood scores.

PiB-PET Acquisition and Processing

Participants underwent simultaneous three-dimensional (3D) PiB-PET and 3D T1-weighted MRI using a 3.0T Biograph mMR (PET-MR) scanner (Siemens, Washington, DC, United States) according to the manufacturer's protocols. Details of PiB-PET imaging acquisition and preprocessing are described elsewhere (Supplementary Material).

The automatic anatomic labeling algorithm and a region combining method (Reiman et al., 2009) were conducted to determine regions of interest (ROIs) and to characterize the PiB retention level in the frontal, lateral parietal, posterior cingulate-precuneus, and lateral temporal regions. The standardized uptake value ratios (SUVRs) were calculated by dividing the mean value for all voxels within each ROI by the mean cerebellar uptake value in the same image. Each participant was classified as cerebral Aβ positive if the SUVR value was >1.4. A global cortical ROI consisting of the four ROIs was defined, and a global Aβ deposition value was generated by dividing the mean value for all voxels of the global cortical ROI by the mean cerebellar uptake value in the same image (Choe et al., 2014).

FDG-PET Acquisition and Processing

Participants also underwent FDG-PET imaging using the same PET-MR machine, as described above. Details of FDG-PET image acquisition and preprocessing are described in the Supplementary Material. AD-signature FDG ROIs including the angular gyri, posterior cingulate cortex, and inferior temporal gyri, which are known to be sensitive to changes associated with AD (Jack et al., 2014, 2015) were determined. AD-signature region cerebral glucose metabolism (AD-CMglu) was defined as a voxel-weighted mean SUVR extracted from the AD-signature FDG ROIs, and AD-signature region neurodegeneration (AD-ND) positivity was defined as AD-CMglu <1.386. Detailed methods used to define the threshold for abnormality of each neurodegeneration biomarker are described in the Supplementary Material.

Statistical Analysis

The associations between CA (independent variable) at each life stage and global Aβ deposition or AD-CMglu (dependent variables) were examined using multiple linear regression analyses controlling for age, sex, years of education, and *APOE4* carrier status as covariates. Multiple logistic regression analyses were conducted to test the association between CA at each life stage (independent variable) and Aβ or AD-ND positivity (independent variables). In this analysis, we also controlled for age, sex, years of education, and *APOE4* carrier status. Sensitivity analyses were conducted using the same analyses, but included only CN subjects to exclude the possibility of recall bias due to MCI. We also performed the same analyses but additionally controlled for geriatric depression using the Geriatric Depression Scale (GDS) (Yesavage et al., 1983), since current depression may influence CA and brain state. We set a *P*-value less than 0.0167 (=0.05/3) as the threshold for statistical significance, given that CA during the three life stages (i.e., CA_{early}, CA_{mid}, and CA_{late}) were explored for AD-related brain changes. In the event that CA significantly influences Aβ-related brain changes, we further explored the moderating effects of *APOE4* using a generalized linear model analysis, including a

CA × *APOE4* interaction term, as well as CA and *APOE4* as independent variables, controlling for age, sex, and education as covariates. In this case, a *P*-value less than 0.05 was indicative of statistical significance. All statistical analyses were conducted using SPSS Statistics version 23.0 (IBM Corp., Armonk, NY, United States).

RESULTS

The characteristics of the study participants are shown in **Table 1**. Both global Aβ deposition and AD-CMglu were weakly correlated with clinical variables. Global Aβ deposition was inversely associated with CERAD total score (Kendall's tau = −0.19, $p < 0.001$) and was positively associated with CDR sum of boxes (Kendall's tau = 0.33, $p < 0.001$). AD-CMglu showed a similar association with CERAD total score (Kendall's tau = 0.16, $p < 0.001$) and was inversely associated with CDR-SOB (Kendall's tau = −0.26, $p < 0.001$). Global Aβ deposition and AD-CMglu were weakly correlated with each other (Kendall's tau = −0.17, $P < 0.001$). CA_{early} was moderately correlated with CA_{mid} (Kendall's tau = 0.52, $P < 0.001$) and CA_{late} (Kendall's tau = 0.43, $P < 0.001$). CA_{mid} and CA_{late} were also moderately correlated (Kendall's tau = 0.51, $P < 0.001$).

Early-Life CA and AD-Related Brain Changes

We observed no association between CA_{early} and global Aβ deposition (**Figure 1A** and **Table 2**). Similarly, no significant association between CA_{early} and Aβ positivity was observed (**Table 3**). In contrast, there was a significant positive association between CA_{early} and AD-CMglu (**Figure 1B** and **Table 2**). We observed a trend for a negative association between CA_{early} and AD-ND positivity, although this was not statistically significant (**Table 3**). We explored moderation effects of *APOE4* on the association between CA_{early} and AD-CMglu, which showed a statistically significant result in the main effect analysis. We observed no CA_{early} × *APOE4* interaction on AD-CMglu (Supplementary Table e-1).

TABLE 1 | Participant characteristics.

Characteristics	All participants
No. of study participants	321
Age, years	69.60 (7.99)
No. of females (%)	180 (56.07)
No. of *ApoE4* carriers (%)[a]	79 (24.61)
Education, year	11.54 (4.69)
MMSE score (maximum, 30)	25.92 (3.35)
GDS score (maximum, 30)	5.53 (5.33)
MCI, no. (%)	67 (20.87)
CA score (maximum, 5)	
Early life	2.24 (0.69)
Midlife	2.37 (0.82)
Late life	2.57 (0.73)
Global cerebral Aβ deposition, SUVR	1.28 (0.37)
Aβ positivity (%)	68 (21.18)
AD-CMglu, SUVR	1.39 (0.13)
AD-ND positivity (%)	151 (47.04)

APOE4, apolipoprotein E ε4; MMSE, Mini-Mental State Examination; GDS, Geriatric Depression Scale; MCI, mild cognitive impairment; CA, cognitive activity; Aβ, amyloid-beta; SUVR, standardized uptake value ratio; AD-CMglu, Alzheimer's disease signature region cerebral glucose metabolism; AD-ND, AD-signature region neurodegeneration. Data are presented as mean (SD) unless otherwise indicated. [a]ApoE4 carriers are the percentage of individuals with at least one APOE4 allele.

Midlife CA and AD-Related Brain Changes

We observed no association between CA_{mid} and global Aβ deposition or AD-CMglu (**Figures 1C,D** and **Table 2**). CA_{mid} was also not associated with Aβ or AD-ND positivity (**Table 3**).

Late-Life CA and AD-Related Brain Changes

We observed a trend-level association between CA_{late} and both global Aβ deposition and AD-CMglu, although this association was not significant (**Figures 1E,F** and **Table 2**). CA_{late} was not associated with Aβ or AD-ND positivity (**Table 3**).

Sensitivity Analysis

Even when the GDS was additionally controlled for age, education, gender, and *APOE4*, the results from the multiple linear or logistic regression analyses were similar (Supplementary Tables e-2, e-3). When the same analyses were conducted for the CN subgroup only, CA_{early} showed trend-level associations with AD-CMglu and AD-ND positivity (Supplementary Tables e-4, e-5), although the association was not statistically significant. We observed no association between CA_{mid} or CA_{late} and any AD-related brain changes. Moreover, because CA_{early} was correlated with CA_{mid} and CA_{late}, we controlled for CA_{early} in addition to age, sex, education, and *APOE4* when analyzing the relationship of CA_{mid} or CA_{late} to AD-related brain changes. As shown in the Supplementary Tables e-6, e-7, the results were almost the same, even after controlling for the effects of CA_{early}.

DISCUSSION

The results of this study generally support the hypothesis that CA during different life stages is differentially associated with cerebral Aβ pathology and AD-related neurodegeneration in non-demented older adults. With regard to the three working hypotheses, our findings supported the first hypothesis: CA_{early} was inversely associated with the degree of AD-related neurodegeneration in late life. In contrast, we could not accept the second hypothesis (i.e., an inverse association between CA_{mid} and cerebral Aβ pathology in late life) or the third (i.e., a significant inverse association between CA_{late} and both cerebral Aβ pathology and AD-related neurodegeneration in late life).

Our study is the first to verify the association between CA_{early} and AD-CMglu in late life, suggesting the presence

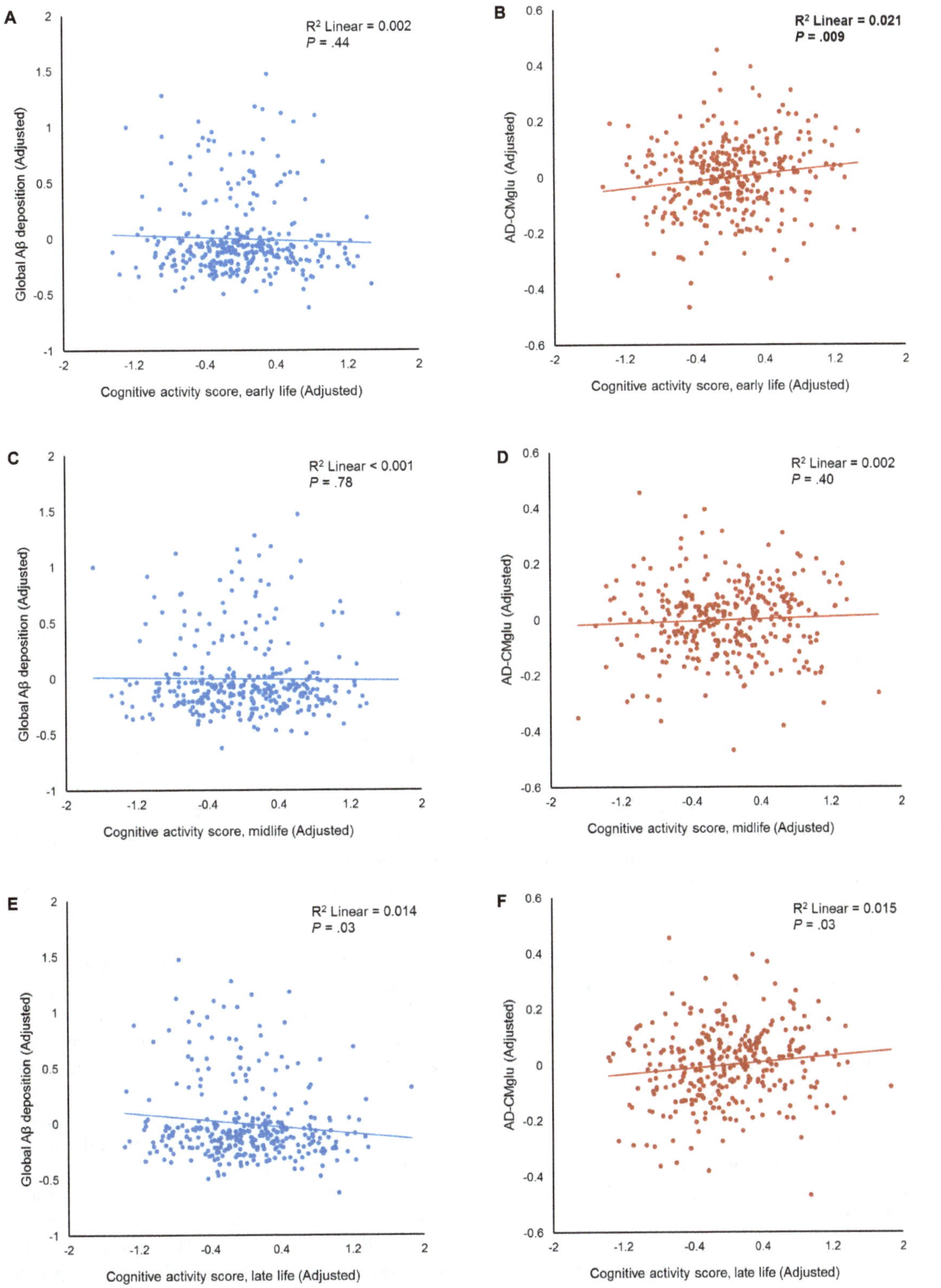

FIGURE 1 | Partial regression plots showing the effect of participating in cognitive activity (CA) during each life period. The results of the independent multiple linear regression model with age, gender, education, and apolipoprotein E ε4 as covariates are presented. **(A,B)** Plots for early-life CA (CA_{early}) and amyloid-beta (Aβ), as well as for Alzheimer's disease signature region cerebral glucose metabolism (AD-CMglu). A significant association was observed between CA_{early} and AD-CMglu, but not Aβ. **(C,D)** Plots for midlife CA (CA_{mid}) and Aβ, as well as for AD-CMglu. **(E,F)** Plots for late-life CA (CA_{late}) and Aβ, as well as for AD-CMglu.

TABLE 2 | Association between cognitive activities (CAs) in each life period and global cerebral amyloid-beta (Aβ) deposition and Alzheimer's disease signature region cerebral glucose metabolism (AD-CMglu).

	B	SE	Beta	*P*	P_B
Global Aβ deposition					
Early life	−0.028	0.036	−0.052	0.44	>0.99
Midlife	−0.009	0.032	−0.020	0.78	>0.99
Late life	−0.072	0.033	−0.142	0.03	0.10
AD-CMglu					
Early life	0.035	0.013	0.180	0.009	0.03
Midlife	0.010	0.012	0.061	0.40	>0.99
Late life	0.028	0.013	0.150	0.03	0.08

Aβ, amyloid-beta; AD-CMglu, Alzheimer's disease signature region cerebral glucose metabolism. The results of the independent multiple linear regression model with age, gender, education, and apolipoprotein E ε4 as covariates are presented. P_B: P-value corrected by Bonferroni's method.

TABLE 3 | Association between cognitive activities in each life period and Aβ and AD-signature region neurodegeneration (AD-ND) positivity.

	Adjusted OR	95% CI	*P*	P_B
Aβ positivity				
Early life	0.840	0.500–1.410	0.51	>0.99
Midlife	0.939	0.594–1.482	0.79	>0.99
Late life	0.786	0.484–1.277	0.33	>0.99
AD-ND positivity				
Early life	0.648	0.427–0.983	0.04	0.13
Midlife	0.790	0.550–1.134	0.20	0.60
Late life	0.712	0.483–1.050	0.09	0.26

OR, odds ratio; CI, confidence interval; Aβ, amyloid-beta; AD-ND, Alzheimer's disease signature region neurodegeneration. The results of the independent multiple logistic regression model with age, gender, education, and apolipoprotein E ε4 as covariates are presented. P_B: P-value corrected by Bonferroni's method.

of a potential mechanism underlying the inverse association between CA_{early} and AD dementia or cognitive decline. Previous studies have reported that childhood CA could reduce cognitive decline (Wilson et al., 2013) and music or foreign language training in early life was associated with a lower risk of MCI or AD dementia (Wilson et al., 2015). Another study showed that a complex occupation could not compensate for low school grades at a young age to prevent dementia, suggesting that early life is a critical period for increasing CR against dementia (Dekhtyar et al., 2016). To the best of our knowledge, no previous human studies have focused on the direct relationship between CA_{early} and brain changes in late life.

The association between CA_{early} and AD-CMglu in late life may be explained by the influence of CA_{early} on brain developmental processes (Chugani et al., 1987; Benes et al., 1994; Paus et al., 1999; Andersen, 2003), such as synaptogenesis and pruning during the early-life period in particular (Tau and Peterson, 2010). As activity-dependent mechanisms could modulate these processes, especially in early life (Bourgeois et al., 1989; Goodman and Shatz, 1993; Hata and Stryker, 1994; Kleim et al., 1996; Baker et al., 2017), it may be that CA_{early} promotes synaptogenesis and/or pruning in humans offers a plausible explanation. Metabolic changes measured by FDG-PET may reflect energy expenditures of these processes (Chugani et al., 1987). Other animal studies also suggest that early-life cognitive enrichment has various protective effects on the brain by increasing neurotrophic factors (Wolf et al., 2006) or gene/protein expression related to synaptic plasticity (Costa et al., 2007). However, the influence of common genetic predisposition cannot be completely excluded when addressing the association between CA_{early} and neurodegeneration in late life. A certain genetic factor may be related to both more CA participation in early life and less neurodegeneration in late life (Fox et al., 2010).

Educational level is associated with the level of CA, regardless of life period (Wilson et al., 2002b, 2013; Barnes et al., 2006; Gidicsin et al., 2015). Our data also show a similar association between years of education and CA_{early} (Kendall's tau = 0.43, $P < 0.001$), CA_{mid} (Kendall's tau = 0.48, $P < 0.001$), and CA_{late} (Kendall's tau = 0.45, $P < 0.001$). A previous report showed that higher-level education, related to early-life enrichment, was associated with reduced age-related alterations of cerebrospinal fluid (CSF) neurodegeneration biomarkers (e.g., CSF total-tau, phosphorylated-tau), but not with amyloid biomarkers (CSF Aβ) (Almeida et al., 2015), similar to our observation for CA_{early}, Aβ pathology, and neurodegeneration. Nevertheless, because the aim of this study was to investigate the differential effect of CA during different life stages on *in vivo* AD pathology, we applied a lifetime CA questionnaire instead of simply using years of education as a measure of CA. In the current study, CA_{early} had a significant inverse relationship with AD-related neurodegeneration, while CA_{mid} and CA_{late} did not, after controlling for the level of education. This finding suggests that CA_{early} itself is potentially protective against late-life neurodegeneration or related cognitive decline, regardless of educational attainment.

An exploratory analysis to investigate the moderating effects of *APOE4* revealed no significant interaction between CA_{early} and *APOE4* on AD-CMglu. This finding may be explained by previous reports indicating that *APOE4*-related cognitive changes generally occur during mid or late life, as opposed to early life (Ruiz et al., 2010; Richter-Schmidinger et al., 2011; Wisdom et al., 2011). A previous meta-analysis of 20 studies also demonstrated that *APOE4* was not associated with cognitive function in young adults, adolescents, or children (Ihle et al., 2012).

Midlife CA was not associated with late-life Aβ deposition, which did not support our second hypothesis. Similar to our current finding, Mayo investigators reported no association between CA_{mid} and late-life Aβ deposition, in general, in non-demented elderly (Vemuri et al., 2016, 2017). They also showed that high CA_{mid} was associated with lower Aβ deposition in highly educated *APOE4* carriers (Vemuri et al., 2016). They proposed that a reverse causality may explain their finding: among highly educated *APOE4* carriers, those with higher Aβ deposition in middle age are most likely to experience subtle cognitive symptoms at that time and, consequently, avoid intellectual activity (Vemuri et al., 2016). We conducted similar analyses for highly educated (>14 years) *APOE4* carriers, but did not find any significant associations between CA_{mid} and Aβ deposition. Such discrepancies may be associated with the time frame for CA_{mid}. We defined CA_{mid} as CA at the age of 40 years, while Mayo investigators measured CA_{mid} at 50–65 years of age. Younger individuals are less likely to be influenced by the reverse causality issue. With respect to neurodegeneration, no association between CA_{mid} and AD-CMglu or AD-ND positivity was observed, which is consistent with previous reports (Vemuri et al., 2016, 2017).

Although not statistically significant, CA_{late} showed a trend association with global Aβ deposition and AD-CMglu. This may be explained by reverse causality: as previously mentioned in the section "Introduction"; elderly individuals with greater AD pathologies may participate in less CA (Jack et al., 2013' Villemagne et al., 2013). This explanation was further supported by the sensitivity analysis conducted for the CN subgroup. In the CN subgroup, no trend level association was observed between CA_{late} and AD-related brain changes, which is consistent with previous reports (Landau et al., 2012; Wirth et al., 2014; Gidicsin et al., 2015).

In a sensitivity analysis, we controlled for the effect of CA_{early} as well as education when analyzing the relationship between CA_{mid} or CA_{late} and global Aβ deposition and AD-CMglu, because CA_{mid} and CA_{late} were correlated with CA_{early}. Controlling for CA_{early} did not change the results, indicating that the negative findings for the relationship of CA_{mid} or CA_{late} with AD-related brain change were significant, regardless of the influence of CA_{early}.

There are several limitations to our study. First, although we used well-validated and reliable questionnaires, retrospective measurements of CA may have a recall bias. Current depression and memory impairment have the potential to affect retrospective measurements based on subjective recall. To mitigate the potential risk, we conducted two sensitivity analyses. We controlled for current depression using the GDS score. This did not change the overall results of our study. Furthermore, the same analyses conducted for the CN group revealed potential associations between CA_{early} and both AD-CMglu and AD-ND positivity, although not statistically significant. Future long-term prospective studies are required to confirm our findings. Second, as for AD-related neurodegeneration, we measured cerebral glucose metabolism by FDG-PET. Although we defined AD-CMglu or AD-ND positivity by applying AD-signature regions showing typical AD-pattern hypometabolism, glucose metabolism may be influenced by non-AD pathologies, such as vascular pathology and non-AD degenerative conditions (Kato et al., 2016). Tau-PET imaging (Saint-Aubert et al., 2016) or CSF phosphorylated tau measurements (Blennow and Hampel, 2003) may provide information to address this issue. Third, we did not consider the influence of potential confounding factors, which may affect the *in vivo* AD pathologies, such as physical activity (Shah et al., 2014), social interaction (Bennett et al., 2006), diet (Berti et al., 2015), oxidative stress (Markesbery, 1997), and various physical conditions, including hypertension, diabetes, obesity, and other chronic illnesses (Chui et al., 2012), although we excluded individuals with serious medical or neurological disorders that may influence mental functioning.

CONCLUSION

Our results support that CA in early life is probably protective against late-life AD-related neurodegeneration, independently of cerebral Aβ pathology. In contrast, CA in midlife and late life appears to have no or limited association with AD-related brain changes, including amyloid pathology and neurodegeneration. With respect to prevention of dementia and cognitive impairment in late life, a cognitively active lifestyle in childhood and early adulthood needs to be more emphasized.

AUTHOR CONTRIBUTIONS

KK and DL designed the study, acquired and interpreted the data, and were major contributors to the writing of the manuscript and critically revising the manuscript for intellectual content. MB, DY, JL, and CK acquired and analyzed the data and helped to draft the manuscript. KK and DY analyzed the imaging data. DL served as the principal investigator and supervised the study. All authors read and approved the final manuscript.

FUNDING

This study was supported by a grant from Ministry of Science and ICT (Grant No. NRF-2014M3C7A1046042).

REFERENCES

Almeida, R. P., Schultz, S. A., Austin, B. P., Boots, E. A., Dowling, N. M., Gleason, C. E., et al. (2015). Effect of cognitive reserve on age-related changes in cerebrospinal fluid biomarkers of Alzheimer disease. *JAMA Neurol.* 72, 699–706. doi: 10.1001/jamaneurol.2015.0098

Andersen, S. L. (2003). Trajectories of brain development: point of vulnerability or window of opportunity? *Neurosci. Biobehav. Rev.* 27, 3–18. doi: 10.1016/s0149-7634(03)00005-8

Arfanakis, K., Wilson, R. S., Barth, C. M., Capuano, A. W., Vasireddi, A., Zhang, S., et al. (2016). Cognitive activity, cognitive function, and brain diffusion characteristics in old age. *Brain Imaging Behav.* 10, 455–463. doi: 10.1007/s11682-015-9405-5

Baker, L. M., Laidlaw, D. H., Cabeen, R., Akbudak, E., Conturo, T. E., Correia, S., et al. (2017). Cognitive reserve moderates the relationship between neuropsychological performance and white matter fiber bundle length in healthy older adults. *Brain Imaging Behav.* 11, 632–639. doi: 10.1007/s11682-016-9540-7

Barnes, L. L., Wilson, R. S., de Leon, C. F., and Bennett, D. A. (2006). The relation of lifetime cognitive activity and lifetime access to resources to late-life cognitive function in older African Americans. *Aging Neuropsychol. Cogn.* 13, 516–528. doi: 10.1080/138255890969519

Benes, F. M., Turtle, M., Khan, Y., and Farol, P. (1994). Myelination of a key relay zone in the hippocampal formation occurs in the human brain during childhood, adolescence, and adulthood. *Arch. Gen. Psychiatry* 51, 477–484.

Bennett, D. A., Schneider, J. A., Tang, Y., Arnold, S. E., and Wilson, R. S. (2006). The effect of social networks on the relation between Alzheimer's disease pathology and level of cognitive function in old people: a longitudinal cohort study. *Lancet Neurol.* 5, 406–412.

Berti, V., Murray, J., Davies, M., Spector, N., Tsui, W. H., Li, Y., et al. (2015). Nutrient patterns and brain biomarkers of Alzheimer's disease in cognitively normal individuals. *J. Nutr. Health Aging* 19, 413–423. doi: 10.1007/s12603-014-0534-0

Blennow, K., and Hampel, H. (2003). CSF markers for incipient Alzheimer's disease. *Lancet Neurol.* 2, 605–613.

Bourgeois, J.-P., Jastreboff, P. J., and Rakic, P. (1989). Synaptogenesis in visual cortex of normal and preterm monkeys: evidence for intrinsic regulation of synaptic overproduction. *Proc. Natl. Acad. Sci. U.S.A.* 86, 4297–4301.

Carlson, M. C., Helms, M. J., Steffens, D. C., Burke, J. R., Potter, G. G., and Plassman, B. L. (2008). Midlife activity predicts risk of dementia in older male twin pairs. *Alzheimers Dement.* 4, 324–331. doi: 10.1016/j.jalz.2008.07.002

Choe, Y. M., Sohn, B. K., Choi, H. J., Byun, M. S., Seo, E. H., Han, J. Y., et al. (2014). Association of homocysteine with hippocampal volume independent of cerebral amyloid and vascular burden. *Neurobiol. Aging* 35, 1519–1525. doi: 10.1016/j.neurobiolaging.2014.01.013

Chugani, H. T., Phelps, M. E., and Mazziotta, J. C. (1987). Positron emission tomography study of human brain functional development. *Ann. Neurol.* 22, 487–497.

Chui, H. C., Zheng, L., Reed, B. R., Vinters, H. V., and Mack, W. J. (2012). Vascular risk factors and Alzheimer's disease: are these risk factors for plaques and tangles or for concomitant vascular pathology that increases the likelihood of dementia? An evidence-based review. *Alzheimers Res. Ther.* 4:1.

Costa, D. A., Cracchiolo, J. R., Bachstetter, A. D., Hughes, T. F., Bales, K. R., Paul, S. M., et al. (2007). Enrichment improves cognition in AD mice by amyloid-related and unrelated mechanisms. *Neurobiol. Aging* 28, 831–844.

Dekhtyar, S., Wang, H.-X., Fratiglioni, L., and Herlitz, A. (2016). Childhood school performance, education and occupational complexity: a life-course study of dementia in the Kungsholmen Project. *Int. J. Epidemiol.* 45, 1207–1215.

Fox, S. E., Levitt, P., and Nelson, C. A. III (2010). How the timing and quality of early experiences influence the development of brain architecture. *Child Dev.* 81, 28–40. doi: 10.1111/j.1467-8624.2009.01380.x

Gidicsin, C. M., Maye, J. E., Locascio, J. J., Pepin, L. C., Philiossaint, M., Becker, J. A., et al. (2015). Cognitive activity relates to cognitive performance but not to Alzheimer disease biomarkers. *Neurology* 85, 48–55. doi: 10.1212/WNL.0000000000001704

Goodman, C. S., and Shatz, C. J. (1993). Developmental mechanisms that generate precise patterns of neuronal connectivity. *Cell* 72, 77–98.

Hata, Y., and Stryker, M. (1994). Control of thalamocortical afferent rearrangement by postsynaptic activity in developing visual cortex. *Science* 265, 1732–1735. doi: 10.1126/science.8085163

Hughes, T. F., Becker, J. T., Lee, C. W., Chang, C. C., and Ganguli, M. (2015). Independent and combined effects of cognitive and physical activity on incident MCI. *Alzheimers Dement.* 11, 1377–1384. doi: 10.1016/j.jalz.2014.11.007

Ihle, A., Bunce, D., and Kliegel, M. (2012). *APOE* ε4 and cognitive function in early life: a meta-analysis. *Neuropsychology* 26, 267–277. doi: 10.1037/a0026769

Jack, C. R., Wiste, H. J., Weigand, S. D., Rocca, W. A., Knopman, D. S., Mielke, M. M., et al. (2014). Age-specific population frequencies of cerebral β-amyloidosis and neurodegeneration among people with normal cognitive function aged 50–89 years: a cross-sectional study. *Lancet Neurol.* 13, 997–1005.

Jack, C. R. Jr., Bennett, D. A., Blennow, K., Carrillo, M. C., Feldman, H. H., Frisoni, G. B., et al. (2016). A/T/N: an unbiased descriptive classification scheme for Alzheimer disease biomarkers. *Neurology* 87, 539–547. doi: 10.1212/WNL.0000000000002923

Jack, C. R. Jr., Wiste, H. J., Lesnick, T. G., Weigand, S. D., Knopman, D. S., Vemuri, P., et al. (2013). Brain β-amyloid load approaches a plateau. *Neurology* 80, 890–896. doi: 10.1212/WNL.0b013e3182840bbe

Jack, C. R. Jr., Wiste, H. J., Weigand, S. D., Knopman, D. S., Mielke, M. M., Vemuri, P., et al. (2015). Different definitions of neurodegeneration produce similar amyloid/neurodegeneration biomarker group findings. *Brain* 138(Pt 12), 3747–3759. doi: 10.1093/brain/awv283

Jansen, W. J., Ossenkoppele, R., Knol, D. L., Tijms, B. M., Scheltens, P., Verhey, F. R., et al. (2015). Prevalence of cerebral amyloid pathology in persons without dementia: a meta-analysis. *JAMA* 313, 1924–1938. doi: 10.1001/jama.2015.4668

Jueptner, M., and Weiller, C. (1995). Does measurement of regional cerebral blood flow reflect synaptic activity?—Implications for PET and fMRI. *Neuroimage* 2, 148–156.

Kato, T., Inui, Y., Nakamura, A., and Ito, K. (2016). Brain fluorodeoxyglucose (FDG) PET in dementia. *Ageing Res. Rev.* 30, 73–84. doi: 10.1016/j.arr.2016.02.003

Kleim, J. A., Lussnig, E., Schwarz, E. R., Comery, T. A., and Greenough, W. T. (1996). Synaptogenesis and Fos expression in the motor cortex of the adult rat after motor skill learning. *J. Neurosci.* 16, 4529–4535.

Kolb, B., and Gibb, R. (2011). Brain plasticity and behaviour in the developing brain. *J. Can. Acad. Child Adolesc. Psychiatry* 20, 265–276.

Lampit, A., Hallock, H., Suo, C., Naismith, S. L., and Valenzuela, M. (2015). Cognitive training-induced short-term functional and long-term structural plastic change is related to gains in global cognition in healthy older adults: a pilot study. *Front. Aging Neurosci.* 7:14. doi: 10.3389/fnagi.2015.00014

Landau, S. M., Marks, S. M., Mormino, E. C., Rabinovici, G. D., Oh, H., O'Neil, J. P., et al. (2012). Association of lifetime cognitive engagement and low β-amyloid deposition. *Arch. Neurol.* 69, 623–629. doi: 10.1001/archneurol.2011.2748

Lee, D. Y., Lee, K. U., Lee, J. H., Kim, K. W., Jhoo, J. H., Kim, S. Y., et al. (2004). A normative study of the CERAD neuropsychological assessment battery in the Korean elderly. *J. Int. Neuropsychol. Soc.* 10, 72–81. doi: 10.1017/S1355617704101094

Lee, J. H., Lee, K. U., Lee, D. Y., Kim, K. W., Jhoo, J. H., Kim, J. H., et al. (2002). Development of the Korean version of the consortium to establish a registry for Alzheimer's Disease assessment packet (CERAD-K): clinical and neuropsychological assessment batteries. *J. Gerontol. B Psychol. Sci. Soc. Sci.* 57, 47–53.

Leuner, B., Kozorovitskiy, Y., Gross, C. G., and Gould, E. (2007). Diminished adult neurogenesis in the marmoset brain precedes old age. *Proc. Natl. Acad. Sci. U.S.A.* 104, 17169–17173. doi: 10.1073/pnas.0708228104

Markesbery, W. R. (1997). Oxidative stress hypothesis in Alzheimer's disease. *Free Radic. Biol. Med.* 23, 134–147.

Marquine, M. J., Segawa, E., Wilson, R. S., Bennett, D. A., and Barnes, L. L. (2012). Association between cognitive activity and cognitive function in older Hispanics. *J. Int. Neuropsychol. Soc.* 18, 1041–1051. doi: 10.1017/S135561771200080X

Paus, T., Zijdenbos, A., Worsley, K., Collins, D. L., Blumenthal, J., Giedd, J. N., et al. (1999). Structural maturation of neural pathways in children and adolescents: in vivo study. *Science* 283, 1908–1911.

Reiman, E. M., Chen, K., Liu, X., Bandy, D., Yu, M., Lee, W., et al. (2009). Fibrillar amyloid-β burden in cognitively normal people at 3 levels of genetic risk for

Alzheimer's disease. *Proc. Natl. Acad. Sci. U.S.A.* 106, 6820–6825. doi: 10.1073/pnas.0900345106

Richter-Schmidinger, T., Alexopoulos, P., Horn, M., Maus, S., Reichel, M., Rhein, C., et al. (2011). Influence of brain-derived neurotrophic-factor and apolipoprotein E genetic variants on hippocampal volume and memory performance in healthy young adults. *J. Neural Transm.* 118, 249–257. doi: 10.1007/s00702-010-0539-8

Ruiz, J. R., Castillo, R., Labayen, I., Moreno, L. A., Fuentes, M. G., Lamuno, D. G., et al. (2010). Individual and combined effects of ApoE and MTHFR 677C/T polymorphisms on cognitive performance in Spanish adolescents: the AVENA study. *J. Pediatr.* 156, 978–984, 984.e1. doi: 10.1016/j.jpeds.2009.12.018

Saint-Aubert, L., Almkvist, O., Chiotis, K., Almeida, R., Wall, A., and Nordberg, A. (2016). Regional tau deposition measured by [18F]THK5317 positron emission tomography is associated to cognition via glucose metabolism in Alzheimer's disease. *Alzheimers Res. Ther.* 8:38. doi: 10.1186/s13195-016-0204-z

Sattler, C., Toro, P., Schonknecht, P., and Schroder, J. (2012). Cognitive activity, education and socioeconomic status as preventive factors for mild cognitive impairment and Alzheimer's disease. *Psychiatry Res.* 196, 90–95. doi: 10.1016/j.psychres.2011.11.012

Shah, T., Verdile, G., Sohrabi, H., Campbell, A., Putland, E., Cheetham, C., et al. (2014). A combination of physical activity and computerized brain training improves verbal memory and increases cerebral glucose metabolism in the elderly. *Transl. Psychiatry* 4:e487. doi: 10.1038/tp.2014.122

Snowball, A., Tachtsidis, I., Popescu, T., Thompson, J., Delazer, M., Zamarian, L., et al. (2013). Long-term enhancement of brain function and cognition using cognitive training and brain stimulation. *Curr. Biol.* 23, 987–992. doi: 10.1016/j.cub.2013.04.045

Sokoloff, L. (1981). Relationships among local functional activity, energy metabolism, and blood flow in the central nervous system. *Fed. Proc.* 40, 2311–2316.

Stern, Y. (2012). Cognitive reserve in ageing and Alzheimer's disease. *Lancet Neurol.* 11, 1006–1012. doi: 10.1016/s1474-4422(12)70191-6

Tau, G. Z., and Peterson, B. S. (2010). Normal development of brain circuits. *Neuropsychopharmacology* 35, 147–168. doi: 10.1038/npp.2009.115

Valenzuela, M. J., Sachdev, P., Wen, W., Chen, X., and Brodaty, H. (2008). Lifespan mental activity predicts diminished rate of hippocampal atrophy. *PLoS One* 3:e2598. doi: 10.1371/journal.pone.0002598

Vemuri, P., Knopman, D. S., Lesnick, T. G., Przybelski, S. A., Mielke, M. M., Graff-Radford, J., et al. (2017). Evaluation of amyloid protective factors and Alzheimer Disease neurodegeneration protective factors in elderly individuals. *JAMA Neurol.* 74, 718–726. doi: 10.1001/jamaneurol.2017.0244

Vemuri, P., Lesnick, T. G., Przybelski, S. A., Knopman, D. S., Machulda, M., Lowe, V. J., et al. (2016). Effect of intellectual enrichment on AD biomarker trajectories: longitudinal imaging study. *Neurology* 86, 1128–1135. doi: 10.1212/WNL.0000000000002490

Vemuri, P., Lesnick, T. G., Przybelski, S. A., Knopman, D. S., Roberts, R. O., Lowe, V. J., et al. (2012). Effect of lifestyle activities on Alzheimer disease biomarkers and cognition. *Ann. Neurol.* 72, 730–738. doi: 10.1002/ana.23665

Villemagne, V. L., Burnham, S., Bourgeat, P., Brown, B., Ellis, K. A., Salvado, O., et al. (2013). Amyloid beta deposition, neurodegeneration, and cognitive decline in sporadic Alzheimer's disease: a prospective cohort study. *Lancet Neurol.* 12, 357–367. doi: 10.1016/S1474-4422(13)70044-9

Wenham, P. R., Newton, C. R., and Price, W. H. (1991). Analysis of apolipoprotein E genotypes by the amplification refractory mutation system. *Clin. Chem.* 37, 241–244.

Wilson, R., Bennett, D., Bienias, J., Aggarwal, N., De Leon, C. M., Morris, M., et al. (2002a). Cognitive activity and incident AD in a population-based sample of older persons. *Neurology* 59, 1910–1914.

Wilson, R. S., Barnes, L. L., Krueger, K. R., Hoganson, G., Bienias, J. L., and Bennett, D. A. (2005). Early and late life cognitive activity and cognitive systems in old age. *J. Int. Neuropsychol. Soc.* 11, 400–407.

Wilson, R. S., Bennett, D. A., Bienias, J. L., Mendes de Leon, C. F., Morris, M. C., and Evans, D. A. (2003). Cognitive activity and cognitive decline in a biracial community population. *Neurology* 61, 812–816.

Wilson, R. S., Boyle, P. A., Yang, J., James, B. D., and Bennett, D. A. (2015). Early life instruction in foreign language and music and incidence of mild cognitive impairment. *Neuropsychology* 29, 292–302. doi: 10.1037/neu0000129

Wilson, R. S., Boyle, P. A., Yu, L., Barnes, L. L., Schneider, J. A., and Bennett, D. A. (2013). Life-span cognitive activity, neuropathologic burden, and cognitive aging. *Neurology* 81, 314–321. doi: 10.1212/WNL.0b013e31829c5e8a

Wilson, R. S., De Leon, C. F. M., Barnes, L. L., Schneider, J. A., Bienias, J. L., Evans, D. A., et al. (2002b). Participation in cognitively stimulating activities and risk of incident Alzheimer disease. *JAMA* 287, 742–748.

Wilson, R. S., Scherr, P. A., Schneider, J. A., Tang, Y., and Bennett, D. A. (2007). Relation of cognitive activity to risk of developing Alzheimer disease. *Neurology* 69, 1911–1920. doi: 10.1212/01.wnl.0000271087.67782.cb

Wilson, R. S., Segawa, E., Boyle, P. A., and Bennett, D. A. (2012). Influence of late-life cognitive activity on cognitive health. *Neurology* 78, 1123–1129. doi: 10.1212/WNL.0b013e31824f8c03

Wirth, M., Villeneuve, S., La Joie, R., Marks, S. M., and Jagust, W. J. (2014). Gene-environment interactions: lifetime cognitive activity, APOE genotype, and β-amyloid burden. *J. Neurosci.* 34, 8612–8617. doi: 10.1523/JNEUROSCI.4612-13.2014

Wisdom, N. M., Callahan, J. L., and Hawkins, K. A. (2011). The effects of apolipoprotein E on non-impaired cognitive functioning: a meta-analysis. *Neurobiol. Aging* 32, 63–74. doi: 10.1016/j.neurobiolaging.2009.02.003

Wolf, S. A., Kronenberg, G., Lehmann, K., Blankenship, A., Overall, R., Staufenbiel, M., et al. (2006). Cognitive and physical activity differently modulate disease progression in the amyloid precursor protein (APP)-23 model of Alzheimer's disease. *Biol. Psychiatry* 60, 1314–1323.

Yesavage, J. A., Brink, T. L., Rose, T. L., Lum, O., Huang, V., Adey, M., et al. (1983). Development and validation of a geriatric depression screening scale - a preliminary-report. *J. Psychiatr. Res.* 17, 37–49. doi: 10.1016/0022-3956(82)90033-4

2

Cerebrovascular-Reactivity Mapping Using MRI: Considerations for Alzheimer's Disease

J. J. Chen[1,2]*

[1] Rotman Research Institute, Baycrest, Toronto, ON, Canada, [2] Department of Medical Biophysics, University of Toronto, Toronto, ON, Canada

***Correspondence:**
J. J. Chen
jchen@research.baycrest.org

Alzheimer's disease (AD) is associated with well-established macrostructural and cellular markers, including localized brain atrophy and deposition of amyloid. However, there is growing recognition of the link between cerebrovascular dysfunction and AD, supported by continuous experimental evidence in the animal and human literature. As a result, neuroimaging studies of AD are increasingly aiming to incorporate vascular measures, exemplified by measures of cerebrovascular reactivity (CVR). CVR is a measure that is rooted in clinical practice, and as non-invasive CVR-mapping techniques become more widely available, routine CVR mapping may open up new avenues of investigation into the development of AD. This review focuses on the use of MRI to map CVR, paying specific attention to recent developments in MRI methodology and on the emerging stimulus-free approaches to CVR mapping. It also summarizes the biological basis for the vascular contribution to AD, and provides critical perspective on the choice of CVR-mapping techniques amongst frail populations.

Keywords: cerebrovascular reactivity (CVR), Alzheimer's disease, APOE, magnetic resonance imaging (MRI), functional MRI (fMRI), carbon dioxide (CO_2), resting-state fMRI, mild-cognitive impairment

BACKGROUND

The brain's energy needs are mainly met by neurovascular regulation of cerebral blood flow (CBF) (Roy and Sherrington, 1890; Duling and Berne, 1970), realized by the neurovascular unit (NVU). The NVU consists of arterial/arteriolar vascular smooth-muscle cells (VMSCs), endothelial cells, neuroglia (notably astrocytes), and pericytes. Pericytes play a crucial role in the formation and functionality of the selectively permeable space that is the blood–brain barrier (BBB), and BBB disruption is a classic marker of vascular dysfunction. Neurovascular dysfunction leads to failure to meet neuronal energy needs, which leads to oxidative stress and eventual neuronal death.

VASCULAR ROLE IN ALZHEIMER'S DISEASE

While the ε4 allele of the apolipoprotein E (APOE) gene is an acknowledged genetic risk factor found in 40–80% of Alzheimer's disease (AD) patients (Strittmatter et al., 1993), and amyloid plaques are a hallmark of AD, an approximated 60–90% of AD patients also exhibit cerebrovascular pathologies (Bell and Zlokovic, 2009), supporting the vascular theory of AD. In brief, the current understanding is that genetic, environmental, and lifestyle factors may all predispose individuals to damage to the NVU (**Figure 1**). Soluble amyloid beta (Aβ), which predates Aβ plaques, deregulates cerebrovascular function by activating a free-radical cascade (Park et al., 2008), leading to compromised microvascular integrity (Dorr et al., 2012), and reduced CBF. Aβ is known to interact with endothelin-1 (Kawanabe and Nauli, 2011) and myocardin (Ramanathan et al., 2015) to promote vascular hypercontractility. Moreover, the cholinergic deficit in AD can result in a reduction of cholinergic input to cortical blood vessels (Claassen and Zhang, 2011). Furthermore, Aβ-mediated pericyte degeneration leads to BBB breakdown, increasing the perivascular accumulation of neurotoxins. The various pathways of vascular dysfunction can lead to increasing vascular tortuosity and decreasing vascular reactivity (Black et al., 2009), compromising Aβ clearance and eventually lead to neuronal death. Paradoxically, tau pathology has been associated with an increase in regional vascular reactivity (Wells et al., 2015), a controversy that is still under investigation.

Irrespective of the specific disease mechanism, vascular deficits have been demonstrated as a promising early indicator of AD. Non-invasive functional magnetic-resonance imaging (MRI) has provided strong evidence that CBF can be used to distinguish between at-risk individuals, patients and normal controls (Johnson et al., 2005). In addition, perfusion deficits have been associated with decreased functional connectivity despite maintained glucose metabolism (Göttler et al., 2018). Interventions to re-establish perfusion have been advocated as a promising preventative treatment (de la Torre, 2016). However, perfusion is a mixture of neuronal and vascular contributions, and unraveling the vascular mechanisms of AD etiology requires a more vascularly specific and routinely adoptable vascular marker. In this respect, there is early evidence that deficits in cerebrovascular reactivity (CVR) are detectable before those in CBF (Yezhuvath et al., 2012). Indeed, this was demonstrated through quantitative cerebrovascular resistance, defined as the ratio of mean-arterial blood pressure to CBF (Yew et al., 2017). Compared to CBF, resistance was found to be more sensitive at distinguishing amyloid-positive from amyloid-negative older populations as well as being more predictive of dementia conversion.

CVR AND MEASUREMENT TECHNIQUES

A recent review by Glodzik et al. (2013) provides an excellent overview of CVR measurement in AD using carbon-dioxide (CO_2) challenges with various imaging modalities. CVR is a vasodilatory or constrictive reaction of a blood vessel to a stimulus. CVR is a well-established indicator of vascular reserve and autoregulatory efficiency. CVR decline has been associated with normal aging (Lu et al., 2011), and is the most reliable neuroimaging predictor of impending cerebrovascular disease (Pillai and Mikulis, 2015).

Vascular Stimulus and CVR

Qualitative CVR information can be gleaned from the functional MRI (fMRI) response to any task (Dumas et al., 2012), but when quantitative CVR values are desired, vascular agents are generally required. Strong CBF responses can be induced by intravascular CO_2 alterations, with CO_2 inspiration thought as the optimal form of stimulus (Fierstra et al., 2013). While breathing and blood flow can both be regulated through the midbrain CO_2 chemoreceptors, CO_2-related blood pH changes are also actively regulated as part of maintaining homeostasis. Thus, hypercapnic challenges, in which the arterial CO_2 content is increased, activate VMSC potassium channels (Ainslie and Duffin, 2009), leading to large CBF increases without a significant concomitant increase in metabolic rate (Chen and Pike, 2010; Jain et al., 2011). In addition, nitric oxide, which is synthesized locally following glutamate receptor activity, has also been implicated in the modulation of vasodilatory effects produced by CO_2 (Iadecola et al., 1994).

End-tidal CO_2 pressure ($PETCO_2$) is an easily measured surrogate for arterial CO_2 ($PaCO_2$) (Battisti-Charbonney et al., 2011). $PETCO_2$ is measured as the peak expired CO_2, typically 35–40 mmHg in healthy individuals, and directly reflects alveolar CO_2. CBF increases by 3–4% per mmHg increase in $PETCO_2$, reaching its highest level when $PETCO_2$ is elevated by 10–20 mmHg above normal resting value (Brugniaux et al., 2007). $PETCO_2$ reductions result in CBF decline by approximately 3% per 1 mmHg change (Ito et al., 2005).

CO_2-Based CVR Mapping Using MRI: Methods

The clinical utility of CO_2-based CVR quantification was established using transcranial Doppler ultrasound (TCD) (Ainslie and Duffin, 2009), positron-emission tomography (Ito et al., 2001) and dynamic X-ray computed tomography (Chen et al., 2006). While fMRI is not the most established method of assessing CVR, it offers marked advantages including richer spatial information and minimal invasiveness (Iannetti and Wise, 2007). CVR has been reliably assessed using CO_2 fMRI in both gray and white matter (Thomas et al., 2014). In the absence of a CO_2 delivery apparatus, breathing challenges such as breath-holding (Bright and Murphy, 2013; Pinto et al., 2016) and cued deep breathing (Bright et al., 2009) have been proposed as alternative ways to modulate intravascular CO_2 (see **Table 1**). A comparison of breath-holding and inhaled-CO_2 approaches reveals important CVR dependence on methodology (Tancredi and Hoge, 2013), but the reproducibility of both approaches has been established in healthy young controls (Kassner et al., 2010; Bright and Murphy, 2013).

CO_2-based CVR measured using fMRI has been widely applied and extensively cross-validated (Herzig et al., 2008). Robust hypercapnia can be induced through manually adjusted administration of blended gases (Cohen et al., 2004), end-tidal forcing (Poulin et al., 1996) or more recently, computerized $PETCO_2$ targeting (Slessarev et al., 2007; Mark et al., 2010). The latter method entails the most lengthy set up but also provides immediate and robust $PETCO_2$ suppression (hypocapnia) (Blockley et al., 2011), and has been proposed as part of a rapid CVR-mapping protocol for routine use (Blockley et al., 2011, 2017).

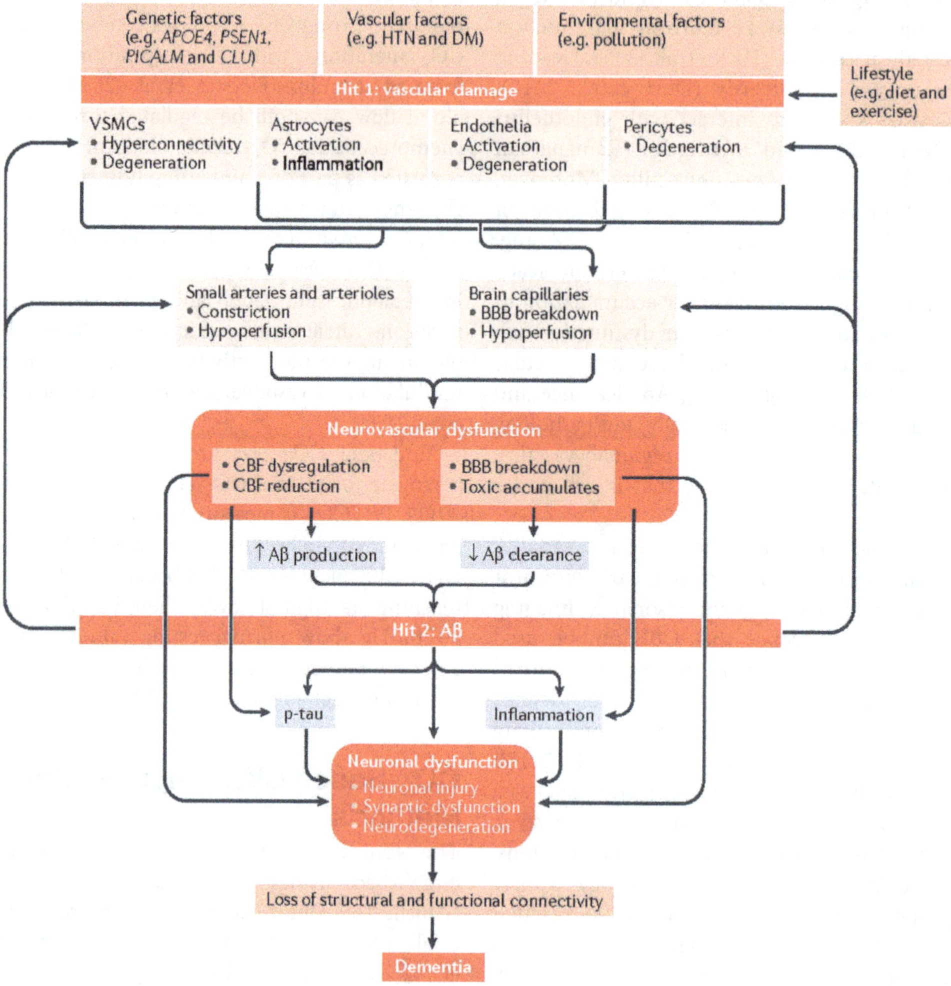

FIGURE 1 | Vascular involvement in AD, as depicted in a "2-hit model" of neurovascular dysfunction. Genetic risk (including due to APOE ε4) predispose individuals to amyloid deposition. Modified from Kisler et al. (2017) with permission.

In the clinical realm, the main considerations in choosing a CVR-mapping methodology are: (1) How to assess CVR in the most non-invasive manner? (2) How to interpret the CVR information?

Consideration for Non-invasiveness

As one of the earliest ways to induce $PETCO_2$ elevation (Ratnatunga and Adiseshiah, 1990), breath-holding typically does not allow the calculation of quantitative CVR, as all participants are assumed to perform breath-holds in similar manners and the actual $PETCO_2$ cannot be monitored during the challenge. The lack of $PETCO_2$ monitoring is particularly concerning, as the actual change in $PETCO_2$ achieved by a breath-hold depends on multiple factors, including the resting metabolic rate of the subject, lung size, recent ventilation history and whether the breath-hold is post-inspiration or post-expiration. Moreover, as typical breath-holds last 15–20 s, there are reports of poor subject compliance (Jahanian et al., 2017), particularly when elderly participants are involved. Despite these drawbacks, breath-holding-based CVR mapping has a key advantage of requiring the least instrumentation, thus allowing it to be implemented in almost any MRI scan session. Ongoing research aims to improve the robustness of breath-hold CVR mapping (Bright and Murphy, 2013), although clinical validation remains far from extensive.

Even less invasive than breath-holding, resting-state fMRI has offered a unique window to glean CVR information. Notably, Kannurpatti et al. (2014) reported a comparison of the resting-state fMRI fluctuation amplitude (voxel-wise temporal standard-deviation) as a CVR surrogate. This type of "unconstrained" or "task-free" CVR protocol does not require cooperation from participants, and is thus a promising direction of research that will likely attract tremendous attention from clinical studies. This topic will be further discussed as part of a proposed future trend.

TABLE 1 | Strengths and weaknesses of various CO_2-based CVR protocols.

Approach	Strengths	Weaknesses
End-tidal forcing	• Accurate targeting of $PETCO_2$ • Can be used to produce complex $PETCO_2$ shapes • Produces quantitative CVR	• Requires complex instrumentation • Feedback mechanism reduces response speed • The hypercapnic challenge may induce discomfort
Prospective targeting	• Accurate targeting of $PETCO_2$ • Feed-forward mechanism enhances response speed • Can be used to produce complex $PETCO_2$ shapes • Produces quantitative CVR	• Requires complex instrumentation • Requires estimation of VO2max • The hypercapnic challenge may induce discomfort
Manually blended gases	• Requires simple instrumentation and set up • Produces quantitative CVR	• $PETCO_2$ response rate depends on ventilation level and cannot be controlled • $PETCO_2$ not actively targeted, so resulting challenge may vary by individual
Breath-holding	• Requires no additional instrumentation	• Actual PETCO2 cannot be measured, so CVR not quantitative • Relationship between breath-hold and $PETCO_2$ depends on numerous factors • Requires active subject cooperation, may vary
Cued deep breathing	• Requires no additional instrumentation	• Actual PETCO2 cannot be measured, so CVR not quantitative • Relationship between deep breathing and $PETCO_2$ depends on numerous factors • Requires active subject cooperation, may vary
Resting state	• Requires little to no additional instrumentation • Requires minimal subject cooperation • Does not induce discomfort • CVR estimated from multiple $PETCO_2$ values instead of block averages	• MRI response to CO_2 is more sensitive to contamination by motion and other artifacts, given the low $PETCO_2$ fluctuation amplitude

Consideration for Data Interpretation

Currently, the de-facto standard protocol to quantitative CVR mapping with MRI remains CO_2 inhalation, notably controlled using computerized targeting (Kassner et al., 2010; Fierstra et al., 2013; Sobczyk et al., 2014, 2015; Poublanc et al., 2015; Sam et al., 2016; Fisher et al., 2017). Despite the complex set up, this approach has been extensively used and validated clinically. The use of modern breathing circuits also allows the CO_2 challenge to follow nearly any shape. However, there has yet to be a consensus as to the level, duration and pattern of $PETCO_2$ perturbation. As different stimulus designs likely have different vaso-stimulating capacities and hence may reveal different CVR patterns, the choice of challenge will be critical, not only in comparing across studies but also across the same individuals over time (Fierstra et al., 2013).

Based on prospective targeting of stepwise $PETCO_2$ changes, researchers at Toronto Western Hospital (TWH) pioneered the use of an uneven task design - one short block followed by longer block (Spano et al., 2013), both typically elevating $PETCO_2$ by 10 mmHg. This design is motivated by the desire to derive more accurate estimates of CVR response time, and

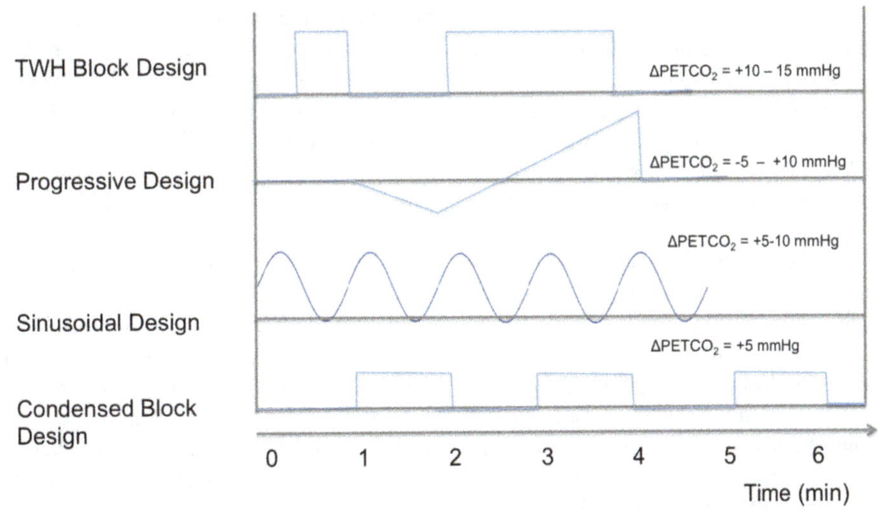

FIGURE 2 | A summary of designs for various $PETCO_2$ challenges in the literature.

(Duffin et al., 2015; Poublanc et al., 2015), which may reflect regional arterial-transit time. Additionally, the same group proposed the use of progressive hypercapnia (CO_2 ramps) (Fisher et al., 2017), in which both hypercapnia and hypocapnia are progressively induced through a ramp stimulus. It has been demonstrated that different segments of the ramp, which resulted in $PETCO_2$ values of 30–50 mmHg, reveal different spatial patterns in CVR that could complement the conventional CVR information (Fisher et al., 2017). Alternatively, the use of a sinusoidal pattern allows direct estimation of response delay (as the phase in the corresponding sinusoidal CVR response), and has allowed the development of a CVR protocol as short as 5 min (Blockley et al., 2017). Such a design makes use of both hypercapnia and hypocapnia for CVR estimation, rendering estimates more robust against biases due to basal vascular tone (Halani et al., 2015). Further reducing scan time is a 1-min blended-gas protocol with 5% CO_2 (Yezhuvath et al., 2009; Blockley et al., 2017), which has compared favorably against longer designs. These stimulation designs are summarized in **Figure 2**, and research is ongoing to validate the unique utility of each design, and it is likely that CVR measurements produced by these various methods are not directly comparable.

Concurrently, the emergence of arterial-spin labeling (ASL) MRI for CBF-based CVR mapping has added a new dimension to the choice of methods. In particular, CBF-based maps, while lower in signal-to-noise ratios (SNRs), can in fact provide more vascular-driven and thus less biased CVR quantification than BOLD fMRI (Halani et al., 2015), as demonstrated by comparisons with TCD (Gao et al., 2013). Great strides have been made in extending the use of ASL-based CVR mapping into aging research (Leoni et al., 2017), and ASL is now ubiquitously used in the study of AD (Alsop et al., 2014).

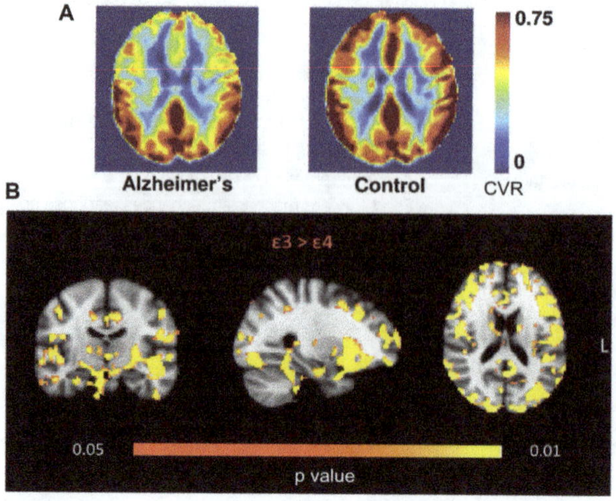

FIGURE 3 | MRI-based CVR maps in AD and APOE gene carriers. **(A)** Frontal, cingular, and insular CVR deficits are found in AD patients. Figure is modified from Yezhuvath et al. (2012) with permission. **(B)** Young ε4 carriers manifest widespread CVR deficits compared to ε3 homozygotes. Figure is modified from Suri et al. (2014) with permission.

AD-ASSOCIATED FINDINGS IN HUMAN CVR MAPPING USING MRI

Cerebrovascular reactivity compromises in the middle-cerebral artery in AD, mainly measured using blended-CO_2 method, is a well-established TCD-based finding (Lee et al., 2007; Sabayan et al., 2012; Viticchi et al., 2012; Hajjar et al., 2015). While the use of MRI-based CVR mapping in AD is still limited, its adoption is on the cusp of expansion due to rapid methodological developments.

Using MRI, such CVR reductions have been localized to the prefrontal, anterior cingulate and insular regions (Yezhuvath et al., 2012). Interestingly, while this pattern overlapped little with that of CBF deficits (found in the temporal and parietal regions), it agreed with the localization of amyloid deposition (Yezhuvath et al., 2012), suggesting that CVR has unique sensitivity to AD pathology (**Figure 3A**). Moreover, cortical and white-matter CVR deficits have been linked to the incidence of leukoaraiosis (Yezhuvath et al., 2012; Sam et al., 2016). Such reductions in CVR echo postmortem observations of vascular dysfunction (Chow et al., 2007), and can be the result of a number of structural changes in the vasculature, including cerebral amyloid angiopathy (CAA), astrocytic end-feet swelling, pericyte degeneration, basement-membrane hypertrophy and endothelial-cell metabolic abnormalities (Hashimura et al., 1991; Miyakawa et al., 1997).

Cerebrovascular reactivity deficits have been discovered amongst young APOE ε4 gene carriers (Hajjar et al., 2015), even when compared to ε3 homozygotes (Suri et al., 2014) (**Figure 3B**). Such deficits are found to be widespread, notably in the prefrontal and parahippocampal regions, bolstering the hypothesis that genetic predisposition to vascular disease contributes to the vulnerability of ε4-carriers to late-life pathology (Kisler et al., 2017).

It is increasingly recognized that vascular deficits may be the most accessible physiological treatment target in the effort to delay dementia onset, and approaches that enhance perfusion have demonstrated potential therapeutic value (de la Torre, 2016). Predicting progression of preclinical AD amongst mild-cognitive impaired (MCI) individuals has been a key research focus. Using breath-hold TCD, the predictive value of CVR (Sato and Morishita, 2013) in terms of MCI-to-AD conversions has been demonstrated (Buratti et al., 2015).

In light of the overwhelming influence of vascular risk factors in AD progression, the lines between vascular deficits in AD and other types of dementia can become blurred in later stages of the disease, as will be discussed in later sections. As a case in point, given the rampant occurrence of CAA amongst suspected AD patients, the vascular dysfunction can produce deleterious oxidative stress that can promote ischemia and accelerate AD progression (Girouard and Iadecola, 2006; Bookheimer and Burggren, 2009). Furthermore, CVR may be a more sensitive early marker of AD severity (Yezhuvath et al., 2012). It is conceivable that a diseased vasculature may sustain normal perfusion but reveal an abnormal response to a stress test such as used in CVR mapping (Fierstra et al., 2013). Nonetheless, as an increasing amount of CVR data is generated using BOLD fMRI, it is also important to note that microvascular CVR is more reflective of AD severity (Jellinger and Attems, 2006), while the BOLD fMRI signal is generally dominated by large-vessels. This is true at clinical field strengths (1.5 or 3 Tesla) and using either gradient- or spin-echo BOLD. ASL, on the other hand, is likely more sensitive to capillaries and arterioles, and should be the most natural alternative for CVR mapping.

There are numerous fMRI studies that report age-related differences in the BOLD response amplitude or extent, but as the BOLD response to neuronal stimuli is intrinsically modulated by CVR, one must be cautioned against interpreting age-related BOLD differences as neuronal differences. This is also true of resting-state fMRI, where functional connectivity has been found to vary with CVR (Golestani et al., 2016a; Lajoie et al., 2017; Chu et al., 2018).

RESEARCH GAPS AND EMERGING TOPICS

As stated earlier, the most commonly reported challenge in acquiring CVR maps in clinical research pertains to the need for subject cooperation. This is true for all of the stimulus designs described thus far, imposing a fundamental limitation on the routine use of CVR mapping amongst patients. Very recently, resting-state methods that do not require CO_2 perturbation have flourished (Golestani et al., 2016b; Jahanian et al., 2017; Liu et al., 2017). Resting-state CVR methods rely on intrinsic fluctuations in the BOLD fMRI signal, and may significantly broaden the accessibility of CVR mapping to clinical researchers. Additionally, beyond the magnitude of CVR, the dynamic features of the fMRI response can also provide useful information. A slowing of the CVR response has been shown to characterize vascular lesions (Poublanc et al., 2015), adding a dimension to the utility of CVR mapping.

The response of the cerebral circulation to a changing arterial CO_2 concentration is not linear - the circulatory response follows a sigmoidal shape, and is greater for hypercapnia than to hypocapnia (Ogoh et al., 2008; Peebles et al., 2008; Rodell et al., 2012). Moreover, it is critical to note that while CVR is traditionally defined as a blood-flow response (as is the case in TCD, PET, and CT), the BOLD signal is not a direct measure of CBF. Rather, BOLD is modulated by CBF, CBV, and baseline oxidative metabolism, not to mention a series of field-dependent physical variables. Thus, the assumption of a linear relationship between the BOLD and CBF responses to CO_2 is likely tenuous. Specifically, it is widely known that the BOLD response varies with CBF in a non-linear fashion (Hoge et al., 1999). This non-linearity is superimposed in the inherently sigmoidal vascular response to CO_2 (Battisti-Charbonney et al., 2011). Such non-linear CVR changes have been demonstrated through a comparison with CBF-based CVR measurements at various vascular baselines (Halani et al., 2015), and may in a small part underlie the BOLD response behavior in the "vascular steal" phenomenon (Sobczyk et al., 2014). This limitation will require careful consideration in the presence of known vascular dysfunction (Battisti-Charbonney et al., 2011).

A critical assumption for CVR mapping is that $PETCO_2$ represents $PaCO_2$. However, $PaCO_2$ is determined by both inhaled CO_2 and the minute ventilation. Low cardiac output can increase alveolar dead space, which would increase the difference between $PaCO_2$ and $PETCO_2$ (Shibutani et al., 1992), leading to underestimations of $PETCO_2$-based CVR. In addition, $PETCO_2$ is shown to overestimate $PaCO_2$ during exercise in young adults, but not in older adults (Williams and Babb, 1997). Moreover, $PETCO_2$-related CVR is known to follow a circadian rhythm, increasing with the level of alertness (Ainslie and Duffin, 2009). These factor contribute to inter-cohort, inter-sessional and inter-subject variability in CVR estimates that must be accounted for when assessing true differences in CVR.

In this regard, an emerging research direction is building normative CVR atlases that allow the significance of CVR deviations to be assessed (Sobczyk et al., 2015). Such atlases would ideally encompass not only quantitative CVR values but also CVR-timing information (van Niftrik et al., 2017). This is a critical step in expanding the clinical utility of CVR maps, and atlases will likely need to be specific to the CO_2 delivery method, stimulation design, study objectives and MRI system used.

The above research gaps pertain not only to AD but to other cerebrovascular diseases also. The increasing awareness of the vascular etiology of various forms of dementia will highlight these limitations and prompt more focused validation studies.

AUTHOR CONTRIBUTIONS

The author confirms being the sole contributor of this work and approved it for publication.

FUNDING

This work was supported by funding from the Canadian Institutes of Health Research (CIHR FRN#126164 and 148398) as well as by the Natural Sciences and Engineering Research Council of Canada (NSERC FRN# 418443).

REFERENCES

Ainslie, P. N., and Duffin, J. (2009). Integration of cerebrovascular CO2 reactivity and chemoreflex control of breathing: mechanisms of regulation, measurement, and interpretation. *Am. J. Physiol. Regul. Integr. Comp. Physiol.* 296, R1473–R1495. doi: 10.1152/ajpregu.91008.2008

Alsop, D. C., Detre, J. A., Golay, X., Gunther, M., Hendrikse, J., Hernandez-Garcia, L., et al. (2014). Recommended implementation of arterial spin-labeled perfusion MRI for clinical applications: a consensus of the ISMRM perfusion study group and the european consortium for ASL in dementia. *Magn. Reson. Med.* doi: 10.1002/mrm.25197 [Epub ahead of print].

Battisti-Charbonney, A., Fisher, J., and Duffin, J. (2011). The cerebrovascular response to carbon dioxide in humans. *J. Physiol.* 589, 3039–3048. doi: 10.1113/jphysiol.2011.206052

Bell, R. D., and Zlokovic, B. V. (2009). Neurovascular mechanisms and blood-brain barrier disorder in Alzheimer's Disease. *Acta Neuropathol.* 118, 103–113. doi: 10.1007/s00401-009-0522-3

Black, S., Gao, F., and Bilbao, J. (2009). Understanding white matter disease: imaging-pathological correlations in vascular cognitive impairment. *Stroke* 3(Suppl.), S48–S52. doi: 10.1161/STROKEAHA.108.537704

Blockley, N. P., Driver, I. D., Francis, S. T., Fisher, J. A., and Gowland, P. A. (2011). An improved method for acquiring cerebrovascular reactivity maps. *Magn. Reson. Med.* 65, 1278–1286. doi: 10.1002/mrm.22719

Blockley, N. P., Harkin, J. W., and Bulte, D. P. (2017). Rapid cerebrovascular reactivity mapping: enabling vascular reactivity information to be routinely acquired. *Neuroimage* 159, 214–223. doi: 10.1016/j.neuroimage.2017.07.048

Bookheimer, S., and Burggren, A. (2009). APOE-4 genotype and neurophysiological vulnerability to Alzheimer's and cognitive aging. *Annu. Rev. Clin. Psychol.* 5, 343–362. doi: 10.1146/annurev.clinpsy.032408.153625

Bright, M. G., Bulte, D. P., Jezzard, P., and Duyn, J. H. (2009). Characterization of regional heterogeneity in cerebrovascular reactivity dynamics using novel hypocapnia task and BOLD fMRI. *Neuroimage* 48, 166–175. doi: 10.1016/j.neuroimage.2009.05.026

Bright, M. G., and Murphy, K. (2013). Reliable quantification of BOLD fMRI cerebrovascular reactivity despite poor breath-hold performance. *Neuroimage* 83, 559–568. doi: 10.1016/j.neuroimage.2013.07.007

Brugniaux, J. V., Hodges, A. N., Hanly, P. J., and Poulin, M. J. (2007). Cerebrovascular responses to altitude. *Respir. Physiol. Neurobiol.* 158, 212–223. doi: 10.1016/j.resp.2007.04.008

Buratti, L., Balestrini, S., Altamura, C., Viticchi, G., Falsetti, L., Luzzi, S., et al. (2015). Markers for the risk of progression from mild cognitive impairment to Alzheimer's Disease. *J. Alzheimer's Dis.* 45, 883–890. doi: 10.3233/JAD-143135

Chen, A., Shyr, M.-H., Chen, T.-Y., Lai, H.-Y., Lin, C.-C., and Yen, P.-S. (2006). Dynamic CT perfusion imaging with acetazolamide challenge for evaluation of patients with unilateral cerebrovascular steno-occlusive disease. *AJNR Am. J. Neuroradiol.* 27, 1876–1881.

Chen, J. J., and Pike, G. B. (2010). Global cerebral oxidative metabolism during hypercapnia and hypocapnia in humans: implications for BOLD fMRI. *J. Cereb. Blood Flow Metab.* 30, 1094–1099. doi: 10.1038/jcbfm.2010.42

Chow, N., Bell, R. D., Deane, R., Streb, J. W., Chen, J., and Brooks, A. (2007). Serum response factor and myocardin mediate arterial hypercontractility and cerebral blood flow dysregulation in Alzheimer's Phenotype. *Proc. Natl. Acad. Sci. U.S.A.* 104, 823–828. doi: 10.1073/pnas.0608251104

Chu, P. P. W., Golestani, A. M., Kwinta, J. B., Khatamian, Y. B., and Chen, J. J. (2018). Characterizing the modulation of resting-state fMRI Metrics by baseline physiology. *Neuroimage* 173, 72–87. doi: 10.1016/j.neuroimage.2018.02.004

Claassen, J. A., and Zhang, R. (2011). Cerebral Autoregulation in Alzheimer's Disease. *J. Cereb. Blood Flow Metab.* 31, 1572–1577. doi: 10.1038/jcbfm.2011.69

Cohen, E. R., Rostrup, E., Sidaros, K., Lund, T. E., Paulson, O. B., Ugurbil, K., et al. (2004). Hypercapnic normalization of BOLD fMRI: comparison across field strengths and pulse sequences. *Neuroimage* 23, 613–624. doi: 10.1016/j.neuroimage.2004.06.021

de la Torre, J. C. (2016). Cerebral perfusion enhancing interventions: a new strategy for the prevention of Alzheimer dementia. *Brain Pathol.* 26, 618–631. doi: 10.1111/bpa.12405

Dorr, A., Sahota, B., Chinta, L. V., Brown, M. E., Lai, A. Y., and Ma, K. (2012). Amyloid-Beta-dependent compromise of microvascular structure and function in a model of Alzheimer's Disease. *Brain* 135, 3039–3050. doi: 10.1093/brain/aws243

Duffin, J., Sobczyk, O., Crawley, A. P., Poublanc, J., Mikulis, D. J., and Fisher, J. A. (2015). The dynamics of cerebrovascular reactivity shown with transfer function analysis. *Neuroimage* 114, 207–216. doi: 10.1016/j.neuroimage.2015.04.029

Duling, B. R., and Berne, R. M. (1970). Longitudinal gradients in periarteriolar oxygen tension: a possible mechanism for the participation of oxygen in local regulation of blood flow. *Circ. Res.* 27, 669–678. doi: 10.1161/01.RES.27.5.669

Dumas, A., Dierksen, G. A., Gurol, M. E., Halpin, A., Martinez-Ramirez, S., Schwab, K., et al. (2012). Functional magnetic resonance imaging detection of vascular reactivity in cerebral amyloid angiopathy. *Ann. Neurol.* 72, 76–81. doi: 10.1002/ana.23566

Fierstra, J., Sobczyk, O., Battisti-Charbonney, A., Mandell, D. M., Poublanc, J., Crawley, A. P., et al. (2013). Measuring cerebrovascular reactivity: what stimulus to use? *J. Physiol.* 591, 5809–5821. doi: 10.1113/jphysiol.2013.259150

Fisher, J. A., Sobczyk, O., Crawley, A., Poublanc, J., Dufort, P., Venkatraghavan, L., et al. (2017). Assessing cerebrovascular reactivity by the pattern of response to progressive hypercapnia. *Hum. Brain Mapp.* doi: 10.1002/hbm.23598 [Epub ahead of print].

Gao, Y.-Z., Zhang, J.-J., Liu, H., Wu, G.-Y., Xiong, L., and Shu, M. (2013). Regional cerebral blood flow and cerebrovascular reactivity in Alzheimer's disease and vascular dementia assessed by arterial spinlabeling magnetic resonance imaging. *Curr. Neurovasc. Res.* 10, 49–53. doi: 10.2174/156720213804806016

Girouard, H., and Iadecola, C. (2006). Neurovascular coupling in the normal brain and in hypertension, stroke, and Alzheimer Disease. *J. Appl. Physiol.* 100, 328–335. doi: 10.1152/japplphysiol.00966.2005

Glodzik, L., Randall, C., Rusinek, H., and de Leon, M. J. (2013). Cerebrovascular reactivity to carbon dioxide in Alzheimer's Disease. *J. Alzheimer's Dis. JAD* 35, 427–440.

Golestani, A. M., Kwinta, J. B., Strother, S. C., Khatamian, Y. B., and Chen, J. J. (2016a). The association between cerebrovascular reactivity and resting-state fMRI functional connectivity in healthy adults: the influence of basal carbon dioxide. *Neuroimage* 132, 301–313. doi: 10.1016/j.neuroimage.2016.02.051

Golestani, A. M., Wei, L. L., and Chen, J. J. (2016b). Quantitative mapping of cerebrovascular reactivity using resting-state BOLD fMRI: validation in healthy adults. *Neuroimage* 138, 147–163. doi: 10.1016/j.neuroimage.2016.05.025

Göttler, J., Preibisch, C., Riederer, I., Pasquini, L., Alexopoulos, P., Bohn, K. P., et al. (2018). Reduced blood oxygenation level dependent connectivity is related to hypoperfusion in Alzheimer's Disease. *J. Cereb. Blood Flow Metab.* doi: 10.1177/0271678X18759182 [Epub ahead of print].

Hajjar, I., Sorond, F., and Lipsitz, L. A. (2015). Apolipoprotein E, carbon dioxide vasoreactivity, and cognition in older adults: effect of hypertension. *J. Am. Geriatr. Soc.* 63, 276–281. doi: 10.1111/jgs.13235

Halani, S., Kwinta, J. B., Golestani, A. M., Khatamian, Y. B., and Chen, J. J. (2015). Comparing cerebrovascular reactivity measured using BOLD and cerebral blood flow MRI: the effect of basal vascular tension on vasodilatory and vasoconstrictive reactivity. *Neuroimage* 110, 110–123. doi: 10.1016/j.neuroimage.2015.01.050

Hashimura, T., Kimura, T., and Miyakawa, T. (1991). Morphological changes of blood vessels in the brain with Alzheimer's Disease. *Jpn. J. Psychiatry Neurol.* 45, 661–665. doi: 10.1111/j.1440-1819.1991.tb01187.x

Herzig, R., Hlustík, P., Skoloudík, D., Sanák, D., Vlachová, I., Herman, M., et al. (2008). Assessment of the cerebral vasomotor reactivity in internal carotid artery occlusion using a transcranial doppler sonography and functional MRI. *J. Neuroimaging* 18, 38–45. doi: 10.1111/j.1552-6569.2007.00168.x

Hoge, R. D., Atkinson, J., Gill, B., Crelier, G. R., Marrett, S., and Pike, G. B. (1999). Investigation of BOLD signal dependence on CBF and CMRO: the deoxyhemoglobin dilution model. *Magn. Reson. Med.* 42, 849–863. doi: 10.1002/(SICI)1522-2594(199911)42:5<849::AID-MRM4>3.0.CO;2-Z

Iadecola, C., Pelligrino, D. A., Moskowitz, M. A., and Lassen, N. A. (1994). Nitric oxide synthase inhibition and cerebrovascular regulation. *J. Cereb. Blood Flow Metab.* 14, 175–192. doi: 10.1038/jcbfm.1994.25

Iannetti, G. D., and Wise, R. G. (2007). BOLD functional MRI in disease and pharmacological studies: room for improvement? *Magn. Reson. Imaging* 25, 978–988. doi: 10.1016/j.mri.2007.03.018

Ito, H., Kanno, I., and Fukuda, H. (2005). Human cerebral circulation: positron emission tomography studies. *Ann. Nucl. Med.* 19, 65–74. doi: 10.1007/BF03027383

Ito, H., Takahashi, K., Hatazawa, J., Kim, S.-G., and Kanno, I. (2001). Changes in human regional cerebral blood flow and cerebral blood volume during visual stimulation measured by positron emission tomography. *J. Cereb. Blood Flow Metab.* 21, 608–612. doi: 10.1097/00004647-200105000-00015

Jahanian, H., Christen, T., Moseley, M. E., Pajewski, N. M., Wright, C. B., Tamura, M. K., et al. (2017). Measuring vascular reactivity with resting-state blood oxygenation level-dependent (BOLD) signal fluctuations: a potential alternative to the breath-holding challenge? *J. Cereb. Blood Flow Metab.* 37, 2526–2538. doi: 10.1177/0271678X16670921

Jain, V., Langham, M. C., Floyd, T. F., Jain, G., Magland, J. F., and Wehrli, F. W. (2011). Rapid magnetic resonance measurement of global cerebral metabolic rate of oxygen consumption in humans during rest and hypercapnia. *J. Cereb. Blood Flow Metab.* 31, 1504–1512. doi: 10.1038/jcbfm.2011.34

Jellinger, K. A., and Attems, J. (2006). Prevalence and impact of cerebrovascular pathology in Alzheimer's Disease and Parkinsonism. *Acta Neurol. Scand.* 114, 38–46. doi: 10.1111/j.1600-0404.2006.00665.x

Johnson, N. A., Jahng, G. H., Weiner, M. W., Miller, B. L., Chui, H. C., Jagust, W. J., et al. (2005). Pattern of cerebral hypoperfusion in Alzheimer Disease and mild cognitive impairment measured with arterial spin-labeling MR imaging: initial experience. *Radiology* 234, 851–859. doi: 10.1148/radiol.2343040197

Kannurpatti, S. S., Motes, M. A., Biswal, B. B., and Rypma, B. (2014). Assessment of unconstrained cerebrovascular reactivity marker for large age-range FMRI studies. *PLoS One* 9:e88751. doi: 10.1371/journal.pone.0088751

Kassner, A., Winter, J. D., Poublanc, J., Mikulis, D. J., and Crawley, A. P. (2010). Blood-Oxygen level dependent MRI measures of cerebrovascular reactivity using a controlled respiratory challenge: reproducibility and gender differences. *J. Magn. Reson. Imaging* 31, 298–304. doi: 10.1002/jmri.22044

Kawanabe, Y., and Nauli, S. M. (2011). Endothelin. *Cell Mol. Life Sci.* 68, 195–203. doi: 10.1007/s00018-010-0518-0

Kisler, K., Nelson, A. R., Montagne, A., and Zlokovic, B. V. (2017). Cerebral blood flow regulation and neurovascular dysfunction in Alzheimer Disease. *Nat. Rev. Neurosci.* 18, 419–434. doi: 10.1038/nrn.2017.48

Lajoie, I., Nugent, S., Debacker, C., Dyson, K., Tancredi, F. B., Badhwar, A., et al. (2017). Application of calibrated fMRI in Alzheimer's Disease. *Neuroimage Clin.* 15, 348–358. doi: 10.1016/j.nicl.2017.05.009

Lee, S.-T., Jung, K.-H., and Lee, Y.-S. (2007). Decreased vasomotor reactivity in Alzheimer's Disease. *J. Clin. Neurol.* 3, 18–23. doi: 10.3988/jcn.2007.3.1.18

Leoni, R. F., Oliveira, I. A., Pontes-Neto, O. M., Santos, A. C., and Leite, J. P. (2017). Cerebral blood flow and vasoreactivity in aging: an arterial spin labeling study. *Braz. J. Med. Biol. Res.* 50:e5670. doi: 10.1590/1414-431X20175670

Liu, P., Li, Y., Pinho, M., Park, D. C., Welch, B. G., and Lu, H. (2017). Cerebrovascular reactivity mapping without gas challenges. *Neuroimage* 146, 320–326. doi: 10.1016/j.neuroimage.2016.11.054

Lu, H., Xu, F., Rodrigue, K. M., Kennedy, K. M., Cheng, Y., Flicker, B., et al. (2011). Alterations in cerebral metabolic rate and blood supply across the adult lifespan. *Cereb. Cortex* 21, 1426–1434. doi: 10.1093/cercor/bhq224

Mark, C. I., Slessarev, M., Ito, S., Han, J., Fisher, J. A., and Pike, G. B. (2010). Precise control of end-tidal carbon dioxide and oxygen improves BOLD and ASL cerebrovascular reactivity measures. *Magn. Reson. Med.* 64, 749–756. doi: 10.1002/mrm.22405

Miyakawa, T., Katsuragi, S., Higuchi, Y., Yamashita, K., Kimura, T., Teraoka, K., et al. (1997). Changes of microvessels in the brain with Alzheimer's Disease. *Ann. N. Y. Acad. Sci.* 826, 428–432. doi: 10.1111/j.1749-6632.1997.tb48497.x

Ogoh, S., Hayashi, N., Inagaki, M., Ainslie, P. N., and Miyamoto, T. (2008). Interaction between the ventilatory and cerebrovascular responses to hypo- and hypercapnia at rest and during exercise. *J. Physiol.* 586, 4327–4338. doi: 10.1113/jphysiol.2008.157073

Park, L., Zhou, P., Pitstick, R., Capone, C., Anrather, J., Norris, E. H., et al. (2008). Nox2-Derived radicals contribute to neurovascular and behavioral dysfunction in mice overexpressing the amyloid precursor protein. *Proc. Natl. Acad. Sci. U.S.A.* 105, 1347–1352. doi: 10.1073/pnas.0711568105

Peebles, K. C., Mark Richards, A., Celi, L., McGrattan, K., Murrell, C. J., and Ainslie, P. N. (2008). Human cerebral arteriovenous vasoactive exchange during alterations in arterial blood gases. *J. Appl. Physiol.* 105, 1060–1068. doi: 10.1152/japplphysiol.90613.2008

Pillai, J. J., and Mikulis, D. J. (2015). Cerebrovascular reactivity mapping: an evolving standard for clinical functional imaging. *AJNR Am. J. Neuroradiol.* 36, 7–13. doi: 10.3174/ajnr.A3941

Pinto, J., Jorge, J., Sousa, I., Vilela, P., and Figueiredo, P. (2016). Fourier modeling of the BOLD response to a breath-hold task: optimization and reproducibility. *Neuroimage* 135, 223–231. doi: 10.1016/j.neuroimage.2016.02.037

Poublanc, J., Crawley, A. P., Sobczyk, O., Montandon, G., Sam, K., Mandell, D. M., et al. (2015). Measuring cerebrovascular reactivity: the dynamic response to a step hypercapnic stimulus. *J. Cereb. Blood Flow Metab.* 35, 1746–1756. doi: 10.1038/jcbfm.2015.114

Poulin, M. J., Liang, P. J., and Robbins, P. A. (1996). Dynamics of the cerebral blood flow response to step changes in end-tidal PCO2 and PO2 in humans. *J. Appl. Physiol.* 81, 1084–1095. doi: 10.1152/jappl.1996.81.3.1084

Ramanathan, A., Nelson, A. R., Sagare, A. P., and Zlokovic, B. V. (2015). Impaired vascular-mediated clearance of brain amyloid beta in Alzheimer's disease: the role, regulation and restoration of LRP1. *Front. Aging Neurosci.* 7:136. doi: 10.3389/fnagi.2015.00136

Ratnatunga, C., and Adiseshiah, M. (1990). Increase in middle cerebral artery velocity on breath holding: a simplified test of cerebral perfusion reserve. *Eur. J. Vasc. Surg.* 4, 519–523. doi: 10.1016/S0950-821X(05)80795-9

Rodell, A. B., Aanerud, J., Braendgaard, H., and Gjedde, A. (2012). Low residual CBF variability in Alzheimer's disease after correction for CO2 effect. *Front. Neuroenerg.* 4:8. doi: 10.3389/fnene.2012.00008

Roy, C. S., and Sherrington, C. S. (1890). On the regulation of the blood supply of the brain. *J. Physiol.* 11, 85–105. doi: 10.1113/jphysiol.1890.sp000321

Sabayan, B., Jansen, S., Oleksik, A. M., van Osch, M. J. P., van Buchem, M. A., van Vliet, P., et al. (2012). Cerebrovascular hemodynamics in Alzheimer's Disease and vascular dementia: a meta-analysis of transcranial doppler studies. *Ageing Res. Rev.* 11, 271–277. doi: 10.1016/j.arr.2011.12.009

Sam, K., Crawley, A. P., Poublanc, J., Conklin, J., Sobczyk, O., Mandell, D. M., et al. (2016). Vascular dysfunction in leukoaraiosis. *AJNR Am. J. Neuroradiol.* 37, 2258–2264. doi: 10.3174/ajnr.A4888

Sato, N., and Morishita, R. (2013). Roles of vascular and metabolic components in cognitive dysfunction of Alzheimer disease: short- and long-term modification by non-genetic risk factors. *Front. Aging Neurosci.* 5:64. doi: 10.3389/fnagi.2013.00064

Shibutani, K., Shirasaki, S., Kubal, K., and Gupte, P. (1992). Changes in cardiac output affect PETCO2 AND CO2 transport during unsteady state in man. *Anesthesiology* 77(Suppl.):A468. doi: 10.1097/00000542-199209001-00468

Slessarev, M., Han, J., Mardimae, A., Prisman, E., Preiss, D., Volgyesi, G., et al. (2007). Prospective targeting and control of end-tidal CO2 and O2 concentrations. *J. Physiol.* 581(Pt 3), 1207–1219.

Sobczyk, O., Battisti-Charbonney, A., Fierstra, J., Mandell, D. M., Poublanc, J., Crawley, A. P., et al. (2014). A conceptual model for CO2-Induced redistribution of cerebral blood flow with experimental confirmation using BOLD MRI. *Neuroimage* 92, 56–68. doi: 10.1016/j.neuroimage.2014.01.051

Sobczyk, O., Battisti-Charbonney, A., Poublanc, J., Crawley, A. P., Sam, K., Fierstra, J., et al. (2015). Assessing cerebrovascular reactivity abnormality by comparison to a reference atlas. *J. Cereb. Blood Flow Metab.* 35, 213–220. doi: 10.1038/jcbfm.2014.184

Spano, V. R., Mandell, D. M., Poublanc, J., Sam, K., Battisti-Charbonney, A., Pucci, O., et al. (2013). CO2 blood oxygen level-dependent MR mapping of cerebrovascular reserve in a clinical population: safety, tolerability, and technical feasibility. *Radiology* 266, 592–598. doi: 10.1148/radiol.12112795

Strittmatter, W. J., Saunders, A. M., Schmechel, D., Pericak-Vance, M., and Enghild Salvesen, G. S. (1993). Apolipoprotein E: high-avidity binding to beta-amyloid and increased frequency of type 4 allele in late-onset familial Alzheimer Disease. *Proc. Natl. Acad. Sci. U.S.A.* 90, 1977–1981. doi: 10.1073/pnas.90.5.1977

Suri, S., Mackay, C. E., Kelly, M. E., Germuska, M., Tunbridge, E. M., Frisoni, G. B., et al. (2014). Reduced cerebrovascular reactivity in young adults carrying the APOE epsilon4 Allele. *Alzheimer's Dement.* 11, 648.e1–657.e1. doi: 10.1016/j.jalz.2014.05.1755

Tancredi, F. B., and Hoge, R. D. (2013). Comparison of cerebral vascular reactivity measures obtained using breath-holding and CO2 inhalation. *J. Cereb. Blood Flow Metab.* 33, 1066–1074. doi: 10.1038/jcbfm.2013.48

Thomas, B. P., Liu, P., Park, D. C., van Osch, M. J., and Lu, H. (2014). Cerebrovascular reactivity in the brain white matter: magnitude, temporal characteristics, and age effects. *J. Cereb. Blood Flow Metab.* 34, 242–247. doi: 10.1038/jcbfm.2013.194

van Niftrik, C. H. B., Piccirelli, M., Bozinov, O., Pangalu, A., Fisher, J. A., Valavanis, A., et al. (2017). Iterative analysis of cerebrovascular reactivity dynamic response by temporal decomposition. *Brain Behav.* 7:e00705. doi: 10.1002/brb3.705

Viticchi, G., Falsetti, L., Vernieri, F., Altamura, C., Bartolini, M., Luzzi, S., et al. (2012). Vascular predictors of cognitive decline in patients with mild cognitive impairment. *Neurobiol. Aging* 33, 1127.e1–1127.e9. doi: 10.1016/j.neurobiolaging.2011.11.027

Wells, J. A., Holmes, H. E., O'Callaghan, J. M., Colgan, N., Ismail, O., Fisher, E. M., et al. (2015). Increased cerebral vascular reactivity in the tau expressing rTg4510 mouse: evidence against the role of tau pathology to impair vascular health in Alzheimer's Disease. *J. Cereb. Blood Flow Metab.* 35, 359–362. doi: 10.1038/jcbfm.2014.224

Williams, J. S., and Babb, T. G. (1997). Differences between estimates and measured PaCO2 during rest and exercise in older subjects. *J. Appl. Physiol.* 83, 312–316. doi: 10.1152/jappl.1997.83.1.312

Yew, B., Nation, D. A., and Alzheimer's Disease Neuroimaging Initiative (2017). Cerebrovascular resistance: effects on cognitive decline, cortical atrophy, and progression to dementia. *Brain* 140, 1987–2001. doi: 10.1093/brain/awx112

Yezhuvath, U. S., Lewis-Amezcua, K., Varghese, R., Xiao, G., and Lu, H. (2009). On the assessment of cerebrovascular reactivity using hypercapnia BOLD MRI. *NMR Biomed.* 22, 779–786. doi: 10.1002/nbm.1392

Yezhuvath, U. S., Uh, J., Cheng, Y., Martin-Cook, K., Weiner, M., Diaz-Arrastia, R., et al. (2012). Forebrain-Dominant deficit in cerebrovascular reactivity in Alzheimer's Disease. *Neurobiol. Aging* 33, 75–82. doi: 10.1016/j.neurobiolaging.2010.02.005

3

Metabolic and Vascular Imaging Biomarkers in Down Syndrome Provide Unique Insights Into Brain Aging and Alzheimer Disease Pathogenesis

Elizabeth Head[1], David K. Powell[2] and Frederick A. Schmitt[3]*

[1] Department of Pharmacology & Nutritional Sciences, Sanders Brown Center on Aging, University of Kentucky, Lexington, KY, United States, [2] Magnetic Resonance Imaging and Spectroscopy Center, Sanders Brown Center on Aging, University of Kentucky, Lexington, KY, United States, [3] Department of Neurology, Sanders Brown Center on Aging, University of Kentucky, Lexington, KY, United States

***Correspondence:**
Elizabeth Head
elizabeth.head@uky.edu

People with Down syndrome (DS) are at high risk for developing Alzheimer disease (AD). Neuropathology consistent with AD is present by 40 years of age and dementia may develop up to a decade later. In this review, we describe metabolic and vascular neuroimaging studies in DS that suggest these functional changes are a key feature of aging, linked to cognitive decline and AD in this vulnerable cohort. FDG-PET imaging in DS suggests systematic reductions in glucose metabolism in posterior cingulate and parietotemporal cortex. Magentic resonance spectroscopy studies show consistent decreases in neuronal health and increased myoinositol, suggesting inflammation. There are few vascular imaging studies in DS suggesting a gap in our knowledge. Future studies would benefit from longitudinal measures and combining various imaging approaches to identify early signs of dementia in DS that may be amenable to intervention.

Keywords: dementia, FDG-PET, hypometabolism, hypermetabolism, myoinositol, MR spectroscopy, T2*, trisomy 21

INTRODUCTION

The life expectancy of people with Down syndrome (DS) continues to increase due to improved health care and management of co-occurring illnesses (Bittles and Glasson, 2004). Consequently there are more people with DS and the population has grown from 49,923 in 1950 to 206, 336 in 2010 (de Graaf et al., 2017). However, mortality rate is higher in people with DS in older ages relative to the general population (Ng et al., 2017) and further, some deaths such as those due to respiratory disorders and epilepsy may be amenable to medical intervention (Hosking et al., 2016). As with the general population, the risk of developing health-related problems increases as people with DS get older. In particular, people with DS are at a high risk of developing cognitive impairment and clinical dementia after the age of 50 years (Zigman et al., 1996; Sinai et al., 2018). Virtually all adults with DS develop the neuropathology for a brain-based Alzheimer disease (AD) diagnosis by the age of 40 years (reviewed in Head et al., 2016). This is thought to be due to the lifelong overexpression of the APP gene on chromosome 21 leading to early onset and rapid accumulation of beta-amyloid (Aβ) with age (Head et al., 2016). Thus, by studying individuals with DS across the lifespan it is possible to identify early biomarkers of AD pathogenesis that may not be feasible in the general population as the age of onset of AD varies tremendously (e.g., 50-over 100 years). As will be discussed later in this review, cerebrovascular pathology may help to accelerate AD in DS and be an important contributor to dementia. Interestingly, a subset of adults with DS never develops dementia even in the presence of this AD pathology (Franceschi et al., 1990; Schupf and Sergievsky, 2002; Head et al., 2012a,b).

Neuroimaging studies help us detect structural, connectivity, activity, neurochemical, and vascular/metabolic functional changes with age and with the development of AD. As the development of AD neuropathology in DS is strongly age-dependent, we can learn about early changes associated with the progression of AD through neuroimaging studies in DS (Neale et al., 2018). These studies not only help us understand aging and AD in people with DS but can translate to our understanding of AD in the general population. For example, Jack and Holtzman (2013) proposed a hypothetical series of biomarker events including neuroimaging outcomes that may occur prior to changes in cognition and be predictive of decline in the general population. For example, Jack and colleagues suggest that Aβ can be detected prior to brain structure changes, which in turn are detectable prior to mild cognitive impairment and dementia. A similar series of biomarker events can be hypothetically applied for people with DS but using age as opposed to the clinical disease stage as the time axis. Whereas in the general population, biomarker changes reflecting progressive AD are plotted as a function of the cognitive continiuum, in DS we can use age as a representative to AD pathogenesis. It is clear from this hypothetical model that neuroimaging can provide early markers of dementia-associated brain changes and the inclusion of vascular or metabolic imaging may play an important role by providing even earlier information regarding AD pathogenesis.

METABOLIC IMAGING BIOMARKERS—FDG-PET

Metabolic imaging using positron emission tomography (PET) has consistently shown reductions in glucose utilization in vulnerable brain regions in sporadic AD (Silverman and Phelps, 2001). In particular, the precuneus, posterior cingulate cortex and posterior parietotemporal lobes may be the earliest site of reduced glucose metabolism (FDG-PET) prior to onset of symptoms (Minoshima et al., 1997). In AD, the extent of cerebral metabolic rate of glucose from FDG-PET studies (CMRglu) is correlated with the severity of dementia (Minoshima et al., 1997). As AD progresses, more brain regions show declines in CMRglu such as the frontal cortex. CMRglu from FDG-PET can also predict AD neuropathology with 84–93% sensitivity and 73% specificity (Silverman et al., 2001; Jagust et al., 2007).

There are relatively few FDG-PET studies in DS with the majority being acquired under resting conditions (**Table 1** summarizes studies since 1983). However the results of these studies have been relatively consistent. First, younger individuals with DS (without dementia) show increased glucose metabolism (Schwartz et al., 1983; Cutler, 1986; Azari et al., 1994a; Haier et al., 2003, 2008; Lengyel et al., 2006; Matthews et al., 2016) relative to age matched controls in all but one study (Schapiro et al., 1992b). The regions that show hypermetabolism include the prefrontal cortex, sensorimotor cortex, thalamus, inferior temporal/entorhinal cortex. Interestingly, increased glucose metabolic rate is associated with decreased gray matter volume in the temporal cortex including the parahippocampus/hippocampus suggesting that hypermetabolism is a compensatory response (Haier et al., 2008). Indeed, autopsy studies of the same brain region in a case series of DS shows evidence of neuronal sprouting positive for tau phosphorylation suggesting a mechanistic basis for increased glucose metabolism in middle age (Head et al., 2003). Other molecular events may also underlie this phenomenon (reviewed in Head et al., 2007).

In contrast, older individuals with DS and particularly those with dementia show hypometabolism in multiple studies (Schwartz et al., 1983; Cutler, 1986; Schapiro et al., 1992a; Azari et al., 1994a,b; Rafii et al., 2015; Sabbagh et al., 2015; Matthews et al., 2016). Brain regions that appear to be systematically affected under either resting or active conditions include the posterior cingulate cortex, hippocampus, parietal and temporal cortex consistent with reports in sporadic AD (Minoshima et al., 1997; Pietrini et al., 1997; Silverman and Phelps, 2001). Further, in a 45 year old female with mosaic/translation DS with clinical signs of early dementia, a pattern of hypometabolism similar to that of sporadic AD was observed (Schapiro et al., 1992a).

Reduced glucose metabolism in older adults with DS and dementia is associated with decreased cortical volumes (Matthews et al., 2016), increased amyloid binding with florbetapir (Matthews et al., 2016) and increased tau binding using AV-1451 (Rafii et al., 2017). Some studies report associations between cognition and glucose metabolism (Haier et al., 2008; Sabbagh et al., 2015; Matthews et al., 2016) but not all (Rafii et al., 2015), with variable results likely due to smaller sample sizes. In one of the only longitudinal studies that was found, Dani and colleagues reported stable glucose metabolic rates over a 7 year period of time unless clinical dementia had evolved (occurred in one person with DS) leading to rapid glucose metabolic decline in parietal and temporal cortices (Dani et al., 1996).

Reductions in glucose metabolism may lead to or reflect neuronal loss, synapse loss, and/or mitochondrial dysfunction. Given that all these events are thought to occur with age and dementia in DS (Head et al., 2016), PET imaging can provide useful information with respect to brain function but there is a clear need for more longitudinal studies that includes measures of cognition. It is also notable that despite the posterior cingulate cortex being an early site of glucose metabolic losses, there are few studies of AD neuropathology in this region in DS. The use of FDG-PET to capture information about metabolism requires the use of intravenous injections of radioactive ligands. This procedure may be problematic for some participants, their families and particularly for those with dementia. However, as an outcome measure that may reflect a rapid response to treatment that is targeting metabolism, FDG-PET has utility. In future, similar outcomes reflecting metabolic changes such as blood flow,

TABLE 1 | Summary of FDG-PET studies in DS (since 1983).

Authors	Date	Resting or active	Cohort	Clinical data	Outcome	References
Schwartz et al.	1983	Resting	$n = 4$ young DS 19–27 years and $n = 1$ aged DS 51 years, $n = 10$ young controls 21–33 years and $n = 8$ aged controls 45–55 years	None	Increased glucose metabolic rate in multiple brain regions in young DS relative to age matched controls whereas the 51 year old showed reduced metabolic rate to young DS controls (but not to old controls).	Schwartz et al., 1983
Cutler	1986	Resting	$n = 10$ DS 19–23 years, $n = 4$ DS 41–64 year (2 were demented) and $n = 14$ young 20–35 year and 19 40–60 year	None	Young and old control groups not different. CMRglu higher by 20–30% in young DS compared to young controls, lower CMRglu in old DS compared to young DS but not different from controls.	Cutler, 1986
Schapiro et al.	1988	Resting	$n = 1$ DS 47 years with autopsy confirmed AD, $n = 13$ non-demented DS, 19–33 years)	General intelligence, visuospatial ability, language and memory	Glucose metabolism was 28% less in the demented DS case involving the parietal and temporal cortex.	Schapiro et al., 1988
Schapiro et al.	1990	Resting	$n = 14$ non-demented DS 25–38 years, $n = 13$ controls 22–38 years.	PPVT	No differences in glucose metabolism in non-demented adults with DS relative to controls.	Schapiro et al., 1990
Horwitz et al.	1990	Resting	$n = 14$ DS < 34 years vs. $n = 24$ controls	None	The correlation between regional rates of glucose metabolism in DS was large and negative for the inferior frontal gyrus including Broca's area whereas in controls this association was positive.	Horwitz et al., 1990
Schapiro et al.	1992	Resting	$n = 20$ DS 19–34 years and 9 older DS, 45–63 years. Controls were $n = 13$ $22 = 39$ years.	Stanford-Binet, PPVT, Digit Span, Block Tapping Span and Object Pointing Span, Memory for Object subtest from DSMSE and recognition memory for designs, grammatic closure and manual expression, Hiskey Nebraska Block Pattery Subtest, WISC-R Block design	No difference in glucose metabolism found between young DS and young controls. DS with dementia had hypometabolism in association cortices (parietal and lateral temporal) and primary neocortex (sensorimotor and occipital). Mosaic/translation person with DS (45 years) with mild dementia showed reduced temporal glucose metabolism.	Schapiro et al., 1992a
Azari et al.	1994	Resting	$n = 14$ DS 26–38 years vs. n-17 controls	Stanford-Binet, DSMSE	DS vs. CTL not different on whole brain CMRglu, DS<CTL in left paracentral, left inferior parietal, anterior cingulate, posterior cingulate, right cerebellum, left cerebellum, DS>CTL left prefrontal, right sensorimotor, right thalamus.	Azari et al., 1994b
Azari et al.	1994	Resting	$n = 15$ Young DS, $n = 10$ older DS without dementia, $n = 4$ DS with dementia and $n = 15$ young controls	Stanford-Binet, DSMSE	All DS with dementia and some of the DS without dementia scans appeared similar to that of AD patterns.	Azari et al., 1994a
Dani et al.	1996	Resting	$n = 12$ non-demented DS 31–59 years, longitudinal evaluation—$n = 2$ (49,50 years) became demented	DSMSE	People with DS who were non-demented did not show changes in glucose metabolism over 7 years. Two people developed dementia after 7 years and showed a rapid decline in glucose metabolism in parietal and temporal regions.	Dani et al., 1996
Pietrini et al.	1997	Resting and audiovisual stimulation	$n = 8$ DS 32–38 years and $n = 8$ DS 43–61 years	Stanford-Binet Intelligence Scale, DSMSE, PPVT	At rest, no differences in glucose metabolism were observed. During stimulation, older subjects with DS showed reduced glucose metabolic rates in parietal and temporal cortex.	Pietrini et al., 1997

(Continued)

TABLE 1 | Continued

Authors	Date	Resting or active	Cohort	Clinical data	Outcome	References
Haier et al.	2003	Continuous performance task	*n* = 17 DS (non-demented 34–55 years), *n*- *n* = 10 moderate AD, *n* = 12 young controls, *n* = 12 old controls)	Wechsler Adult Intelligence Scale III, DSDS, DMR, MMSE (for AD)	DS and AD participants had lower glucose metabolic rates relative to each of their control groups in the posterior cingulate. DS had higher GMR in inferior temporal/entorhinal cortex where AD subjects had lower GMR. Non-demented people with DS showed hypermetabolism as a compensatory response.	Haier et al., 2003
Lengyel et al.	2006	Resting	*n* = 11 DS (5–24 years) and *n* = 9 control (4–24 years)	None	Glucose metabolic rate was higher in DS relative to controls in 6 regions: left medial temporal gyrus, left precentral and inferior frontal gyri, anterior cingulate gyri.	Lengyel et al., 2006
Haier et al.	2008	Continuous performance task	*n* = 19 non-demented DS 34–52 years	DMR	Higher glucose metabolic rate was associated with decreased gray matter volume in temporal cortex including the parahippocampus/hippocampus, in the thalamus, caudate, and frontal lobe. Results consistent with a compensatory response.	Haier et al., 2008
Rafii et al.	2015	Resting	*n* = 12 non-demented DS (30–60 years)	CANTAB, RBANS, VABS, Observer Memory Questionnaire-Parent Form, Anxiety Depression and Mood Scale, Cambridge Examination for Mental Disorders of Older People with Down's syndrome and other with Intellectual Disability, Dalton Dyspraxia scale, Goodenough-Harris Draw-A-Person Test	People with DS over 39 years age of showed consistent hypometabolism by clinical read. No correlations with cognition.	Rafii et al., 2015
Sabbagh et al.	2015	Resting	*n* = 5 DS with AD, 12 non-demented DS and 9 normal controls	DMR, MMSE, BPT, SIB and VABS	DS with AD showed hypometabolism in posterior cingulate, lateral parietal, and temporal and frontal regions. Non-demented and demented DS had lower glucose metabolic rates in additional frontal regions compared with controls.	Sabbagh et al., 2015
Matthews et al.	2016		*n* = 12 non-demented DS (32–61 years), *n* = 12 normal, *n* = 12 early MCI, *n* = 12 late MCI, *n* = 12 AD and *n* = 12 and controls from ADNI	VABS	Posterior cingulate cortex and hippocampus showed hypometabolism in DS relative to controls. Lower glucose metabolic rate was observed in regions showing volumetric losses (mid cingulate, anterior cingulate, paracentral lobule, and hippocampus). Hypermetabolism was observed with preserved volume in the prefrontal cortex but reduced volume in occipital cortex. Patterns of glucose metabolism and volume losses corresponded to amyloid burden (florbetapir) and cognition.	Matthews et al., 2016

(Continued)

TABLE 1 | Continued

Authors	Date	Resting or active	Cohort	Clinical data	Outcome	References
Rafii et al.	2017	Resting	$n = 12$ non-demented DS 30–60 years, $n = 12$ normal older adults, $n = 12$ AD	CANTAB, RBANS, VABS, Observer Memory Questionnaire-Parent Form, Anxiety Depression and Mood Scale, Cambridge Examination for Mental Disorders of Older People with Down's syndrome and other with Intellectual Disability, Dalton Dyspraxia scale, Goodenough-Harris Draw-A-Person Test	Areas with lower glucose metabolic rates were associated with tau accumulation by PET (F-AV-1451).	Rafii et al., 2017
Lao et al.	2018	Resting	$n = 16$ non-demented DS (Avg age 35 years—PiB negative), $n = 5$ non-demented DS (Avg age 47 years—PiB positive), $n = 3$ demented DS (Avg age 49 years)	PPVT	Glucose metabolism was reduced in the parietal cortex with increased PiB (amyloid) binding. Glucose metabolism was negatively associated with age (frontal, parietal, and temporal cortex). No correlation between striatal binding for PiB (amyloid) and glucose metabolism.	Lao et al., 2018

CMRglu, glucose cerebral metabolic rate; GMR, glucose metabolic rate; PPVT, Peabody Picture Vocabulary Test; DSMSE, Down syndrome mental state examination; WISC, Wechsler Intelligence Scale for Children; DSDS, Dementia scale for Down syndrome; DMR, dementia questionnaire for mentally retarded persons; RBANS, Repeatable Battery for the Assessment of Neuropsychological status; CANTAB, Cambridge Neuropsychological Test Automated Battery; VABS, Vineland Adaptive Behavior Scale; BPT, Brief Praxis Test; SIB, severe impairment battery.

may be obtainable using relatively short MR protocols such as arterial spin labeling (7 min). Further, as will be discussed next, magnetic resonance spectroscopy, which is also a relatively short protocol (5 min) that may be useful for a broader spectrum of participants can provide specific metabolic markers that could help dissect the different neuronal/glial pathways that signal onset of dementia.

METABOLIC IMAGING BIOMARKERS—MRS

Proton magnetic resonance spectroscopy (^{1}H-MRS) has been widely used to characterize the neurochemistry of brain health and disease. In particular, the neuronal markers of N-acetylaspartate (NAA) and glutamate-glutamine complex (Glx) decrease, and the glial marker of myo-inositol (MI) increases, both correlate with clinical variables in aging and AD (Parnetti et al., 1997; Lin and Rothman, 2014). It is thought that lower levels of NAA or Glx reflects neuronal loss or injury; neuroinflammation is associated with activated astrocytes and microglial cells leading to increased MI (Chang et al., 2013). The ratio of NAA to MI can also be used to distinguish non-demented from demented people (cf. Lin et al., 2005).

In DS, there have been several studies using MRS with assessments done for posterior cingulate cortex, hippocampus, frontal cortex, occipital cortex, and parietal cortex with comparisons to age matched controls (**Table 2**). Decreased NAA and increased MI is observed relatively consistently across studies in non-demented adults with DS compared with age matched non-DS controls (Shonk and Ross, 1995; Berry et al., 1999; Huang et al., 1999; Beacher et al., 2005; Lamar et al., 2011; Lin et al., 2016) with a few exceptions (Murata et al., 1993; Smigielska-Kuzia et al., 2010). Hippocampal Glx was not different in people with DS from controls (Tan et al., 2014). It may not be surprising that MI levels are generally higher in people with DS as the MI cotransporter (SLC5A3) gene is on chromosome 21 and is overexpressed in DS (Berry et al., 1995). Further, synaptojanin 1 (gene also on chromosome 21) can lead to increased gliosis (Herrera et al., 2009) and thus possibly, higher MI levels.

With age, older people with DS show higher MI and lower NAA than younger people with DS. MI was higher in the occipital and parietal cortex of older DS subjects relative to younger people with DS (Huang et al., 1999). In the hippocampus of older adults with dementia with DS, MI is also higher and NAA lower when compared to non-demented people with DS (Lamar et al., 2011) but Glx is unchanged (Tan et al., 2014). In the posterior cingulate cortex, MI was not significantly different in people with DS who were demented compared with those who were not demented, but NAA was significantly decreased (Lin et al., 2016). However, there is a case report of an individual with DS who was demented showing higher MI and lower NAA relative to non-demented DS individuals (Shonk and Ross, 1995). Further increases in MI reported in some studies with aging and dementia may reflect

TABLE 2 | Summary of MRS studies in DS (since 1993).

Authors	Date	Brain Region	Cohort	Clinical data	Outcome	References
Murata et al.	1993	white matter around the anterior horn of the lateral ventricle of frontal cortex	$n = 18$ DS 20–40 years, $n = 15$ controls (avg age 35.8 years)	Koh's Block-Design Test, Goodenough's Draw a Man Test	No differences in NAA noted across the groups nor as a function of age. MI was not analyzed. Note, many of these DS participants were institutionalized and controls were physicians and staff members. Two people with DS were mosaic.	Murata et al., 1993
Shonk & Ross	1995	N/A	$n = 23$ non-demented DS (age unknown), $n = 1$ demented DS (age unknown)	Unknown	MI was elevated in non-demented people with DS relative to controls and further elevated in DS with dementia. NAA was decreased in the DS with dementia participant.	Shonk and Ross, 1995
Huang et al.	1999	parietal and occipital cortex	$n = 8$ young DS 28–39 years, n-11 non-demented older DS 42–62 years, $n = 8$ young controls 22–39 years and $n = 9$ old controls 40–64 years	None	MI was 50% higher in occipital and parietal cortex of adults with DS relative to controls. Older DS subjects had higher MI than younger DS subjects. NAA was lower in older DS and controls relative to younger controls but not exacerbated in DS.	Huang et al., 1999
Berry et al.	1999	corpus striatum	$n = 14$, 1.2–13.6 years DS and n-13 1.3–11.7 year old controls	None	MI was significantly higher (28%) in basal ganglia of DS relative to controls. Choline containing compounds were significantly lower in DS relative to controls.	Berry et al., 1999
Beacher et al.	2005	Hippocampus	$n = 38$, 18–66 years non-demented DS and $n = 42$, 19–66 controls	CAMCOG	Hippocampal MI was higher in DS than controls. In DS, hippocampal MI correlated with cognition.	Beacher et al., 2005
Smigielska-Kuzia et al.	2007	Frontal cortex	$n = 14$ non-demented DS 7–17 years, $n = 20$ controls	None	Signficantly decreased Glx and NAA observed in DS relative to controls.	Smigielska-Kuzia and Sobaniec, 2007
Smigielska-Kuzia et al.	2010	Temporal lobes	$n = 20$ DS 3–15 years and $n = 20$ controls 6–15 years	None	Glx was not different between the DS and control groups. NAA and MI was significantly lower in DS relative to controls. GABA was also lower in DS.	Smigielska-Kuzia et al., 2010
Lamar et al.	2011	Hippocampus	$n = 35$ demented people with DS (Avg age = 52.8 years), $n = 18$ non-demented DS (Avg age 47.2 years) and $n = 13$ controls (Avg age 50.6 years), $n = 39$ sporadic AD (Avg age 76.8 years)	CAMDEX	MI was significantly higher in DS with dementia relative to non-demented DS (13% higher) and controls (19% higher).NAA was significantly reduced in DS with dementia relative to DS without dementia (11%) but was similar to controls. DS with dementia MI was significannlty higher relative to sporadic AD.	Lamar et al., 2011
Tan et al.	2014	Hippocampus	$n = 35$ non-demented DS (Avg age 35 years), $n = 11$ demented DS (Avg age 52 years) and $n = 39$ controls (Avg age 35 years)	CAMCOG	No differences in Glx across the 3 groups nor correlation with cognition.	Tan et al., 2014
Lin et al.	2016	Posterior Cingulate Cortex	$n = 22$ non-demented DS (Avg age 46.7 years), $n = 5$ demented DS (Avg age 53.7 years), $n = 15$ control (Avg age 47.8 years)	SIB, BPT, DMR	NAA reduced in DS with dementia relative to controls and non-demented DS groups. MI increased in DS relative to controls but not further increased with DS and dementia. Higher NAA levels associated with cognition (i.e. better performance associated with more NAA).	Lin et al., 2016

DMR, dementia questionnaire for mentally retarded persons; BPT, Brief Praxis Test; SIB, severe impairment battery; CAMDEX, Cambridge Mental Disorders of the Elderly Examination; CAMCOG, Cambridge Cognitive Examination.

increased neuroinflammation that has been observed with aging in DS (Wilcock, 2012).

Thus, MRS provides novel information and unique signatures for DS (e.g., higher MI) but also may be amenable to future treatment studies as metabolic outcomes measured by MRS may be rapidly modifiable as opposed to outcomes reflecting brain structure. Comparing MRS outcomes in different affected brain regions in people with DS (e.g., comparing hippocampus, frontal cortex, cingulate cortex) may provide novel links between the presence of *in vivo* amyloid by PET imaging and glial/neuronal consequences. For example, as amyloid PiB binding increases with age, how does NAA or MI decrease or increase correspondingly? These studies may lead us to novel interventions in future for DS with outcome measures and a further examination of the link between MRS outcomes, brain region, and cognition will be useful in future.

VASCULAR IMAGING BIOMARKERS

Cerebrovascular pathology occurs in over 85% of autopsy cases presenting with AD neuropathology and is associated with impaired cognition (Arvanitakis et al., 2016). One form of this pathology, cerebral amyloid angiopathy (CAA) is present in near all brains of people with AD (Viswanathan and Greenberg, 2011). Thus, there is an increasing recognition that along with the development of Aβ plaques and neurofibrillary tangles, vascular neuropathology may also affect cognition and the progression of dementia (White et al., 2002). Interestingly, in DS, there is significant cerebrovascular neuropathology in the form of CAA, primarily due to the overexpression of APP and Aβ (Ikeda et al., 1994; Iwatsubo et al., 1995; Mendel et al., 2010; Head et al., 2017; Zis and Strydom, 2018).

Extensive CAA is associated with microhemorrhages and strokes in general (Arvanitakis et al., 2017; Banerjee et al., 2017) although in DS, stroke is relatively rare (Buss et al., 2016). Nonetheless, CAA may have a significant impact on blood vessel function. CAA can lead to deficits in cerebrovascular regulation (Grinberg et al., 2012) and reduced blood flow may lead to impaired perivascular clearance of Aβ. Impaired clearance will in turn lead to additional accumulation of Aβ (Banerjee et al., 2017).

Neuroimaging of CAA is typically by GRE or T2*-weighted MRI (Fazekas et al., 1999). There is only one neuroimaging study using T2* to observe the extent of CAA *in vivo* in older adults with DS (Carmona-Iragui et al., 2017). CAA was observed in 31% of cognitively impaired people with DS, which is similar to early onset AD (38%) and higher than sporadic AD (12%). In addition, 15.4% of people with DS had evidence of intracerebral hemorrhages. Thus, CAA is a consistent feature of aging and dementia in DS and may serve as a future target for clinical trials.

While PET-based studies in DS show metabolic differences that mirror AD in the general population, changes in blood flow may also be seen in DS. For example, single photon emission computed tomography (SPECT) patterns in younger individuals with DS reveal perfusion changes in temporal, parietal, and occipital regions (Kao et al., 1993) that are also reminiscent of those seen in AD (DeKosky et al., 1990). However, these regional differences in perfusion may reflect the added impact of CAA-associated or other cerebrovascular mechanisms in DS.

Cerebrovascular dysfunction measured *in vivo* may be critical for understanding not only the aging process and progression to AD in DS but treatment that rely on and are also relatively short MR protocols (T2*~7 min, FLAIR~4.5 min) (**Figure 1**). Immunotherapy trials in patients with AD suggest that cerebrovascular adverse effects can occur and are visualized with FLAIR (Sperling et al., 2012). The possibility of a similar outcome in DS is as yet unknown. Intervention studies that target Aβ or other pathways may be less effective in people with DS with significant cerebrovascular pathology and can confound the opportunity to observe benefits in clinical trials. Characterizing the extent of cerebrovascular pathology may serve as an exclusion/inclusion criteria or included as a covariate so as not to obscure positive clinical outcomes.

DEVELOPMENTAL DIFFERENCES AND CAVEATS WITH NEUROIMAGING IN DS

Structural differences in childhood and early adulthood suggest that some brain regions (e.g.,) are smaller in people with DS whereas others (parahippocampal gyrus) may be larger (Kesslak et al., 1994; Teipel and Hampel, 2006). It will be important to consider additional volumetric tissue losses using structural MRI when interpreting reductions in vascular flow or metabolic outcomes. Additional atrophy occurs with aging in DS and with the development of dementia with posterior cingulate, parietal, temporal, and frontal regions being affected (summarized nicely in Neale et al., 2018).

In studies of people with DS, sample sizes are typically smaller. This is due to challenges with recruitment, the ability of people to be scanned (e.g., fear) or to stay motionless (movement artifacts, people with dementia; Neale et al., 2018). Obesity or being overweight can lead to discomfort in the scanner and in some cases, may preclude a person from participating. The neck and facial structure of people with DS also can lead to discomfort in the prone position. For these situations, there are methods to provide additional padding and support along with frequent pauses in the procedures. Unfortunately, in many studies this leads to small sample sizes of demented individuals with DS, which may skew our results. Anxiolytics can be helpful when obtaining structural images but may interfere with functional measures. In our own experiences, we have found that repeated visits leads to greater successes with our volunteers participating in the scanning procedures and the option of anxiolytics has been helpful. Age of the participant also influences success with scanning. Estimates from our cohort suggest that a full set of images (MPRAGE, FLAIR, T2*, ASL, MRS, DTI ~50 min), 92% of people 25–37 years, 82% of 37–50 year olds and 40% of 50–65 year olds can be successfully scanned (unpublished observations from the University of Kentucky Down syndrome and Aging study). However, there are fewer sets of full imaging protocols we can acquire with increasing age as our participants may not be able to stay in the scanner as long as we require.

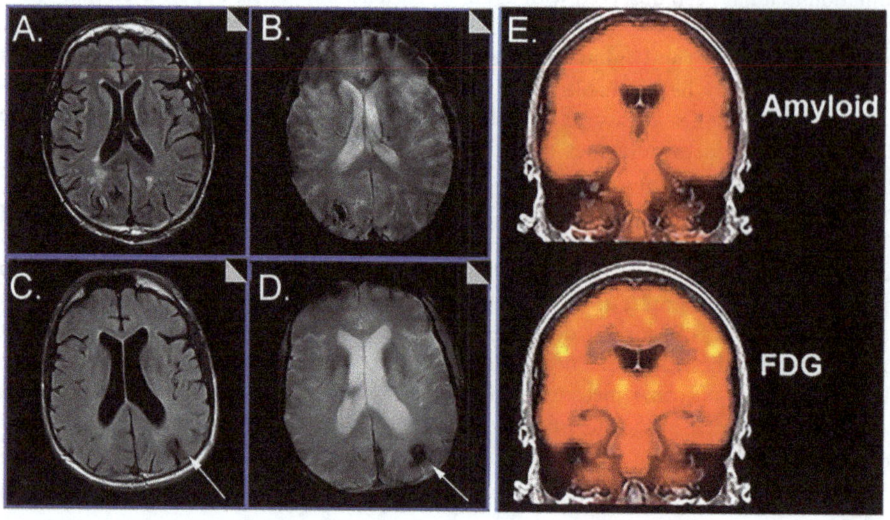

FIGURE 1 | Representative examples of neuroimaging protocols acquired in Down syndrome. Panels **(A–D)** show MR imaging in a 57 year old male and 59 year old male imaged with T2* **(A, C)** and FLAIR **(B, D)** showing the presence of microbleeds. Arrows distinguish edema and hemosiderin positive microbleeds. Panel **(E)** shows examples of amyloid PiB-PET imaging (top) and FDG-PET imaging (bottom). Images from **(A–D)** were modified from Figure 5 with permission of Elsevier Press (Head et al., 2018). Images from **(E)** were modified from Figure 1 reproduced with permission from Dr. M. Rafii and under the Creative Commons Attribution License (CC BY) (Rafii et al., 2015).

SUMMARY AND FUTURE DIRECTIONS

Longitudinal studies in virtually all of the imaging parameters discussed here are critical. There are few longitudinal studies of metabolic and vascular neuroimaging changes with age in DS. In studies of structural imaging some show progressive atrophy (reviewed in Neale et al., 2018). Over a 3 year period of time, studies in non-demented adults with DS report an increasing number of individuals developing amyloid by PET (PiB binding) and those with existing amyloid binding showed an increasing number of brain regions affected along with increased accumulation within affected brain regions (Hartley et al., 2017; Lao et al., 2017; also reviewed in Neale et al., 2018) (**Figure 1**). It is interesting to note that PiB tends to bind more mature amyloid deposits (LeVine et al., 2017) *in vitro* consistent with the typical age of onset of PiB binding in DS being after 40 years of age. In summary, neuroimaging is a powerful tool to detect structural, metabolic and vascular changes with age and dementia in DS but there are still important gaps in our knowledge remaining. Feasibility concerns may be overcome with the use of mock scanners, increasing sample sizes (based upon estimates of scan success as a function of age and dementia) and reducing scan times. Given that neuroimaging outcomes could be critically important in future clinical trials, it will be important to encourage further studies for people with DS.

AUTHOR CONTRIBUTIONS

All authors listed have made a substantial, direct, and intellectual contribution to the work, and approved it for publication.

ACKNOWLEDGMENTS

The authors are supported by NIH/NICHD R01HD064993. The authors thank Dr. M. Rafii for kindly allowing us to reproduce the figure of Amyloid and FDG PET imaging.

REFERENCES

Arvanitakis, Z., Capuano, A. W., Leurgans, S. E., Bennett, D. A., and Schneider, J. A. (2016). Relation of cerebral vessel disease to Alzheimer's disease dementia and cognitive function in elderly people: a cross-sectional study. *Lancet Neurol.* 15, 934–943. doi: 10.1016/S1474-4422(16)30029-1

Arvanitakis, Z., Capuano, A. W., Leurgans, S. E., Buchman, A. S., Bennett, D. A., and Schneider, J. A. (2017). The relationship of cerebral vessel pathology to brain microinfarcts. *Brain Pathol.* 27, 77–85. doi: 10.1111/bpa.12365

Azari, N. P., Horwitz, B., Pettigrew, K. D., Grady, C. L., Haxby, J. V., Giacometti, K. R., et al. (1994a). Abnormal pattern of cerebral glucose metabolic rates involving language areas in young adults with Down syndrome. *Brain Lang.* 46,1–20. doi: 10.1006/brln.1994.1001

Azari, N. P., Pettigrew, K. D., Pietrini, P., Horwitz, B., and Schapiro, M. B. (1994b). Detection of an Alzheimer disease pattern of cerebral metabolism in Down syndrome. *Dementia* 5, 69–78. doi: 10.1159/000106700

Banerjee, G., Carare, R., Cordonnier, C., Greenberg, S. M., Schneider, J. A., Smith, E. E., et al. (2017). The increasing impact of cerebral amyloid angiopathy: essential new insights for clinical practice. *J. Neurol. Neurosurg. Psychiatr.* 88, 982–994. doi: 10.1136/jnnp-2016-314697

Beacher, F., Simmons, A., Daly, E., Prasher, V., Adams, C., Margallo-Lana, M. L., et al. (2005). Hippocampal myo-inositol and cognitive ability in adults with Down syndrome: an *in vivo* proton magnetic resonance spectroscopy study. *Arch. Gen. Psychiatry* 62, 1360–1365. doi: 10.1001/archpsyc.62.12.1360

Berry, G. T., Mallee, J. J., Kwon, H. M., Rim, J. S., Mulla, W. R., Muenke, M., et al. (1995). The human osmoregulatory Na^+/myo-inositol cotransporter gene

SLC5A3): molecular cloning and localization to chromosome 21. *Genomics* 25, 507–513. doi: 10.1016/0888-7543(95)80052-N

Berry, G. T., Wang, Z. J., Dreha, S. F., Finucane, B. M., and Zimmerman, R. A. (1999). *In vivo* brain myo-inositol levels in children with Down syndrome. *J. Pediatr.* 135, 94–97. doi: 10.1016/S0022-3476(99)70334-3

Bittles, A. H., and Glasson, E. J. (2004). Clinical, social, and ethical implications of changing life expectancy in Down syndrome. *Dev. Med. Child Neurol.* 46, 282–286. doi: 10.1111/j.1469-8749.2004.tb00483.x

Buss, L., Fisher, E., Hardy, J., Nizetic, D., Groet, J., Pulford, L., et al. (2016). Intracerebral haemorrhage in Down syndrome: protected or predisposed? *F1000Res.* 5:F1000 Faculty Rev-876. doi: 10.12688/f1000research.7819.1

Carmona-Iragui, M., Balasa, M., Benejam, B., Alcolea, D., Fernández, S., Videla, L. et al. (2017). Cerebral amyloid angiopathy in Down syndrome and sporadic and autosomal-dominant Alzheimer's disease. *Alzheimers. Dement.* 13, 1251–1260. doi: 10.1016/j.jalz.2017.03.007

Chang, L., Munsaka, S. M., Kraft-Terry, S., and Ernst, T. (2013). Magnetic resonance spectroscopy to assess neuroinflammation and neuropathic pain. *J. Neuroimmune Pharmacol.* 8, 576–593. doi: 10.1007/s11481-013-9460-x

Cutler, N. R. (1986). Cerebral metabolism as measured with positron emission tomography (PET) and [18F] 2-deoxy-D-glucose: healthy aging, Alzheimer's disease and Down syndrome. *Prog. Neuropsychopharmacol. Biol. Psychiatry* 10, 309–321. doi: 10.1016/0278-5846(86)90010-2

Dani, A., Pietrini, P., Furey, M. L., McIntosh, A. R., Grady, C. L., Horwitz, B., et al. (1996). Brain cognition and metabolism in Down syndrome adults in association with development of dementia. *Neuroreport* 7, 2933–2936. doi: 10.1097/00001756-199611250-00026

de Graaf, G., Buckley, F., and Skotko, B. G. (2017). Estimation of the number of people with Down syndrome in the United States. *Genet. Med.* 19, 439–447. doi: 10.1038/gim.2016.127

DeKosky, S. T., Shih, W. J., Schmitt, F. A., Coupal, J., and Kirkpatrick, C. (1990). Assessing utility of single photon emission computed tomography (SPECT) scan in Alzheimer disease: correlation with cognitive severity. *Alzheimer Dis. Assoc. Disord.* 4, 14–23. doi: 10.1097/00002093-199040100-00002

Fazekas, F., Kleinert, R., Roob, G., Kleinert, G., Kapeller, P., Schmidt, R., et al. (1999). Histopathologic analysis of foci of signal loss on gradient-echo T2*-weighted MR images in patients with spontaneous intracerebral hemorrhage: evidence of microangiopathy-related microbleeds. *AJNR Am. J. Neuroradiol.* 20, 637–642.

Franceschi, M., Comola, M., Piattoni, F., Gualandri, W., and Canal, N. (1990). Prevalence of dementia in adult patients with trisomy 21. *Am. J. Med. Genet.* 7, 306–308. doi: 10.1002/ajmg.1320370760

Grinberg, L. T., Korczyn, A. D., and Heinsen, H. (2012). Cerebral amyloid angiopathy impact on endothelium. *Exp. Gerontol.* 47, 838–842. doi: 10.1016/j.exger.2012.08.005

Haier, R. J., Alkire, M. T., White, N. S., Uncapher, M. R., Head, E., Lott, I. T., et al. (2003). Temporal cortex hypermetabolism in Down syndrome prior to the onset of dementia. *Neurology* 61, 1673–1679. doi: 10.1212/01.WNL.0000098935.36984.25

Haier, R. J., Head, K., Head, E., and Lott, I. T. (2008). Neuroimaging of individuals with Down's syndrome at-risk for dementia: evidence for possible compensatory events. *Neuroimage* 39, 1324–1332. doi: 10.1016/j.neuroimage.2007.09.064

Hartley, S. L., Handen, B. L., Devenny, D., Mihaila, I., Hardison, R., Lao, P. J., et al. (2017). Cognitive decline and brain amyloid-beta accumulation across 3 years in adults with Down syndrome. *Neurobiol. Aging* 58, 68–76. doi: 10.1016/j.neurobiolaging.2017.05.019

Head, E., Helman, A. M., Powell, D., and Schmitt, F. A. (2018). Down syndrome, beta-amyloid and neuroimaging. *Free Radic. Biol. Med.* 114, 102–109. doi: 10.1016/j.freeradbiomed.2017.09.013

Head, E., Lott, I. T., Hof, P. R., Bouras, C., Su, J. H., Kim, R., et al. (2003). Parallel compensatory and pathological events associated with tau pathology in middle aged individuals with down syndrome. *J. Neuropath. Exp. Neurol.* 62, 917–926. doi: 10.1093/jnen/62.9.917

Head, E., Lott, I. T., Patterson, D., Doran, E., and Haier, R. J. (2007). Possible compensatory events in adult Down syndrome brain prior to the development of Alzheimer disease neuropathology: targets for nonpharmacological intervention. *J. Alzheimers. Dis.* 11, 61–76. doi: 10.3233/JAD-2007-11110

Head, E., Lott, I. T., Wilcock, D. M., and Lemere, C. A. (2016). Aging in Down Syndrome and the Development of Alzheimer's Disease Neuropathology. *Curr. Alzheimer Res.* 13, 18–29. doi: 10.2174/1567205012666151020114607

Head, E., Phelan, M. J., Doran, E., Kim, R. C., Poon, W. W., Schmitt, F. A., et al. (2017). Cerebrovascular pathology in Down syndrome and Alzheimer disease. *Acta Neuropathol. Commun.* 5:93. doi: 10.1186/s40478-017-0499-4

Head, E., Powell, D., Gold, B. T., and Schmitt, F. A. (2012a). Alzheimer's disease in Down syndrome. *Eur. J. Neurodegenerative Dis.* 1, 353–364.

Head, E., Silverman, W., Patterson, D., and Lott, I. T. (2012b). Aging and down syndrome. *Curr. Gerontol. Geriatr. Res.* 2012:412536. doi: 10.1155/2012/412536

Herrera, F., Chen, Q., Fischer, W. H., Maher, P., and Schubert, D. R. (2009). Synaptojanin-1 plays a key role in astrogliogenesis: possible relevance for Down's syndrome. *Cell Death Differ.* 16, 910–920. doi: 10.1038/cdd.2009.24

Horwitz, B., Schapiro, M. B., Grady, C. L., and Rapoport, S. I. (1990). Cerebral metabolic pattern in young adult Down's syndrome subjects: altered intercorrelations between regional rates of glucose utilization. *J. Ment. Defic. Res.* 34 (Pt 3), 237–252. doi: 10.1111/j.1365-2788.1990.tb01535.x

Hosking, F. J., Carey, I. M., Shah, S. M., Harris, T., DeWilde, S., Beighton, C., et al. (2016). Mortality among adults with intellectual disability in england: comparisons with the general population. *Am. J. Public Health* 106, 1483–1490. doi: 10.2105/AJPH.2016.303240

Huang, W., Alexander, G. E., Daly, E. M., Shetty, H. U., Krasuski, J. S., Rapoport, S. I., et al. (1999). High brain myo-inositol levels in the predementia phase of Alzheimer's disease in adults with Down's syndrome: a 1H MRS study. *Am. J. Psychiatry* 156, 1879–1886.

Ikeda, S., Tokuda, T., Yanagisawa, N., Kametani, F., Ohshima, T., and Allsop, D. (1994). Variability of beta-amyloid protein deposited lesions in Down's syndrome brains. *Tohoku J. Exp. Med.* 174, 189–198. doi: 10.1620/tjem.174.189

Iwatsubo, T., Mann, D. M., Odaka, A., Suzuki, N., and Ihara, Y. (1995). Amyloid beta protein (A beta) deposition: a beta 42(43) precedes A beta 40 in Down syndrome. *Ann. Neurol.* 37, 294–299. doi: 10.1002/ana.410370305

Jack, C. R., and Holtzman, D. M. (2013). Biomarker modeling of Alzheimer's disease. *Neuron* 80, 1347–1358. doi: 10.1016/j.neuron.2013.12.003

Jagust, W., Reed, B., Mungas, D., Ellis, W., and Decarli, C. (2007). What does fluorodeoxyglucose PET imaging add to a clinical diagnosis of dementia? *Neurology* 69, 871–877. doi: 10.1212/01.wnl.0000269790.05105.16

Kao, C. H., Wang, P. Y., Wang, S. J., Chou, K. T., Hsu, C. Y., Lin, W. Y., et al. (1993). Regional cerebral blood flow of Alzheimer's disease-like pattern in young patients with Down's syndrome detected by 99Tcm-HMPAO brain SPECT. *Nucl. Med. Commun.* 14, 47–51. doi: 10.1097/00006231-199301000-00010

Kesslak, J. P., Nagata, S. F., Lott, I., and Nalcioglu, O. (1994). Magnetic resonance imaging analysis of age-related changes in the brains of individuals with Down's syndrome. *Neurology* 44, 1039–1045. doi: 10.1212/WNL.44.6.1039

Lamar, M., Foy, C. M., Beacher, F., Daly, E., Poppe, M., Archer, N., et al. (2011). Down syndrome with and without dementia: an *in vivo* proton magnetic resonance spectroscopy study with implications for Alzheimer's disease. *Neuroimage* 57, 63–68. doi: 10.1016/j.neuroimage.2011.03.073

Lao, P. J., Handen, B. L., Betthauser, T. J., Mihaila, I., Hartley, S. L., Cohen, A. D., et al. (2018). Alzheimer-Like Pattern of hypometabolism emerges with elevated amyloid-beta burden in down syndrome. *J. Alzheimers. Dis.* 61, 631–644. doi: 10.3233/JAD-170720

Lao, P. J., Handen, B. L., Betthauser, T. J., Mihaila, I., Hartley, S. L., Cohen, A. D., et al. (2017). Longitudinal changes in amyloid positron emission tomography and volumetric magnetic resonance imaging in the nondemented Down syndrome population. *Alzheimer's Dementia* 9, 1–9. doi: 10.1016/j.dadm.2017.05.001

Lengyel, Z., Balogh, E., Emri, M., Szikszai, E., Kollar, J., Sikula, J., et al. (2006). Pattern of increased cerebral FDG uptake in down syndrome patients. *Pediatr. Neurol.* 34, 270–275. doi: 10.1016/j.pediatrneurol.2005.08.035

LeVine, H. 3rd, Spielmann, H. P., Matveev, S., Cauvi, F. M., Murphy, M. P., Beckett, T. L., et al. (2017). Down syndrome: age-dependence of PiB binding in postmortem frontal cortex across the lifespan. *Neurobiol. Aging* 54, 163–169. doi: 10.1016/j.neurobiolaging.2017.03.005

Lin, A. L., and Rothman, D. L. (2014). What have novel imaging techniques revealed about metabolism in the aging brain? *Future Neurol.* 9, 341–354. doi: 10.2217/fnl.14.13

Lin, A. L., Powell, D., Caban-Holt, A., Jicha, G., Robertson, W., Gold, B. T., et al. (2016). ^{1}**H**-MRS metabolites in adults with Down syndrome: effects of dementia. *NeuroImage Clin.* 11, 728–735. doi: 10.1016/j.nicl.2016.06.001

Lin, A., Ross, B. D., Harris, K., and Wong, W. (2005). Efficacy of proton magnetic resonance spectroscopy in neurological diagnosis and neurotherapeutic decision making. *NeuroRx* 2, 197–214. doi: 10.1602/neurorx.2.2.197

Matthews, D. C., Lukic, A. S., Andrews, R. D., Marendic, B., Brewer, J., Rissman, R. A., et al. (2016). Dissociation of Down syndrome and Alzheimer's disease effects with imaging. *Alzheimers Dement* 2, 69–81. doi: 10.1016/j.trci.2016.02.004

Mendel, T., Bertrand, E., Szpak, G. M., Stepien, T., and Wierzba-Bobrowicz, T. (2010). Cerebral amyloid angiopathy as a cause of an extensive brain hemorrhage in adult patient with Down's syndrome - a case report. *Folia Neuropathol.* 48, 206–211.

Minoshima, S., Giordani, B., Berent, S., Frey, K. A., Foster, N. L., and Kuhl, D. E. (1997). Metabolic reduction in the posterior cingulate cortex in very early Alzheimer's disease. *Ann. Neurol.* 42, 85–94. doi: 10.1002/ana.410420114

Murata, T., Koshino, Y., Omori, M., Murata, I., Nishio, M., Horie, T., et al. (1993). *In vivo* proton magnetic resonance spectroscopy study on premature aging in adult Down's syndrome. *Biol. Psychiatry* 34, 290–297. doi: 10.1016/0006-3223(93)90086-S

Neale, N., Padilla, C., Fonseca, L. M., Holland, T., and Zaman, S. (2018). Neuroimaging and other modalities to assess Alzheimer's disease in Down syndrome. *NeuroImage Clin.* 17, 263–271. doi: 10.1016/j.nicl.2017.10.022

Ng, N., Flygare Wallen, E., and Ahlstrom, G. (2017). Mortality patterns and risk among older men and women with intellectual disability: a Swedish national retrospective cohort study. *BMC Geriatr.* 17:269. doi: 10.1186/s12877-017-0665-3

Parnetti, L., Tarducci, R., Presciutti, O., Lowenthal, D. T., Pippi, M., Palumbo, B., et al. (1997). Proton magnetic resonance spectroscopy can differentiate Alzheimer's disease from normal aging. *Mech. Ageing Dev.* 97, 9–14. doi: 10.1016/S0047-6374(97)01877-0

Pietrini, P., Dani, A., Furey, M. L., Alexander, G. E., Freo, U., Grady, C. L., et al. (1997). Low glucose metabolism during brain stimulation in older Down's syndrome subjects at risk for Alzheimer's disease prior to dementia. *Am. J. Psychiatry* 154, 1063–1069. doi: 10.1176/ajp.154.8.1063

Rafii, M. S., Lukic, A. S., Andrews, R. D., Brewer, J., Rissman, R. A., Strother, S. C., et al. (2017). PET Imaging of Tau Pathology and Relationship to Amyloid, Longitudinal, MRI and Cognitive Change in Down Syndrome: results From the Down Syndrome Biomarker Initiative (DSBI). *J. Alzheimers Dis.* 60, 439–450. doi: 10.3233/JAD-170390

Rafii, M. S., Wishnek, H., Brewer, J. B., Donohue, M. C., Ness, S., Mobley, W. C., et al. (2015). The down syndrome biomarker initiative (DSBI) pilot: proof of concept for deep phenotyping of Alzheimer's disease biomarkers in down syndrome. *Front. Behav. Neurosci.* 9:239. doi: 10.3389/fnbeh.2015.00239

Sabbagh, M. N., Chen, K., Rogers, J., Fleisher, A. S., Liebsack, C., Bandy, D., et al. (2015). Florbetapir, PET, FDG PET, and MRI in Down syndrome individuals with and without Alzheimer's dementia. *Alzheimers Dement* 11, 994–1004. doi: 10.1016/j.jalz.2015.01.006

Schapiro, M. B., Azari, N. P., Grady, C. L., Haxby, J. V., and Horwitz, B. (1992a). Down syndrome: differentiating mental retardation and dementia with brain imaging techniques. *Prog. Clin. Biol. Res.* 379, 103–122.

Schapiro, M. B., Ball, M. J., Grady, C. L., Haxby, J. V., Kaye, J. A., and Rapoport, S. I. (1988). Dementia in Down's syndrome: cerebral glucose utilization, neuropsychological assessment, and neuropathology. *Neurology* 38, 938–942. doi: 10.1212/WNL.38.6.938

Schapiro, M. B., Grady, C. L., Kumar, A., Herscovitch, P., Haxby, J. V., Moore, A. M., et al. (1990). Regional cerebral glucose metabolism is normal in young adults with Down syndrome. *J. Cereb. Blood Flow Metab.* 10, 199–206. doi: 10.1038/jcbfm.1990.35

Schapiro, M. B., Haxby, J. V., and Grady, C. L. (1992b). Nature of mental retardation and dementia in Down syndrome: study with PET, CT, and neuropsychology. *Neurobiol. Aging* 13, 723–734. doi: 10.1016/0197-4580(92)90096-G

Schupf, N., and Sergievsky, G. H. (2002). Genetic and host factors for dementia in Down's syndrome. *Br. J. Psychiatry* 180, 405–410. doi: 10.1192/bjp.180.5.405

Schwartz, M., Duara, R., Haxby, J., Grady, C., White, B. J., Kessler, R. M., et al. (1983). Down's syndrome in adults: brain metabolism. *Science* 221, 781–783. doi: 10.1126/science.6224294

Shonk, T., and Ross, B. D. (1995). Role of increased cerebral myo-inositol in the dementia of Down syndrome. *Magn. Reson. Med.* 33, 858–861. doi: 10.1002/mrm.1910330619

Silverman, D. H., and Phelps, M. E. (2001). Application of positron emission tomography for evaluation of metabolism and blood flow in human brain: normal development, aging, dementia, and stroke. *Mol. Genet. Metab.* 74, 128–138. doi: 10.1006/mgme.2001.3236

Silverman, D. H., Small, G. W., Chang, C. Y., Lu, C. S., Kung De Aburto, M. A., Chen, Wm et al. (2001). Positron emission tomography in evaluation of dementia: regional brain metabolism and long-term outcome. *JAMA* 286, 2120–2127. doi: 10.1001/jama.286.17.2120

Sinai, A., Mokrysz, C., Bernal, J., Bohnen, I., Bonell, S., Courtenay, K., et al. (2018). Predictors of age of diagnosis and survival of Alzheimer's Disease in down syndrome. *J. Alzheimers. Dis.* 61, 717–728. doi: 10.3233/JAD-170624

Smigielska-Kuzia, J., and Sobaniec, W. (2007). Brain metabolic profile obtained by proton magnetic resonance spectroscopy HMRS in children with Down syndrome. *Adv. Med. Sci.* 52(Suppl. 1), 183–187.

Smigielska-Kuzia, J., Bockowski, L., Sobaniec, W., Kulak, W., and Sendrowski, K. (2010). Amino acid metabolic processes in the temporal lobes assessed by proton magnetic resonance spectroscopy (^{1}H MRS) in children with Down syndrome. *Pharmacol. Rep.* 63, 1070–1077. doi: 10.1016/S1734-1140(10)70369-8

Sperling, R., Salloway, S., Brooks, D. J., Tampieri, D., Barakos, J., Fox, N. C., et al. (2012). Amyloid-related imaging abnormalities in patients with Alzheimer's disease treated with bapineuzumab: a retrospective analysis. *Lancet Neurol.* 11, 241–249. doi: 10.1016/S1474-4422(12) 70015-7

Tan, G. M., Beacher, F., Daly, E., Horder, J., Prasher, V., Hanney, M. L., et al. (2014). Hippocampal glutamate-glutamine (Glx) in adults with Down syndrome: a preliminary study using *in vivo* proton magnetic resonance spectroscopy (^{1}H MRS). *J. Neurodev. Disord.* 6:42. doi: 10.1186/1866-1955-6-42

Teipel, S. J., and Hampel, H. (2006). Neuroanatomy of Down syndrome *in vivo*: a model of preclinical Alzheimer's disease. *Behav. Genet.* 36, 405–415. doi: 10.1007/s10519-006-9047-x

Viswanathan, A., and Greenberg, S. M. (2011). Cerebral amyloid angiopathy in the elderly. *Ann. Neurol.* 70, 871–880. doi: 10.1002/ana.22516

White, L., Petrovitch, H., Hardman, J., Nelson, J., Davis, D. G., Ross, G. W., et al. (2002). Cerebrovascular pathology and dementia in autopsied Honolulu-Asia Aging Study participants. *Ann. N. Y. Acad. Sci.* 977, 9–23. doi: 10.1111/j.1749-6632.2002.tb04794.x

Wilcock, D. M. (2012). Neuroinflammation in the aging down syndrome brain; lessons from Alzheimer's disease. *Curr. Gerontol. Geriatr. Res.* 2012:170276. doi: 10.1155/2012/170276

Zigman, W. B., Schupf, N., Sersen, E., and Silverman, W. (1996). Prevalence of dementia in adults with and without Down syndrome. *Am. J. Ment. Retard.* 100, 403–412.

Zis, P., and Strydom, A. (2018). Clinical aspects and biomarkers of Alzheimer's disease in Down syndrome. *Free Radic. Biol. Med.* 114, 3–9. doi: 10.1016/j.freeradbiomed.2017.08.024

4

Small Vessel Disease on Neuroimaging in a 75-Year-Old Cohort (PIVUS): Comparison with Cognitive and Executive Tests

Ruta Nylander[1], Lena Kilander[2], Håkan Ahlström[1], Lars Lind[3] and Elna-Marie Larsson[1]*

[1]Department of Surgical Sciences, Radiology, Uppsala University, Uppsala, Sweden, [2]Department of Public Health and Caring Sciences, Geriatrics, Uppsala University, Uppsala, Sweden, [3]Department of Medical Sciences, Uppsala University, Uppsala, Sweden

Correspondence:
Ruta Nylander
ruta.nylander@radiol.uu.se

Background and Purpose: Signs of small vessel disease (SVD) are commonly seen on magnetic resonance imaging (MRI) of the brain in cognitively healthy elderly individuals, and the clinical relevance of these are often unclear. We have previously described three different MRI manifestations of SVD as well as cerebral perfusion in a longitudinal study of non-demented 75-year-old subjects. The purpose of the present study was to evaluate the relationship of these findings to cognition and executive function at age 75 and changes after 5 years.

Methods: In all, 406 subjects from the Prospective Investigation of the Vasculature in Uppsala Seniors (PIVUS) study were examined with MRI of the brain at age 75 years. Two-hundred and fifty of the subjects were re-examined 5 years later. White matter hyperintensities (WMHs) and lacunar infarcts (LIs) were assessed on both occasions, but microbleeds (MBs) and perfusion only at age 75. Cognitive function was screened by the Mini Mental State Examination (MMSE). Trail Making Test A and B (TMT-A and TMT-B) were performed at baseline and at follow-up at age 80.

Results: At baseline, 93% performed >27 points in the MMSE. The TMT-B at age 75 was significantly related to WMH visual scoring after adjustment for sex, education and cerebrovascular disease risk factors (+80 s (95% CI 0.3–161 s), $P < 0.05$ for grade 2–3 vs. grade 0). Neither MMSE nor TMT-A was significantly related to WMH scoring. There was no relation between any test performance and WMH volume, white matter volume, number of MBs or brain perfusion at age 75. Subjects who had sustained a new LI ($n = 26$) showed a greater increase of the time to perform TMT-A at the 5-year follow-up (+25 s vs. +4 s in LI-free subjects, $P = 0.003$). Changes in MMSE or TMT-A and -B test performance between ages 75 and 80 were not related to changes in WMH scoring or volume during the 5 years follow-up, or to brain perfusion at age 75.

Conclusion: In this cognitively healthy community-based population, moderate-severe WMHs and incident LIs on brain MRI in individuals aged 75–80 years were associated with a mild impairment of processing speed and executive function.

Keywords: small vessel disease, magnetic resonance imaging, perfusion, white matter hyperintensities, lacunar infarct, cognitive tests

INTRODUCTION

Cerebral small vessel disease (SVD) is a common process in the ageing brain, which affects small vessels, including arterioles, capillaries and small veins. SVD predicts stroke, cognitive impairment and depression, and is believed to contribute to approximately 45% of all dementia disorders (Wardlaw et al., 2013b). Multiple and complex pathogenetic mechanisms cause ischemic changes, enlarged perivascular spaces, cerebral microbleeds (MBs) and brain atrophy (Wardlaw et al., 2013a). The resulting brain parenchymal changes detectible by neuroimaging can be regarded as markers of SVD (Pantoni, 2010; de Guio et al., 2016). On magnetic resonance imaging (MRI), these markers are seen as white matter hyperintensities (WMHs) of presumed vascular origin, small subcortical infarcts, lacunar infarcts (LIs), cerebral MBs, prominent perivascular spaces (PVS) and cerebral atrophy (Pantoni, 2010; Wardlaw et al., 2013a).

WMHs are seen on MRI as focal or confluent/more extensive signal changes. They may be located in the periventricular and/or subcortical white matter. LIs evolve into small (3–15 mm) cavities/lacunes in the deep gray or white matter (Wardlaw et al., 2013a). MBs, due to small intramural and perivascular hemeorrhages, are seen on susceptibility-weighted MRI due to residual hemosiderin in macrophages located around small vessels (Pantoni, 2010; Wardlaw et al., 2013b). Perivascular spaces are fluid-filled spaces around small vessels and are detected on MRI when they are enlarged. Brain atrophy that occurs with ageing can be general or focal and has been shown to be associated with the severity of SVD (Wardlaw et al., 2013a).

MRI provides objective information not only on manifestations and progression of changes in the brain parenchyma, but it also allows evaluation of cerebral perfusion. Atherosclerosis and non-atherosclerotic diffuse atheropathy in SVD may produce chronic hypoperfusion, which progresses with increasing age (Pantoni, 2010; Chutinet et al., 2012). Several studies show an association between decreased cerebral perfusion and cognitive decline (Leeuwis et al., 2016; Lou et al., 2016; Zlatar et al., 2016).

Cognitive impairment due to vascular or neurodegenerative dementia disorders develops slowly over several years or decades. In early stages, a subtle cognitive impairment may be reported by the patient or family members but is not always detectable by cognitive tests. The Mini Mental-State Examination (MMSE) is the most widely used cognitive screening instrument, measuring mainly verbal and memory functions. The Trail Making Tests A and B (TMT-A, TMT-B) examine executive functions, including the ability to maintain attention, speed of processing and set-shifting/mental flexibility, mainly reflecting subcortico-frontal functions and cerebrovascular lesions (Conti et al., 2015).

Signs of SVD are often seen on magnetic imaging (MRI) of the brain in cognitively healthy elderly and are highly age-related (Ylikoski et al., 1995; Wardlaw et al., 2015). On a group basis, these changes are associated with lower cognitive and executive performance speed, as shown in several previously reviewed studies of cohorts of different sizes (Debette et al., 2010; Kloppenborg et al., 2014; Wardlaw et al., 2015). One of these studies reviewed 33 cross-sectional and 14 longitudinal studies focused on WMH and cognition (Kloppenborg et al., 2014). However, the clinical role of these imaging findings is often difficult to translate to the individual patient. An association between progression of SVD and decline of general cognitive function and processing speed has also been reported (Debette et al., 2010; Kloppenborg et al., 2014). However, longitudinal results from previous studies are not clear-cut due to different selection of the subjects: many patients in cohorts from Memory Clinics will decline over time; other cohorts have subjective cognitive impairment; some cohorts are healthy community-based samples (Debette et al., 2010; Kloppenborg et al., 2014) others have a wide age range. Studies on the relation between SVD and cognition, including not only WMH but also infarcts and MBs in stroke- and dementia-free subjects between age 75 and 80 years are sparse.

We have previously described three different MRI manifestations of SVD as well as cerebral perfusion in a longitudinal study of non-demented 75-year-old subjects (Nylander, 2017; Nylander et al., 2018). The aim of the present study was to evaluate how cognitive performance on MMSE and TMT-A and -B is related to the WMH, LI, MBs and cerebral perfusion on MRI in a prospective community-based population of cognitively healthy individuals of the same age. We also assessed the evolution over 5 years.

MATERIALS AND METHODS

Ethics Statement

The Regional Ethical Review Board in Uppsala, Sweden, approved the study and all subjects provided written informed consent.

Study Population

Within the Prospective Investigation of the Vasculature in Uppsala Seniors (PIVUS) study, 406 subjects at the age of 75 years were randomly selected to be examined with MRI of the brain. The subjects had been recruited from the population register of the municipality. MRI was repeated after 5 years in 250 of the 406 subjects who agreed to participate in a follow-up study. Uppsala University Hospital and the primary care in Uppsala County use the same electronic medical records system. All available charts from out-patient and in-patient care of the included individuals were reviewed until each subject reached the age of 80 and all dementia diagnoses were noted. Clinical diagnoses of vascular dementia (VAD), Alzheimer's disease (AD), Parkinson's disease dementia (PDD) and unspecified dementia (UNS; cases lacking sufficient information) were verified by one of the authors (Ronnemaa et al., 2011).

Morphological MRI

MRI of the brain had been performed on a 1.5 Tesla MRI system (Gyroscan Intera, Philips Medical Systems, the Netherlands). At ages 75 and 80 years, the protocol included sagittal 3-dimensional (3D) T1-weighted (TR 8.6 ms, TE 4 ms, slice thickness 1.2 mm, pixel size 0.94 × 0.94 mm) and transverse proton density and T2-weighted turbo spin echo images (TR 3000 ms, TE 21 and 100 ms, slice thickness 3 mm, pixel size 0.94 × 0.94 mm) as described previously (Nylander et al., 2015). In the 75-year-old cohort, a T2*-weighted sequence for evaluation of MBs was also performed.

WMHs were scored using the visual Leukoaraiosis And DISability (LADIS) rating scale, which is a modification of the widely used Fazekas scale (Inzitari et al., 2009). The scale has three grades where grade three indicates the most severe changes (**Figure 1**). LIs were defined as hypointense foci (3–15 mm size) on 3D T1-weighted images (Nylander et al., 2018).

Perfusion MRI

Cerebral perfusion MRI was performed using DSC MRI with contrast agent injection in the 75-year-old subjects and analyzed in our previous study. (Nylander, 2017; Nylander et al., 2018). Perfusion MRI was not repeated in the 80-year-old subjects due to patient age and potential risk of contrast-induced nephropathy.

Cognitive Tests

The MMSE, the TMT-A and TMT-B were administered at baseline and follow-up.

The MMSE includes 11 questions, requires only 5–10 min to perform, and is a composite test mainly of memory and verbal functions (Folstein et al., 1975). The TMT-A requires subjects to draw lines connecting the numbers 1–25 unevenly distributed on a sheet of paper, as fast as possible and provides information on visual search and speed of processing (Tombaugh, 2004). The TMT-B is more complex than the TMT-A since the subject is asked to draw lines as fast as possible alternating between numbers (1–13) and letters (A–L) in the right order, testing the ability to shift attention and action, i.e., mental flexibility or executive functions. The score on each part represents the time in seconds required to complete the task, and a higher score means a slower performance. The maximum time was set to 180 s for the TMT-A and to 600 s for the TMT-B.

Cardiovascular Risk Factors/Markers

Recordings of cerebrovascular risk factors were available at both ages (Nylander et al., 2015). Systolic and diastolic blood pressure, smoking, diabetes mellitus, serum total cholesterol and body mass index (BMI) were used for adjustment of statistical analyses.

Data Analysis and Visual Image Evaluation

WMHs were assessed qualitatively (visual scoring grade 1–3, where 3 is most severe) and quantitatively (semi-automatic volume calculation), and brain tissue segmentation was performed automatically as described previously (Nylander et al., 2018). As previously described LIs and MBs were assessed visually, and the perfusion maps were evaluated with regard to regional and supratentorial rCBF (Nylander et al., 2018).

The WMH volume was analyzed at ages 75 and 80 years using the CASCADE software (ki.se/en/nvs/cascade; Damangir et al., 2012; Cover et al., 2016; Nylander et al., 2018).

CBF maps were calculated, and regional values relative to the cerebellum were used for the analyses (Nylander et al., 2018).

Statistical Analysis

STATA14 (Stata Inc., College Station, TX, USA) was used for calculations. $P < 0.05$ was regarded as significant.

The relationships between the cognitive function tests and markers of cerebral SVD at age 75 (cross-sectional) were evaluated with Tobit regression (since all three tests were censored at high levels). The models were adjusted for sex, education level, baseline systolic blood pressure, HDL and LDL cholesterol, BMI, smoking and diabetes.

The relationships between changes in the cognitive function tests and changes in markers of cerebral SVD over 5 years (longitudinal) were evaluated with mixed models with a random intercept. Also, these models were adjusted for sex, education level, baseline systolic blood pressure, HDL and LDL cholesterol, BMI, smoking and diabetes.

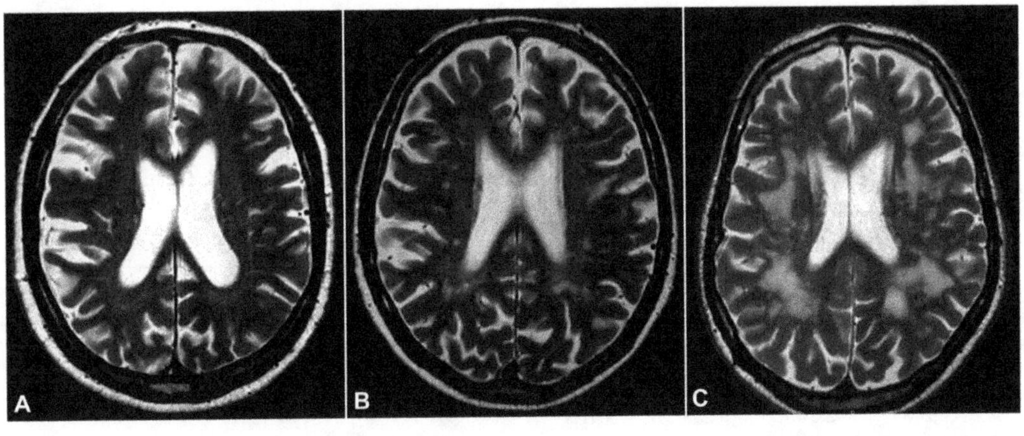

FIGURE 1 | White matter hyperintensities (WMHs). T2-weighted magnetic resonance imaging (MRI) of the brain in three of our subjects, showing three grades of severity according to the Leukoaraiosis And DISability (LADIS) visual scoring scale (modified Fazekas scale): **(A)**, mild; **(B)**, moderate; **(C)**, severe.

RESULTS

An overview of cardiovascular risk factors, imaging findings and cognitive tests at age 75 and 80 are shown in **Tables 1, 2**.

Findings at Age 75

At baseline, none of the individuals had a dementia diagnosis, and 93% performed >27 points in the MMSE, i.e., the vast majority had no cognitive impairment (**Table 1**).

Moderate or severe (grades 2 or 3) WMHs were found in 162 (40%) of the 406 subjects at age 75 (Nylander et al., 2018).

Out of 406 subjects, 89 (22%) had one or more LIs and only a few had cortical infarcts, 56 (14%) had MBs (Nylander et al., 2015).

The time to perform TMT-B at age 75 was significantly related to WMH visual scoring after adjustment for sex, education, baseline systolic blood pressure, HDL and LDL cholesterol, BMI, smoking and diabetes (+80 s for WMH grades 2 and 3 vs. grade 0 (95% CI 0.3–161 s), $P < 0.05$; **Figure 2**). Neither MMSE nor TMT-A was significantly related to WMH scoring. None of the three cognitive tests was significantly related to WMH volume, WM volume, number of MBs, total brain perfusion, WM perfusion or to perfusion in specific brain areas.

TABLE 1 | Description of the population at baseline.

	Data at age 75	
Characteristics	***N***	**Mean (SD)**
SBP (mmHg)	406	148.1 (18.8)
DBP (mmHg)	406	76.0 (9.8)
Blood sugar (mmol/L)	406	5.2 (1.4)
Cholesterol (mmol/L)	406	5.4 (1.1)
WMH score	406	1.5 (0.7)
GM volume (ml)	404	564.8 (49.5)
WM volume (ml)	404	465.3 (58.7)
WMHs volume (ml)	396	10.5 (5.2)
Number of microbleeds	406	0.5 (3.0)
MMSE (points)	398	29 (1.4)
TMT-A (s)	394	57 (22)
TMT-B (s)	392	170 (117)

SBP, systolic blood pressure; DBP, diastolic blood pressure; WMHs, white matter hyperintensities; GM, gray matter; WM, white matter; MMSE, mini mental state examination test; TMT-A, trail making test A; TMT-B, trail making test B.

TABLE 2 | Description of the population who returned for follow-up after 5 years.

	Data at age 75		Data at age 80	
Characteristics	***N***	**Mean (SD)**	***N***	**Mean (SD)**
SBP (mmHg)	252	147.8 (18.8)	251	146.9 (18.4)
DBP (mmHg)	252	75.5 (10.0)	251	73.5 (9.4)
Blood sugar (mmol/L)	252	5.2 (1.4)	248	5.3 (1.6)
Cholesterol (mmol/L)	252	5.5 (1.1)	251	5.2 (1.1)
WMH score	252	1.4 (0.7)	252	1.5 (0.7)
GM volume (ml)	252	568.9 (51.1)	231	554.5 (52.4)
WM volume (ml)	252	466.1 (59.7)	231	453.2 (59.1)
WMHs volume (ml)	246	10.1 (4.7)	229	11.9 (5.7)
Number of microbleeds	252	0.5 (3.0)	n/a	n/a
MMSE (points)	250	28.8 (1.2)	242	28 (1.9)
TMT-A (s)	248	53.8 (17.6)	239	60 (30)
TMT-B (s)	247	142.8 (87.2)	237	150 (77)

SBP, systolic blood pressure; DBP, diastolic blood pressure; WMHs, white matter hyperintensities; GM, gray matter; WM, white matter; MMSE, mini mental state examination test; TMT-A, trail making test A; TMT-B, trail making test B.

Changes in Cognitive Performance Between Age 75 and Years Compared With Changes of MRI Findings

After 5 years, there was progression of WMH volume, WMH scoring and LIs.

The 26 subjects who developed a new LI during the 5-year follow-up showed a greater increase of the time to perform TMT-A over 5 years than those who did not develop any LIs (n = 224; +25 s vs. +4 s, P = 0.003) after adjustment for sex, education level, baseline systolic blood pressure, HDL and LDL cholesterol, BMI, smoking and diabetes (**Figure 3** and **Table 3**). The same trend was seen with regard to the TMT-B (but not the

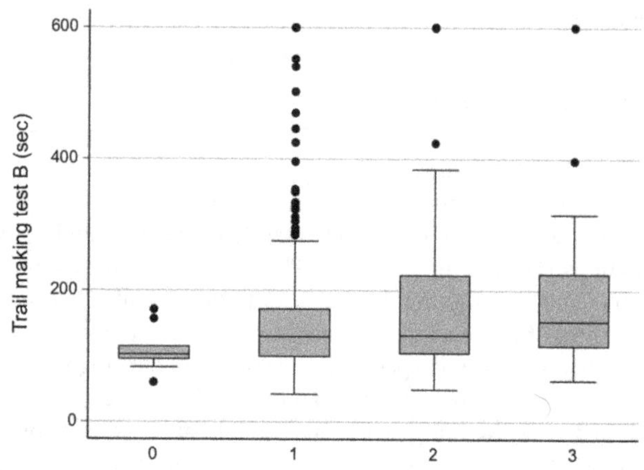

FIGURE 2 | LADIS score vs. Trail Making Test B (TMT-B) results at age 75 years (n = 392).

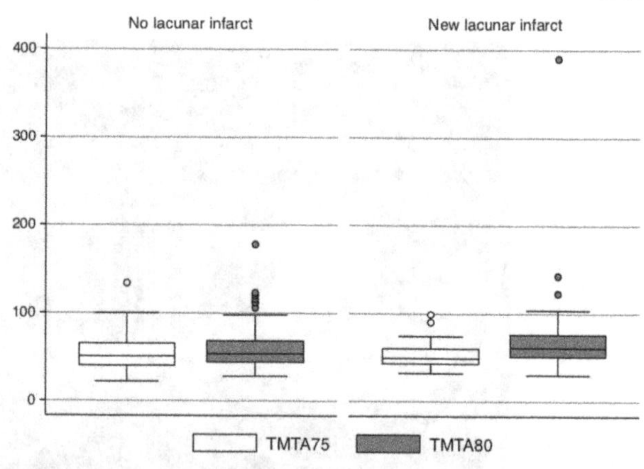

FIGURE 3 | Subjects (n = 26) who developed a new lacunar infarct (LI) during the 5-year follow-up compared with those (n = 168) without new LI vs. time to perform TMT-A at age 75 and 80.

MMSE); however, this trend was not significant (+24 s vs. +2 s, $P = 0.24$, $n = 172$).

There was no significant association between changes in the MMSE, TMT-A or TMT-B and changes in WMH scoring or volume during 5 years' follow-up and not to total brain perfusion, WM perfusion or regional perfusion at age 75.

During the 5-year follow-up, clinically diagnosed dementia disorders of different types were found in 18 subjects. Their baseline WMH grades and baseline MMSE are shown in **Table 4**. Only two of these subjects with incident dementia participated in the follow-up. Non-participants at age 80 performed markedly slower in the TMT-B at baseline (mean 216 s (SD 144) vs. 143 s (SD 87) s in participants).

DISCUSSION

In this community-based population of dementia-free 75 year-old subjects, WMH grade 2–3 was neither associated with impaired performance in global cognition, as measured by the MMSE nor with incident dementia.

WMH grade 2–3 was associated with mildly impaired executive function, as measured by time to perform the TMT-B at baseline. No association was found in the longitudinal data, probably due to a selective loss at follow-up (**Table 1**).

This finding is consistent with other studies, showing that WMHs mainly affect executive function (Debette et al., 2010; Kloppenborg et al., 2014). Re-evaluation 5 years later did not capture any deterioration in the TMT-A or TMT-B over time associated with WMHs.

During follow-up, incident LIs were associated with slowing of the performance on the TMT-A.

Our results indicate that a majority of healthy elderly subjects with moderate-severe WMHs will not experience any significant decline in cognitive and executive function between age 75 and 80 years. However, our cohort is assumable healthier than a general population. Only 7% had less than 28 points on MMSE at the baseline and during follow–up the incidence of LIs and cognitive decline was low.

TABLE 3 | Description of the 26 subjects who gained lacunar infarcts between age 75 and 80.

	Data at age 75		Data at age 80	
Characteristics	***N***	**Mean (SD)**	***N***	**Mean (SD)**
SBP (mmHg)	26	156.9 (20.0)	26	154.7 (15.3)
DBP (mmHg)	26	76.4 (11.3)	26	77.1 (8.2)
Blood sugar (mmol/L)	26	4.9 (0.6)	26	5.3 (1.2)
Cholesterol (mmol/L)	26	5.9 (1.1)	26	5.4 (1.1)
WMH score	26	1.7 (0.6)	26	1.7 (0.7)
GM volume (ml)	26	584.1 (40.3)	24	578.2 (44.9)
WM volume (ml)	26	487.4 (44.9)	24	468.6 (44.2)
WMHs volume (ml)	26	11.0 (4.4)	24	14.1 (6.3)
Number of microbleeds	26	0.4 (0.2)	n/a	n/a
MMSE (points)	25	28.4 (1.4)	25	28.2 (2.3)
TMT-A (s)	25	54.3 (16.7)	25	79.6 (69.6)
TMT-B (s)	25	140.9 (103.1)	24	162.1 (82.4)

SBP, systolic blood pressure; DBP, diastolic blood pressure; WMHs, white matter hyperintensities; GM, gray matter; WM, white matter; MMSE, mini mental state examination test; TMT-A, trail making test A; TMT-B, trail making test B.

WMHs and Cognition

Several previous studies have described an association between WMHs and cognitive deterioration in high-risk subjects, such as patients referred to a Memory clinic (Benedictus et al., 2015), patients with subjective cognitive impairment (de Groot et al., 2001), or subjects with clinically manifest cerebrovascular disease (Ihle-Hansen et al., 2012), or the LADIS Study where the participants had a higher prevalence of WMHs at baseline (van der Flier et al., 2005; Inzitari et al., 2009; Pantoni et al., 2015).

In patients with subjective cognitive decline, WMHs were reported to be associated with progression of subjective cognitive failures (de Groot et al., 2001), and with a higher risk of incident mild cognitive impairment or dementia (Benedictus et al., 2015). Further, both WMH and cognitive decline are highly age-related. A cognitively intact population of 80 year-olds (Boyle et al., 2016), i.e., older than our subjects, and with high WMH volume, had a 2.7 times higher risk of developing MCI compared to those with low WMH volume. There are several cross-sectional and longitudinal population-based studies on healthy subjects, mainly younger than 80 years, that used a similar study design as ours (Schmidt et al., 2005; Kramer et al., 2007; Smith et al., 2008; van Dijk et al., 2008; Debette and Markus, 2010; Debette et al., 2010; Inaba et al., 2011; Kloppenborg et al., 2014) and the majority, but not all (Schmidt et al., 2005) found an association with impaired global cognition, affecting processing speed and executive function more than memory. However, considering publication bias, all negative studies may not have been published.

The MMSE is the most common screening instrument for cognitive disorders, with focus on verbal function, memory, orientation and calculation (Folstein et al., 1975). The TMT-A measures attention and perceptual speed and the TMT-B examines executive functions, as it also requires cognitive

TABLE 4 | Dementia diagnosis, LADIS score and MMSE at baseline in the subjects who were diagnosed with dementia between age 75 and 80 years.

	Data at age 75	
Diagnosis type	**LADIS score**	**MMSE (seconds)**
UNS	3	28
VAD	2	28
AD	2	29
AD	2	25
UNS	3	27
AD	2	29
UNS	1	28
VAD	2	27
UNS	2	28
AD	1	24
UNS	1	28
LBD	1	26
AD	3	Not available
UNS	2	27
AD	2	25
UNS	2	26
VAD	1	26
AD	2	26

UNS, unspecified dementia; VAD, vascular dementia; AD, Alzheimer's disease; LBD, Lewy body dementia.

flexibility (Sörös et al., 2015). Impaired performance in these tests is common in patients with a previous TIA or stroke (Ihle-Hansen et al., 2012; Sörös et al., 2015) in contrast to preserved global cognition as measured by the MMSE.

In a recent review, the TMTs were recognized as two of the most frequently used instruments in testing executive function in stroke patients (Conti et al., 2015). Further, we have previously shown in a cohort of stroke-free elderly men that impaired performance in the TMT-B (in contrast to TMT-A or the MMSE) was an independent predictor of subsequent brain infarction (Wiberg et al., 2010). Hence, performance in the TMT-B seems to be a sensitive marker of both clinical overt and subclinical cerebrovascular disease.

The cross-sectional association between WMH grade 2–3 and impaired results in the TMT-B is in agreement with several studies that have shown a relationship between WMH and impaired executive function including processing speed, commonly assessed by the TMTs, the Stroop Test, the Digit span and the Letter Digit Substitution, among others (Prins et al., 2005; Kramer et al., 2007; Wiberg et al., 2010; Benedictus et al., 2015; Conti et al., 2015; Dong et al., 2015; Boyle et al., 2016). Impaired executive function mirrors subcortico-frontal dysfunction and is consistent with the localization of WMHs.

LI and Cognition

LIs as a part of SVD have previously been reported to be associated with a higher risk of dementia, mainly in individuals with WMHs, cortical atrophy and recurrent strokes (Loeb et al., 1992). In the LADIS study, progression of LIs showed an association with cognitive impairment, mostly in processing speed and executive function (Jokinen et al., 2011). This is in agreement with our study, showing that appearance of new LIs was associated with a slower speed in the TMT-A during the 5-year observation period.

WMHs and LIs were independently associated with a decline of general cognitive function in the LADIS study (Pantoni et al., 2015), which used the MMSE and a modified AD Assessment scale (ADAS) for 633 independently living elderly subjects (van der Flier et al., 2005). Also, the longitudinal evaluation in the LADIS study showed a significantly steeper decline of cognitive function and showed a risk of developing dementia and medial temporal atrophy in patients with a combination of severe WMH and lacunas, independently of age, sex or education (Pantoni et al., 2015).

MB and Cognition

Cerebral MBs are part of SVD, and the number of MBs increases with age. Recent longitudinal studies showed that MBs have an impact on cognitive impairment, which varies with their location in the brain (van Norden et al., 2011; Poels et al., 2012). In the Rotterdam study, a higher number of MBs was associated with a lower MMSE score and worse performance on tests of information processing speed and motor speed. The presence of lobar MBs was associated with worse performance on tests measuring cognitive function even after adjustments for vascular risk factors and other imaging markers of SVD (Poels et al., 2012). In our study, the number of MBs was not significantly related to cognitive tests at the age of 75, which is not in agreement with these findings. The Rotterdam study stated that the location (lobar) and number of MBs are related to cognitive decline: a higher number of MBs was associated with lower results on a cognitive test (Poels et al., 2012). However, in our sample only 14% (56 of 406 subjects) had MBs, and most of them had less than five MBs. The MRI markers of SVD, WMHs, LIs and MBs have in other studies been shown to be independently associated with cognitive decline and dementia (van der Flier et al., 2005; Jokinen et al., 2011; Østergaard et al., 2016).

Perfusion and Cognition

Our findings did not show a significant relationship between cerebral perfusion and cognitive functions at age 75, neither in total nor regionally. This is in line with a recent study of non-demented patients showing that cognitive function was stronger associated with white matter integrity than with perfusion (Zhong et al., 2017). In contrast, another study showed an association between reduced cerebral blood flow velocity in the middle cerebral artery, more severe WMH and cognitive impairment (Alosco et al., 2013). In a study of patients with hypertension, higher white matter lesion volume was related to regional decrease of perfusion within areas of WMHs but not to a reduction of general perfusion (van Dalen et al., 2016). Cerebral perfusion can be measured by MRI in different ways, but the dynamic susceptibility contrast (DSC) technique used in our study has so far been most commonly used. However, arterial spin labeling (ASL) perfusion without contrast agent injection and with the possibility to obtain absolute CBF-values is increasingly used, especially for research studies (van Dalen et al., 2016).

Strengths and Limitations

Our study population was a community-based sample of cognitively healthy 75-year-old subjects and we were able to repeat the MRI scans at the age of 80 in 62%. The study participants in this cohort were of the same age, and this homogeneity means that the confounding effect of age, which is strongly associated with WMHs, was minimized without requiring further adjustment in multivariable regression models.

The relative reduction of the sample size at follow-up was a limitation: 38% was lost due to different diseases and/or unknown conditions, which affects the conclusions.

The observation period was only 5 years. Longer follow-up periods, expanding the age and sample size, may reveal further progression of SVD in association with cognitive decline.

To determine cognitive function, the MMSE was used to get a composite cognitive assessment, and the TMT-A (process speed), and TMT-B (executive function) were used in both cohorts. For further investigations, a wider range of tests on memory, language and executive function with greater sensitivity to early decline would be preferable.

Both quantitative and qualitative techniques for the detection of WMHs have limitations. However, visual rating scales may not always provide the same results as the measurement of absolute lesion volume (van Straaten et al., 2006), and we have used both methods in the present study.

We found no association between rCBF and cognitive tests. The physiological variability of rCBF may be too large to reveal small differences among participants on DSC perfusion. No perfusion study was performed at age 80 years (due to patient age and potential risk of contrast-induced nephropathy), which prevented comparison of perfusion over time. Also, the DSC perfusion method only provides relative values.

Our study focused on MRI manifestations of SVD and their relationship to cognitive impairment. However, synergistic effect between these changes and concomitant diseases including stroke and neurodegenerative disorders may also be of importance.

CONCLUSION

Executive function, as measured by the TMT-B, at age 75 was significantly related to WMH score. In the longitudinal part of this study, progression of LIs over 5 years was associated with impaired performance in the TMT-A.

No other significant associations were found but cannot be excluded because of the reduced size of the cohort (250 of the original 406) at follow-up.

Thus, SVD on MRI is not only an incidental finding related to normal ageing. Moderate-severe WMHs or new LIs on MRI of the brain in elderly individuals may be considered potential risk factors for decline in cognitive function. However, according to our results, it shall also be noted that the vast majority of 75 year olds with moderate to severe WMHs will not experience a significant decline in cognitive or executive function during the next few years.

AUTHOR CONTRIBUTIONS

LL, HA: substantial contribution to the conception of the work. E-ML and LK: design of the work. RN and EML: acquisition and analysis. LL and LK: interpretation of data for the work. RN: drafting the work. LL, LK, E-ML and RN: revising it critically for important intellectual content. RN, LK, HA, LL and E-ML: final approval of the version to be published and agreement to be accountable for all aspects of the work ensuring the questions related to the accuracy or integrity of any part of the work are appropriately investigated and resolved by all authors.

ACKNOWLEDGMENTS

I would like to acknowledge all those who collaborated in and assisted me in the endeavor of my thesis "Magnetic resonance imaging markers of cerebral small vessel disease in an elderly population-association with cardiovascular disease and cognitive function," (Nylander, 2017; Summaries of Uppsala Dissertation from the Faculty of Medicine 1327, Uppsala University), which included a preliminary version of the present article. The thesis is cited and referenced accordingly in the Reference list.

REFERENCES

Alosco, M. L., Brickman, A. M., Spitznagel, M. B., Garcia, S. L., Narkhede, A., Griffith, E. Y., et al. (2013). Cerebral perfusion is associated with white matter hyperintensities in older adults with heart failure. *Congest. Heart Fail.* 19, E29–E34. doi: 10.1111/chf.12025

Benedictus, M. R., van Harten, A. C., Leeuwis, A. E., Koene, T., Scheltens, P., Barkhof, F., et al. (2015). White matter hyperintensities relate to clinical progression in subjective cognitive decline. *Stroke* 46, 2661–2664. doi: 10.1161/STROKEAHA.115.009475

Boyle, P. A., Yu, L., Fleischman, D. A., Leurgans, S., Yang, J., Wilson, R. S., et al. (2016). White matter hyperintensities, incident mild cognitive impairment and cognitive decline in old age. *Ann. Clin. Transl. Neurol.* 3, 791–800. doi: 10.1002/acn3.343

Chutinet, A., Biffi, A., Kanakis, A., Fitzpatrick, K. M., Furie, K. L., and Rost, N. S. (2012). Severity of leukoaraiosis in large vessel atherosclerotic disease. *AJNR Am. J. Neuroradiol.* 33, 1591–1595. doi: 10.3174/ajnr.A3015

Conti, J., Sterr, A., Brucki, S. M., and Conforto, A. B. (2015). Diversity of approaches in assessment of executive functions in stroke: limited evidence? *eNeurologicalSci* 1, 12–20. doi: 10.1016/j.ensci.2015.08.002

Cover, K. S., van Schijndel, R. A., Versteeg, A., Leung, K. K., Mulder, E. R., Jong, R. A., et al. (2016). Reproducibility of hippocampal atrophy rates measured with manual, FreeSurfer, AdaBoost, FSL/FIRST and the MAPS-HBSI methods in Alzheimer's disease. *Psychiatry Res. Neuroimaging* 252, 26–35. doi: 10.1016/j.pscychresns.2016.04.006

Damangir, S., Manzouri, A., Oppedal, K., Carlsson, S., Firbank, M. J., Sonnesyn, H., et al. (2012). Multispectral MRI segmentation of age related white matter changes using a cascade of support vector machines. *J. Neurol. Sci.* 322, 211–216. doi: 10.1016/j.jns.2012.07.064

de Groot, J. C., de Leeuw, F. E., Oudkerk, M., Hofman, A., Jolles, J., and Breteler, M. M. (2001). Cerebral white matter lesions and subjective cognitive dysfunction: the Rotterdam Scan Study. *Neurology* 56, 1539–1545. doi: 10.1212/WNL.56.11.1539

de Guio, F., Jouvent, E., Biessels, G. J., Black, S. E., Brayne, C., Chen, C., et al. (2016). Reproducibility and variability of quantitative magnetic resonance imaging markers in cerebral small vessel disease. *J. Cereb. Blood Flow Metab.* 36, 1319–1337. doi: 10.1177/0271678X16647396

Debette, S., Beiser, A., DeCarli, C., Au, R., Himali, J. J., Kelly-Hayes, M., et al. (2010). Association of MRI markers of vascular brain injury with incident stroke, mild cognitive impairment, dementia and mortality: the Framingham Offspring Study. *Stroke* 41, 600–606. doi: 10.1161/STROKEAHA.109.570044

Debette, S., and Markus, H. S. (2010). The clinical importance of white matter hyperintensities on brain magnetic resonance imaging: systematic review and meta-analysis. *BMJ* 341:c3666. doi: 10.1136/bmj.c3666

Dong, C., Nabizadeh, N., Caunca, M., Cheung, Y. K., Rundek, T., Elkind, M. S., et al. (2015). Cognitive correlates of white matter lesion load and brain atrophy: the Northern Manhattan Study. *Neurology* 85, 441–449. doi: 10.1212/WNL.0000000000001716

Folstein, M. F., Folstein, S. E., and McHugh, P. R. (1975). "Mini-mental state". A practical method for grading the cognitive state of patients for the clinician. *J. Psychiatr. Res.* 12, 189–198. doi: 10.1016/0022-3956(75)90026-6

Ihle-Hansen, H., Thommessen, B., Fagerland, M. W., Wyller, T. B., Engedal, K., Oksengård, A. R., et al. (2012). Impact of white matter lesions on cognition in stroke patients free from pre-stroke cognitive impairment: a one-year follow-up study. *Dement. Geriatr. Cogn. Dis. Extra* 2, 38–47. doi: 10.1159/000336817

Inaba, M., White, L., Bell, C., Chen, R., Petrovitch, H., Launer, L., et al. (2011). White matter lesions on brain magnetic resonance imaging scan and 5-year cognitive decline: the Honolulu-Asia aging study. *J. Am. Geriatr. Soc.* 59, 1484–1489. doi: 10.1111/j.1532-5415.2011.03490.x

Inzitari, D., Pracucci, G., Poggesi, A., Carlucci, G., Barkhof, F., Chabriat, H., et al. (2009). Changes in white matter as determinant of global functional decline in older independent outpatients: three year follow-up of LADIS (leukoaraiosis and disability) study cohort. *BMJ* 339:b2477. doi: 10.1136/bmj.b2477

Jokinen, H., Gouw, A. A., Madureira, S., Ylikoski, R., van Straaten, E. C., van der Flier, W. M., et al. (2011). Incident lacunes influence cognitive decline: the LADIS study. *Neurology* 76, 1872–1878. doi: 10.1212/WNL.0b013e31821d752f

Kloppenborg, R. P., Nederkoorn, P. J., Geerlings, M. I., and van den Berg, E. (2014). Presence and progression of white matter hyperintensities and cognition: a meta-analysis. *Neurology* 82, 2127–2138. doi: 10.1212/WNL.0000000000000505

Kramer, J. H., Mungas, D., Reed, B. R., Wetzel, M. E., Burnett, M. M., Miller, B. L., et al. (2007). Longitudinal MRI and cognitive change in healthy elderly. *Neuropsychology* 21, 412–418. doi: 10.1037/0894-4105.21.4.412

Leeuwis, A. E., Benedictus, M. R., Kuijer, J. P., Binnewijzend, M. A., Hooghiemstra, A. M., Verfaillie, S. C., et al. (2016). Lower cerebral blood flow is associated with impairment in multiple cognitive domains in Alzheimer's disease. *Alzheimers Dement.* 13, 531–540. doi: 10.1016/j.jalz.2016.08.013

Loeb, C., Gandolfo, C., Croce, R., and Conti, I. (1992). Dementia associated with lacunar infarctions. *Stroke* 2, 1225–1229. doi: 10.1161/01.str.23.9.1225

Lou, W., Shi, L., Wong, A., Chu, W. C., Mok, V. C., and Wang, D. (2016). Changes of cerebral perfusion and functional brain network organization in patients with mild cognitive impairment. *J. Alzheimers Dis.* 54, 397–409. doi: 10.3233/JAD-160201

Nylander, R. (2017). *Magnetic Resonance Imaging Markers of Cerebral Small Vessel Disease in an Elderly Population-Association with Cardiovascular Disease and Cognitive Function.* Uppsala: Acta Universitatis Upsaliens.

Nylander, R., Fahlström, M., Rostrup, E., Kullberg, J., Damangir, S., Ahlstrom, H., et al. (2018). Quantitative and qualitative MRI evaluation of cerebral small vessel disease in an elderly population: a longitudinal study. *Acta Radiol.* 59, 612–618. doi: 10.1177/0284185117727567

Nylander, R., Lind, L., Wikstrom, J., Lindahl, B., Venge, P., Larsson, A., et al. (2015). Relation between cardiovascular disease risk markers and brain infarcts detected by magnetic resonance imaging in an elderly population. *J. Stroke Cerebrovasc. Dis.* 24, 312–318. doi: 10.1016/j.jstrokecerebrovasdis.2014.08.027

Østergaard, L., Engedal, T. S., Moreton, F., Hansen, M. B., Wardlaw, J. M., Dalkara, T., et al. (2016). Cerebral small vessel disease: capillary pathways to stroke and cognitive decline. *J. Cereb. Blood Flow Metab.* 36, 302–325. doi: 10.1177/0271678X15606723

Pantoni, L. (2010). Cerebral small vessel disease: from pathogenesis and clinical characteristics to therapeutic challenges. *Lancet Neurol.* 9, 689–701. doi: 10.1016/S1474-4422(10)70104-6

Pantoni, L., Fierini, F., Poggesi, A., and LADIS Study Group. (2015). Impact of cerebral white matter changes on functionality in older adults: an overview of the LADIS Study results and future directions. *Geriatr. Gerontol. Int.* 15, 10–16. doi: 10.1111/ggi.12665

Poels, M. M., Ikram, M. A., van der Lugt, A., Hofman, A., Niessen, W. J., Krestin, G. P., et al. (2012). Cerebral microbleeds are associated with worse cognitive function: the Rotterdam Scan Study. *Neurology* 78, 326–333. doi: 10.1212/WNL.0b013e3182452928

Prins, N. D., van Dijk, E. J., den Heijer, T., Vermeer, S. E., Jolles, J., Koudstaal, P. J., et al. (2005). Cerebral small-vessel disease and decline in information processing speed, executive function and memory. *Brain* 128, 2034–2041. doi: 10.1093/brain/awh553

Ronnemaa, E., Zethelius, B., Lannfelt, L., and Kilander, L. (2011). Vascular risk factors and dementia: 40-year follow-up of a population-based cohort. *Dement. Geriatr. Cogn. Disord.* 31, 460–466. doi: 10.1159/000330020

Schmidt, R., Ropele, S., Enzinger, C., Petrovic, K., Smith, S., Schmidt, H., et al. (2005). White matter lesion progression, brain atrophy and cognitive decline: the Austrian stroke prevention study. *Ann. Neurol.* 58, 610–616. doi: 10.1002/ana.20630

Smith, E. E., Egorova, S., Blacker, D., Killiany, R. J., Muzikansky, A., Dickerson, B. C., et al. (2008). Magnetic resonance imaging white matter hyperintensities and brain volume in the prediction of mild cognitive impairment and dementia. *Arch. Neurol.* 65, 94–100. doi: 10.1001/archneurol.2007.23

Sörös, P., Harnadek, M., Blake, T., Hachinski, V., and Chan, R. (2015). Executive dysfunction in patients with transient ischemic attack and minor stroke. *J. Neurol. Sci.* 354, 17–20. doi: 10.1016/j.jns.2015.04.022

Tombaugh, T. N. (2004). Trail Making Test A and B: normative data stratified by age and education. *Arch. Clin. Neuropsychol.* 19, 203–214. doi: 10.1016/s0887-6177(03)00039-8

van Dalen, J. W., Mutsaerts, H. J., Nederveen, A. J., Vrenken, H., Steenwijk, M. D., Caan, M. W., et al. (2016). White matter hyperintensity volume and cerebral perfusion in older individuals with hypertension using arterial spin-labeling. *AJNR Am. J. Neuroradiol.* 37, 1824–1830. doi: 10.3174/ajnr.a4828

van der Flier, W. M., van Straaten, E. C., Barkhof, F., Verdelho, A., Madureira, S., Pantoni, L., et al. (2005). Small vessel disease and general cognitive function in nondisabled elderly: the LADIS study. *Stroke* 36, 2116–2120. doi: 10.1161/01.STR.0000179092.59909.42

van Dijk, E. J., Prins, N. D., Vrooman, H. A., Hofman, A., Koudstaal, P. J., and Breteler, M. M. (2008). Progression of cerebral small vessel disease in relation to risk factors and cognitive consequences: rotterdam Scan study. *Stroke* 39, 2712–2719. doi: 10.1161/STROKEAHA.107.513176

van Norden, A. G., van den Berg, H. A., de Laat, K. F., Gons, R. A., van Dijk, E. J., and de Leeuw, F. E. (2011). Frontal and temporal microbleeds are related to cognitive function: the Radboud University Nijmegen Diffusion Tensor and Magnetic Resonance Cohort (RUN DMC) study. *Stroke* 42, 3382–3386. doi: 10.1161/STROKEAHA.111.629634

van Straaten, E. C., Fazekas, F., Rostrup, E., Scheltens, P., Schmidt, R., Pantoni, L., et al. (2006). Impact of white matter hyperintensities scoring method on correlations with clinical data: the LADIS study. *Stroke* 37, 836–840. doi: 10.1161/01.STR.0000202585.26325.74

Wardlaw, J. M., Smith, E. E., Biessels, G. J., Cordonnier, C., Fazekas, F., Frayne, R., et al. (2013a). Neuroimaging standards for research into small vessel disease and its contribution to ageing and neurodegeneration. *Lancet Neurol.* 12, 822–838. doi: 10.1016/S1474-4422(13)70124-8

Wardlaw, J. M., Smith, C., and Dichgans, M. (2013b). Mechanisms of sporadic cerebral small vessel disease: insights from neuroimaging. *Lancet Neurol.* 12, 483–497. doi: 10.1016/S1474-4422(13)70060-7

Wardlaw, J. M., Valdés Hernández, M. C., and Muñoz-Maniega, S. (2015). What are white matter hyperintensities made of? Relevance to vascular cognitive impairment. *J. Am. Heart Assoc.* 4:001140. doi: 10.1161/JAHA.114.001140

Wiberg, B., Lind, L., Kilander, L., Zethelius, B., Sundelof, J. E., and Sundstrom, J. (2010). Cognitive function and risk of stroke in elderly men. *Neurology* 74, 379–385. doi: 10.1212/WNL.0b013e3181ccc516

Ylikoski, A., Erkinjuntti, T., Raininko, R., Sarna, S., Sulkava, R., and Tilvis, R. (1995). White matter hyperintensities on MRI in the neurologically nondiseased elderly. Analysis of cohorts of consecutive subjects aged 55 to 85 years living at home. *Stroke* 26, 1171–1177. doi: 10.1161/01.STR.26.7.1171

Zhong, G., Zhang, R., Jiaerken, Y., Yu, X., Zhou, Y., Liu, C., et al. (2017). Better correlation of cognitive function to white matter integrity than to blood supply in subjects with leukoaraiosis. *Front. Aging Neurosci.* 9:185. doi: 10.3389/fnagi.2017.00185

Zlatar, Z. Z., Bischoff-Grethe, A., Hays, C. C., Liu, T. T., Meloy, M. J., Rissman, R. A., et al. (2016). Higher brain perfusion may not support memory functions in cognitively normal carriers of the ApoE epsilon4 allele compared to non-carriers. *Front. Aging Neurosci.* 8:151. doi: 10.3389/fnagi.2016.00151

5

Decreased Complexity in Alzheimer's Disease: Resting-State fMRI Evidence of Brain Entropy Mapping

Bin Wang[1, 2†], *Yan Niu*[1†], *Liwen Miao*[1], *Rui Cao*[1], *Pengfei Yan*[1], *Hao Guo*[1], *Dandan Li*[1], *Yuxiang Guo*[1], *Tianyi Yan*[3, 4*], *Jinglong Wu*[5, 6], *Jie Xiang*[1*], and *Hui Zhang*[2*]

[1] *College of Computer Science and Technology, Taiyuan University of Technology, Taiyuan, China,* [2] *Department of Radiology, First Hospital of Shanxi Medical University, Taiyuan, China,* [3] *School of Life Science, Beijing Institute of Technology, Beijing, China,* [4] *Key Laboratory of Convergence Medical Engineering System and Healthcare Technology, Ministry of Industry and Information Technology, Beijing Institute of Technology, Beijing, China,* [5] *Key Laboratory of Biomimetic Robots and Systems, Ministry of Education, Beijing Institute of Technology, Beijing, China,* [6] *Graduate School of Natural Science and Technology, Okayama University, Okayama, Japan*

***Correspondence:**
Jie Xiang
xiangjie@tyut.edu.cn
Tianyi Yan
yantianyi@bit.edu.cn
Hui Zhang
zhanghui_mr@163.com

† co-first authors.

‡ The data used in preparation of this article were obtained from the Alzheimer's Disease Neuroimaging Initiative (ADNI) database (adni.loni.usc.edu). As such, the investigators within the ADNI contributed to the design and implementation of the ADNI and/or provided data but did not participate in analysis or writing of this report. A complete listing of the ADNI investigators can be found at https://adni.loni.usc.edu/wp-content/uploads/how_to_apply/ADNI_Acknowledgement_List.pdf

Alzheimer's disease (AD) is a frequently observed, irreversible brain function disorder among elderly individuals. Resting-state functional magnetic resonance imaging (rs-fMRI) has been introduced as an alternative approach to assessing brain functional abnormalities in AD patients. However, alterations in the brain rs-fMRI signal complexities in mild cognitive impairment (MCI) and AD patients remain unclear. Here, we described the novel application of permutation entropy (PE) to investigate the abnormal complexity of rs-fMRI signals in MCI and AD patients. The rs-fMRI signals of 30 normal controls (NCs), 33 early MCI (EMCI), 32 late MCI (LMCI), and 29 AD patients were obtained from the Alzheimer's disease Neuroimaging Initiative (ADNI) database. After preprocessing, whole-brain entropy maps of the four groups were extracted and subjected to Gaussian smoothing. We performed a one-way analysis of variance (ANOVA) on the brain entropy maps of the four groups. The results after adjusting for age and sex differences together revealed that the patients with AD exhibited lower complexity than did the MCI and NC controls. We found five clusters that exhibited significant differences and were distributed primarily in the occipital, frontal, and temporal lobes. The average PE of the five clusters exhibited a decreasing trend from MCI to AD. The AD group exhibited the least complexity. Additionally, the average PE of the five clusters was significantly positively correlated with the Mini-Mental State Examination (MMSE) scores and significantly negatively correlated with Functional Assessment Questionnaire (FAQ) scores and global Clinical Dementia Rating (CDR) scores in the patient groups. Significant correlations were also found between the PE and regional homogeneity (ReHo) in the patient groups. These results indicated that declines in PE might be related to changes in regional functional homogeneity in AD. These findings suggested that complexity analyses using PE in rs-fMRI signals can provide important information about the fMRI characteristics of cognitive impairments in MCI and AD.

Keywords: Alzheimer's disease, mild cognitive impairment, resting-state functional magnetic resonance imaging, permutation entropy, complexity

INTRODUCTION

Alzheimer's disease (AD) is a neurodegenerative disease that is characterized by declines in cognition and memory (Brookmeyer et al., 2007). The neuropathology of AD is characterized by neuronal loss and the appearance of neuritic plaques containing amyloid-β-peptide and neurofibrillary tangles (Haass and Selkoe, 2007). And these changes lead to abnormal brain function in AD (Cho et al., 2013). Mild cognitive impairment (MCI) is an intermediate state between normal aging and AD and is associated with a high risk of progression to AD (Petersen and Negash, 2008). Several neuroimaging techniques, including magnetic resonance imaging (MRI), blood oxygenation level-dependent (BOLD) functional MRI (fMRI), and positron emission tomography (PET), have been explored to study brain function in AD (Lebedeva et al., 2017; Li et al., 2017). Usually, the brain function of AD patients is weakened including problems storing and retrieving information due to the destruction of neurons in parts of the patient's brain. Then, AD affects the brain areas involved in language and reasoning. Eventually, the most notable characteristic of AD on MRI is cerebral atrophy in the medial temporal lobe, hippocampus, right temporal lobe, precuneus, cingulate gyrus, and inferior frontal cortex (Möller et al., 2013). The changes in these brain regions suggest that they are relevant for the loss of functionality in patients with dementia. A differential diagnosis for the types of dementia should be attempted. Recently, resting-state fMRI (rs-fMRI) has been introduced as an alternative approach for studying brain functional abnormalities in AD (Gusnard and Raichle, 2001; Fox and Raichle, 2007).

Based on its structure and function, the human brain is one of the most complex information processing systems. Complexity can be defined as the difficulties that arise when describing or predicting a signal. Normal physiology requires a complex network to effectively control function. Lipsitz and Goldberger (Lipsitz, 1992, 2004) argued that with aging and disease, losses of complexity occur in the dynamics of many integrated physiological processes of an organism. The development of the concept of complexity has focused on measuring regularity using various metrics that are based on non-linear time series analysis. Lyapunov exponents (Wolf et al., 1985) and correlation dimensions (Broock et al., 1996) have been used to characterize non-linear dynamics, but they require large data sets (Eckmann and Ruelle, 1992) and assume that the time series is stationary (Grassberger and Procaccia, 1983), which is typically inappropriate for biological data. Entropy measures the randomness and predictability of a stochastic process and generally increases with greater randomness; i.e., lower entropy indicates lower signal complexity.

Previous research has noted decreased complexity in the EEG and MEG signals of aging and diseased brains. Gomez et al. used approximate entropy (ApEn) and sample entropy (SampEn) to analyze MEG signals and found that the signals were less complex and more regular in AD patients than in control subjects (Gómez and Hornero, 2009; Gomez et al., 2010). Recent EEG studies have explored event-related multiscale entropy (MSE) measures as features for effectively discriminating between normal aging, MCI, and AD and found decreasing complexity with the severity of cognitive decline (McBride et al., 2014a,b). These findings indicate decreases in the EEG and MEG signal complexities of AD and MCI patients.

Entropy is a commonly used metric for the measurement of brain complexity. Permutation entropy (PE) is a new method that is used to measure the irregularity of non-stationary time series (Bandt and Pompe, 2002). PE considers only the ranks of the samples and not their metrics. As an ordinal measure, PE has some advantages over other commonly used entropy measures, such as ApEn (Pincus, 1991) and SampEn (Richman and Moorman, 2000), including its simplicity, low complexity in computation without further model assumptions, and robustness in the presence of observational and dynamical noise (Zanin et al., 2012). PE has been used in EEG signal studies of human absence epilepsy (Ferlazzo et al., 2014), typical absences (Li et al., 2014), MCI (Timothy et al., 2014), and AD (Morabito et al., 2012). These studies suggest that PE is a useful tool for the study of abnormalities of brain complexity.

Few studies have performed complexity analyses of rs-fMRI signals (Liu et al., 2013; Sokunbi et al., 2013). To the best of our knowledge, PE has not been applied to the complexity study of rs-fMRI signals. Some fMRI studies have found that complexity decreases in gray and white matter and some brain regions with normal aging (Liu et al., 2013; Sokunbi et al., 2015). Compared with normal controls (NCs), AD patients exhibit a greater decrease in cognitive ability and memory. EEG studies have demonstrated that declining brain function is associated with decreased complexity in the brains of AD patients (McBride et al., 2014a,b). Liu et al. found that cognitive impairment was associated with decreased complexity of the fMRI signals in the gray matter and brain regions in a familial AD group (Liu et al., 2013). However, the alterations in the complexities of rs-fMRI signals in MCI and AD patients remain unclear.

In the present study, an analysis of PE complexity was performed using rs-fMRI signals of NC, early MCI (EMCI), late MCI (LMCI), and AD subjects from the Alzheimer's disease neuroimaging initiative (ADNI, http://adni.loni.usc.edu/) database. First, PE brain maps of the four groups were extracted and subjected to Gaussian smoothing. One-way analysis of variance (ANOVA) was performed to identify the significantly different clusters. Then, the average PEs of the selected regions of interest (ROIs) were analyzed. Finally, Pearson's correlations between the average PEs of ROIs for each participant and each of the Mini-Mental State Examination (MMSE), Functional Assessment Questionnaire (FAQ) and global Clinical Dementia Rating (CDR) scores were analyzed. Moreover, we examined the relationships between regional homogeneity (ReHo) and PE in AD and MCI patients. ReHo is suitable for exploring resting-state functional homogeneity (Zang et al., 2004). A larger ReHo value indicates higher regional synchronization. We also examined the relationships between glucose metabolism on FDG-PET and PE in AD and MCI patients. Finally, we examined the gray matter volumes in the four groups using a voxel-based morphometry (VBM) method and studied the relationship between the gray matter volumes and PEs in the patient groups.

The objective of our study was to determine the alterations of complexity in MCI and AD patients from brain entropy maps based on rs-fMRI data. We also found that these alterations were related to the changes in regional synchronization present in MCI and AD compared with NCs.

MATERIALS AND METHODS

Participants

All of the subjects were selected from the ADNI (ADNI-2) database. The ADNI aims to study the pathogenesis and prevention of AD by analyzing various medical imaging data.

A total of 124 subjects were selected, and the data from each subject consisted of 140 functional volumes from the database according to disease type (AD, LMCI, EMCI, and NC). The subjects included 29 AD patients (average age of 72.33 years, 18 females), 32 LMCI patients (average age of 72.57 years, 13 females), 33 EMCI patients (average age of 72.01 years, 16 females), and 30 NC subjects (average age of 74.18 years, 19 females; **Table 1**). The AD patients had MMSE scores of 14–26, the LMCI patients had MMSE scores of 23–28, the EMCI patients had MMSE scores of 24–30, and the NC subjects, who did not exhibit depression or dementia, had MMSE scores of 24–30. The FAQ is a measure of the ability to perform 10 high-level skills used in daily tasks (shopping, preparing meals, handling finances, and understanding current events), each of which is rated by a knowledgeable informant. The total score ranges from 0 to 50, and higher scores indicating poorer functional performance. The AD patients had FAQ scores of 3–28, the LMCI patients had FAQ scores of 0–18, the EMCI patients had FAQ scores of 0–12, and the NC subjects had FAQ scores of 0–3. The global CDR scores are discrete values of 0, 0.5, and 1 that indicate no dementia, mild dementia, and dementia, respectively. All AD patients had a global CDR of 0.5 or 1, the LMCI and EMCI patients had global CDR scores of 0.5, and the NC subjects had a global CDR score of 0.

Data Acquisition

All subjects were scanned in a three-tesla (3T) scanner. During the resting-state scans, the subjects were asked to keep their eyes closed (Jack et al., 2008). Functional and structural MRI data were collected with the following parameters: field strength = 3.0; manufacturer = Philips Medical Systems; slice thickness = 3.3; repetition time (TR) = 3,000 ms; echo time (TE) = 30 ms; flip angle = 80°; and slice number = 48.

TABLE 1 | Demographic and clinical information of the participants.

Group	NC	EMCI	LMCI	AD	*P*-value
Age (years)[a]	74.18 ± 5.96	72.01 ± 5.87	72.57 ± 8.16	72.33 ± 7.26	0.505
Sex (M/F)	11/19	17/16	19/13	11/18	0.732
MMSE[b]	28.9 ± 1.7	27.59 ± 2.02	26.96 ± 2.69	21.0 ± 3.5	<0.001
FAQ[c]	0.14 ± 0.44	3.03 ± 4.50	4.07 ± 4.70	15 ± 7.47	<0.001
CDR[d]	0	0.5	0.5	0.84 ± 0.23	<0.001

[a,b,c,d]Values represent the mean ± standard deviation.

MMSE, Mini-Mental State Examination; FAQ, Functional Assessment Questionnaire; CDR, Clinical Dementia Rating.

FDG-PET images were acquired at a variety of scanners nationwide using either a 30-min six-frame scan or a static 30-min single-frame scan acquired 30–60 min post-injection (details are available at https://adni.loni.usc.edu/wp-content/uploads/2010/05/ADNI2_PET_Tech_Manual_0142011.pdf).

Data Preprocessing

The preprocessing of rs-fMRI data was performed using the Data Processing Assistant for Resting-State fMRI (DPARSF) toolbox (Chao-Gan and Yu-Feng, 2010) and the SPM8 package (http://www.fil.ion.ucl.ac.uk/spm). Briefly, the preprocessing steps were as follows: the first 10 volumes of the functional images during the participant's adaptation to the circumstances were discarded; slice-timing correction was performed according to the last slice; the images were realigned for head movement compensation using a six-parameter rigid-body spatial transformation because excessive head motion may induce large artifacts in fMRI time series; the images were normalized to the Montreal Neurological Institute (MNI) space; and finally, the signal drift was removed using a linear model. Additionally, spatial smoothing of the brain PE maps was performed to reduce the white noise and suppress the effects due to residual differences during inter-subject averaging using an 8-mm full-width at half maximum (FWHM) smoothing kernel (Sokunbi et al., 2015). Notably, PE complexity was accomplished by voxel-based analysis to explore regional differences, and smoothing before a PE calculation will greatly increase the regional similarity (Chao-Gan and Yu-Feng, 2010). A recent study involving fuzzy approximate entropy analysis of rs-fMRI signals performed the smoothing after the entropy calculation (Sokunbi et al., 2015). Moreover, the ReHo explores the functional homogeneity of resting-state fMRI data (Zang et al., 2004), which might provide convenience in the potential explanation of PE. Thus, we calculated the ReHo after preprocessing. Then, the ReHo of the brain was smoothed with an 8-mm FWHM smoothing kernel.

Some studies have shown that the removal of nuisance signals had influence on the results (Chao-Gan and Yu-Feng, 2010; Wang et al., 2014). We also tried to remove the effect of nuisance covariates, including the global signal, the motion parameters, the cerebrospinal fluid (CSF), and the white matter signals. The detailed data processing, statistical analyses, and results were presented in Presentation 1 (Supplementary Material).

The analysis of the gray matter volume was performed according to the VBM protocol using DPARSF (Chao-Gan and Yu-Feng, 2010). This process primarily consisted of segmentation and normalization. First, each subject's MRI data were segmented into gray matter, white matter and cerebrospinal fluid (CSF). Subsequently, diffeomorphic anatomical registration using exponential lie algebra (DARTEL) was applied to normalize the gray matter images and iteratively create the template. The subjects' gray matter images were registered to new templates for each iteration. Then, the normalized gray matter images were multiplied to preserve the absolute volume of the gray matter in the subjects' native spaces. Finally, all gray matter images were smoothed with an 8-mm FWHM Gaussian kernel.

Preprocessing of the FDG-PET scans was performed using the SPM8 package (http://www.fil.ion.ucl.ac.uk/spm). Dynamic scans were registered to the mean frame and averaged to create a single average image. Then, the images were normalized to the MNI space (voxel size: 3 × 3 × 3). Next, spatial smoothing was performed using a Gaussian smoothing kernel with FWHM of [8 8 8]. Therefore, each voxel time series was standardized to a mean of zero and a standard deviation of unity to allow the data sets to be compared. The scans were intensity-normalized using a whole-cerebellum reference region to create standardized uptake value ratio (SUVR) images.

PE Algorithm

The basic principle of PE is that it does not consider the specific values of the data; rather, PE is based on the comparison of adjacent data points in the time domain. The algorithm is described below.

Given a time series $x(i), i = 1, 2, ..., N$, a vector composed of the m-th subsequent values is constructed as follows:

$$\left.\begin{aligned} X(1) &= \{x(1), x(1+l), \cdots, x(1+(m-1)l)\} \\ &\vdots \\ X(i) &= \{x(i), x(i+l), \cdots, x(i+(m-1)l)\} \\ &\vdots \\ X(N-(m-1)l) &= \{x(N-(m-1)l), \\ &\quad x(N-(m-2)l), \cdots, x(N)\} \end{aligned}\right\} \tag{1}$$

where m is the embedding dimension, and l is the delay time.

The vector $X(i)$ can be rearranged in an ascending order as follows:

$$X(i) = \{x(i+(j_1-1)l) \leq x(i+(j_2-1)l) \leq \cdots \leq x(i+(j_m-1)l)\} \tag{2}$$

where $j = 1, 2, \cdots, m$. Note that if two values are equal (here, $x(i+(j_1-1)l) = x(i+(j_2-1)l)$), they are ordered according to the size of the j_1, j_2 value, such that $x(i+(j_1-1)l) \leq x(i+(j_2-1)l)$ when $j_1 < j_2$. Then we can obtain a set of symbol sequences by each raw of it that the reconstructed matrix of any time series, where the symbol sequences just like $S(g) = \{j_1, j_2, \cdots, j_m\}, (g = 1, 2, \cdots k, k \leq m!)$, where the k means the objectively quantity of $\{j_1, j_2, \cdots, j_m\}$. So, any vector $X(i)$ is uniquely mapped into $(1, 2, \cdots, m)$ or $(2, 1, \cdots, m) \cdots$ or $(m, m-1, \cdots, 1)$ in total $m!$ possible symbol sequences and $S(g)$ is one of them. Then, let the probability distribution of the distinct symbols be $P_g(g = 1, 2, \cdots k)$. The PE is defined as the Shannon entropy for the k distinct symbols:

$$PE = -\sum_{g=1}^{k} P_g \ln P_g \tag{3}$$

Be aware, PE reaches its maximum $\ln(m!)$ when $p_g = 1/m!$. Therefore, PE is standardized by $\ln(m!)$:

$$PE_s = PE/\ln(m!) \tag{4}$$

Obviously, the range of PE_s is $0 \leq PE_s \leq 1$.

PE_s is the local order structure of the time series. A large PE value indicates a more random time series, whereas a small PE value indicates that the time series is regular.

Computation of PE

In the calculation of PE, three parameter values must be considered and set, including the length of the time series N, the embedding dimension m and the time delay l. Bandt et al. (Bandt and Pompe, 2002) suggested that the embedding dimension should range from 3 to 7 because if the value is too small, the reconstructed sequence contains too few states; therefore, the algorithm loses its meaning and validity and cannot detect the dynamic mutation of the time series. However, if the value is too large, the phase space reconstruction will homogenize the time series, the calculation will be time consuming, and subtle changes in the sequence will not be reflected. The time delay l has little influence on the entropy of the time series (Mateos et al., 2014). To allow every possible order pattern of dimension m to occur in a time series of length N, the condition $m! \leq N-(m-1)l$ must hold. Moreover, to avoid undersampling, $N \geq m! + (m-1)l$ is required. Therefore, we need to choose $N \geq (m+1)!$. For $N = 130$, an obviously unsatisfying complexity estimation is obtained when $m \geq 5$. To satisfy this condition, we therefore chose a low dimension, i.e., $m = 4$, when calculating the permutation entropy. In the present study, we chose $m = 4, l = 1$ for calculation and analysis (Li et al., 2014).

Statistical Analyses

The first statistical tests were performed using the rs-fMRI Data Analysis Toolkit (REST 1.8) (Song et al., 2011). One-way ANOVA was performed to examine differences among the four groups (NC, EMCI, LMCI, and AD). Clusters that were significantly different after adjusting for age and sex differences were selected by setting $P < 0.005$ with a Gaussian random fields (GRF) correction.

The DPARSF toolbox was used to define the ROIs to extract the average PE, ReHo, and PDG-PET values according to the peak MNI coordinates (XYZ), and the radius of the spheres was 8 mm.

The subsequent statistical tests were performed using Statistical Package for Social Sciences (SPSS 20.0; New York, NY, USA) software. The averages PEs of the ROIs of each subject were obtained and one-way ANOVA was performed to examine the differences among the four groups. The relationships between the PE and the clinical measurements of MMSE, FAQ, and CDR were analyzed using Pearson's correlations in the patient groups.

Pearson's correlation analyses of the PE with the ReHo and FDG-PET data were performed in the patient groups using SPSS. Moreover, we also performed correlation analyses between the PEs and the gray matter volumes in the patient groups.

RESULTS

Demographic and Clinical Data

The demographic and clinical data for each group were summarized in **Table 1**. The means (±*SD*) were presented for the baseline clinical tests. The results of one-way ANOVAs revealed significant effects of group on the MMSE ($F = 40.924, P < 0.001$), FAQ ($F = 61.810$, $P < 0.001$), and the CDR ($F = 238.31$, $P < 0.001$) scores but not sex ($F = 0.431$; $P = 0.732$) or age ($F = 0.785$; $P = 0.505$). Note that a higher FAQ score represents greater impairment, whereas a lower MMSE represents greater impairment. The MMSE scores were significantly lower in the MCI ($t = -3.302$, $P = 0.002$) and AD ($t = -9.333$, $P < 0.001$) groups than in the NC group. The FAQ scores were significantly higher in the MCI ($t = 5.642$, $P < 0.001$) and AD groups ($t = 12.625$, $P < 0.001$) than in the NC group. The CDR scores were significantly higher in the MCI ($t = 7.687$, $P < 0.001$) and AD groups ($t = 28.436$, $P < 0.001$) than in the NC group.

rs-fMRI PE Brain Maps

We extracted the mean PEs of the whole brain, gray matter (GM), white matter (WM), and cerebral spinal fluid (CSF). There were differences in the GM ($F = 2.711$, $P = 0.048$) and WM ($F = 2.792$, $P = 0.043$) but no differences in the whole brain ($F = 1.713$, $P = 0.168$) or CSF ($F = 1.183$, $P = 0.319$) among the four groups. The results of the one-way ANOVAs were presented in **Figure 1**. At the regional levels, five clusters were found to exhibit significant differences in PE among the four groups, as illustrated in **Figure 2**. The complexity differences among the four groups were mainly observed in the temporal, occipital, and frontal lobes. The results after removing the effect of nuisance covariates showed the complexity differences were mainly observed in the frontal lobes (Presentation 1 in Supplementary Material).

ROI Analysis

In addition to the brain regions at the peak points, other significant brain regions that accounted for a large proportion were also extracted. We obtained eight ROIs from five clusters for the next analysis as presented in **Table 2**. The average PE values were extracted according to the peak MNI coordinates of the ROIs, and the sphere radius was 8 mm. Specifically, as presented in **Table 2**, the following regions exhibited significant differences: the right inferior temporal gyrus (ITG.R), the left middle frontal gyrus (MFG.L), the left superior frontal gyrus (SFGdor.L), the left anterior cingulate and paracingulate gyri (ACG.L), the right cuneus (CUN.R) and left cuneus (CUN.L), the right middle occipital gyrus (MOG.R), and the right superior occipital gyrus (SOG.R). In particular, five peak MNI coordinate regions (ITG.R, MFG.L, ACG.L, CUN.R, and MOG.R) exhibited statistically significant differences ($F > 8.13$, $p < 0.005$, corrected). The results of one-way ANOVAs revealed significant effects of group in eight brain regions that exhibited significantly decreased complexity in the AD group compared with the MCI groups and the NC group ($t > 2.909$, $P < 0.01$). Compared with the NC, decreased complexity was also found in the left cuneus in the MCI group ($P = 0.04$, one-tailed uncorrected). **Figure 3** illustrated that the PE values were lowest in the AD patients in all of the clusters. Specifically, four brain regions (ITG.R, MFG.L, ACG.L, and MOG.R) exhibited significant differences between the AD patients and the other groups. After removing the effect of nuisance covariates, five clusters were also found decreased complexity in the AD group compared with the MCI groups and the NC group (Presentation 1 in Supplementary Material).

Relationships between PE and Clinical Measurements

The MMSE score is the most widely used brief screening measure of cognition. First, we performed correlation analyses of the MMSE scores with the mean PEs of the whole brain, WM, GM, and CSF in the patient groups (EMCI+LMCI+AD) and found that only the GM ($r = 0.227$, $P = 0.032$) and WM ($r = 0.210$, $P = 0.049$) PEs exhibited positive correlations. We also examined the correlations of the MMSE scores with the PEs of the eight ROIs in the pooled patient groups (EMCI+LMCI+AD). The results were presented in **Table 3**. The eight ROIs exhibited significant positive correlations between the PEs and MMSE scores ($r > 0.212$, $P < 0.046$) with the MFG.L and MOG.R showing strong positive correlations ($r > 0.414$, $P < 0.001$). A higher MMSE score indicates higher cognitive ability.

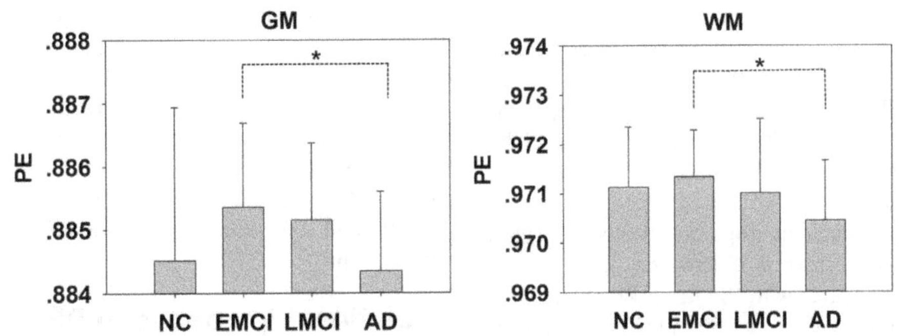

FIGURE 1 | Mean PE values of the gray matter (GM) and white matter (WM) in the NC, EMCI, LMCI, and AD subjects. Significant differences between pairs of groups after Bonferroni correction ($P < 0.05$) are indicated. $^{*}P < 0.05$. The error bars indicate the *SD*s.

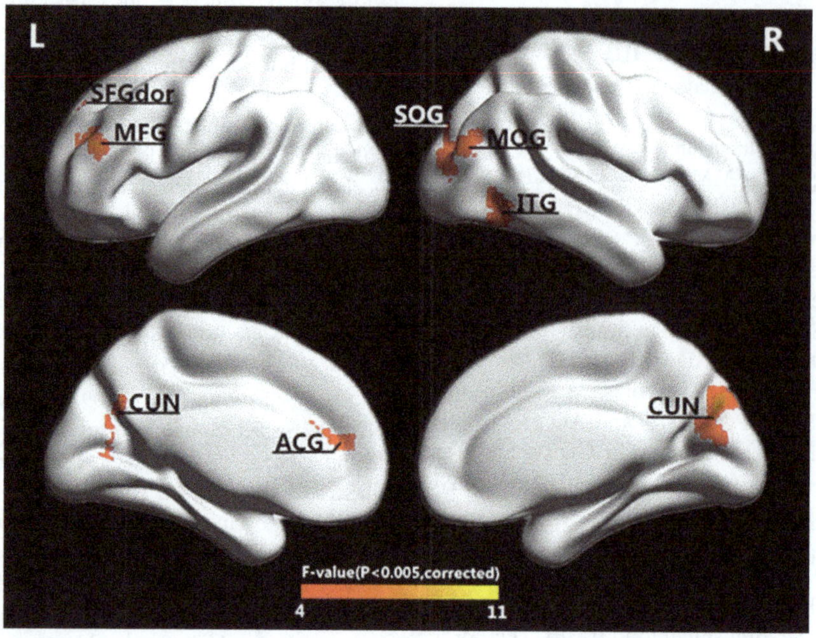

FIGURE 2 | Surface-rendered images showed the differences between the control and patient groups after adjusting for age and sex. The regions showed exhibited different complexities among the four groups. See **Table 2** for a complete list of these regions (threshold $P < 0.005$, GRF corrected).

TABLE 2 | Characteristics of the brain regions that were significantly different among the four groups.

Brain region	AAL.Abbr	Peak MNI (X, Y, Z)	Cluster voxels	Voxel F value
Inferior temporal gyrus	ITG.R	(51, 63, 15)	117	8.15
Middle frontal gyrus	MFG.L	(−33, 41, 24)	278	10.82
Superior frontal gyrus	SFGdor.L			
Anterior cingulate gyrus	ACG.L	(−12, 44, 15)	59	8.13
Right cuneus	CUN.R	(12, 78, 30)	126	8.61
Left cuneus	CUN.L			
Middle occipital gyrus	MOG.R	(45, 78, 21)	201	8.42
Superior occipital gyrus	SOG.R			

The location coordinates are those of the peak significance in each region ($P < 0.005$, GRF corrected).

The FAQ is more closely tied to functionally relevant abilities, such as accomplishing everyday tasks required for independent living. There were no correlations of the FAQ scores with the mean PEs of the whole brain, WM, GM, or CSF in patient groups. The PEs of seven ROIs exhibited strong negative correlations with the FAQ scores ($r < -0.213$, $P < 0.045$), whereas the CUN.L ROI did not (**Table 3**). A higher FAQ score indicates poorer functional performance.

The CDR has been validated neuropathologically particularly in terms of the presence or absence of dementia. There were no correlations of the CDR scores with the mean PE of the whole brain or the PEs of the WM, GM, or CSF in the patient groups. The PEs of six ROIs exhibited strong negative correlations with the CDR scores ($r < -0.211$, $P < 0.047$), whereas the PEs of the CUN.L and CUN.R did not (**Table 3**). A higher CDR score indicates the presence of dementia.

In addition, the correlation analyses were performed between the PE and the clinical measurements in the four groups and consistent significant correlations were found (Table S1). We also found the significant correlations between the PE and the clinical measurements in the patient groups and in the four groups after removing the effect of nuisance covariates (Presentation 1 in Supplementary Material).

Relationships between PE and ReHo

We extracted the ReHos of 8 ROIs according to the peak MNI coordinates (**Table 2**), and the sphere radius was 8 mm. We explored the relationship between PE and ReHo in the pooled groups (EMCI+LMCI+AD). The results were presented in **Table 4**. The GM ($r = -0.347$, $P = 0.001$), WM ($r = -0.537$, $P < 0.001$) and three ROIs (ITG.R, MFG.L, and MOG.R) exhibited significant negative correlations between the PE and ReHo in the patients groups. And the results after removing the effect of nuisance covariates showed that the inferior and middle frontal gyrus exhibited negative correlations between the PE and ReHo in the patient groups (Presentation 1 in Supplementary Material). The results illustrated that high regional spontaneous activities may be associated with a decrease in complexity.

Correlation analyses in the four groups (NC+EMCI+LMCI+AD) were also performed between the PE and ReHo (Table S2). Consistent significant correlations were found.

Relationships between PE and the Gray Matter Volume, FDG-PET

We extracted the gray matter volumes of eight ROIs according to the peak MNI coordinates, and the sphere radius was 8 mm. Then, we explored the relationships between the PEs and the

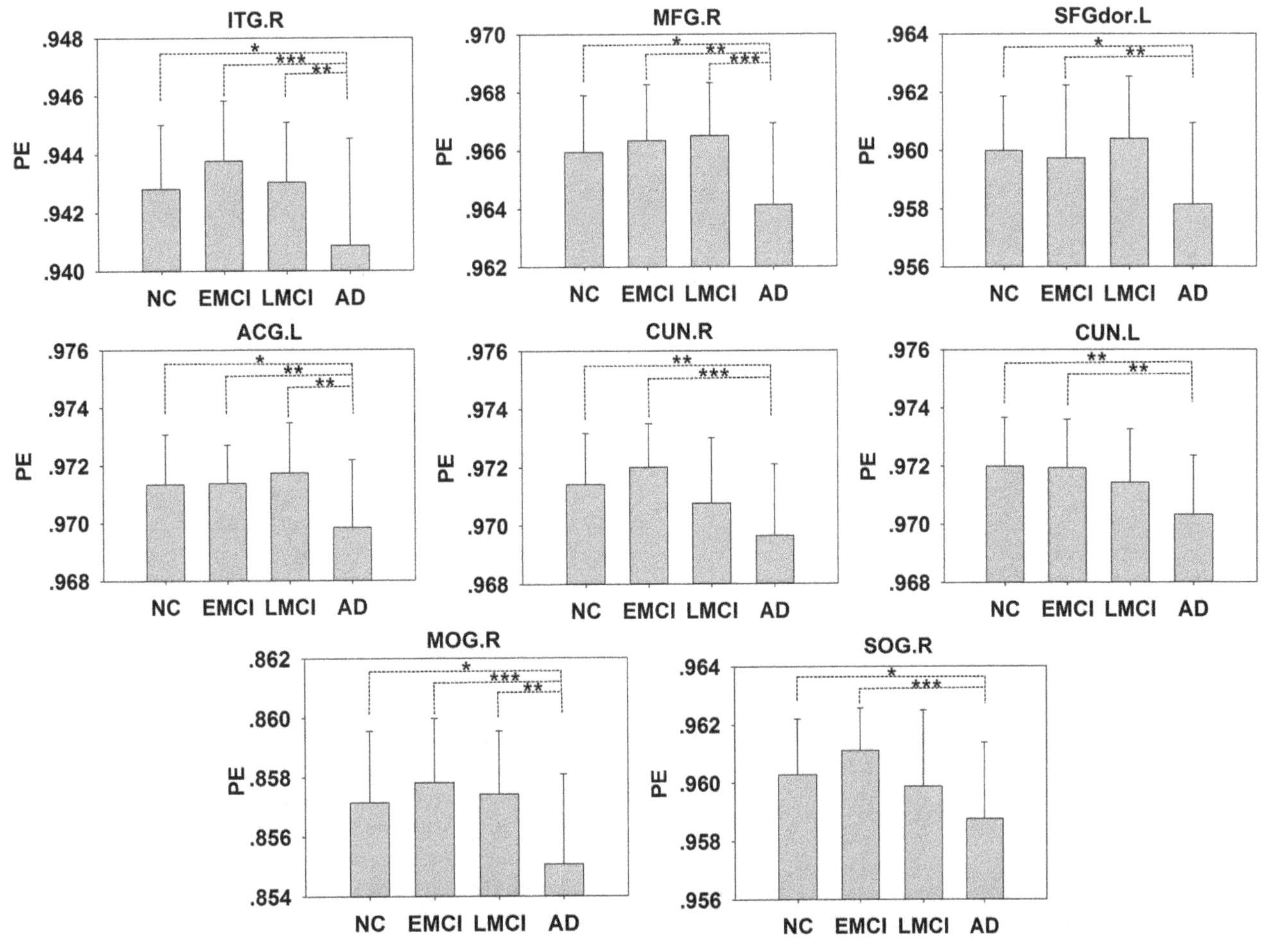

FIGURE 3 | The PE values of the NC, EMCI, LMCI, and AD subjects. Significant differences between pairs of groups after Bonferroni correction ($P < 0.05$) are indicated. *$P < 0.05$, **$P < 0.01$, ***$P < 0.001$. The error bars indicate the *SDs*.

gray matter volumes in the patient groups. The results were presented in **Table 4**. The SOG.R exhibited a positive correlation ($r = 0.200$, $P = 0.053$) between the PE and the gray matter volume in the patient groups. Correlation analyses in the four groups (NC+EMCI+LMCI+AD) were also performed between the PE and gray matter volume, and the SOG.R exhibited a significant positive correlation ($r = 0.210$, $P = 0.010$) between the PE and the gray matter volume (Table S2). And the right middle frontal gyrus exhibited a positive correlation ($r = 0.270$, $P = 0.008$) between the PE and the gray matter volume after removing the effect of nuisance covariates (Presentation 1 in Supplementary Material).

Finally, the FDG-PET data of the eight ROIs from the same group of subjects were extracted. Pearson's correlation analyses of the PE and FDG-PET data were performed in the pooled groups (EMCI+LMCI+AD). Two significant correlations were detected (**Table 4**). The MOG.R ($r = 0.419$, $P < 0.001$) and ITG.R ($r = 0.273$, $P = 0.019$) exhibited significant positive correlations between the PE and FDG-PET data. The correlation analyses in the four groups (NC+EMCI+LMCI+AD) produced consistent results (Table S2).

DISCUSSION

This study reported the global and regional differences in PE between patients and controls. The significant differences were mainly distributed in the occipital, frontal, and temporal lobes. In the ROI analysis, the AD patients exhibited significantly lower values (lower complexities) than the healthy controls and MCI groups. To identify the continuous distribution of the AD symptoms, we conducted correlation analyses of the PE values and the clinical MMSE, FAQ and CDR scores, all of which revealed an increasing symptom load with decreasing brain activity complexity. We also extracted the regional homogeneities (ReHos) of eight ROIs and performed correlation analyses between the PEs and ReHos, and significant correlations were observed. Additionally, we extracted the FDG-PET data from eight ROIs and performed correlation analyses between the PE and the FDG-PET data. Significant positive correlations between the PE and FDG-PET data were observed in the ITG.R and MOG.R in the patient groups. A positive correlation was found between the PE and the gray matter volume in the patient groups. To summarize, we found significantly decreased complexity in

TABLE 3 | Results of the correlation analyses between the PE maps and the MMSE, FAQ, and CDR scores in the patient groups (EMCI+LMCI+AD).

Brain region Abbr.	MMSE (r, P)	FAQ (r, P)	CDR(r, P)
ITG.R	0.312, 0.003**	−0.223, 0.036*	−0.259, 0.014*
MFG.L	0.429, <0.001***	−0.290, 0.006**	−0.345, 0.001***
SFGdor.L	0.294, 0.005**	−0.337, 0.001***	−0.365, <0.001***
ACG.L	0.317, 0.002**	−0.216, 0.042*	−0.355, 0.001***
CUN.R	0.349, 0.001***	−0.213, 0.045*	−0.144, 0.177
CUN.L	0.212, 0.046*	−0.125, 0.243	−0.120, 0.262
MOG.R	0.414, <0.001***	−0.326, 0.002**	−0.339, 0.001**
SOG.R	0.349, 0.001***	−0.288, 0.006**	−0.211, 0.047*
GM	0.227, 0.032*	−0.139, 0.193	−0.159, 0.137
WM	0.210, 0.049*	−0.112, 0.298	−0.111, 0.302

*In the table, r is the Pearson correlation coefficient, and P indicates the level of statistical significance. *P < 0.05, **P < 0.01, ***P < 0.001. GM, Gray Matter; WM, White Matter.*

TABLE 4 | Results of the correlation analyses between the PE maps and the ReHo, gray matter volume, and FDG-PET values in the patient groups (EMCI+LMCI+AD).

Brain region Abbr.	ReHo (r, P)	GMV (r, P)	FDG-PET (r, P)
ITG.R	−0.414, <0.001***	−0.020, 0.845	0.273, 0.019*
MFG.L	−0.369, <0.001***	0.081, 0.440	0.027, 0.819
SFGdor.L	−0.179, 0.084	0.074, 0.480	0.043, 0.716
ACG.L	−0.012, 0.909	0.089, 0.391	0.096, 0.417
CUN.R	−0.032, 0.757	0.046, 0.661	0.009, 0.939
CUN.L	−0.020, 0.847	−0.141, 0.175	0.113, 0.341
MOG.R	−0.195, 0.049*	0.040, 0.705	0.419, <0.001***
SOG.R	−0.068, 0.515	0.200, 0.053*	0.118, 0.320
GM	−0.347, 0.001***	0.039, 0.736	0.092, 0.438
WM	−0.537, <0.001***	–	0.078, 0.509

*In the table, r is the Pearson correlation coefficient, and P indicates the level of statistical significance. *P < 0.05, ***P < 0.001. GMV, Gray Matter Volume; GM, Gray Matter; WM, White Matter.*

the AD patients, and the results were related to the results of the ReHo analysis.

Applications of PE for Analyzing the Complexity of Neural Signals in the Brain

The PE method measures the irregularity of non-stationary time series, and there have been a number of practical applications of complexity measures using EEG data (Li et al., 2007, 2014; Bruzzo et al., 2008). A study demonstrated that the PE can track the dynamical changes of EEG data (Li et al., 2007). Li et al. utilized PE to predict the changes in EEG signals during absence seizures and provided evidence that the three different seizure phases in absence epilepsy can be effectively distinguished (Li et al., 2014). Mammone et al. evaluated PE data extracted from different electrodes in patients with typical absences and healthy subjects (Mammone et al., 2012). Another study used PE as a feature for effectively discriminating between normal aging, MCI, and AD participants (McBride et al., 2014a). In this study, using the PE method, we found decreased complexity in the MCI and AD patients. These findings demonstrated that PE can measure the complexity of neural signals in the brain and disclose abnormalities of the brain in disease states.

In addition to PE, other entropy methods have been used to explore the complexity of fMRI signals. For example, Liu et al. explored the complexity of normal aging using approximate entropy and found that gray and white matter decreased in complexity with normal aging (Liu et al., 2013). Sokunbi MO and co-workers applied approximate entropy, sample entropy, and fuzzy entropy to complexity analyses of the fMRI data in diseases (i.e., schizophrenia and ADHD) and found alterations in complexity compared with normal people (Sokunbi et al., 2013, 2014). We found significantly decreased complexity in MCI and AD patients using the PE analysis that revealed increasing symptom load with decreasing complexity of the brain. We also applied these entropy methods to ADNI datasets, but the differences among the four groups were not significant (results not shown). Compared with other entropy methods, we thought the PE method had the advantages of placing a continuous time series into a symbolic sequence, entailing a faster calculation speed and being more accurate for complexity estimations (Unakafova et al., 2013). Therefore, PE seems to be a useful tool for identifying abnormalities in brain function.

Decreased Complexity in AD

From our results, decreases in complexity were associated with AD. We found decreased complexity in the mean whole-brain PEs of the gray matter and white matter in AD compared with EMCI (**Figure 1**). One study of the complexity of rs-fMRI data found cognitive impairment was associated with decreases in the gray matter of a familial AD group (Liu et al., 2013). At the regional level, five clusters were found to exhibit significantly decreased complexity in the AD group compared with the MCI and NC groups, and these clusters were mainly distributed in the occipital, frontal, and temporal lobes. Compared with the NCs, decreased complexity was also found in the CUN.L in the MCI group ($P = 0.08$). These regions are mainly involved in short-term memory processing, visual recognition memory, rational thought processes and higher-level functions, basic visual processing, and motion perception (Goldman, 2013; de Schotten et al., 2014). The complexities of these brain regions in the patient groups decreased, and the brain function may also have been damaged. Liu et al. reported decreased complexities in some brain regions (i.e., the STG, ACG, CUN) in a complexity study of rs-fMRI signals in familial AD (Liu et al., 2013). Studies of EEG signals in AD and MCI patients also have reported results similar to ours. For example, Labate et al. (2012). measured dynamic EEG signal complexity in AD subjects using PE and found that the severity of disease was reflected in the dynamic complexity, and complexity reductions were present in the frontal and occipital areas (Labate et al., 2012). Timothy et al. found that in the frontal and temporal regions, the PEs of EEG recordings in an MCI group were significantly lower than those of controls (Timothy et al., 2014). The MMSE score has been demonstrated to be effective for the cognitive screening of the elderly and might help differentiate between AD and MCI, and the FAQ and CDR are frequently used indices of cognitive decline. **Table 3** presents the positive correlations between of the PE with the MMSE in patients and the negative correlations of the PE with the FAQ and CDR. These findings indicated that lower MMSE and higher FAQ and CDR scores were observed in MCI and AD patient groups who exhibited lower complexity and cognitive decline.

These findings were supported by the decrease-in-complexity hypothesis of Lipsitz and Goldberger, which suggested that physiological diseases were associated with a generalized loss of complexity in the dynamics of healthy systems and hypothesizes that such a loss of complexity led to an impaired ability to adapt to physiological stress, that in turn results in functional loss and deficits (Lipsitz, 1992, 2004). These results indicated that AD patients demonstrated decreased complex behavioral output and suggested that AD patients had decreased brain complexity, resulting in cognitive decline.

Potential Explanations for the Decreased Complexity in AD

AD is characterized by the presence of neuritic plaques and neurofibrillary tangles and is accompanied by the loss of cortical neurons and synapses. These changes lead to cognitive and behavioral disturbances. Brain atrophy and the loss of cells are major changes in the AD brain. We examined the relationships between PE and the gray matter volume and glucose metabolism in patient groups. We found that the SOG exhibited a positive correlation between the PE and the gray matter volume, and two ROIs (i.e., the ITG and MOG) exhibited significant positive correlations between glucose metabolism and complexity. The SOG has been indicated in the gray matter atrophy in AD (Guo et al., 2010; Ouyang et al., 2015). Many studies have also found low cerebral glucose metabolism in some brain regions (i.e., the ITG and MOG) in AD and MCI (Castellano et al., 2015; Firbank et al., 2016). Because the related areas we found were few and not particularly significant, gray matter atrophy and decreased glucose metabolism may be indirect evidence for decreased complexity in AD.

A reliable explanation has been found for the decreased complexity of fMRI signals in AD. High regional functional homogeneity led to lower complexity. Functional homogeneity was measured by ReHo, which calculates the coherence of the BOLD signal in a given voxel with those of its nearest neighbors. In this study, we found significant negative correlations in the gray matter, white matter and some brain regions (i.e., the ITG, MFG, and MOG) between the PE and ReHo in the patient groups. He et al. investigated the pattern of regional coherence in AD patients using the ReHo index and found that the ReHo indices increased in the occipital (MOG and SOG) and temporal lobes (ITG), and significant negative correlations with the MMSE scores were presented in the MFG and CUN (He et al., 2007). These findings reflected the high homogeneity and low complexity in some brain areas in MCI and AD patients and may be helpful in the development of disease diagnoses.

Limitations

There were several limitations to our research. A limitation of this study was that the nuisance covariates had influence on PE of fMRI signals. We found that differences between groups became smaller, after removing the effect of nuisance covariates. However, similar to the main result, significantly decreased complexities were found in frontal lobe in the AD group compared with the MCI groups and the NC group with weak statistical threshold ($P < 0.01$, uncorrected). According to these results, we speculated that the PE of fMRI signals might reflect the changes in complexity of brain activity and a fraction of nuisance signals. In addition, we also found the significant correlations between the PE and clinical measurements ReHo, gray matter volume, showing that the PE could reflect the abnormal brain activity of AD to a certain extent. The weak statistical threshold may be associated with the small sample size and unfavorable results after removing the nuisance signal. In the future research, we will take full account of the nuisance signals and improving the PE algorithm to measure the alterations in the complexity of brain activity more effectively.

Moreover, a limitation of the study was about the detailed information of subjects. Recent studies have demonstrated that age, sex, years of education, lifestyle, cardiovascular diseases, and risk factors (e.g., smoking and hypertension) were associated with cognitive decline and AD (Santos et al., 2014; Wirth et al., 2014). In this study, the data selected from the ADNI database, which did not publicly provide data about the risk factors related to AD. Another limitation was the number of time points of the fMRI data. According the PE algorithm, larger values of the embedding dimension contain more states of the reconstructed sequence. In this study, we chose $m = 4$, and there were 24 states. One hundred thirty time points might be inadequate for evaluating the abnormal complexity of fMRI signals in AD.

CONCLUSIONS

Our analysis represents a novel implementation of temporal signal entropy (PE) to investigate the changes in the complexity of 4D fMRI brain signals in MCI and AD patients compared with healthy controls. We found decreased complexity in the AD group and found that the decreased complexity was significantly correlated with clinical measurements (i.e., the FAQ, MMSE, and CDR) in the patient groups. Furthermore, we also found a significant correlation between the PE and ReHo in the patient groups. These findings suggest that the complexity analysis of fMRI data using PE can provide important information about the fMRI characteristics of cognitively impaired conditions that can lead to AD. We suggest that PE is a useful and easily obtainable measure for identifying changes in AD brain dynamics. Future efforts will focus on increasing the fMRI database and applying the PE approach to other neurodegenerative diseases.

AUTHOR CONTRIBUTIONS

BW and YN are co-first authors and completed the entire study of the experiment and writing. LM, RC, PY, HG, DL, and YG revised the manuscript. TY, JW, and HZ provided advice and guidance. JX provided the research ideas.

ACKNOWLEDGMENTS

This project was supported by the National Natural Science Foundation of China (61503272, 61305142, 61373101, and 81471752), the Natural Science Foundation of Shanxi (2015021090), a project funded by the China Postdoctoral Science Foundation (2016M601287), the Shanxi Provincial Foundation for Returned Scholars, China (2016-037); Beijing Municipal Science & Technology Commission (Z161100002616020) and the Scientific Research Foundation for Returned Overseas Chinese Scholars.

Data collection and sharing for this project was funded by the Alzheimer's Disease Neuroimaging Initiative (ADNI) (National Institutes of Health Grant U01 AG024904) and DOD ADNI (Department of Defense award number W81XWH-12-2-0012). ADNI is funded by the National Institute on Aging and the National Institute of Biomedical Imaging and Bioengineering and through generous contributions from the following: AbbVie, Alzheimer's Association; Alzheimer's Drug Discovery Foundation; Araclon Biotech; BioClinica, Inc.; Biogen; Bristol-Myers Squibb Company; CereSpir, Inc.; Cogstate; Eisai Inc.; Elan Pharmaceuticals, Inc.; Eli Lilly and Company; EuroImmun; F. Hoffmann-La Roche Ltd and its affiliated company Genentech, Inc.; Fujirebio; GE Healthcare; IXICO Ltd.; Janssen Alzheimer Immunotherapy Research & Development, LLC.; Johnson & Johnson Pharmaceutical Research & Development LLC.; Lumosity; Lundbeck; Merck & Co., Inc.; Meso Scale Diagnostics, LLC.; NeuroRx Research; Neurotrack Technologies; Novartis Pharmaceuticals Corporation; Pfizer Inc.; Piramal Imaging; Servier; Takeda Pharmaceutical Company; and Transition Therapeutics. The Canadian Institutes of Health Research provides funds to support ADNI clinical sites in Canada. Private sector contributions are facilitated by the Foundation for the National Institutes of Health (www.fnih.org). The grantee organization is the Northern California Institute for Research and Education, and the study is coordinated by the Alzheimer's Therapeutic Research Institute at the University of Southern California. ADNI data are disseminated by the Laboratory for Neuro Imaging at the University of Southern California.

SUPPLEMENTARY MATERIAL

REFERENCES

Bandt, C., and Pompe, B. (2002). Permutation entropy: a natural complexity measure for time series. *Phys. Rev. Lett.* 88:174102. doi: 10.1103/PhysRevLett.88.174102

Broock, W. A., Scheinkman, J. A., Dechert, W. D., and LeBaron, B. (1996). A test for independence based on the correlation dimension. *Econ. Rev.* 15, 197–235. doi: 10.1080/07474939608800353

Brookmeyer, R., Johnson, E., Ziegler-Graham, K., and Arrighi, H. M. (2007). Forecasting the global burden of Alzheimer's disease. *Alzheimers Dement.* 3, 186–191. doi: 10.1016/j.jalz.2007.04.381

Bruzzo, A. A., Gesierich, B., Santi, M., Tassinari, C. A., Birbaumer, N., and Rubboli, G. (2008). Permutation entropy to detect vigilance changes and preictal states from scalp EEG in epileptic patients. A preliminary study. *Neurol. Sci.* 29, 3–9. doi: 10.1007/s10072-008-0851-3

Castellano, C.-A., Nugent, S., Paquet, N., Tremblay, S., Bocti, C., Lacombe, G., et al. (2015). Lower brain 18F-fluorodeoxyglucose uptake but normal 11C-acetoacetate metabolism in mild Alzheimer's disease dementia. *J. Alzheimers Dis.* 43, 1343–1353. doi: 10.3233/JAD-141074

Chao-Gan, Y., and Yu-Feng, Z. (2010). DPARSF: a MATLAB toolbox for "pipeline" data analysis of resting-state fMRI. *Front. Syst. Neurosci.* 4:13. doi: 10.3389/fnsys.2010.00013

Cho, H., Jeon, S., Kang, S. J., Lee, J.-M., Lee, J.-H., Kim, G. H., et al. (2013). Longitudinal changes of cortical thickness in early- versus late-onset Alzheimer's disease. *Neurobiol. Aging* 34, 1921.e1929–e1915. doi: 10.1016/j.neurobiolaging.2013.01.004

de Schotten, M. T., Urbanski, M., Valabregue, R., Bayle, D. J., and Volle, E. (2014). Subdivision of the occipital lobes: an anatomical and functional MRI connectivity study. *Cortex* 56, 121–137. doi: 10.1016/j.cortex.2012.12.007

Eckmann, J. P., and Ruelle, D. (1992). Fundamental limitations for estimating dimensions and Lyapunov exponents in dynamical systems. *Phys. D Nonlinear Phenomena* 56, 185–187. doi: 10.1016/0167-2789(92)90023-G

Ferlazzo, E., Mammone, N., Cianci, V., Gasparini, S., Gambardella, A., Labate, A., et al. (2014). Permutation entropy of scalp EEG: a tool to investigate epilepsies: suggestions from absence epilepsies. *Clin. Neurophysiol.* 125, 13–20. doi: 10.1016/j.clinph.2013.06.023

Firbank, M., Lloyd, J., Williams, E., Barber, R., Colloby, S., Barnett, N., et al. (2016). An evidence based algorithm for the utility of FDG-PET for diagnosing Alzheimer's disease according to presence of medial temporal lobe atrophy. *Brit. J. Psychiatry* 208, 491–496. doi: 10.1192/bjp.bp.114.160804

Fox, M. D., and Raichle, M. E. (2007). Spontaneous fluctuations in brain activity observed with functional magnetic resonance imaging. *Nat. Rev. Neurosci.* 8, 700–711. doi: 10.1038/nrn2201

Goldman, B. (2013). *Scienxtists Pinpoint Brain's Area for Numeral Recognition.* Stanford, CA: Stanford School of Medicine.

Gomez, C., Abasolo, D., Poza, J., and FernáNdez, A. (2010). MEG analysis in Alzheimer's disease computing approximate entropy for different frequency bands. *Conf. Proc. IEEE Eng. Med. Biol. Soc.* 2010, 2379–2382. doi: 10.1109/IEMBS.2010.5627236

Gómez, C., and Hornero, R. (2009). Entropy and complexity analyses in Alzheimer's disease: an MEG study. *Open Biomed. Eng. J.* 4, 223–235. doi: 10.2174/1874120701004010223

Grassberger, P., and Procaccia, I. (1983). Characterization of strange attractors. *Phys. Rev. Lett. A.* 50, 346–349. doi: 10.1103/PhysRevLett.50.346

Guo, X., Wang, Z., Li, K., Li, Z., Qi, Z., Jin, Z., et al. (2010). Voxel-based assessment of gray and white matter volumes in Alzheimer's disease. *Neurosci. Lett.* 468, 146–150. doi: 10.1016/j.neulet.2009.10.086

Gusnard, D. A., and Raichle, M. E. (2001). Searching for a baseline: functional imaging and the resting human brain. *Nat. Rev. Neurosci.* 2, 685–694. doi: 10.1038/35094500

Haass, C., and Selkoe, D. J. (2007). Soluble protein oligomers in neurodegeneration: lessons from the Alzheimer's amyloid β-peptide. *Nat. Rev. Mol. Cell Biol.* 8, 101–112. doi: 10.1038/nrm2101

He, Y., Wang, L., Zang, Y., Tian, L., Zhang, X., Li, K., et al. (2007). Regional coherence changes in the early stages of Alzheimer's disease: a combined structural and resting-state functional MRI study. *Neuroimage* 35, 488–500. doi: 10.1016/j.neuroimage.2006.11.042

Jack, C. R., Bernstein, M. A., Fox, N. C., Thompson, P., Alexander, G., Harvey, D., et al. (2008). The Alzheimer's disease neuroimaging initiative (ADNI): MRI methods. *J. Magn. Res. Imaging* 27, 685–691. doi: 10.1002/jmri.21049

Labate, D., Palamara, I., Occhiuto, G., Morabito, G., La Foresta, F., and Morabito, F. (2012). "Complexity analysis of Alzheimer disease EEG data through multiscale permutation entropy," in *Proceedings of the 7th International Workshop on Biosignal Interpretation (BSI2012)* (Como).

Lebedeva, A. K., Westman, E., Borza, T., Beyer, M. K., Engedal, K., Aarsland, D., et al. (2017). MRI-based classification models in prediction of mild cognitive impairment and dementia in late-life depression. *Front. Aging Neurosci.* 9:13. doi: 10.3389/fnagi.2017.00013

Li, H., Jia, X., Qi, Z., Fan, X., Ma, T., Ni, H., et al. (2017). Altered Functional connectivity of the basal nucleus of meynert in mild cognitive impairment: a resting-state fMRI study. *Front. Aging Neurosci.* 9:127. doi: 10.3389/fnagi.2017.00127

Li, J., Yan, J., Liu, X., and Ouyang, G. (2014). Using permutation entropy to measure the changes in EEG signals during absence seizures. *Entropy* 16, 3049–3061. doi: 10.3390/e16063049

Li, X., Ouyang, G., and Richards, D. A. (2007). Predictability analysis of absence seizures with permutation entropy. *Epilepsy Res.* 77, 70–74. doi: 10.1016/j.eplepsyres.2007.08.002

Lipsitz, L. A. (1992). A loss of complexity and aging. Potential application of fractal and chaos theory to senescence. *JAMA* 267, 1806–1809. doi: 10.1001/jama.1992.03480130122036

Lipsitz, L. A. (2004). Physiological complexity, aging, and the path to frailty. *Sci. Aging Knowl. Environ.* 2004:pe16. doi: 10.1126/sageke.2004.16.pe16

Liu, C. Y., Krishnan, A. P., Yan, L., Smith, R. X., Kilroy, E., Alger, J. R., et al. (2013). Complexity and synchronicity of resting state blood oxygenation level-dependent (BOLD) functional MRI in normal aging and cognitive decline. *J. Magn. Reson. Imaging* 38, 36–45. doi: 10.1002/jmri.23961

Mammone, N., Labate, D., Lay-Ekuakille, A., and Morabito, F. C. (2012). Analysis of absence seizure generation using EEG spatial-temporal regularity measures. *Int. J. Neural Syst.* 22:1250024. doi: 10.1142/S0129065712500244

Mateos, D., Diaz, J. M., and Lamberti, P. W. (2014). Permutation entropy applied to the characterization of the clinical evolution of epileptic patients under pharmacologicaltreatment. *Entropy* 16, 5668–5676. doi: 10.3390/e16115668

McBride, J., Zhao, X., Munro, N., Jicha, G., Smith, C., and Jiang, Y. (2014a). "EEG multiscale entropy dynamics in mild cognitive impairment and early Alzheimer's disease," in *Proceedings of the Biomedical Science and Engineering Center Conference (BSEC), 2014 Annual Oak Ridge National Laboratory* (Oak Ridge, TN: IEEE), 1–4.

McBride, J., Zhao, X., Munro, N., Smith, C., Jicha, G., Hively, L., et al. (2014b). Spectral and complexity analysis of scalp eeg characteristics for mild cognitive impairment and early Alzheimer's disease. *Comput. Methods Progr. Biomed* 114, 153–163. doi: 10.1016/j.cmpb.2014.01.019

Möller, C., Vrenken, H., Jiskoot, L., Versteeg, A., Barkhof, F., Scheltens, P., et al. (2013). Different patterns of gray matter atrophy in early- and late-onset Alzheimer's disease. *Neurobiol. Aging* 34, 2014–2022. doi: 10.1016/j.neurobiolaging.2013.02.013

Morabito, F. C., Labate, D., La Foresta, F., Bramanti, A., Morabito, G., and Palamara, I. (2012). Multivariate multi-scale permutation entropy for complexity analysis of Alzheimer's disease, EEG. *Entropy* 14, 1186–1202. doi: 10.3390/e14071186

Ouyang, X., Chen, K., Yao, L., Hu, B., Wu, X., Ye, Q., et al. (2015). Simultaneous changes in gray matter volume and white matter fractional anisotropy in Alzheimer's disease revealed by multimodal CCA and joint ICA. *Neuroscience* 301, 553–562. doi: 10.1016/j.neuroscience.2015.06.031

Petersen, R. C., and Negash, S. (2008). Mild cognitive impairment: an overview. *CNS Spectr.* 13, 45–53. doi: 10.1017/S1092852900016151

Pincus, S. M. (1991). Approximate entropy as a measure of system complexity. *Proc. Natl. Acad. Sci. U.S.A.* 88, 2297–2301. doi: 10.1073/pnas.88.6.2297

Richman, J. S., and Moorman, J. R. (2000). Physiological time-series analysis using approximate entropy and sample entropy. *Am. J. Heart Circ. Physiol.* 278, H2039–H2049.

Santos, N. C., Costa, P. S., Cunha, P., Portugal-Nunes, C., Amorim, L., Cotter, J., et al. (2014). Clinical, physical and lifestyle variables and relationship with cognition and mood in aging: a cross-sectional analysis of distinct educational groups. *Fron. Aging Neurosci.* 6:21. doi: 10.3389/fnagi.2014.00021

Sokunbi, M. O., Cameron, G. G., Ahearn, T. S., Murray, A. D., and Staff, R. T. (2015). Fuzzy approximate entropy analysis of resting state fMRI signal complexity across the adult life span. *Med. Eng. Phys.* 37, 1082–1090. doi: 10.1016/j.medengphy.2015.09.001

Sokunbi, M. O., Fung, W., Sawlani, V., Choppin, S., Linden, D. E., and Thome, J. (2013). Resting state fMRI entropy probes complexity of brain activity in adults with ADHD. *Psychiatry Res. Neuroimaging* 214, 341–348. doi: 10.1016/j.pscychresns.2013.10.001

Sokunbi, M. O., Gradin, V. B., Waiter, G. D., Cameron, G. G., Ahearn, T. S., Murray, A. D., et al. (2014). Nonlinear complexity analysis of brain fMRI signals in schizophrenia. *PLoS ONE* 9:e95146. doi: 10.1371/journal.pone.0095146

Song, X. W., Dong, Z. Y., Long, X. Y., Li, S. F., Zuo, X. N., Zhu, C. Z., et al. (2011). REST: a toolkit for resting-state functional magnetic resonance imaging data processing. *PLoS ONE* 6:e25031. doi: 10.1371/journal.pone.0025031

Timothy, L. T., Krishna, B. M., Menon, M. K., and Nair, U. (2014). *Permutation Entropy Analysis of EEG of Mild Cognitive Impairment Patients During Memory Activation Task.* Berlin: Springer International Publishing.

Unakafova, V. A., Unakafov, A. M., and Keller, K. (2013). An approach to comparing Kolmogorov-Sinai and permutation entropy. *Eur. Phys. J. Spec. Top.* 222, 353–361. doi: 10.1140/epjst/e2013-01846-7

Wang, Z., Li, Y., Childress, A. R., and Detre, J. A. (2014). Brain entropy mapping using fMRI. *PLoS ONE* 9:e89948. doi: 10.1371/journal.pone.0089948

Wirth, M., Haase, C. M., Villeneuve, S., Vogel, J., and Jagust, W. J. (2014). Neuroprotective pathways: lifestyle activity, brain pathology, and cognition in cognitively normal older adults. *Neurobiol. Aging* 35, 1873–1882. doi: 10.1016/j.neurobiolaging.2014.02.015

Wolf, A., Swift, J. B., Swinney, H. L., and Vastano, J. A. (1985). Determining Lyapunov exponents from a time series. *Phys. D* 16, 285–317. doi: 10.1016/0167-2789(85)90011-9

Zang, Y., Jiang, T., Lu, Y., He, Y., and Tian, L. (2004). Regional homogeneity approach to fMRI data analysis. *Neuroimage* 22, 394–400. doi: 10.1016/j.neuroimage.2003.12.030

Zanin, M., Zunino, L., Rosso, O. A., and Papo, D. (2012). Permutation entropy and its main biomedical and econophysics applications: a review. *Entropy* 14, 1553–1577. doi: 10.3390/e14081553

6

Reduced Dynamic Coupling Between Spontaneous BOLD-CBF Fluctuations in Older Adults: A Dual-Echo pCASL Study

Piero Chiacchiaretta [1,2]*, *Francesco Cerritelli* [1,2,3], *Giovanna Bubbico* [1,2], *Mauro Gianni Perrucci* [1,2] and *Antonio Ferretti* [1,2]

[1] Department of Neuroscience, Imaging and Clinical Sciences, Università degli Studi G. d'Annunzio Chieti e Pescara, Chieti, Italy, [2] Institute for Advanced Biomedical Technologies (ITAB), Università degli Studi G. d'Annunzio Chieti e Pescara, Chieti, Italy, [3] Clinical-Based Human Research Department—C.O.M.E. Collaboration ONLUS, Pescara, Italy

***Correspondence:**
Piero Chiacchiaretta
p.chiacchiaretta@unich.it

Measurement of the dynamic coupling between spontaneous Blood Oxygenation Level Dependent (BOLD) and cerebral blood flow (CBF) fluctuations has been recently proposed as a method to probe resting-state brain physiology. Here we investigated how the dynamic BOLD-CBF coupling during resting-state is affected by aging. Fifteen young subjects and 17 healthy elderlies were studied using a dual-echo pCASL sequence. We found that the dynamic BOLD-CBF coupling was markedly reduced in elderlies, in particular in the left supramarginal gyrus, an area known to be involved in verbal working memory and episodic memory. Moreover, correcting for temporal shift between BOLD and CBF timecourses resulted in an increased correlation of the two signals for both groups, but with a larger increase for elderlies. However, even after temporal shift correction, a significantly decreased correlation was still observed for elderlies in the left supramarginal gyrus, indicating that the age-related dynamic BOLD-CBF uncoupling in this region is more pronounced and can be only partially explained with a simple time-shift between the two signals. Interestingly, these results were observed in a group of elderlies with normal cognitive functions, suggesting that the study of dynamic BOLD-CBF coupling during resting-state is a promising technique, potentially able to provide early biomarkers of functional changes in the aging brain.

Keywords: aging, arterial spin labeling, BOLD-CBF coupling, fMRI, resting-state

INTRODUCTION

Since the first observation that spontaneous Blood Oxygenation Level Dependent (BOLD) signal fluctuations in the left and right motor cortex are correlated in the absence of a task (Biswal et al., 1995), resting-state fMRI has witnessed an exponential growth of interest.

Since it does not require any task, resting-state fMRI is particularly attractive for studies on patients, children and elderlies, reducing problems related to participant's compliance or intersubject variability due to task performance. Indeed, there is an increasing number of investigations using resting-state fMRI as a sensitive biomarker to study normal and pathological aging (D'Esposito et al., 1999; Fox and Greicius, 2010; Brier et al., 2014; Gardini et al., 2014; Li et al., 2015; Vecchio et al., 2015; Esposito et al., 2018).

Most fMRI studies are based on the BOLD technique (Bandettini et al., 1992; Kwong et al., 1992; Ogawa et al., 1992) which offers a large sensitivity and easy of implementation. However, due to the complex nature of the BOLD effect, the quantitative interpretation of this fMRI signal can be problematic. Indeed, the BOLD signal change is modulated by local variations in deoxyhemoglobin content stemming from changes in cerebral blood flow (CBF), cerebral blood volume (CBV) and cerebral metabolic rate of oxygen consumption ($CMRO_2$) induced by neuronal activation or vascular challenges (Buxton, 2012). Depending on the complex interplay of these variables, the magnitude and dynamics of the BOLD signal change may not always reflect the underlying change in neuronal activity or the variation of a specific hemodynamic/metabolic quantity (Ances et al., 2008; Buxton, 2010; Griffeth and Buxton, 2011; Moradi et al., 2012). This limitation is especially important in studies comparing populations with different neurovascular properties (Liu, 2013). In particular, this issue has been largely recognized when comparing elderly vs. young adults since significant vascular changes are known to occur during adult life (O'Rourke and Hashimoto, 2007; Samanez-Larkin and D'Esposito, 2008; Chen et al., 2011; Lu et al., 2011; Gauthier and Hoge, 2013; De Vis et al., 2015).

To overcome the problem of BOLD signal ambiguity, the acquisition of concurrent BOLD and CBF data from arterial spin labeling (ASL) sequences has been proposed in an early biophysical model that allows the calculation of fractional changes of the different hemodynamic and metabolic variables involved in brain activation (Davis et al., 1998). ASL uses magnetically labeled arterial blood water as an endogenous tracer (Detre et al., 1992) and can quantify both baseline levels and activity induced variation of regional CBF. The Davis model is currently applied with different strategies, usually requiring additional calibration measurements based on gas challenges (Davis et al., 1998; Hoge et al., 1999; Chiarelli et al., 2007) and has been expanded to allow the measurement of absolute $CMRO_2$ changes or baseline levels of oxygen consumption (Bulte et al., 2012; Gauthier et al., 2012; Wise et al., 2013; Germuska and Bulte, 2014; Germuska et al., 2016). Although gas challenges might be less tolerated by patients or elderlies, applications of these techniques to aging studies have been recently reported (Mohtasib et al., 2012; Hutchison et al., 2013; Liu et al., 2013; De Vis et al., 2015; Garrett et al., 2017). Alternative calibration techniques without gas administration have also been proposed based on particular MRI acquisition sequences or breath-hold tasks (Kastrup et al., 1999; Fujita et al., 2006; Bulte et al., 2009; Blockley et al., 2012, 2015). Nevertheless, the calibrated BOLD technique has been mostly applied and validated in studies using block paradigms, and its extension to more dynamic experimental designs is not straightforward (Kida et al., 2006; Simon and Buxton, 2015).

In this regard, however, the combined acquisition of BOLD and CBF data using ASL has recently attracted increasing interest to study brain function, even without calibration measurements (Chen et al., 2015; Simon and Buxton, 2015; Storti et al., 2017).

Indeed, although CBF is still an indirect measurement of cerebral metabolism and neuronal activity, it constitutes a well defined and fundamental physiological process that is altered in different pathologies and with physiological aging. Furthermore, despite ASL has lower sensitivity compared to BOLD, it can extend the study of resting-state brain function beyond that of functional connectivity, allowing quantitative CBF measurements and the investigation of BOLD-CBF coupling when the two signals are acquired simultaneously. In particular, the possibility to capture spontaneous fluctuations of cerebral blood flow with ASL has recently received an increasing attention (De Luca et al., 2006; Chuang et al., 2008; Fukunaga et al., 2008; Zou et al., 2009; Viviani et al., 2011; Liang et al., 2014; Tak et al., 2014; Chen et al., 2015; Fernández-Seara et al., 2015; Jann et al., 2015).

This is an appealing application of concurrent BOLD and CBF dynamic data acquisition, potentially able to offer insights on mechanisms underlying resting-state brain functioning and physiology. In this regard, recent evidence demonstrated that the resting-state dynamic relationship between BOLD and CBF is approximately linear across the brain (Fukunaga et al., 2008; Wu et al., 2009), with a significantly stronger coupling between spontaneous BOLD and CBF fluctuations within the major nodes of established resting-state networks (Tak et al., 2014; Cohen et al., 2017). Noteworthy, the study of BOLD-CBF dynamic coupling during resting-state could offer innovative metrics to assess brain health (Chen et al., 2015), in addition to the more commonly used functional connectivity metrics. However, to the best of our knowledge, no investigation based on this method has been performed on aging so far.

In the present study we investigated how the dynamic BOLD-CBF coupling during resting-state is affected by aging. Specifically, we compared a group of healthy elderlies with a group of young subjects, addressing between-group differences in: (i) the linear correlation between the two signals; and (ii) the effect on the calculated correlation when introducing a relative temporal shift between BOLD and CBF timecourses.

MATERIALS AND METHODS

Fifteen healthy young adults (Young: mean age = 26.4, SD = 4.2) and 17 healthy elderlies (Elderly: mean age = 63.4, SD = 8.1) were included in the study. All individuals were right-handed, gave their written informed consent according to the Declaration of Helsinki (World Medical Association Declaration of Helsinki, 1997) and all procedures were approved by the Ethics Committee for Biomedical Research of the provinces of Chieti and Pescara and the "G. D'Annunzio" University of Chieti and Pescara. None of the participants reported a history of neurological or psychiatric disease, or used psychopharmacological drugs. Subjects with any drug or alcohol abuse within the previous 6 months were also excluded to avoid confounding effects on the fMRI signal. Other exclusion criteria included implanted metals, pregnancy and abnormal findings in their structural brain MRI. Mild forms of hypertension and hyperlipidemia were accepted. Six older adults used antihypertensive medication.

Elderlies were screened with Mini Mental State Examination (MMSE; Folstein et al., 1975) to evaluate the global cognitive status (reported score range of included subjects: 25.5 ÷ 28.9), Babcock story test to evaluate prose memory (reported score range: 5.2 ÷ 8.8 for immediate recall, 2.5 ÷ 8.6 for delayed recall), and the Frontal Assessment Battery (FAB) to assess global executive functions (reported score range: 14.7 ÷ 18.3). Young group was screened using the Trail Making Test to evaluate sustained visuo-spatial attention (reported score range: 5.5s ÷ 48.8), MMSE (27.7 ÷ 29.3), Babcock story test (7.2 ÷ 8.9 for immediate recall, 5.1 ÷ 8.8 for delayed recall) and FAB (15.1 ÷ 18.9). Statistical between-groups comparisons were performed with parametric or non-parametric tests, depending on normality distribution verified using the Shapiro test. A significant between-group difference was observed for MMSE ($p = 0.03$, Wilcoxon test), whereas Babcock and FAB tests did not reveal significant effects ($p = 0.19$ and $p = 0.43$ respectively, unpaired t-tests).

All participants were required to refrain from caffeine, alcohol and nicotine for at least 6 h before the MRI session.

MRI was performed with a 3T Philips Achieva scanner (Philips Medical Systems, Best, Netherlands), using a whole-body radiofrequency coil for signal excitation and an 8-channel phased-array head coil for signal reception.

Subjects were instructed to keep their eyes closed and not to engage in structured thoughts during acquisition.

Resting-state CBF and BOLD data were simultaneously acquired with a dual-echo pseudo-continuous ASL (pCASL) sequence (Dai et al., 2008) with the following parameters: TR/TE1/TE2: 3500/10/28 ms, FOV 230 mm × 230 mm, matrix 64 × 64, voxel size 3.6 mm × 3.6 mm × 5 mm, SENSE factor 2.3, 19 slices acquired in ascending order, 90 dynamics. The label duration was 1650 ms and the postlabel delay was 1000 ms.

Baseline perfusion was measured using a pCASL sequence optimizing the labeling parameters for a reliable quantification of CBF for both young and elderly subjects (Alsop et al., 2015): TR/TE 4269/10 ms, FOV 230 mm × 230 mm, matrix 64 × 64, voxel size 3.6 mm × 3.6 mm × 5 mm, SENSE factor 2.3, 19 slices acquired in ascending order, 60 dynamics. The label duration was 1750 ms and the postlabel delay was 1900 ms. Background suppression pulses at 2110 ms and 3260 ms after start of labeling were used. The labeling plane of the pCASL sequences was positioned 85 mm below the AC-PC line, according to recent guidelines (Aslan et al., 2010; Alsop et al., 2015). An equilibrium magnetization image (M_0) was also acquired with scan parameters identical to the pCASL sequence (same matrix and readout) but using a long TR (10,000 ms) and without labeling or background suppression pulses.

A high resolution structural volume was finally acquired via a 3D fast field echo T1-weighted sequence with the following parameters: 1 mm isotropic voxel size, TR/TE = 8.1/3.7 ms, flip angle = 8°, 160 sections, SENSE factor = 2.

During fMRI, physiological signals related to respiratory and cardiac cycles were registered using a pneumatic belt strapped around the upper abdomen and a pulse oximeter placed on a finger of the right hand, respectively. Respiratory and cardiac data were both sampled at 100 Hz and stored in a logfile for each run.

Resting state pCASL fMRI data were analyzed using AFNI (Cox et al., 2006[1]) and custom-written software implemented in Python[2]. First, the dual-echo pCASL data were split into four EPI timeseries, corresponding to label and control images for acquisitions at TE1 and TE2.

Then, initial preprocessing was performed for both echoes on the label and control ASL images separately (Restom et al., 2006; Wang et al., 2008) according to the following steps:

(i) RETROICOR was applied to remove signal fluctuations related to cardiac and respiratory cycles (Glover et al., 2000);
(ii) slice-timing correction using sinc interpolation;
(iii) motion correction was performed using rigid body registration to realign all time frames to a base image represented by the first label/control volume (dummy scans prevented the need to discard the first few volumes). A summary statistic of motion was defined as the root mean square (RMS) of the six realignment parameters (three translations and three rotations), in order to inspect for EPI timeseries affected by excessive motion. One elderly subject exceeded an RMS value of 1.5 mm for both label and control images and was discarded from further analysis. Further motion assessment was performed considering the RMS value of the differentiated EPI timeseries (DVARS) within a whole brain spatial mask (Power et al., 2012, 2014). The run-averaged DVARS metrics was then compared across groups using ANOVA in order to characterize potential motion effects not accounted for by spatial registration and regression of motion parameters;
(iv) an additional coregistration was performed to minimize effects of the spatial offset between label and control timeseries caused by possible head motion between the reference control image and the reference label image. The corresponding spatial transformation was determined using the mutual information-based approach (Studholme et al., 1998) which is much less sensitive to the labeling related signal intensity differences that could be interpreted by the standard rigid body motion correction algorithm as apparent head motion between label and control images (Friston et al., 1995; Woods et al., 1998).

After these steps, the coregistration matrix between the structural data set and the preprocessed timeseries was determined using an affine transformation.

Then, additional preprocessing was performed using ANATICOR (Jo et al., 2010). Briefly, we first obtained individual masks of large ventricles and white matter from the structural scans segmentation using FreeSurfer[3]. The white matter mask was slightly eroded (one functional voxel) to prevent partial volume effects that might include signal from gray matter voxels in the mask. This step was not performed for the CSF mask, since with the functional voxel size used in this study the eroded

[1] afni.nimh.nih.gov/afni
[2] http://www.python.org
[3] http://surfer.nmr.mgh.harvard.edu

CSF mask would not contain enough voxels in most subjects. Then, for each run, a global nuisance regressor was obtained extracting the EPI average time course within the ventricle mask and local nuisance regressors were obtained calculating for each gray matter voxel the average signal time course for all white matter voxels within a 3 cm radius (Jo et al., 2010). These nuisance regressors and the six regressors derived from motion parameters were removed from the EPI timeseries using AFNI's @ANATICOR.

At this stage, pCASL time series with interleaved control and label volumes were rebuilt using the preprocessed data. These preprocessed pCASL data were then temporal filtered to separate CBF and BOLD signals (Chuang et al., 2008). Briefly, the ASL time series can be view as the sum of a component with a rapid modulation reflecting the alternating control and label images, and a component that is not modulated by the labeling process, reflecting slower BOLD weighted signal variations. An high-pass filtering with a cut-off frequency corresponding to 1/4TR has been demonstrated to be effective in retaining the modulated component while minimizing the BOLD contamination (Chuang et al., 2008; Tak et al., 2014). Note that this high-pass filtering does not restrict the CBF timeseries to the high frequency band since the CBF signal is derived afterward from the difference between subsequent scans (i.e., control—label). Specifically, CBF timeseries were obtained from TE1 data by high-pass filtering the corresponding preprocessed pCASL signal (>0.071 Hz, corresponding to 1/4TR), multiplying it by $\cos[\pi(n-1)]$ (where n is the frame number), and then summing together every two images. BOLD timeseries were obtained from TE2 data by low-pass filtering (<0.071 Hz) the corresponding preprocessed pCASL signal and then summing together every two images.

After these processing procedures, both BOLD and CBF data were spatially normalized using Advanced Normalization Tools (ANTs; Avants et al., 2009). Briefly, the individual T1-weighted anatomical images of young and elderly subjects were first bias corrected using the N4ITK algorithm (Tustison et al., 2010) and then used to create a study specific template encompassing the age range in our study (Avants et al., 2010). Non-brain removal was also performed using BET (Smith, 2002) and a nonlinear warping of the resulting template to the MNI standard space (3 mm isotropic spatial resolution) was computed using symmetric diffeomorphic image normalization (Avants et al., 2008). Finally, BOLD and CBF data were spatial smoothed (6 mm FWHM) and band-pass filtered (0.01–0.071 Hz).

After these preprocessing procedures, linear correlation (Pearson r) between BOLD and CBF timeseries was calculated for each voxel to obtain individual maps representing the BOLD-CBF coupling during resting-state. In this step no time-shift was introduced between the two timecourses and the resulting correlation coefficients were indicated as r_0. Random effects group maps (one sample t-test) were then obtained after individual r_0 to z-Fisher transform for Young and Elderly separately and then compared between groups (two-sample unpaired t-test). Group maps were thresholded at $p < 0.05$, FDR corrected.

In a second step, the cross-correlation between BOLD and CBF timecourses was calculated again after introducing a variable time-shift τ in the BOLD signal (eq.1), following previous work (Fukunaga et al., 2008; Tak et al., 2014). In this calculation, both BOLD (t) and CBF (t) were first upsampled to a resolution of 100 ms using sync interpolation as implemented in the AFNI program *3Dtshift*. The maximum correlation value (r_{max}) was retained for τ ranging between ±7 s (with a 350 ms step). Then, after transforming individual r_{max} to z-Fisher, the random effects group maps were calculated again for Young and Elderly and compared between groups.

$$r_{\max} = \max_{\tau} \sum_{t} BOLD(t+\tau)CBF(t) \qquad -7s < \tau < 7s \quad (1)$$

Note that previous studies mostly considered the r_{max} approach, in order to maximize the statistical significance of correlation by correcting for potential temporal mismatch between the two hemodynamic signals (Fukunaga et al., 2008; Tak et al., 2014). Here we investigated both r_0 and r_{max} and in particular how the two groups compare with respect to these metrics. Our choice was motivated by the fact that the temporal mismatch between BOLD and CBF might be group dependent (due to e.g., age-related vascular effects). A quantitative estimation of the effect of time-shift correction on the correlation coefficient was performed in selected regions of interest (ROIs) as follows.

We focused on ROIs in the default mode network (DMN) and frontoparietal network (FPN) that are the two most investigated brain networks. In order to allow the definition of ROIs independent from the previous analysis, independent component analysis (ICA) was performed, using a probabilistic algorithm (Beckmann and Smith, 2004) as implemented in the MELODIC tool of FSL (FMRIB Software Library). Briefly, individual functional datasets were first temporally concatenated across subjects, groups (Young and Elderly) and modalities (BOLD and CBF) to form a single 4D data set to be used as input for the probabilistic ICA algorithm. The number of components was fixed to 20. Dual-regression (Beckmann et al., 2009) was then used to identify individual spatial maps for each independent component to be used as input for the second-level group analysis. In this calculation random-effects group statistical maps were obtained for each component using permutation-based non-parametric testing (5000 permutations; Nichols and Holmes, 2002). Multiple comparisons correction was addressed applying a cluster-based threshold of $Z > 2.3$ and a family-wise-error (FWE) corrected cluster significance of $p < 0.01$ for the suprathreshold clusters. Using these group maps, the DMN and FPN were easily identified from their characteristic spatial pattern, including posterior cingulate cortex, bilateral angular gyrus and ventromedial prefrontal cortex for DMN, bilateral inferior parietal lobe and bilateral middle frontal gyrus for FPN. For our ROIs definition we pooled BOLD and CBF data because a high degree of spatial overlap has been shown for the two modalities in both resting state and task paradigms (Mayhew et al., 2014; Jann et al., 2015). Furthermore, in order to consider gray matter voxels only, a binary mask was defined by averaging the normalized individual gray matter masks obtained from the FreeSurfer segmentation and thresholding at 0.3 (Jann et al., 2015). The final masks representing the investigated ROIs were defined multiplying this binary mask with the ICA clusters.

Then, mean r_0 and r_{max} values were extracted from these ROIs and the $r_{max} - r_0$ difference was compared between groups (two-sample unpaired t-test). Correction for multiple comparisons was performed using FDR. We expect this difference to be larger for elderlies due to an increased time-shift between BOLD and CBF timecourses, possibly reflecting age related modifications of vascular response.

In addition, we computed the resting state fluctuation amplitude (RSFA; Kannurpatti and Biswal, 2008) for both BOLD and CBF timeseries in Elderly and Young, using the AFNI program *3dRSFC*. The corresponding values were extracted from our ROIs and compared between groups (two-sample unpaired t-tests with correction for multiple comparisons using FDR). This analysis aimed at evaluating the impact of potential age dependent differences in the amplitude of resting state BOLD and CBF fluctuations on the observed linear correlation between the two signals, since a reduced fluctuation amplitude could lead to a decreased correlation coefficient in presence of noise (Liu, 2013).

Finally, we also extracted regional perfusion values from quantitative CBF maps provided by the background suppressed ASL data and a single compartment model (Buxton et al., 1998; Alsop et al., 2015):

$$CBF = \frac{6000\lambda(SI_c - SI_L)e^{\frac{PLD}{T_{1A}}}}{2\alpha\alpha_{inv}T_{1A}M_0\left(1 - e^{-\frac{\tau}{T_{1A}}}\right)} \quad [\text{ml}/100\,\text{g}/\,\text{min}] \quad (2)$$

Where λ is the blood-brain partition coefficient (0.9 ml/g), SI_C and SI_L are the means over time of the control and label images respectively, PLD is the slice-dependent post label delay (1900–2800 ms), T_{1A} is the longitudinal relaxation time of arterial blood (1650 ms at 3T), α is the labeling efficiency (0.85; Alsop et al., 2015), α_{inv} is a correction factor for the background suppression (0.83; van Osch et al., 2009), M_0 is the equilibrium magnetization signal, and τ is the label duration (1750 ms).

RESULTS

Random effects group maps obtained using the z-Fisher transformed voxelwise correlation (r_0, see "Materials and Methods" section) between BOLD and CBF timeseries during resting state are shown in **Figure 1A** for the two groups. In

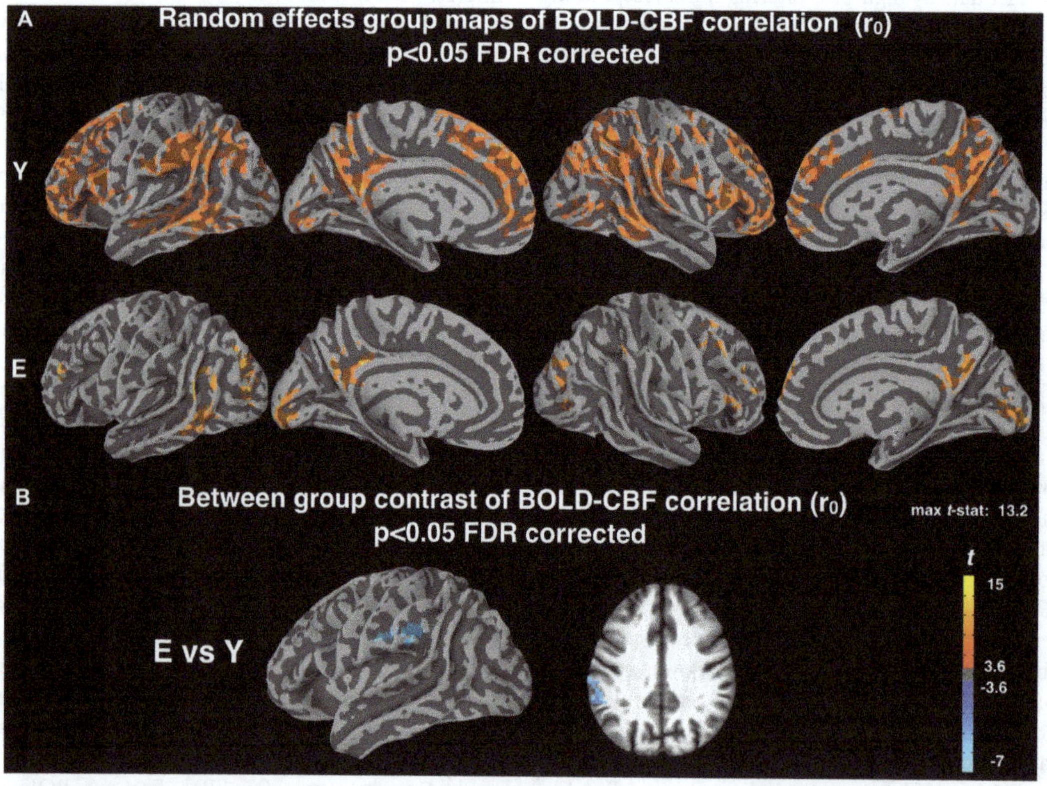

FIGURE 1 | (A) Random effect group maps showing the dynamic coupling between spontaneous blood oxygenation level dependent (BOLD) and cerebral blood flow (CBF) fluctuations for Young (Y) and Elderly (E) groups when potential time shifts between the two signals were not compensated for (r_0, see "Materials and Methods" section). **(B)** Between-group contrast comparing the dynamic coupling between spontaneous BOLD and CBF fluctuations for Y and E, using r_0 values. A significant age related decrease of BOLD-CBF coupling is observed in the left supramarginal gyrus (MNI coordinates: −59, −34, 33). The statistical maps were thresholded at $p < 0.05$ (corrected for multiple comparisons using FDR) and superimposed on the partially inflated study specific template.

young subjects, a significant correlation between spontaneous fluctuations of BOLD and CBF signals was observed in most cortical areas, whereas in elderly subjects this correlation was markedly reduced (mean r_0 values in significant areas were 0.24 ± 0.03 for Young and 0.18 ± 0.04 for Elderly). The BOLD-CBF coupling was stronger in medial, parietal and frontal regions, which are part of well-established resting state brain networks. No significant correlation was observed in white matter or other brain structures. The voxelwise contrast between groups showed a significantly lower correlation for elderly subjects in the left supramarginal gyrus (MNI coordinates: −59, −34, 33; **Figure 1B**).

Random effects group maps obtained with the z-Fisher transformed maximum voxelwise correlation between BOLD and CBF timeseries (r_{max}, obtained introducing a temporal shift between the two signals as described in "Materials and Methods" section) are reported in **Figure 2A**. As expected, the number of cortical voxels showing a significant coupling increased for both groups. Interestingly, this increase was more pronounced for Elderly (mean r_{max} values in significant areas were 0.32 ± 0.02 for Young and 0.30 ± 0.03 for Elderly). However, the voxelwise contrast between groups still showed a significantly lower correlation for elderly subjects in the left supramarginal gyrus (MNI coordinates: −58, −36, 34; **Figure 2B**), in a cluster of voxels largely overlapping with that observed in **Figure 1B**.

DMN and FPN were easily identified in the ICA results, with one component showing the typical DMN pattern, one component showing the left FPN and another component the right FPN (**Figure 3**). The results of the ROI approach for the selected regions in DMN and FPN are reported in **Figure 4A**. The comparison of the $r_{max} - r_0$ difference between groups showed significantly larger values for Elderly in all ROIs, indicating a more pronounced effect of time-shift corrections on the linear correlation between BOLD and CBF timecourses in elderly subjects. An effect size estimate (Cohen's *d*) was also computed for the between-group comparison of the $r_{max} - r_0$ difference in these ROIs. The observed values were quite large, ranging from 0.78 to 1.24.

A larger $r_{max} - r_0$ difference for Elderly with respect to Young was also observed in the supramarginal gyrus, without reaching statistical significance (**Figure 4B**, values extracted from a mask obtained pooling the clusters in **Figures 1B**, **2A**). The time-shift

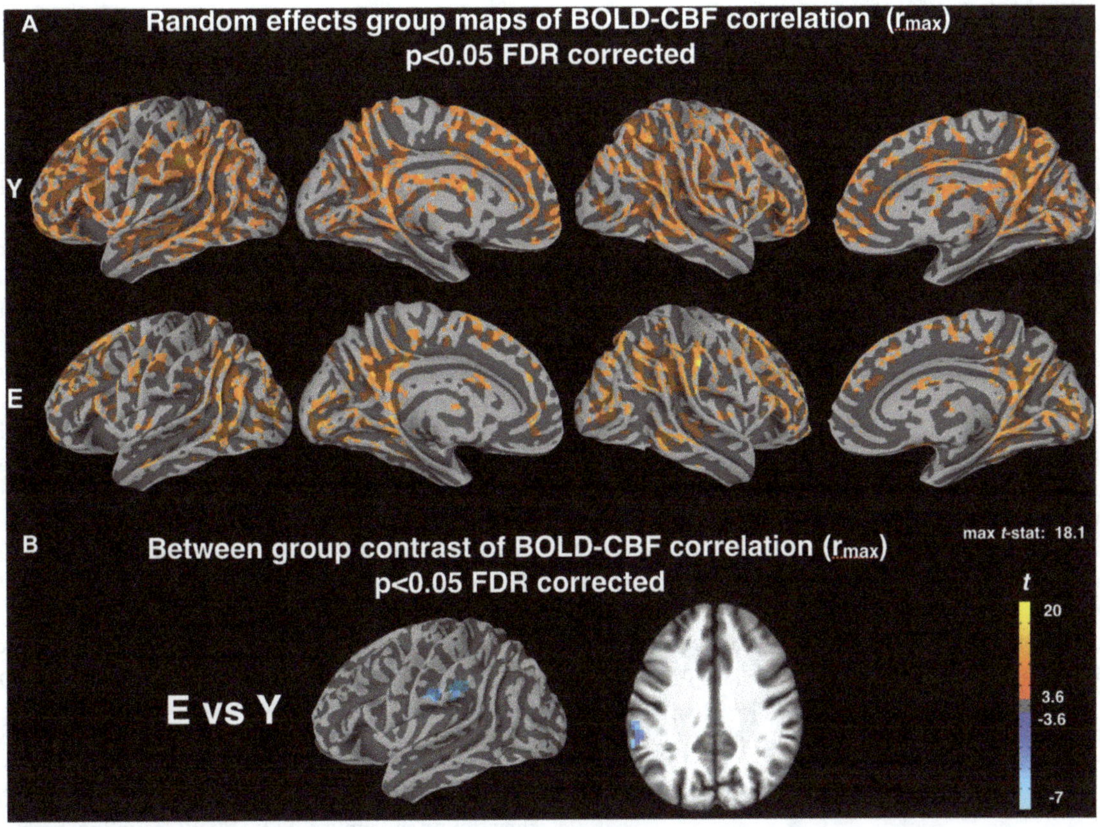

FIGURE 2 | (A) Random effect group maps showing the dynamic coupling between spontaneous BOLD and CBF fluctuations for Y and E groups when potential time shifts between the two signals were compensated for (r_{max}, see "Materials and Methods" section). **(B)** Between-group contrast comparing the dynamic coupling between spontaneous BOLD and CBF fluctuations for Y and E, using r_{max} values. Note that a significant age related decrease of BOLD-CBF coupling is observed in the left supramarginal gyrus (MNI coordinates: −58, −36, 34) even after temporal shift correction, in a cluster of voxels largely overlapping with that observed in **Figure 1B**. The statistical maps were thresholded at $p < 0.05$ (corrected for multiple comparisons using FDR) and superimposed on the partially inflated study specific template.

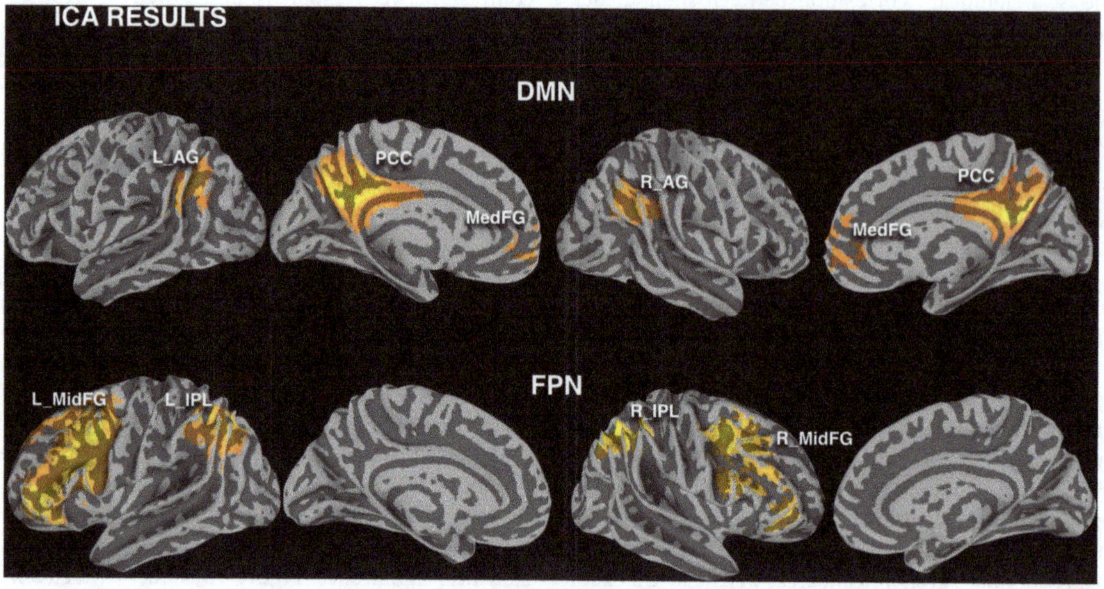

FIGURE 3 | Investigated nodes of default mode network (DMN) and frontoparietal network (FPN), defined with independent component analysis (ICA) calculated pooling the two groups and modalities (FWE corrected cluster significance of $p < 0.01$). Regions of interest (ROIs) were defined masking these clusters with a gray matter binary mask (L_AG/R_AG, left/right angular gyrus; PCC, posterior cingulate cortex; Med_FG, medial frontal gyrus; L_IPL/R_IPL, left/right inferior parietal lobule; L_MidFG/R_MidFG, left/right middle frontal gyrus).

parameters in the different ROIs ranged from −1.12 s to −1.81 s for Elderly and from −0.4 s to −1.4 s for Young. The between-group difference was significant in the right angular gyrus (−1.8 s for Elderly and −0.5 s for Young, $p < 0.03$, unpaired *t*-test), indicating an increased delay of BOLD dynamics (with respect to CBF) in elderlies.

The baseline CBF values showed the well known age related decrease for all the investigated regions (**Figure 3**). However, no significant correlation of the BOLD-CBF coupling with baseline CBF values was observed across subjects, for either Elderly or Young groups.

The control analysis on the amplitude of resting state low frequency fluctuations revealed that RSFA values in these regions did not change significantly with age, except for the BOLD-RSFA in the frontal regions of FPN (**Figure 4A**). However, no region showed a significant across-subjects correlation of the values of BOLD-CBF coupling with BOLD-RSFA or CBF-RSFA values, for either Elderly or Young groups.

The comparison of the run-averaged DVARS metrics did not show statistically significant differences across groups for either control or label images ($F_{(2,120)} = 1.29$; $p = 0.26$). Additional control analysis showed no significant correlation of DVARS values with the BOLD-CBF coupling for either Elderly or Young groups.

DISCUSSION

The present results showed that in young subjects spontaneous BOLD and CBF fluctuations are significantly synchronized in most cortical areas and especially within the major nodes of prominent resting-state networks, confirming previous evidence (Tak et al., 2014, 2015; Chen et al., 2015). As a new finding, this resting-state BOLD-CBF dynamic coupling was reduced in elderly individuals, especially in the left supramarginal gyrus. Moreover, this decrease was not related to a reduced amplitude of either BOLD or CBF spontaneous fluctuations. Furthermore, elderlies showed a larger increase in the correlation coefficient after the introduction of a relative time-shift between BOLD and CBF timecourses.

Recently, an increasing evidence that intrinsic CBF fluctuations are a major contributor to the resting state BOLD signal has been reported. Indeed, different studies showed a high level of spatial overlap between connectivity maps obtained from BOLD and CBF timecourses (Viviani et al., 2011; Jann et al., 2015). Moreover, a set of studies investigated the dynamic relationship between spontaneous CBF and BOLD fluctuations (Fukunaga et al., 2008; Wu et al., 2009; Tak et al., 2014, 2015; Chen et al., 2015; Cohen et al., 2017). Fukunaga et al. (2008) were the first to investigate the dynamic coupling between BOLD and perfusion fluctuations during resting state, showing that the two signals are correlated in most part of the cortex, with little involvement of white matter and cerebrospinal fluid. Furthermore, using the BOLD/perfusion ratio to target resting state oxidative metabolism fluctuations, they found a similar BOLD/CBF coupling with respect to a visual task induced brain activity, adding evidence to a metabolic/neuronal origin of spontaneous BOLD and CBF fluctuations. In a subsequent work, Wu et al. (2009) obtained functional connectivity maps using $CMRO_2$ time series derived from simultaneous BOLD and CBF time series acquired with ASL. Although the $CMRO_2$ time courses were estimated

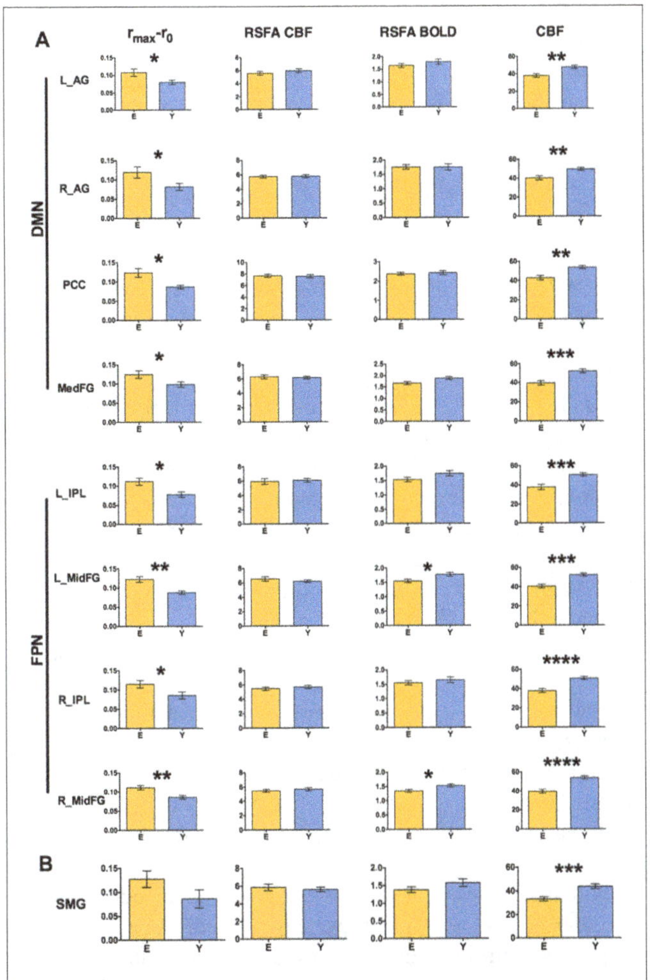

FIGURE 4 | (A) Between-group comparison of $r_{max} - r_0$ values, resting state fluctuation amplitudes (RSFAs) and baseline perfusion values extracted in ROIs of **Figure 3** (two-sample unpaired *t*-test; $^*p < 0.05$ FDR corrected, $^{**}p < 0.01$ FDR corrected, $^{***}p < 0.001$ FDR corrected, $^{****}p < 0.0005$ FDR corrected). **(B)** The same values extracted from the ROI obtained pooling the two clusters in **Figures 1B, 2B** and masking with gray matter. Error bars are standard errors.

assuming the steady-state biophysical BOLD model, that might have some limitations in a more dynamical situation (Simon and Buxton, 2015), the strong similarity observed by Wu et al. (2009) between functional connectivity maps obtained from BOLD, CBF and $CMRO_2$ time courses added further evidence to a significant BOLD-CBF coupling during resting state. In a recent work the study of dynamic BOLD-CBF relationship during resting state was addressed with significant methodological improvements, including physiological noise correction in the tag and control ASL images and taking into account the influence of global cardiac fluctuations (Tak et al., 2014). This work demonstrated that the resting-state BOLD-CBF coupling strength, although varying across the brain, was stronger in the gray matter and in particular in the major nodes of well-established functional networks. Moreover, the BOLD-CBF coupling observed by Tak and collaborators was significantly reduced in voxels associated with a high macrovascular content, suggesting that the component of spontaneous BOLD signal fluctuations that is more directly driven by dynamic CBF fluctuations is more likely related to neuronal activity, which is known to modulate the microvascular response.

Keeping in line with previous evidence, our results confirm that in young individuals spontaneous BOLD and CBF fluctuations are significantly synchronized in most cortical areas and especially in regions of the major resting state networks. As a new finding, we observed a general age-related decrease of the BOLD-CBF dynamic coupling during resting state across cortical areas. The between-group voxelwise contrast showed that this decrease was statistically significant in a cluster of voxels in the left supramarginal gyrus.

Slight discrepancies between BOLD and CBF dynamics have been previously reported even in young subjects using e.g., visual or motor stimuli (Obata et al., 2004; Cavusoglu et al., 2012). These discrepancies can be expected, due to possible temporal uncoupling of the involved physiological responses (i.e., CBF, CBV and $CMRO_2$) that have a competing effect on the BOLD signal amplitude. Indeed, a temporal uncoupling of e.g., CBF and venous CBV has been proposed in early models trying to explain BOLD signal transients like the post-stimulus undershoot or the initial overshoot during long stimulation blocks (Buxton et al., 1998, 2004; Buxton, 2012). Although a neuronal contribution to these transients has been recognized (Sadaghiani et al., 2009; Mullinger et al., 2014, 2017), there is increasing evidence that vascular mechanisms related to delayed compliance of venous vessels play an important role as well (Chen and Pike, 2009; Havlicek et al., 2017). In particular, a recent work suggests that the venous CBV response can be an order of magnitude slower than either CBF or $CMRO_2$ (Simon and Buxton, 2015).

Despite the specific physiological mechanisms responsible for the decreased BOLD-CBF dynamic coupling that we observed in elderly cannot be determined using the present data alone, it could be argued that increased vessel stiffening due to age (Podlutsky et al., 2010; Trott et al., 2011; Csiszár et al., 2015; Tsvetanov et al., 2015; Chiarelli et al., 2017; Tan et al., 2017; Tarantini et al., 2017; Toth et al., 2017) can lead to increased delay in venous compliance, thus introducing further temporal discrepancies between BOLD and CBF timecourses. Animal studies also showed that modifications of vessel compliance with age decrease the ratio of CBV to CBF responses (Dubeau et al., 2011; Desjardins et al., 2014) that in turn would also affect the BOLD response. Moreover, the ratio of CBV to CBF response is also reflected in the Grubb's parameter (Grubb et al., 1974) that is involved in calibrated BOLD models. Importantly, this parameter has been shown to vary not only with aging (Dubeau et al., 2011) but also during different phases of functional stimulation, leading to transient relationships between CBF, CBV and BOLD changes (Kida et al., 2006), suggesting a possible effect on BOLD-CBF coupling. The potential role of delayed vessel compliance is also supported by our second finding, i.e., that introducing a time-shift correction between BOLD and CBF signals has more effect for elderlies than for young subjects in increasing the calculated correlation coefficient. However, even with time-shift correction, the left supramarginal gyrus showed a significant between-group difference in the voxelwise contrast, indicating that the dynamic uncoupling of BOLD and CBF timecourses in this region is more affected by the aging process and can be only partially explained with a simple time-shift between the two signals. Interestingly, different neuroimaging and transcranial magnetic stimulation studies reported that the left supramarginal gyrus is involved in verbal working memory and episodic memory (Romero et al., 2006; Koelsch et al., 2009; Deschamps et al., 2014; Thakral et al., 2017), which are functions known to be impaired with age. Considering that our investigated population was selected among healthy elderlies that did not show a compromised performance in memory tests, our results acquire an increased interest. Indeed, the observed age related differences in the dynamic BOLD-CBF coupling could be considered a potential biomarker that might anticipate changes in neuronal function. In this regard, this type of index could be spatially more specific than e.g., age-related decrease of baseline perfusion that we and others (Parkes et al., 2004; Ambarki et al., 2015; De Vis et al., 2015) clearly observed in most cortical areas. However, we are aware that a full validation of this hypothesis would require additional data, with a larger sample size and possibly longitudinal studies.

Potential Limitations and Caveats

As in all studies using dynamic ASL to assess brain function, a major concern is minimizing BOLD contamination of the CBF signal. We addressed this issue by using the short echo time data (which have minimal sensitivity to the BOLD effect) and by high pass filtering the ASL signal followed by demodulation to derive the CBF timecourse (Chuang et al., 2008). This approach can be considered a generalization of previously proposed methods like e.g., sinc interpolation (Liu and Wong, 2005), with similar efficiency in removing BOLD contamination from the perfusion timeseries. Another important concern in resting state fMRI studies is the physiological noise due to cardiac and respiratory activity. While different methods of noise cleanup have been established for the BOLD signal (for a review see; Murphy et al., 2013; Liu, 2016), there is scarce evidence on the application of similar procedures to ASL. We chose the approach using RETROICOR to correct time-locked effects of cardiac and respiratory fluctuations on the EPI signal of label and control separately (Restom et al., 2006). Indeed, modeling the effect of the cardiac and respiratory cycles on the derived CBF weighted timeseries had minimal effect on signal quality (Restom et al., 2006). However, as observed by the same authors, future approaches using additional information such as end tidal carbon dioxide measurements could allow improved modeling of the effect of physiological noise on the perfusion timecourses, extending previous work on BOLD (Wise et al., 2004). An additional source of noise in the fMRI signals is represented by head motion, that has been shown to introduce spurious correlations in functional networks investigated in resting state BOLD studies (Power et al., 2012). This issue is particularly important when comparing different populations that could differ in the amount of head motion, like e.g healthy subjects vs. patients or young subjects vs. elderlies and censoring procedures have been proposed, in addition to regression of motion parameters, to mitigate these effects in resting state BOLD timeseries (Power et al., 2014). Again, the extension of these methods to CBF timeseries is not straightforward because the perfusion information is carried by the difference image between label and control that should be censored in pairs, thus strongly reducing the number of usable timepoints. However, motion parameters derived during preprocessing of label and control images did not differ significantly between groups in our data, suggesting a negligible effect of motion on the observed results.

In addition to noise concerns, potential between-group differences in BOLD and/or CBF signal fluctuation amplitude could also affect the calculated correlations. Indeed, while from a mathematical point of view the linear correlation of two timecourses is not affected by the amplitude of the signals, in presence of noise a reduced fluctuation amplitude could lead to a decreased correlation coefficient (Liu, 2013). However, the two groups showed comparable levels of signal fluctuations for both BOLD and CBF in the majority of investigated ROIs, suggesting no bias related to this issue. Even in the two regions showing a significant decrease of BOLD fluctuations in elderlies, any significant correlation of RSFA with BOLD-CBF correlation was observed. A reduced fluctuation amplitude in elderlies could have been expected due to gray matter atrophy. In this regard, the observation of similar fluctuation amplitudes of the functional signals in the two groups also helps to mitigate the concern of potential confounds due to the presence of atrophy in elderlies that could have biased our results.

Potential biases in the results could also be introduced by the six older adults using antihypertensive medication that would possibly alter the hemodynamic response in these subjects. In our group of subjects a control analysis revealed similar BOLD-CBF coupling when comparing this hypertensive subgroup with the other elderlies, with no significant differences. Nevertheless, future studies should address this issue using larger sample sizes.

A further concern could be raised regarding the postlabel delay (1000 ms for the first slice) used for the study of dynamic BOLD-CBF coupling that can be too short to ensure a complete delivery of the bolus to the tissue at the time of acquisition, in particular for elderlies. However, while this is an important issue for absolute CBF quantification, short postlabel delays are often used or even recommended for functional applications of ASL because offer a larger sensitivity and temporal resolution without introducing bright spots in activation maps due to large vessel contribution or introducing distortions of timecourses (Gonzalez-At et al., 2000; Zappe et al., 2008). In contrast, for the quantification of baseline CBF, we used a longer postlabel delay (1900 ms for the first slice), following current guidelines for both young and healthy elderlies (Alsop et al., 2015).

Finally, another limitation of the study could arise from the small sample size, potentially resulting in a low statistical power. Indeed, despite statistical significance was obtained for the between-group comparison of our main metrics of interest, future studies with larger sample size possibly including elderlies with impaired cognitive functions would allow further assessment of the significance of our findings.

CONCLUSION

In this study we observed an age-related decrease of the temporal correlation between the BOLD and CBF spontaneous fluctuations in the cortex. Interestingly, when compensating for potential time-shifts between the two signals, the increase of the correlation coefficient was larger for elderlies. However a significant between-group difference was observed in the left supramargynal gyrus even after time-shift correction, suggesting a more pronounced age-related BOLD-CBF uncoupling in this area. These results suggest that the study of dynamic coupling between spontaneous BOLD-CBF fluctuations using the simultaneous acquisition of the two signals with ASL is a promising technique to study-resting state brain function in aging and disease.

AUTHOR CONTRIBUTIONS

PC and AF: conceived and designed the study and wrote the article. FC and GB: enrolled and tested the subjects. PC and MGP: performed the experiments. PC: implemented AFNI and Python scripts. PC, FC and AF: performed the analyses.

REFERENCES

Alsop, D. C., Detre, J. A., Golay, X., Günther, M., Hendrikse, J., Hernandez-Garcia, L., et al. (2015). Recommended implementation of arterial spin-labeled perfusion MRI for clinical applications: a consensus of the ISMRM perfusion study group and the European consortium for ASL in dementia. *Magn. Reson. Med.* 73, 102–116. doi: 10.1002/mrm.25197

Ambarki, K., Wahlin, A., Zarrinkoob, L., Wirestam, R., Petr, J., Malm, J., et al. (2015). Accuracy of parenchymal cerebral blood flow measurements using pseudocontinuous arterial spin-labeling in healthy volunteers. *Am. J. Neuroradiol.* 36, 1816–1821. doi: 10.3174/ajnr.A4367

Ances, B. M., Leontiev, O., Perthen, J. E., Liang, C., Lansing, A. E., and Buxton, R. B. (2008). Regional differences in the coupling of cerebral blood flow and oxygen metabolism changes in response to activation: implications for BOLD-fMRI. *Neuroimage* 39, 1510–1521. doi: 10.1016/j.neuroimage.2007.11.015

Aslan, S., Xu, F., Wang, P. L., Uh, J., Yezhuvath, U. S., van Osch, M., et al. (2010). Estimation of labeling efficiency in pseudocontinuous arterial spin labeling. *Magn. Reson. Med.* 63, 765–771. doi: 10.1002/mrm.22245

Avants, B. B., Cook, P., Pluta, J., Duda, J. T., Rao, H., Giannetta, J., et al. (2009). Multivariate diffeomorphic analysis of longitudinal increase in white matter directionality and decrease in cortical thickness between ages 14 and 18. *Neuroimage* 47:S105. doi: 10.1016/s1053-8119(09)70918-8

Avants, B. B., Epstein, C., Grossman, M., and Gee, J. (2008). Symmetric diffeomorphic image registration with cross-correlation: evaluating automated labeling of elderly and neurodegenerative brain. *Med. Image Anal.* 12, 26–41. doi: 10.1016/j.media.2007.06.004

Avants, B. B., Yushkevich, P., Pluta, J., Minkoff, D., Korczykowski, M., Detre, J., et al. (2010). The optimal template effect in hippocampus studies of diseased populations. *Neuroimage* 49, 2457–2466. doi: 10.1016/j.neuroimage.2009.09.062

Bandettini, P. A., Wong, E. C., Hinks, R. S., Tikofsky, R. S., and Hyde, J. S. (1992). Time course EPI of human brain function during task activation. *Magn. Reson. Med.* 25, 390–397. doi: 10.1002/mrm.1910250220

Beckmann, C. F., Mackay, C. E., Filippini, N., and Smith, S. M. (2009). Group comparison of resting-state FMRI data using multi-subject ICA and dual regression. *Neuroimage* 47:S148. doi: 10.1016/s1053-8119(09)71511-3

Beckmann, C. F., and Smith, S. M. (2004). Probabilistic independent component analysis for functional magnetic resonance imaging. *IEEE Trans. Med. Imaging* 23, 137–152. doi: 10.1109/tmi.2003.822821

Biswal, B., Yetkin, F. Z., Haughton, V. M., and Hyde, J. S. (1995). Functional connectivity in the motor cortex of resting human brain using echo-planar MRI. *Magn. Reson. Med.* 34, 537–541. doi: 10.1002/mrm.1910340409

Blockley, N. P., Griffeth, V. E. M., and Buxton, R. B. (2012). A general analysis of calibrated BOLD methodology for measuring $CMRO_2$ responses: comparison of a new approach with existing methods. *Neuroimage* 60, 279–289. doi: 10.1016/j.neuroimage.2011.11.081

Blockley, N. P., Griffeth, V. E. M., Simon, A. B., Dubowitz, D. J., and Buxton, R. B. (2015). Calibrating the BOLD response without administering gases: comparison of hypercapnia calibration with calibration using an asymmetric spin echo. *Neuroimage* 104, 423–429. doi: 10.1016/j.neuroimage.2014.09.061

Brier, M. R., Thomas, J. B., and Ances, B. M. (2014). Network dysfunction in Alzheimer's disease: refining the disconnection hypothesis. *Brain Connect.* 4, 299–311. doi: 10.1089/brain.2014.0236

Bulte, D. P., Drescher, K., and Jezzard, P. (2009). Comparison of hypercapnia-based calibration techniques for measurement of cerebral oxygen metabolism with MRI. *Magn. Reson. Med.* 61, 391–398. doi: 10.1002/mrm.21862

Bulte, D. P., Kelly, M., Germuska, M., Xie, J., Chappell, M. A., Okell, T. W., et al. (2012). Quantitative measurement of cerebral physiology using respiratory-calibrated MRI. *Neuroimage* 60, 582–591. doi: 10.1016/j.neuroimage.2011.12.017

Buxton, R. B. (2010). Interpreting oxygenation-based neuroimaging signals: the importance and the challenge of understanding brain oxygen metabolism. *Front. Neuroenergetics* 2:8. doi: 10.3389/fnene.2010.00008

Buxton, R. B. (2012). Dynamic models of BOLD contrast. *Neuroimage* 62, 953–961. doi: 10.1016/j.neuroimage.2012.01.012

Buxton, R. B., Frank, L. R., Wong, E. C., Siewert, B., Warach, S., and Edelman, R. R. (1998). A general kinetic model for quantitative perfusion imaging with arterial spin labeling. *Magn. Reson. Med.* 40, 383–396. doi: 10.1002/mrm.1910400308

Buxton, R. B., Uludağ, K., Dubowitz, D. J., and Liu, T. T. (2004). Modeling the hemodynamic response to brain activation. *Neuroimage* 23, S220–S233. doi: 10.1016/j.neuroimage.2004.07.013

Cavusoglu, M., Bartels, A., Yesilyurt, B., and Uludağ, K. (2012). Retinotopic maps and hemodynamic delays in the human visual cortex measured using arterial spin labeling. *Neuroimage* 59, 4044–4054. doi: 10.1016/j.neuroimage.2011.10.056

Chen, J. J., Jann, K., and Wang, D. J. J. (2015). Characterizing resting-state brain function using arterial spin labeling. *Brain Connect.* 5, 527–542. doi: 10.1089/brain.2015.0344

Chen, J. J., and Pike, G. B. (2009). Origins of the BOLD post-stimulus undershoot. *Neuroimage* 46, 559–568. doi: 10.1016/j.neuroimage.2009.03.015

Chen, J. J., Rosas, H. D., and Salat, D. H. (2011). Age-associated reductions in cerebral blood flow are independent from regional atrophy. *Neuroimage* 55, 468–478. doi: 10.1016/j.neuroimage.2010.12.032

Chiarelli, P. A., Bulte, D. P., Wise, R., Gallichan, D., and Jezzard, P. (2007). A calibration method for quantitative BOLD fMRI based on hyperoxia. *Neuroimage* 37, 808–820. doi: 10.1016/j.neuroimage.2007.05.033

Chiarelli, A. M., Fletcher, M. A., Tan, C. H., Low, K. A., Maclin, E. L., Zimmerman, B., et al. (2017). Individual differences in regional cortical volumes across the life span are associated with regional optical measures of arterial elasticity. *Neuroimage* 162, 199–213. doi: 10.1016/j.neuroimage.2017.08.064

Chuang, K.-H., van Gelderen, P., Merkle, H., Bodurka, J., Ikonomidou, V. N., Koretsky, A. P., et al. (2008). Mapping resting-state functional connectivity using perfusion MRI. *Neuroimage* 40, 1595–1605. doi: 10.1016/j.neuroimage.2008.01.006

Cohen, A. D., Nencka, A. S., Lebel, R. M., and Wang, Y. (2017). Multiband multi-echo imaging of simultaneous oxygenation and flow timeseries for resting state connectivity. *PLoS One* 12:e0169253. doi: 10.1371/journal.pone.0169253

Csiszár, A., Csiszar, A., Pinto, J. T., Gautam, T., Kleusch, C., Hoffmann, B., et al. (2015). Resveratrol encapsulated in novel fusogenic liposomes activates Nrf2 and attenuates oxidative stress in cerebromicrovascular endothelial cells from aged rats. *J. Gerontol. A Biol. Sci. Med. Sci.* 70, 303–313. doi: 10.1093/gerona/glu029

Dai, W., Garcia, D., de Bazelaire, C., and Alsop, D. C. (2008). Continuous flow-driven inversion for arterial spin labeling using pulsed radio frequency and gradient fields. *Magn. Reson. Med.* 60, 1488–1497. doi: 10.1002/mrm.21790

Davis, T. L., Kwong, K. K., Weisskoff, R. M., and Rosen, B. R. (1998). Calibrated functional MRI: mapping the dynamics of oxidative metabolism. *Proc. Natl. Acad. Sci. U S A* 95, 1834–1839. doi: 10.1073/pnas.95.4.1834

De Luca, M., Beckmann, C. F., De Stefano, N., Matthews, P. M., and Smith, S. M. (2006). fMRI resting state networks define distinct modes of long-distance interactions in the human brain. *Neuroimage* 29, 1359–1367. doi: 10.1016/j.neuroimage.2005.08.035

De Vis, J. B., Hendrikse, J., Bhogal, A., Adams, A., Kappelle, L. J., and Petersen, E. T. (2015). Age-related changes in brain hemodynamics; A calibrated MRI study. *Hum. Brain Mapp.* 36, 3973–3987. doi: 10.1002/hbm.22891

Deschamps, I., Baum, S. R., and Gracco, V. L. (2014). On the role of the supramarginal gyrus in phonological processing and verbal working memory: evidence from rTMS studies. *Neuropsychologia* 53, 39–46. doi: 10.1016/j.neuropsychologia.2013.10.015

Desjardins, M., Berti, R., Pouliot, P., Dubeau, S., and Lesage, F. (2014). Multimodal study of the hemodynamic response to hypercapnia in anesthetized aged rats. *Neurosci. Lett.* 563, 33–37. doi: 10.1016/j.neulet.2014.01.027

D'Esposito, M., Zarahn, E., Aguirre, G. K., and Neuroimage, B. R. (1999). The effect of normal aging on the coupling of neural activity to the bold hemodynamic response. *Neuroimage* 10, 6–14. doi: 10.1006/nimg.1999.0444

Detre, J. A., Leigh, J. S., Williams, D. S., and Koretsky, A. P. (1992). Perfusion imaging. *Magn. Reson. Med.* 23, 37–45. doi: 10.1002/mrm.1910230106

Dubeau, S., Ferland, G., Gaudreau, P., Beaumont, E., and Lesage, F. (2011). Cerebrovascular hemodynamic correlates of aging in the Lou/c rat: a model of healthy aging. *Neuroimage* 56, 1892–1901. doi: 10.1016/j.neuroimage.2011.03.076

Esposito, R., Cieri, F., Chiacchiaretta, P., Cera, N., Lauriola, M., Di Giannantonio, M., et al. (2018). Modifications in resting state functional anticorrelation between default mode network and dorsal attention network: comparison among young adults, healthy elders and mild cognitive impairment patients. *Brain Imaging Behav.* 12, 127–141. doi: 10.1007/s11682-017-9686-y

Fernández-Seara, M. A., Mengual, E., Vidorreta, M., Castellanos, G., Irigoyen, J., Erro, E., et al. (2015). Resting state functional connectivity of the subthalamic nucleus in Parkinson's disease assessed using arterial spin-labeled perfusion fMRI. *Hum. Brain Mapp.* 36, 1937–1950. doi: 10.1002/hbm.22747

Folstein, M. F., Folstein, S. E., and McHugh, P. R. (1975). "Mini-mental state". A practical method for grading the cognitive state of patients for the clinician. *J. Psychiatr. Res.* 12, 189–198. doi: 10.1016/0022-3956(75)90026-6

Fox, M. D., and Greicius, M. (2010). Clinical applications of resting state functional connectivity. *Front. Syst. Neurosci.* 4:19. doi: 10.3389/fnsys.2010.00019

Friston, K. J., Ashburner, J., Frith, C. D., Poline, J. B., Heather, J. D., and Frackowiak, R. S. J. (1995). Spatial registration and normalization of images. *Hum. Brain Mapp.* 3, 165–189. doi: 10.1002/hbm.460030303

Fujita, N., Matsumoto, K., Tanaka, H., Watanabe, Y., and Murase, K. (2006). Quantitative study of changes in oxidative metabolism during visual stimulation using absolute relaxation rates. *NMR Biomed.* 19, 60–68. doi: 10.1002/nbm.1001

Fukunaga, M., Horovitz, S. G., de Zwart, J. A., van Gelderen, P., Balkin, T. J., Braun, A. R., et al. (2008). Metabolic origin of bold signal fluctuations in the absence of stimuli. *J. Cereb. Blood Flow Metab.* 28, 1377–1387. doi: 10.1038/jcbfm.2008.25

Gardini, S., Sambataro, F., Cuetos, F., Fasano, F., Marchi, M., Crisi, G., et al. (2014). Increased default mode network functional connectivity in mild cognitive impairment: a detrimental brain mechanism associated with poor semantic memory performance. *Alzheimers Dement.* 10, P823–P824. doi: 10.1016/j.jalz.2014.05.1623

Garrett, D. D., Lindenberger, U., Hoge, R. D., and Gauthier, C. J. (2017). Age differences in brain signal variability are robust to multiple vascular controls. *Sci. Rep.* 7:10149. doi: 10.1038/s41598-017-09752-7

Gauthier, C. J., Desjardins-Crépeau, L., Madjar, C., Bherer, L., and Hoge, R. D. (2012). Absolute quantification of resting oxygen metabolism and metabolic reactivity during functional activation using QUO2 MRI. *Neuroimage* 63, 1353–1363. doi: 10.1016/j.neuroimage.2012.07.065

Gauthier, C. J., and Hoge, R. D. (2013). A generalized procedure for calibrated MRI incorporating hyperoxia and hypercapnia. *Hum. Brain Mapp.* 34, 1053–1069. doi: 10.1002/hbm.21495

Germuska, M., and Bulte, D. P. (2014). MRI measurement of oxygen extraction fraction, mean vessel size and cerebral blood volume using serial hyperoxia and hypercapnia. *Neuroimage* 92, 132–142. doi: 10.1016/j.neuroimage.2014.02.002

Germuska, M., Merola, A., Murphy, K., Babic, A., Richmond, L., Khot, S., et al. (2016). A forward modelling approach for the estimation of oxygen extraction fraction by calibrated fMRI. *Neuroimage* 139, 313–323. doi: 10.1016/j.neuroimage.2016.06.004

Glover, G. H., Li, T. Q., and Ress, D. (2000). Image-based method for retrospective correction of physiological motion effects in fMRI: RETROICOR. *Magn. Reson. Med.* 44, 162–167. doi: 10.1002/1522-2594(200007)44:1<162::aid-mrm23>3.3.co;2-5

Gonzalez-At, J. B., Alsop, D. C., and Detre, J. A. (2000). Cerebral perfusion and arterial transit time changes during task activation determined with continuous arterial spin labeling. *Magn. Reson. Med.* 43, 739–746. doi: 10.1002/(sici)1522-2594(200005)43:5<739::aid-mrm17>3.0.co;2-2

Griffeth, V. E. M., and Buxton, R. B. (2011). A theoretical framework for estimating cerebral oxygen metabolism changes using the calibrated-BOLD method: modeling the effects of blood volume distribution, hematocrit, oxygen extraction fraction, and tissue signal properties on the BOLD signal. *Neuroimage* 58, 198–212. doi: 10.1016/j.neuroimage.2011.05.077

Grubb, R. L. Jr., Raichle, M. E., Eichling, J. O., and Ter-Pogossian, N. M. (1974). The effects of changes in $PaCO_2$ on cerebral blood volume, blood flow, and vascular mean transit time. *Stroke* 5, 630–639. doi: 10.1161/01.str.5.5.630

Havlicek, M., Ivanov, D., Poser, B. A., and Uludağ, K. (2017). Echo-time dependence of the BOLD response transients—A window into brain functional physiology. *Neuroimage* 159, 355–370. doi: 10.1016/j.neuroimage.2017.07.034

Hoge, R. D., Atkinson, J., Gill, B., Crelier, G. R. R., Marrett, S., and Pike, G. B. (1999). Investigation of BOLD signal dependence on cerebral blood flow and oxygen consumption: the deoxyhemoglobin dilution model. *Magn. Reson. Med.* 42, 849–863. doi: 10.1002/(sici)1522-2594(199911)42:5<849::aid-mrm4>3.0.co;2-z

Hutchison, J. L., Lu, H., and Cortex, B. R. C. (2013). Neural mechanisms of age-related slowing: the $\Delta CBF/\Delta CMRO_2$ ratio mediates age-differences in BOLD signal and human performance. *Cereb. Cortex* 23, 2337–2346. doi: 10.1093/cercor/bhs233

Jann, K., Hernandez, L. M., Beck-Pancer, D., McCarron, R., Smith, R. X., Dapretto, M., et al. (2015). Altered resting perfusion and functional connectivity of default mode network in youth with autism spectrum disorder. *Brain Behav.* 5:e00358. doi: 10.1002/brb3.358

Jo, H. J., Saad, Z. S., Simmons, W. K., Milbury, L. A., and Cox, R. W. (2010). Mapping sources of correlation in resting state FMRI, with artifact detection and removal. *Neuroimage* 52, 571–582. doi: 10.1016/j.neuroimage.2010.04.246

Kannurpatti, S. S., and Biswal, B. B. (2008). Detection and scaling of task-induced fMRI-BOLD response using resting state fluctuations. *Neuroimage* 40, 1567–1574. doi: 10.1016/j.neuroimage.2007.09.040

Kastrup, A., Krüger, G., Glover, G. H., and Moseley, M. E. (1999). Assessment of cerebral oxidative metabolism with breath holding and fMRI. *Magn. Reson. Med.* 42, 608–611. doi: 10.1002/(sici)1522-2594(199909)42:3<608::aid-mrm26>3.3.co;2-9

Kida, I., Rothman, D. L., and Hyder, F. (2006). Dynamics of changes in blood flow, volume, and oxygenation: implications for dynamic functional magnetic resonance imaging calibration. *J. Cereb. Blood Flow Metab.* 27, 690–696. doi: 10.1038/sj.jcbfm.9600409

Koelsch, S., Schulze, K., Sammler, D., Fritz, T., Müller, K., and Gruber, O. (2009). Functional architecture of verbal and tonal working memory: an FMRI study. *Hum. Brain Mapp.* 30, 859–873. doi: 10.1002/hbm.20550

Kwong, K. K., Belliveau, J. W., Chesler, D. A., Goldberg, I. E., Weisskoff, R. M., Poncelet, B. P., et al. (1992). Dynamic magnetic resonance imaging of human brain activity during primary sensory stimulation. *Proc. Natl. Acad. Sci. U S A* 89, 5675–5679. doi: 10.1073/pnas.89.12.5675

Li, H.-J., Hou, X.-H., Liu, H.-H., Yue, C.-L., He, Y., and Zuo, X.-N. (2015). Toward systems neuroscience in mild cognitive impairment and Alzheimer's disease: a meta-analysis of 75 fMRI studies. *Hum. Brain Mapp.* 36, 1217–1232. doi: 10.1002/hbm.22689

Liang, X., Connelly, A., and Calamante, F. (2014). Graph analysis of resting-state ASL perfusion MRI data: nonlinear correlations among CBF and network metrics. *Neuroimage* 87, 265–275. doi: 10.1016/j.neuroimage.2013.11.013

Liu, T. T. (2013). Neurovascular factors in resting-state functional MRI. *Neuroimage* 80, 339–348. doi: 10.1016/j.neuroimage.2013.04.071

Liu, T. T. (2016). Noise contributions to the fMRI signal: an overview. *Neuroimage* 143, 141–151. doi: 10.1016/j.neuroimage.2016.09.008

Liu, P., Hebrank, A. C., Rodrigue, K. M., Kennedy, K. M., Section, J., Park, D. C., et al. (2013). Age-related differences in memory-encoding fMRI responses after accounting for decline in vascular reactivity. *Neuroimage* 78, 415–425. doi: 10.1016/j.neuroimage.2013.04.053

Liu, T. T., and Wong, E. C. (2005). A signal processing model for arterial spin labeling functional MRI. *Neuroimage* 24, 207–215. doi: 10.1016/j.neuroimage.2004.09.047

Lu, H., Xu, F., Rodrigue, K. M., Kennedy, K. M., Cheng, Y., Flicker, B., et al. (2011). Alterations in cerebral metabolic rate and blood supply across the adult lifespan. *Cereb. Cortex* 21, 1426–1434. doi: 10.1093/cercor/bhQ234

Mayhew, S. D., Mullinger, K. J., Bagshaw, A. P., Bowtell, R., and Francis, S. T. (2014). Investigating intrinsic connectivity networks using simultaneous BOLD and CBF measurements. *Neuroimage* 99, 111–121. doi: 10.1016/j.neuroimage.2014.05.042

Mohtasib, R. S., Lumley, G., Goodwin, J. A., Emsley, H. C. A., Sluming, V., and Parkes, L. M. (2012). Calibrated fMRI during a cognitive Stroop task reveals reduced metabolic response with increasing age. *Neuroimage* 59, 1143–1151. doi: 10.1016/j.neuroimage.2011.07.092

Moradi, F., Buračas, G. T., and Buxton, R. B. (2012). Attention strongly increases oxygen metabolic response to stimulus in primary visual cortex. *Neuroimage* 59, 601–607. doi: 10.1016/j.neuroimage.2011.07.078

Mullinger, K. J., Cherukara, M. T., Buxton, R. B., Francis, S. T., and Mayhew, S. D. (2017). Post-stimulus fMRI and EEG responses: evidence for a neuronal origin hypothesised to be inhibitory. *Neuroimage* 157, 388–399. doi: 10.1016/j.neuroimage.2017.06.020

Mullinger, K. J., Mayhew, S. D., Bagshaw, A. P., Bowtell, R., and Francis, S. T. (2014). Evidence that the negative BOLD response is neuronal in origin: a simultaneous EEG-BOLD-CBF study in humans. *Neuroimage* 94, 263–274. doi: 10.1016/j.neuroimage.2014.02.029

Murphy, K., Birn, R. M., and Bandettini, P. A. (2013). Resting-state fMRI confounds and cleanup. *Neuroimage* 80, 349–359. doi: 10.1016/j.neuroimage.2013.04.001

Nichols, T. E., and Holmes, A. P. (2002). Nonparametric permutation tests for functional neuroimaging: a primer with examples. *Hum. Brain Mapp.* 15, 1–25. doi: 10.1002/hbm.1058

O'Rourke, M. F., and Hashimoto, J. (2007). Mechanical factors in arterial aging: a clinical perspective. *J. Am. Coll. Cardiol.* 50, 1–13. doi: 10.1016/j.jacc.2006.12.050

Obata, T., Liu, T. T., Miller, K. L., Luh, W. M., Wong, E. C., Frank, L. R., et al. (2004). Discrepancies between BOLD and flow dynamics in primary and supplementary motor areas: application of the balloon model to the interpretation of BOLD transients. *Neuroimage* 21, 144–153. doi: 10.1016/j.neuroimage.2003.08.040

Ogawa, S., Tank, D. W., Menon, R., Ellermann, J. M., Kim, S. G., Merkle, H., et al. (1992). Intrinsic signal changes accompanying sensory stimulation: functional brain mapping with magnetic resonance imaging. *Proc. Natl. Acad. Sci. U S A* 89, 5951–5955. doi: 10.1073/pnas.89.13.5951

Parkes, L. M., Rashid, W., Chard, D. T., and Tofts, P. S. (2004). Normal cerebral perfusion measurements using arterial spin labeling: reproducibility, stability, and age and gender effects. *Magn. Reson. Med.* 51, 736–743. doi: 10.1002/mrm.20023

Podlutsky, A., Ballabh, P., and Csiszar, A. (2010). Oxidative stress and endothelial dysfunction in pulmonary arteries of aged rats. *Am. J. Physiol. Heart Circ. Physiol.* 298, H346–H351. doi: 10.1152/ajpheart.00972.2009

Power, J. D., Barnes, K. A., Snyder, A. Z., Schlaggar, B. L., and Petersen, S. E. (2012). Spurious but systematic correlations in functional connectivity MRI networks arise from subject motion. *Neuroimage* 59, 2142–2154. doi: 10.1016/j.neuroimage.2011.10.018

Power, J. D., Mitra, A., Laumann, T. O., Snyder, A. Z., Schlaggar, B. L., and Petersen, S. E. (2014). Methods to detect, characterize and remove motion artifact in resting state fMRI. *Neuroimage* 84, 320–341. doi: 10.1016/j.neuroimage.2013.08.048

Restom, K., Behzadi, Y., and Liu, T. T. (2006). Physiological noise reduction for arterial spin labeling functional MRI. *Neuroimage* 31, 1104–1115. doi: 10.1016/j.neuroimage.2006.01.026

Romero, L., Walsh, V., and Papagno, C. (2006). The neural correlates of phonological short-term memory: a repetitive transcranial magnetic stimulation study. *J. Cogn. Neurosci.* 18, 1147–1155. doi: 10.1162/jocn.2006.18.7.1147

Sadaghiani, S., Uğurbil, K., and Uludağ, K. (2009). Neural activity-induced modulation of BOLD poststimulus undershoot independent of the positive signal. *Magn. Reson. Imaging* 27, 1030–1038. doi: 10.1016/j.mri.2009.04.003

Samanez-Larkin, G. R., and D'Esposito, M. (2008). Group comparisons: imaging the aging brain. *Soc. Cogn. Affect. Neurosci.* 3, 290–297. doi: 10.1093/scan/nsn029

Simon, A. B., and Buxton, R. B. (2015). Understanding the dynamic relationship between cerebral blood flow and the BOLD signal: implications for quantitative functional MRI. *Neuroimage* 116, 158–167. doi: 10.1016/j.neuroimage.2015.03.080

Smith, S. M. (2002). Fast robust automated brain extraction. *Hum. Brain Mapp.* 17, 143–155. doi: 10.1002/hbm.10062

Storti, S. F., Boscolo Galazzo, I., Montemezzi, S., Menegaz, G., and Pizzini, F. B. (2017). Dual-echo ASL contributes to decrypting the link between functional connectivity and cerebral blow flow. *Hum. Brain Mapp.* 38, 5831–5844. doi: 10.1002/hbm.23804

Studholme, C., Hawkes, D. J., and Hill, D. L. (1998). "Normalized entropy measure for multimodality image alignment," in *SPIE The International Society for Optical Engineering*, ed. K. M. Hanson (San Diego, CA: Medical Imaging), 132–143.

Tak, S., Polimeni, J. R., Wang, D. J. J., Yan, L., and Chen, J. J. (2015). Associations of resting-state fmri functional connectivity with flow-BOLD coupling and regional vasculature. *Brain Connect.* 5, 137–146. doi: 10.1089/brain.2014.0299

Tak, S., Wang, D. J. J., Polimeni, J. R., Yan, L., and Chen, J. J. (2014). Dynamic and static contributions of the cerebrovasculature to the resting-state BOLD signal. *Neuroimage* 84, 672–680. doi: 10.1016/j.neuroimage.2013.09.057

Tan, C. H., Low, K. A., Kong, T., Fletcher, M. A., Zimmerman, B., Maclin, E. L., et al. (2017). Mapping cerebral pulse pressure and arterial compliance over the adult lifespan with optical imaging. *PLoS One* 12:e0171305. doi: 10.1371/journal.pone.0171305

Tarantini, S., Tran, C. H. T., Gordon, G. R., Ungvari, Z., and Csiszar, A. (2017). Impaired neurovascular coupling in aging and Alzheimer's disease: contribution of astrocyte dysfunction and endothelial impairment to cognitive decline. *Exp. Gerontol.* 94, 52–58. doi: 10.1016/j.exger.2016.11.004

Thakral, P. P., Madore, K. P., and Schacter, D. L. (2017). A role for the left angular gyrus in episodic simulation and memory. *J. Neurosci.* 37, 8142–8149. doi: 10.1523/JNEUROSCI.1319-17.2017

Toth, P., Tarantini, S., Csiszar, A., and Ungvari, Z. (2017). Functional vascular contributions to cognitive impairment and dementia: mechanisms and consequences of cerebral autoregulatory dysfunction, endothelial impairment and neurovascular uncoupling in aging. *Am. J. Physiol. Heart Circ. Physiol.* 312, H1–H20. doi: 10.1152/ajpheart.00581.2016

Trott, D. W., Seawright, J. W., Luttrell, M. J., and Woodman, C. R. (2011). NAD(P)H oxidase-derived reactive oxygen species contribute to age-related impairments of endothelium-dependent dilation in rat soleus feed arteries. *J. Appl. Physiol.* 110, 1171–1180. doi: 10.1152/japplphysiol.01037.2010

Tsvetanov, K. A., Henson, R. N. A., Tyler, L. K., Davis, S. W., Shafto, M. A., Taylor, J. R., et al. (2015). The effect of ageing on fMRI: correction for the confounding effects of vascular reactivity evaluated by joint fMRI and MEG in 335 adults. *Hum. Brain Mapp.* 36, 2248–2269. doi: 10.1002/hbm.22768

Tustison, N. J., Avants, B. B., Cook, P. A., Zheng, Y., Egan, A., Yushkevich, P. A., et al. (2010). N4ITK: improved N3 bias correction. *IEEE Trans. Med. Imaging* 29, 1310–1320. doi: 10.1109/TMI.2010.2046908

van Osch, M. J. P., Teeuwisse, W. M., van Walderveen, M. A. A., Hendrikse, J., Kies, D. A., and van Buchem, M. A.. (2009). Can arterial spin labeling detect white matter perfusion signal? *Magn. Reson. Med.* 62, 165–173. doi: 10.1002/mrm.22002

Vecchio, F., Miraglia, F., Curcio, G., Altavilla, R., Scrascia, F., Giambattistelli, F., et al. (2015). Cortical brain connectivity evaluated by graph theory in dementia: a correlation study between functional and structural data. *J. Alzheimers Dis.* 45, 745–756. doi: 10.3233/JAD-142484

Viviani, R., Messina, I., and Walter, M. (2011). Resting state functional connectivity in perfusion imaging: correlation maps with BOLD connectivity and resting state perfusion. *PLoS One* 6:e27050. doi: 10.1371/journal.pone.0027050

Wang, Z., Aguirre, G. K., Rao, H., Wang, J., Fernández-Seara, M. A., Childress, A. R., et al. (2008). Empirical optimization of ASL data analysis using an ASL data processing toolbox: ASLtbx. *Magn. Reson. Imaging* 26, 261–269. doi: 10.1016/j.mri.2007.07.003

Wise, R. G., Harris, A. D., Stone, A. J., and Murphy, K. (2013). Measurement of OEF and absolute $CMRO_2$: MRI-based methods using interleaved and combined hypercapnia and hyperoxia. *Neuroimage* 83, 135–147. doi: 10.1016/j.neuroimage.2013.06.008

Wise, R. G., Ide, K., Poulin, M. J., and Tracey, I. (2004). Resting fluctuations in arterial carbon dioxide induce significant low frequency variations in BOLD signal. *Neuroimage* 21, 1652–1664. doi: 10.1016/j.neuroimage.2003.11.025

Woods, R. P., Grafton, S. T., Holmes, C. J., Cherry, S. R., and Mazziotta, J. C. (1998). Automated image registration: I. general methods and intrasubject, intramodality validation. *J. Comput. Assist. Tomogr.* 22, 139–152. doi: 10.1097/00004728-199801000-00027

Wu, C. W., Gu, H., Lu, H., Stein, E. A., Chen, J.-H., and Yang, Y. (2009). Mapping functional connectivity based on synchronized $CMRO_2$ fluctuations during the resting state. *Neuroimage* 45, 694–701. doi: 10.1016/j.neuroimage.2008.12.066

Zappe, A. C., Pfeuffer, J., Merkle, H., Logothetis, N. K., and Goense, J. B. M. (2008). The effect of labeling parameters on perfusion-based fMRI in nonhuman primates. *J. Cereb. Blood Flow Metab.* 28, 640–652. doi: 10.1038/sj.jcbfm.9600564

Zou, Q., Wu, C. W., Stein, E. A., Zang, Y., and Yang, Y. (2009). Static and dynamic characteristics of cerebral blood flow during the resting state. *Neuroimage* 48, 515–524. doi: 10.1016/j.neuroimage.2009.07.006

7

Insulin Resistance and Alzheimer's Disease: Bioenergetic Linkages

Bryan J. Neth and Suzanne Craft*

Department of Internal Medicine, Section on Gerontology and Geriatric Medicine, Wake Forest School of Medicine, Winston-Salem, NC, United States

***Correspondence:**
Bryan J. Neth
bneth@wakehealth.edu

Metabolic dysfunction is a well-established feature of Alzheimer's disease (AD), evidenced by brain glucose hypometabolism that can be observed potentially decades prior to the development of AD symptoms. Furthermore, there is mounting support for an association between metabolic disease and the development of AD and related dementias. Individuals with insulin resistance, type 2 diabetes mellitus (T2D), hyperlipidemia, obesity, or other metabolic disease may have increased risk for the development of AD and similar conditions, such as vascular dementia. This association may in part be due to the systemic mitochondrial dysfunction that is common to these pathologies. Accumulating evidence suggests that mitochondrial dysfunction is a significant feature of AD and may play a fundamental role in its pathogenesis. In fact, aging itself presents a unique challenge due to inherent mitochondrial dysfunction and prevalence of chronic metabolic disease. Despite the progress made in understanding the pathogenesis of AD and in the development of potential therapies, at present we remain without a disease-modifying treatment. In this review, we will discuss insulin resistance as a contributing factor to the pathogenesis of AD, as well as the metabolic and bioenergetic disruptions linking insulin resistance and AD. We will also focus on potential neuroimaging tools for the study of the metabolic dysfunction commonly seen in AD with hopes of developing therapeutic and preventative targets.

Keywords: Alzheimer's disease, insulin resistance, bioenergetic shift, ketone body, inflammation, metabolism, positron emission tomography

INTRODUCTION AND OVERVIEW

Alzheimer's disease (AD) is a fatal neurodegenerative disorder that afflicts an estimated 5.3 million people in the United States. Due to socioeconomic forces such as an aging population, the prevalence of AD is projected to nearly triple to about 13.8 million Americans at an annual cost of greater than $1 trillion by 2050 (Alzheimer's Association, 2015). AD consists of two forms; familial or early-onset AD (FAD), which constitutes less than 5% of all AD cases and is normally diagnosed prior to the age of 65 years, with clear genetic risk through inherited mutations in three main genes: amyloid precursor protein (APP), presenilin 1 (PSEN1) and presenilin 2 (PSEN2; Selkoe, 1996). Sporadic or late-onset-AD (LOAD) makes up the great majority of all AD cases and is usually diagnosed after the age of 65 years. The most prominent risk factor for the development of LOAD is advanced age and indeed the incidence of AD increases with advancing age.

Although several genetic risk factors for LOAD have been identified, the most significant of these is the Apolipoprotein-E-epsilon-4 allele (APOE4), which is an isoform of the APOE gene that plays a role in cholesterol and beta-amyloid peptide (Aβ) homeostasis (Genin et al., 2011; Karch et al., 2012; Alzheimer's Association, 2015).

AD is characterized by a progressive deterioration in cognition with significant impairments in memory, executive function and behavioral/personality changes. Neuropathologic hallmarks of AD include neuritic plaques and neurofibrillary tangles that are initially seen in the medial temporal lobes and eventually extend throughout the cortex (Braak and Braak, 1991; Braak et al., 2006). Additional misfolded proteins, including TAR DNA binding protein 43 (TDP-43) positive inclusions may be found in brains of individuals with AD (Amador-Ortiz et al., 2007). The leading hypothesis concerning the pathogenesis of AD is the Amyloid Cascade Hypothesis, which postulates that Aβ plays a central role in AD pathology leading to oxidative injury, synaptic/neuronal dysfunction and eventual neurodegeneration (Hardy and Higgins, 1992; Hardy and Selkoe, 2002). The clinical path of AD may be viewed as a continuum with an extended asymptomatic stage without cognitive or behavioral symptoms, but with documentable changes in brain pathological processes—with ultimate progression to mild cognitive impairment (MCI) and eventually dementia with cognitive and functional decline (Sperling et al., 2011).

Central metabolic dysfunction is a well-established feature of AD, evidenced by brain glucose hypometabolism that can be observed potentially decades prior to the development of AD symptoms (Reiman et al., 1996; Small et al., 2000; Sperling et al., 2011). Furthermore, there is mounting support for an association between metabolic disease and the development of AD and related dementias (Whitmer et al., 2008; Craft, 2009). Individuals with insulin resistance, type 2 diabetes mellitus (T2D), hyperlipidemia, obesity, or other metabolic disease may have increased risk for the development of AD and similar conditions, such as vascular dementia (Craft, 2009; Di Paolo and Kim, 2011). This association may in part be due to the systemic mitochondrial dysfunction that is common to these pathologies (Lesnefsky et al., 2001; Lowell and Shulman, 2005; Madamanchi and Runge, 2007; Johri and Beal, 2012). Accumulating evidence suggests that mitochondrial dysfunction is a significant feature of AD and may play a fundamental role in its pathogenesis (Yao et al., 2010; Yao and Brinton, 2011; Chaturvedi and Beal, 2013). In fact, aging itself presents a unique challenge due to inherent mitochondrial dysfunction and prevalence of chronic metabolic disease (Mammucari and Rizzuto, 2010; Cui et al., 2012).

Despite the progress made in understanding the pathogenesis of AD and in the development of potential therapies, at present we remain without a disease-modifying treatment (Armstrong, 2011; Schneider et al., 2011a,b; Howard et al., 2012; Doody et al., 2014; Salloway et al., 2014). In this review, we will discuss insulin resistance as a contributing factor to the pathogenesis of AD, as well as the metabolic and bioenergetic disruptions linking insulin resistance and AD. We will close with a review of potential tools for the study of the metabolic dysfunction commonly seen in AD.

METABOLIC PATHWAYS TO ALZHEIMER'S DISEASE: INSULIN RESISTANCE

Overview of Insulin in the Brain

Insulin is a peptide hormone secreted principally by pancreatic beta cells with well-characterized functions in glucose/lipid metabolism, vascular regulation, and cell growth (Saltiel and Kahn, 2001; Muniyappa et al., 2007). Mounting evidence suggests that insulin plays a vital role in the central nervous system (CNS; Craft and Watson, 2004; Ketterer et al., 2011; Liu et al., 2011; Banks et al., 2012; Correia et al., 2012; Duarte et al., 2012; Cholerton et al., 2013; Craft et al., 2013; Blázquez et al., 2014). Insulin readily crosses the Blood Brain Barrier (BBB) through a saturable, receptor-mediated process (Baskin et al., 1987; Baura et al., 1993; Banks et al., 1997a,b; Woods et al., 2003). Moreover, several regions in the brain (hypothalamus, choroid plexus, etc.) may serve as a more rapid site of entry for peripheral insulin into the CNS (Baskin et al., 1987). There is continuing debate concerning production of insulin within CNS. Studies in animal models have described presence of insulin mRNA in various brain regions (Banks et al., 2012; Duarte et al., 2012). Clinical studies have described the presence of C-peptide, which is secreted at the time of insulin production in pancreatic beta cells, in cerebrospinal fluid (CSF; Ghasemi et al., 2013b; Blázquez et al., 2014). However, this too may be from the pancreas and not produced within the CNS.

Insulin exerts its action through binding to the insulin receptor (IR) with two different isoforms (IR-A and IR-B). IR-A is found in the adult nervous system and has a higher affinity for insulin than IR-B, which is found mainly is adipose tissue, hepatic tissue, and skeletal muscle (Zhao W.-Q. et al., 2004; Dou et al., 2005; Watson and Craft, 2006; Banks et al., 2012; Ghasemi et al., 2013b). However, a recent study has reported IR-B expression in astrocytes (Garwood et al., 2015), with a potential role in mediating insulin and insulin-like growth factor (IGF) function in the CNS. It is important to note that insulin-like growth factor-1 and 2 (IGF-1, IGF-2) can also bind at the IR, but at decreased affinity than insulin (Banks et al., 2012; Kleinridders et al., 2014). IRs are tyrosine kinases with alpha and beta subunits. Once insulin or other substrates are bound, the alpha subunit promotes autophosphorylation of tyrosine residues on the beta subunits leading to the recruitment of scaffolding proteins, mainly IR substrates 1 and 2 (IRS-1 and IRS-2). IRS-1, 2 ultimately connect insulin to two significant signal transduction pathways: the PI3K/Akt pathway, largely responsible for metabolic effects, lipid/protein synthesis and the Ras/ERK pathway which modulates cell growth, survival, and gene expression (De Felice and Ferreira, 2014; Kleinridders et al., 2014). IRs are located in both neurons and glia (Abbott et al., 1999). These receptors are selectively distributed throughout the brain, with higher concentrations in the olfactory bulb, cerebral cortex, hippocampus, hypothalamus, amygdala, and septum—regions of strategic importance for feeding and cognition (Havrankova et al., 1978a,b; Baskin et al., 1987; Unger et al., 1991). Similar to IR, IGF-1 receptors (IGF1-R) are also tyrosine kinases binding IGF-1/2 and insulin. Interestingly, both IR and IGF1-R can form hybrids of either heterodimers or homodimers with each other. The ultimate downstream effects depend on the ligand and type/location of receptor. Likewise, the affinity of the ligand also depends on the receptor type. The distribution of IR, IGF1-R, and their hybrids are regionally specific within the CNS (Kleinridders, 2016; Cai et al., 2017). Refer to a recent review by Kleinridders (2016) for a more comprehensive understanding of IR and IGF-1 receptors in the brain.

Insulin and Cognition

An acute elevation of peripheral insulin (generally in response to an increase in exogenous or endogenous glucose) promotes insulin transport across the BBB into the CNS, thus facilitating its role for a variety of important brain functions (Woods et al., 2003; Kleinridders et al., 2014). The regional localization of IR in the hippocampus (Werther et al., 1987) suggests that insulin may influence memory, one of the main tasks supported by the hippocampus and closely connected structures. Intracerebroventricular administration of insulin in rats has been shown to improve passive avoidance and spatial memory (Park et al., 2000; Haj-ali et al., 2009). Clinical studies utilizing acute intravenous administration of insulin with maintenance of euglycemia have described enhanced performance in verbal memory (Craft et al., 1996, 1999, 2003; Kern et al., 2001). Similar memory improvement has been observed following administration of intranasal insulin (Benedict et al., 2004, 2008; Stockhorst et al., 2004; Reger et al., 2006, 2008; Craft et al., 2012; Schiöth et al., 2012; Claxton et al., 2013, 2015; Freiherr et al., 2013; Novak et al., 2014); these studies will be reviewed in detail below. In total, the above work forms a strong foundation for insulin's role in memory, one of the key cognitive domains affected by AD.

Intriguingly, the process of learning may modify IR expression and function throughout specific brain regions (Zhao et al., 1999; Zhao W.-Q. et al., 2004; Agrawal et al., 2011). In rats, spatial memory training has been shown to upregulate IR mRNA in the hippocampal CA1 region and dentate gyrus and lead to increased accumulation of IR protein within the hippocampus. Moreover, training increased insulin-stimulated tyrosine phosphorylation of the IR *in vitro* in trained animals (Zhao et al., 1999). These results suggest that learning itself may influence both IR concentration and insulin signaling in the hippocampus and potentially other brain regions. It is likely that insulin plays a key role in learning and memory given IR localization in the hippocampus, IR changes in the hippocampus secondary to spatial learning, and improvements in memory secondary to insulin administration in both animal models and human studies. Although it is not entirely clear how insulin exerts its action on cognition, several mechanisms likely contribute.

Insulin and Cerebral Glucose Metabolism

One such mechanism by which insulin may influence cognition is by affecting cerebral energy metabolism. The importance of glucose in the CNS is demonstrated by the disproportionate metabolic rate of the brain relative most organs and tissues. While the brain only makes up 2% of the average body weight, it utilizes about 25% of the body's glucose and 20% of the body's oxygen to meet metabolic demand (Attwell and Laughlin, 2001; Bélanger et al., 2011). The energy derived from glucose metabolism is used to maintain neuronal ion gradients and cell membrane lipid remodeling, among other processes (Attwell and Laughlin, 2001). Insulin undoubtedly is crucial for peripheral energy metabolism in adipose tissue, hepatic tissue, and skeletal muscle (Saltiel and Kahn, 2001). Until recently brain (glucose) metabolism has largely been thought of as insulin-independent. Yet, recent research has highlighted an important role of insulin in cerebral/peripheral metabolism and other functions (Banks et al., 2012; Blázquez et al., 2014).

Bingham et al. (2002) reported increased cerebral glucose metabolism after restoration of basal levels of insulin in metabolically healthy participants. Metabolic changes were most apparent in cortical areas. This work indicates that normal basal levels of peripheral insulin may play an important role in the maintenance of cerebral glucose metabolism. In a recent study of adults with metabolic dysfunction, Hirvonen et al. (2011) reported increased glucose metabolism on ^{18}F-fluorodeoxyglucose (FDG) Positron Emission Tomography (PET) imaging after a hyperinsulinemic clamp procedure. Interestingly, glucose metabolism was not affected by the hyperinsulinemic condition in metabolically healthy participants (Hirvonen et al., 2011). These results support the view that insulin may modify cerebral glucose metabolism, and that effects may differ depending upon metabolic status.

Insulin likely exerts regional effects on cerebral glucose metabolism due to the localized distribution of glucose transporters (GLUTs; Schulingkamp et al., 2000; Reagan et al., 2001). A recent review by Shah et al. (2012) discusses the role of these transporters in brain disease, with a focus on AD and diabetes. The insulin independent GLUT1 and GLUT3 were traditionally believed to be the sole cerebral GLUTs (Lund-Andersen, 1979). These GLUTs are expressed at the BBB and within neurons and glia (Devraj et al., 2011; Shah et al., 2012). However, it is now apparent that insulin-responsive GLUTs, such as GLUT4 and GLUT8, are also localized within specific brain regions such as the hippocampus, cerebellum, sensorimotor cortex, hypothalamus and pituitary (Brant et al., 1993; Livingstone et al., 1995; El Messari et al., 1998; Apelt et al., 1999; Reagan et al., 2001; Shah et al., 2012). Insulin has been reported to increase cerebral GLUT4 expression and translocation (Piroli et al., 2007). Importantly, insulin-responsive GLUT4 and GLUT8 are co-localized to regions that express IR and insulin (Apelt et al., 1999; Schulingkamp et al., 2000). Our understanding of cerebral glucose metabolism continues to expand, with new insights supporting the role of insulin in mediating at least some portion of cerebral glucose metabolism, which likely impacts cognitive processes including learning and memory.

Other Actions

In addition to insulin's function in cerebral glucose metabolism, another mechanism by which it may impact the brain is its influence on long-term potentiation (LTP; Zhao and Alkon, 2001). In particular, insulin has been reported to affect the expression of N-methyl-D-aspartate (NMDA) receptors (Skeberdis et al., 2001). Furthermore, insulin has been shown to modulate levels of the neurotransmitters, acetylcholine and norepinephrine, which have been shown to influence cognition (Figlewicz et al., 1993; Kopf and Baratti, 1999). Insulin also serves other important functions through actions in the brain such as neuroprotective effects as well as mediation of vascular function through nitric oxide (NO) and endothelin-1 (Banks et al., 2012; Katakam et al., 2012; Blázquez et al., 2014). The importance of insulin's role in the CNS is becoming increasingly clear as converging evidence demonstrates that disrupted insulin signaling (insulin resistance) may promote neurodegenerative disorders, such as AD (Craft, 2007, 2009; Neumann et al., 2008; Cholerton et al., 2011; Correia et al., 2012; Chen and Zhong, 2013; Ghasemi et al., 2013b; Blázquez et al., 2014; De Felice and Ferreira, 2014; Sridhar et al., 2015).

Overview of Insulin Resistance

Insulin resistance occurs when insulin binding to its receptors has diminished effects. Although this term is most commonly applied to decreased glucose clearance from the blood and entry into target tissues (Reaven, 1983, 2003; DeFronzo et al., 1992), it can also refer to insulin's ability to engage its canonical signaling network in any target tissue. In the periphery this resistance is accompanied by increased release of insulin from the pancreas to meet the demand of chronically elevated levels of glucose and/or increased amount of adipose tissue that requires insulin for its glucose metabolism (DeFronzo et al., 1992). Prolonged elevation of systemic insulin may ultimately lead to a dysfunction in insulin signaling (DeFronzo, 2010). This chronic elevation in peripheral insulin levels also impacts central insulin availability and function. Insulin's passage through the BBB is transporter-mediated (Banks et al., 2012). In a healthy state, an acute, transient rise in peripheral insulin leads to an increase in CNS insulin, where it enters the brain. Chronic peripheral hyperinsulinemia leads to the downregulation of insulin transporters at the BBB, which in turn decreases the amount of insulin that may enter brain (Wallum et al., 1987; Schwartz et al., 1990; Banks et al., 2012). This CNS insulin deficiency may potentially lead to impairments in memory, neuroprotective effects, synaptic transmission, as well as likely contributing to the development of neurodegenerative disease (Craft and Watson, 2004; Craft, 2007; Cholerton et al., 2011; Correia et al., 2012; Ghasemi et al., 2013a; Blázquez et al., 2014; De Felice and Ferreira, 2014; De Felice and Lourenco, 2015). Importantly, negative impacts of insulin resistance occur years prior to the development of clinically defined diabetes (Roriz-Filho et al., 2009). Early defects in insulin signaling may be associated with pathologic brain changes even decades before clinical symptoms of the disease (Roriz-Filho et al., 2009). Moreover, patients may not appreciate significant symptoms until the disease process has already exerted a negative, and potentially irreversible impact on peripheral tissues and the brain (Sperling et al., 2011; Sridhar et al., 2015).

Impact of Insulin Resistance on the Brain

In a metabolically healthy state, an acute elevation of insulin levels has a beneficial impact on cognitive function. However, chronically elevated insulin greatly diminishes insulin's end-organ effects (Neumann et al., 2008). Evidence supporting this include impaired learning in animal models of T2D and in humans with the disorder (Greenwood and Winocur, 2001). Vanhanen et al. (1998) described lower scores on the Bushcke Selective Reminding Task (verbal learning and memory) in older adults with impaired glucose tolerance. Insulin resistance also impacts brain structure and function corresponding with changes in brain volumes and cerebral glucose metabolism. Convit et al. (2003) described lower hippocampal volumes in older adults with impaired glucose tolerance, which were also associated with lower scores on delayed recall of a logical memory task. Similarly, a study by Kerti et al. (2013) reported that adults with higher fasting glucose and HbA1c had lower delayed recall, learning, and memory consolidation utilizing the Rey Auditory Verbal Learning Test. Higher fasting glucose and HbA1c also correlated with lower hippocampal volume and altered hippocampal microstructure as determined by Mean Diffusivity, a Diffusion Tensor Imaging (DTI) metric (Kerti et al., 2013). Further analysis in this group suggested that the beneficial effects of lower blood glucose on learning and memory could in part be explained by the hippocampal changes described in the study (Kerti et al., 2013). Moreover, we have previously reported that older adults with insulin resistance (pre-diabetes or diabetes without treatment) showed AD-like patterns of reduced brain glucose metabolism, as quantified with FDG PET imaging. Glucose hypometabolism was most apparent in frontal, parietotemporal, and cingulate cortices (Baker et al., 2011). This finding is profound in that it provides evidence that insulin resistance affects similar brain areas as AD, supporting the view that insulin resistance may promote neurodegenerative disease. Diabetes has been shown to be a strong predictor of cognitive decline in older adults (Yaffe et al., 2004, 2006; Cheng et al., 2012; Biessels et al., 2014). In fact, those with diabetes may be twice as likely to experience a decline in cognition over 5 years relative to those without the disorder (Tilvis et al., 2004). Likewise, several epidemiologic studies have described an association between insulin resistance and cognitive impairment and/or the development of dementia in older adults (Hassing et al., 2004; Yaffe et al., 2004; Strachan, 2011; Cheng et al., 2012). Cognitive impairment is not restricted to changes in learning and memory, but also other domains. For example, Abbatecola et al. (2004) showed that insulin resistance was associated with longer time to complete Trail Making Test—Part B. The Trail Making Test is a task of processing speed, cognitive flexibility and visual motor skills and has sensitivity for a variety of disorders negatively affecting cognition (Bowie and Harvey, 2006). Given current evidence insulin resistance must be considered an important risk factor for cognitive decline.

Research in humans is largely supported by work in animal models of insulin resistance, describing its negative impact on cognitive performance. Stranahan et al. (2008) demonstrated that a high-saturated fat diet supplemented with high fructose corn syrup-laden water, as a proxy for a "Western Diet," led to worse performance on a spatial memory (water-maze) task relative to control animals and reduced LTP after 8 months on diet. Rats on a high saturated fat diet developed insulin resistance, which was accompanied by lower concentrations of hippocampal brain-derived neurotrophic factor (BDNF; Stranahan et al., 2008). These results provide evidence supporting the profound impact that insulin resistance may have on the mammalian brain, an in particular on the hippocampus, one of the primary brain regions implicated in AD pathology.

In summary, work in both humans and animal models suggest that insulin resistance has detrimental effects on cognition, most notably learning and memory. Given the vital influence of insulin resistance on brain, it is important to further understand the metabolic pathways that may be impacted in such conditions, as well as how these pathways related to AD and other neurodegenerative disorders.

BIOENERGETIC DISRUPTIONS IN INSULIN RESISTANT STATE RELEVANT TO ALZHEIMER'S DISEASE

Although the pathogenesis of insulin resistance and AD are yet to be fully elucidated, both share common pathologic features, supporting the notion that systemic insulin resistance may ultimately promote AD. Common features of an insulin resistant state and AD include inflammation, dyslipidemia, amyloidogenesis and overt bioenergetic dysfunction.

Inflammation and Vascular Dysfunction

Chronic inflammation is detrimental to the body and brain (Blasko et al., 2004; Khansari et al., 2009; Schwartz and Baruch, 2014), with elevated levels of inflammatory cytokines and chemokines reported in AD and insulin resistance (Blum-Degen et al., 1995; Pradhan et al., 2001; Kubaszek et al., 2003; Swardfager et al., 2010). Not surprisingly, chronic low-level inflammation in adipose tissue has been hypothesized to contribute to the pathogenesis of insulin resistance (Festa et al., 2000; Akash et al., 2013). A type of inflammatory cell, the adipose tissue macrophage, may be a central player in perpetuating the inflammatory cascade that ultimately leads to insulin resistance and T2D (Lee, 2013). Inflammation has been a feature commonly identified in studies of AD and other neurodegenerative disorders (Akiyama et al., 2000; Amor et al., 2010; Wyss-Coray and Rogers, 2012). Inflammatory cytokines are commonly elevated in the plasma and CSF of Alzheimer's patients (Blum-Degen et al., 1995; Swardfager et al., 2010). Furthermore, research has explored the role of other inflammatory mediators in AD with focus on BBB and vascular integrity (Ryu and McLarnon, 2009; Takeda et al., 2013).

A powerful mediator of inflammation and vascular dysfunction common to both insulin resistance and AD are advanced glycation end products (AGEs), which are glycated proteins and lipids formed through non-enzymatic glycosylation after exposure to glucose (Singh et al., 2001). There are increased AGEs in adults with insulin resistance and diabetes relative to healthy controls (Goldin et al., 2006; Unoki et al., 2007; Unoki and Yamagishi, 2008; Yamagishi et al., 2012). Accumulation of AGEs may exert negative effects on tissues. For example, AGE binding to its target, the receptor for advanced glycation end products (RAGE), promotes upregulation of nuclear factor-kappa beta (NF-κβ), which is a transcription factor and crucial mediator of inflammation (Goldin et al., 2006). AGEs may block the production of NO in the endothelium, thereby mitigating its vasodilatory effects. Moreover, a complex of AGE-RAGE may interfere with vascular structure, making it permeable to macromolecule invasion and resultant pathology (Goldin et al., 2006). Wautier et al. (1996) reported that inhibition of RAGE prevents the AGE-related changes in vascular permeability within diabetic rats. This research suggests that a prominent feature in individuals with insulin resistance (AGE) may propagate an inflammatory cascade and vascular injury. AGEs are also more elevated in adults with AD than age-matched controls and may ultimately contribute to AD pathology (Sasaki et al., 1998; Srikanth et al., 2011). AGEs have been discovered in amyloid-containing senile plaques, tau-containing neurofibrillary tangles, neurons and glia (Lüth et al., 2005). Glycation of Aβ has been shown to enhance its aggregation (Sasaki et al., 1998) AGEs have been reported to stimulate tau hyperphosphorylation, which is attenuated with inhibition of RAGE in rats (Lüth et al., 2005). Moreover, AGEs stimulate similar oxidative stress, inflammation, and vascular pathology in the brain as that found in the periphery (Ramasamy et al., 2005).

Dyslipidemia

Insulin is an important mediator of lipid metabolism, and a core feature of insulin resistance is dyslipidemia (DeFronzo and Ferrannini, 1991; Savage et al., 2007). Lipids and cholesterol constitute a significant portion of the brain mass, with continual turnover, especially at synapses and cellular connections (Robinson et al., 1992; Purdon et al., 2002). Impaired lipid metabolism may therefore have a profound impact on the brain and contribute to neurologic disease. The characteristic lipid profile of chronic insulin resistance includes elevated free fatty acids (FFA), which inhibit the insulin-related suppression of very low density lipoprotein (VLDL) secretion by the liver (DeFronzo and Ferrannini, 1991). This contributes to an altered lipid balance with elevated VLDL and other lipids, which may perpetuate an insulin resistant state (DeFronzo and Ferrannini, 1991; Kamagate et al., 2008). Higher low density lipoprotein (LDL) and lower high density lipoprotein (HDL) levels are known cardiovascular risk factors, and could play a role in development of AD-related amyloid deposition, potentially due to the impact of cholesterol on Aβ processing within the brain (Reitz, 2013; Berti et al., 2015).

Furthermore, various genetic studies including genome-wide association studies (GWAS) have identified several genes involved with lipid and cholesterol metabolism as increasing risk for AD. Most notably is Apolipoprotein-E (APOE), followed by Apolipoprotein-J (APOJ or Clusterin, CLU), ATP-binding cassette subfamily A member 7 (ABCA7) and sortilin-like receptor (SORL1; Reitz, 2013). Although our understanding of dyslipidemia, cholesterol metabolism and its relation to AD is incomplete, it seems plausible that altered states of systemic lipid metabolism may contribute to pathologic brain changes seen in the disease. A study by Reed et al. (2014) reported that higher levels of LDL and lower levels of HDL were associated with higher amount of amyloid concentration as determined by Pittsburgh Compound B (PiB) PET imaging. These results suggest a potential association between dyslipidemia and cardiovascular risk and the accumulation of cerebral amyloid, which may in turn be mediated by insulin resistance as well as other causes of disturbed lipid metabolism, such as carriage of the APOE4 allele. Intriguingly, a recent study suggests that carriage of an APOE4 allele may contribute to diminished IR signaling by directly interacting with the IR, impairing its trafficking and ultimately leading to the IR being trapped within endosomes (Zhao et al., 2017). This may provide novel insight into the role of APOE and its relation to insulin signaling, thus explaining the differential response to intranasal insulin in APOE4 carriers (Reger et al., 2006; Claxton et al., 2013, 2015).

Amyloidogenesis

Both AD and T2D are amyloidogenic conditions; Aβ (1–40 and 1–42) is found at increased concentrations in AD and amylin (islet amyloid polypeptide, IAPP) is found at elevated levels within insulin resistant states (Cooper et al., 1989; Hardy and Higgins, 1992; Lim et al., 2010). Amylin accumulates primarily in the pancreas, which may potentiate the development of T2D and worsening insulin resistance as pancreatic beta cells become depleted (Cooper et al., 1989; Jackson et al., 2013). Recent studies have also described amylin accumulation in other tissues throughout the body, including in cerebral vasculature and brain parenchyma (Despa et al., 2012; Jackson et al., 2013; Srodulski et al., 2014). Jackson et al. (2013) described the accumulation of oligomeric amylin and amylin plaques in the temporal lobes, vasculature and perivascular spaces of older adults with T2D, but not in age-matched controls. A similar pattern of amylin deposition was found in the cerebral vessels and brain parenchyma of adults with AD, even in the absence of T2D. Co-localized amylin and Aβ deposition were also observed (Jackson et al., 2013). These results suggest that amylin may have a pathologic impact on the brain and contribute to metabolic risk for AD. It is becoming increasingly clear that the amylin and Aβ may not be mutually exclusive. Research suggests that amylin may indeed contribute to the accumulation of Aβ in AD through seeding effects (Yan et al., 2014; Oskarsson et al., 2015). Yet, further research into this Aβ-amylin interaction must be performed in order to fully understand the molecular link between these two amyloidogenic molecules.

Furthermore, insulin has been shown to impact Aβ, which has traditionally been implicated in the pathogenesis of AD (Hardy and Higgins, 1992; Hardy and Selkoe, 2002). Evidence in animal models suggests that brain insulin deficiency may lead to increased formation of Aβ due to the upregulation of APP and beta-secretase 1 (BACE1), which are involved in formation of Aβ (Devi et al., 2012). *In vitro* studies have reported that insulin impacts amount of Aβ. For example, in neuronal cultures insulin stimulates the release of intracellular Aβ (1–40 and 1–42) into the extracellular space. Trafficking of intracellular Aβ and APP is accelerated as they are transported from the Golgi/trans-Golgi network to the plasma membrane (Gasparini et al., 2001). An insulin resistant state would interfere with this action of insulin and reduce trafficking of Aβ out of the cell.

A significant factor in Aβ degradation is the metalloprotease insulin-degrading enzyme (IDE; Cook et al., 2003; Farris et al., 2003; Zhao L. et al., 2004). IDE is highly expressed in tissue throughout the body, including brain, liver, skeletal muscle and kidney (Authier et al., 1996). Importantly, IDE has been described to facilitate the breakdown of both insulin and Aβ (Kurochkin and Goto, 1994; McDermott and Gibson, 1997; Qiu et al., 1998; Sudoh et al., 2002; Zhao L. et al., 2004). The IDE-dependent degradation of Aβ has been shown to occur through a PI3K-dependent mechanism (Zhao L. et al., 2004). Thus, an early insulin-resistant state (with higher levels of circulating insulin) may contribute to the accumulation of Aβ due to competition for IDE (Qiu et al., 1998; Roriz-Filho et al., 2009; Bosco et al., 2011). Research in AD mouse models has further solidified the role of insulin resistance in IDE-related amyloid pathology. Tg2576 mice with diet-induced insulin resistance had increased production of Aβ (1–40 and 1–42) in the brain relative to Tg2576 mice without insulin resistance. Interestingly, these results were associated with an increased gamma-secretase activity and decreased IDE activity (Ho et al., 2004). Moreover, IDE knockout mice have been shown to have a reduced breakdown of cerebral Aβ and insulin (Pérez et al., 2000; Cook et al., 2003; Farris et al., 2003). These results suggest that insulin resistance may independently contribute to amyloid production and exacerbate an already amyloidogenic state, such as AD.

Chronically elevated peripheral insulin may lead to lower levels of insulin within the CNS (Wallum et al., 1987; Schwartz et al., 1990; Banks et al., 2012). Initially cerebral levels of insulin may be increased (as with the periphery), yet insulin eventually decreases as BBB transport is reduced and amyloid accumulates, promoting central insulin resistance (Banks et al., 1997b). This process may negatively impact insulin's functions in the brain and the clearance of Aβ. Patients with AD have been shown to have lower insulin in the CSF, elevated insulin in the blood, and a lower CSF:Plasma insulin ratio relative to healthy controls (Craft et al., 1998). Furthermore, increased peripheral insulin concentration may interrupt breakdown of Aβ after being transported out of the brain as well as by interfering with its exit from the brain. A potential mediator of these effects is LDL receptor-related protein (LRP-1). Tamaki et al. (2007) reported that insulin mediates the hepatic uptake of circulating Aβ (1–40) from the blood by increasing LRP-1 expression on hepatic cellular plasma membranes. This process is dose-dependent and reversed with administration of an LRP-1 inhibitor (Tamaki et al., 2007). LRP-1 has also been shown to contribute to Aβ (1–40) transport across the BBB to the peripheral circulation (Ito et al., 2006). These results suggest that insulin resistance may contribute to the accumulation of amyloid species due to impaired clearance from the brain to the periphery where it may be cleared by the liver. Both decreased removal of Aβ from the CNS and reduced degradation of Aβ once it reaches the periphery may contribute to the clogging of a peripheral Aβ "sink." Thus, the pattern of high peripheral insulin levels and low brain insulin levels may increase risk for AD and ultimately help exacerbate disease pathology.

Additional mechanisms may relate insulin resistance to AD pathology. For example, the soluble form of Aβ is able to bind to the IR, and has been shown to disrupt insulin signaling and activation of three kinases in primary hippocampal neurons (Townsend et al., 2007). Specifically, Aβ was shown to act through diminishing insulin-induced autophosphorylation (Townsend et al., 2007). Moreover, a study by Zhang et al. (2013) suggests that Aβ promotes hepatic insulin resistance through JAK2 signaling. Taken together these results infer that over accumulation of Aβ may promote impaired insulin signaling that could further propagate disease pathology. Synaptotoxic effects also link Aβ and insulin. Synapse loss is an early event in AD pathology, which may be promoted by soluble Aβ oligomers (Selkoe, 2002; Scheff et al., 2006). Insulin has been shown to prevent binding of Aβ to synapses, thus minimizing synaptic damage (De Felice et al., 2009). Insulin has also been shown to diminish formation of Aβ oligomers, which is likely protective against Aβ oligomer-related damage (Lee et al., 2009). This research suggests that a pathologic hallmark of AD initiated by Aβ oligomers may be mitigated by insulin administration. Inflammation, dyslipidemia, and amyloidogenesis are each prominent features linking insulin resistance and AD. Yet, one of the most important connections between the two pathologies is the inherent bioenergetic dysfunction that is common to each.

Bioenergetic Dysfunction in Insulin Resistance and Alzheimer's Disease

Another common feature of AD and insulin resistance is mitochondrial dysfunction, which is supported by several key findings (Lowell and Shulman, 2005; Kim et al., 2008; Szendroedi et al., 2011; Johri and Beal, 2012; Chaturvedi and Beal, 2013). First, enzymes involved in energy metabolism are differentially regulated in AD. Lower activity of the pyruvate dehydrogenase (PDH) and alpha-ketoglutarate dehydrogenase (AKGDH) complexes has been reported in AD (Park et al., 1999; Blass, 2000; Starkov et al., 2004). These enzymes are fundamental for cellular respiration, with PDH being particularly important for linking glycolytic metabolism to the Kreb's cycle. Like many bioenergetic enzymes, both may be affected by the accumulation of oxidative moieties leading to decreased enzyme efficiency and ultimate production of reactive oxygen species (ROS) and further oxidative stress (Wei and Lee, 2002).

Second, mitochondrial function in adults with AD may be affected by the accumulation of Aβ, which seems to be at least partly mediated by Aβ-binding-alcohol-dehydrogenase (ABAD; Yao et al., 2011; Chaturvedi and Beal, 2013). Specifically, Aβ has been shown to inhibit activity of complexes II and IV of the electron transport chain (ETC) and lead to increased production of ROS (Swerdlow et al., 2010; Yao et al., 2011; Chaturvedi and Beal, 2013). Reduced activity of complex IV, also known as cytochrome c oxidase (COX), has been widely reported in platelets as well as within the brain, which supports the view of AD being a systemic disorder (Parker et al., 1990; Cardoso et al., 2004). Aβ and APP have been implicated in the disruption of mitochondrial dynamics (fission/fusion), contributing to the mitochondrial dysfunction seen in AD (Wang et al., 2008, 2009; Chaturvedi and Beal, 2013).

Additionally, Aβ has been shown to impair mitochondrial calcium homeostasis, which may lead to disruption of mitochondrial permeability transition pore and eventually cell death (Bezprozvanny and Mattson, 2008; Reddy, 2009). Insulin has also been described to impact intracellular calcium homeostasis. A recent study by the Thibault lab reported that acute insulin administration decreases calcium transients ultimately affecting the function of intracellular calcium channels (Maimaiti et al., 2017). Understanding this relationship is necessary, as higher levels of intracellular calcium may consequently disrupt physiologic glucose metabolism in the brain; potentially promoting further pathology (Pancani et al., 2011).

Epidemiological evidence has described parental history of AD as being an important predisposition to developing the disease (Fratiglioni et al., 1993). The risk may be more prominent for maternal than paternal history and lead to AD-related brain changes, even in cognitively normal adults (Edland et al., 1996; Mosconi et al., 2007, 2009a). As mitochondrial DNA (mtDNA) is inherited from the mother, any maternal genetic predispositions for bioenergetic disturbances may be passed down leading to increased risk for disease (Taylor and Turnbull, 2005).

Even prior to the first articles concerning an Amyloid Cascade Hypothesis of AD (Hardy and Higgins, 1992), evidence described mitochondrial/bioenergetic disturbances in AD (Sims et al., 1987; Parker et al., 1990; Blass and Gibson, 1991). Blass (2000) described a Mitochondrial Spiral as contributing significantly to AD pathogenesis. Three main points were discussed: reduced brain (glucose) metabolism, oxidative stress and calcium dysregulation. Deficiencies in either of these domains may ultimately led to disruption in the others—contributing to the pathogenesis of AD (Blass, 2000). Swerdlow and Khan (2004) proposed a Mitochondrial Cascade Hypothesis of sporadic AD. This theory of AD pathogenesis identifies the mitochondria and mitochondrial dysfunction as a central mediator in the development of LOAD. The inheritance of genes important for bioenergetic processes combined with various environmental influences throughout life could lead to the pathological changes associated with AD. One such environmental influence is insulin resistance. The impaired energy metabolism seen in insulin resistance may catalyze the bioenergetic deficits that contribute to the mitochondrial dysfunction seen in AD (Correia et al., 2012;

Montgomery and Turner, 2015). Disrupted insulin signaling leads to impaired energy metabolism, likely affecting the bioenergetic machinery working to maintain an adequate supply of energy for bodily function. There is still debate whether insulin resistance leads to mitochondrial dysfunction, if mitochondrial dysfunction contributes to insulin resistance, or if they mutually impact each other (Montgomery and Turner, 2015). Regardless of causality, mitochondrial dysfunction is fundamental feature of insulin resistance. Thus, insulin resistance may either promote or intensify the bioenergetic dysfunction already apparent in AD.

CEREBRAL METABOLISM AND THE BIOENERGETIC SHIFT IN ALZHEIMER'S DISEASE

Given the systemic metabolic dysfunction seen in AD potentially promoted by insulin resistance, it is important to understand the various metabolic fuels that may be used by the brain and how our current knowledge of brain metabolism is limited by the study of mainly one of these fuels. In this section, we will also discuss a potential bioenergetic shift in brain metabolism in AD and how this may be visualized with neuroimaging techniques prior to significant disease pathology.

Metabolic Fuels

Several sources of energy may be utilized in the production of adenosine triphosphate (ATP) that is required for many physiologic processes (Wallace et al., 2010). It is well established that glucose is the primary source of brain metabolic energy for healthy individuals. The interaction between neurons and glia, especially astrocytes, is fundamental for brain energy metabolism (Pellerin et al., 2007; Bélanger et al., 2011); and must be appreciated when interpreting results of cerebral metabolic studies. Glucose may be metabolized into pyruvate and lactate, via erobic and anerobic glycolysis, both of which have received attention concerning their roles in brain metabolism (Gonzalez et al., 2005; Boumezbeur et al., 2010; Barros, 2013). Furthermore, accumulating evidence describes the importance of erobic glycolysis in brain function (Vaishnavi et al., 2010; Vlassenko et al., 2010).

When glucose is in excess it is stored as glycogen, which is largely stored in the liver for systemic use and in the skeletal and cardiac muscle for local utilization (Shulman et al., 1990; Roden et al., 1996). However, glycogen has also been found within brain astrocytes (Brown and Ransom, 2007). There is debate to how long these stores may provide energy for the brain. Yet, astrocytic stores likely make glycogen an important source of cerebral fuel in times of need.

In addition to glucose and its derivatives, other sources may be used as metabolic fuels. Beta-oxidation of fatty acids may be a significant source of fuel for systemic energy metabolism, especially at times when glucose and glycogen reserves are depleted or within states of diminished glucose metabolism (Cahill, 2006). Even though fatty acids may cross the BBB, they are not the preferred alternate substrate to glucose for brain metabolism. Schonfeld and Reiser suggest that fatty acids may be less efficient with a slower rate of oxidation than glucose and ketone bodies, while being associated with higher rates of oxidative stress (Schönfeld and Reiser, 2013).

Ketone bodies (acetoacetate (AcAc), beta-hydroxybutyrate (BHB) and acetone) or KB are mainly synthesized in the liver as a result of beta-oxidation of fatty acids and are the primary alternative fuel to glucose in brain metabolism (Garber et al., 1974). They are released in marginal amounts in healthy individuals, and in times of fast or on a high fat ketogenic diet levels are increased compensating for decreased glucose metabolism (Cahill, 2006). Ketone bodies are more efficient than glucose relative to the amount of oxygen needed to carry out oxidative metabolism (Cahill, 2006). The lower amount of oxygen required for KB metabolism not only conserves the use of a vital resource (especially in hypoxic states), but it leads to decreased generation of ROS that may promote cellular damage and eventual cell death. Furthermore, increased KB metabolism may lead to an improved glucose metabolism, which may add to the efficacy of a therapy aimed at ketosis (Roy et al., 2012). In states where circulating KB are elevated, transporters regulating their flux into the BBB are upregulated. These monocarboxylate transporters (MCTs) are known to transport various substrates depending on their class, including: KB, lactate, pyruvate and thyroid hormone (Halestrap and Wilson, 2012).

In the brain, MCTs are found in the cell membranes of neurons and glia in addition to the BBB. Even though KB only marginally contribute to brain metabolism under basal conditions in a healthy individual, they may constitute over 60% of brain energy metabolism during the fasted state, and help mitigate decreased glucose metabolism (Morris, 2005). There are three main determinants of KB use by the brain: concentration of KB in the blood, transport across the BBB via MCTs, and cerebral activity of enzymes used in KB metabolism (Morris, 2005). KBs become a significant source of metabolic fuel as their plasma concentration increases. After transport across the BBB, research suggests that the rate-limiting factor in the utilization of KB is activity of catalytic enzymes that may regionally vary throughout the brain (Morris, 2005). However, other research describes the rate-limiting step after acute KB administration as transport across the BBB (Blomqvist et al., 2002). MCTs on the BBB are upregulated in states of chronic ketosis (Halestrap and Wilson, 2012). With an acute administration of KB, MCT density on the BBB may be the rate-limiting step for the ability of KB to be used in brain metabolism, while in a chronic state of ketosis the environment is adapted to a state of decreased glucose metabolism and may be dependent on the ketolytic metabolic machinery.

Brain Hypermetabolism in Alzheimer's Disease and Related Disorders

One of the most prominent features of the underlying mitochondrial and metabolic abnormalities in AD may be brain glucose hypometabolism. Disrupted cerebral glucose metabolism is visible using FDG PET and one of the earliest pathologic events in AD (Mosconi, 2005; Mosconi et al., 2008; Sperling et al., 2011). The hypometabolic pattern seen in AD is fairly characteristic. Metabolic declines are first found in the parietal-temporal area, posterior cingulate cortices and medial temporal lobes. Hypometabolism eventually progresses to the frontal lobes, subcortical areas and the cerebellum (Mosconi et al., 2009b). This may occur more than a decade prior to clinical onset of AD and is most evident in individuals that carry an APOE4 allele or with a positive family history (especially maternal history) of dementia (Mosconi et al., 2009b; Cunnane et al., 2011; Sperling et al., 2011). However, in recent years mounting evidence has described a state of reactive or compensatory glucose hypermetabolism in AD as well as Parkinson's, Huntington's and other neurologic diseases (Gilman et al., 1990; Haier et al., 2003; Borghammer et al., 2012; Cistaro et al., 2012; Lee et al., 2012; Ashraf et al., 2015).

Ashraf et al. (2015) reported cortical glucose hypermetabolism in individuals with amnestic MCI. Glucose hypermetabolism was found in amyloid (11C-PiB PET) negative (n = 4) and amyloid positive (n = 1) participants. Opposing results were seen in participants with the highest amyloid load (n = 5), which were found to have cortical glucose hypometabolism. Interestingly, amyloid negative participants with glucose hypermetabolism did not convert to AD within an 18-month follow-up, while amyloid positive participants (n = 4) did convert to AD within the same time period (Ashraf et al., 2015). Results from this study suggest that cerebral glucose hypermetabolism may precede glucose hypometabolism in the earliest stages of AD pathology.

Findings of compensatory hypermetabolism in a clinical population with MCI/AD have been supported by evidence describing a similar cerebral metabolic profile in AD mouse models. In the APP/PS1 mouse model of AD, Poisnel et al. (2012) found cortical and hippocampal glucose hypermetabolism in APP/PS1 mice relative to controls at 12 months. Moreover, the group used autoradiography to show that the increased glucose uptake was generally limited to areas near amyloid plaque accumulation (Poisnel et al., 2012). Similar results have been found in the 5xFAD (Rojas et al., 2013) and Tg2576 mouse models of AD (Luo et al., 2012).

Cerebral glucose hypermetabolism has also been described in several other neurologic disorders, commonly preceding a state of impaired glucose metabolism in a disease-specific manner. In Huntington's disease (HD), relative cerebral glucose hypermetabolism has been described in several brain areas including the thalamus, while hypometabolism was seen in the striatum (Lee et al., 2012). In Parkinson's disease (PD), hypermetabolism has been found in the globus pallidus externus and other subcortical areas. This contrasts the near-global cortical hypometabolism seen in PD (Borghammer et al., 2012). Patients with bulbar and spinal-onset Amyotrophic Lateral Sclerosis (ALS) had higher glucose metabolism on FDG PET than controls in several regions of interest (ROIs), including the amygdala, midbrain, pons, and cerebellum. While lower glucose metabolism was found in frontal/parietal lobes in those with bulbar-onset alS relative to spinal-onset patients and controls (Cistaro et al., 2012). In Down Syndrome, inferior temporal lobe and entorhinal cortex hypermetabolism has been reported prior to the onset of dementia, which may be a compensatory response to early pathologic changes (Haier et al., 2003, 2008). Similar evidence has been found in the study of Friedreich's ataxia, where glucose hypermetabolism was reported in those with early disease. An apparent glucose hypometabolic state was associated with further progression of the clinical condition. This difference between hypermetabolic to hypometabolic state was noted by authors to be regionally specific (Gilman et al., 1990). In theory, similar metabolic changes could occur in a disease-specific pattern in any disorder of the CNS with significant neurodegenerative pathology.

Intriguingly, cerebral energy metabolism may be impacted by systemic metabolic disease without clinically defined neuropathology. In Willette et al. (2015a) examined the relationship of systemic insulin resistance (HOMA-IR) and cerebral glucose metabolism. They found a higher degree of insulin resistance was related to lower glucose metabolism in AD ROIs. Conversely, in participants with MCI that eventually progressed to AD, higher HOMA-IR was associated with glucose hypermetabolism in the medial temporal lobes and hippocampus (Willette et al., 2015a,b). These results suggest that there may be a differential cerebral metabolic response throughout the clinical spectrum of AD and highlight the importance of studying the relation of brain metabolism to systemic metabolic risk factors. Moreover, our lab has previously reported that older adults with insulin resistance showed AD-like patterns of reduced brain glucose metabolism, as quantified with FDG PET imaging. Glucose hypometabolism was most apparent in frontal, parietotemporal, and cingulate cortices (Baker et al., 2011). This suggests that insulin resistance may promote AD-related changes in brain in those at-risk for the disorder.

Although underlying synaptic dysfunction and neuronal degeneration likely promotes decreased glucose utilization in the brain (cerebral glucose hypometabolism on FDG PET imaging) there is still debate as to whether an inherent glucose hypometabolism causes the early pathologic changes seen in AD and related disorders. A review by Cunnane et al. (2011) explores this topic by offering several mechanisms by which glucose hypometabolism may contribute to AD-related pathology. Potential mechanisms described include tau hyperphosphorylation resulting from lower glucose availability, decreased glycolytic enzyme activity—with a potential impact on cholinergic neurotransmission, and brain microvascular changes that may disrupt glucose influx into the brain (Cunnane et al., 2011). Yet, another potential mediator of the AD-related brain glucose changes may be a bioenergetic shift in metabolism from glucose-based to KB-based.

Brain Bioenergetic Shifts and Alzheimer's Disease Pathogenesis

The notion of a bioenergetic shift in energy metabolism in AD has been described in the literature spurred by observations concerning the metabolic deficits commonly seen in the disorder—especially glucose hypometabolism, mitochondrial dysfunction and oxidative stress (Kadish et al., 2009; Yao et al., 2011). Important work has come from Roberta Brinton and colleagues, who have described brain changes resulting from a potential bioenergetic shift, with special interest in how this shift is impacted by estrogen (Brinton, 2008a,b; Yao et al., 2009, 2010, 2011, 2012; Yao and Brinton, 2012; Ding et al., 2013a,b). Evidence using a female triple transgenic AD mouse model (3xTg-AD) and non-transgenic mice describes an upregulation of succinyl-CoA:3-ketoacid coenzyme A transferase (SCOT) and hydroxyacyl-coenzyme A dehydrogenase (HADH) during reproductive senescence (Yao et al., 2010). SCOT is an important enzyme for KB energy metabolism, while HADH is an enzyme with a role in the beta-oxidation of fatty acids (Fukao et al., 1997; Houten and Wanders, 2010). Notably, this upregulation of SCOT and HADH occurred concurrent with the decreased activity of PDH, an important enzyme in glucose energy metabolism (Yao et al., 2010). When coupled with an apparent inefficiency of glucose metabolism in AD, an upregulation of genes involved in KB (and fatty acid) metabolism strongly supports a bioenergetic shift phenomenon.

In a state where glucose metabolism is disrupted, it would be beneficial to increase the fraction of metabolism that is contributed by an alternate source of fuel. Genes involved in KB and fatty acid metabolism would be upregulated, while genes driving glycolytic metabolism may be downregulated. However, even with a change in metabolic machinery favoring KB and fatty acid metabolism, if the newly preferred metabolic fuel is not supplied through diet then it must come another source. When exogenous glucose supply is low in a healthy adult, glucose is derived from the breakdown of stored glycogen and through gluconeogenesis (Cahill, 2006). If glycogen stores are depleted and the amount of gluconeogenesis is not sufficient to meet energy demands, then the use of fats, KB, and even amino acids (in later stages) are utilized as fuel by the body (Cahill, 2006). If an individual is progressing through a systemic bioenergetic shift in which the preferred brain fuel substrate are KB and there is an inadequate supply of this fuel through exogenous intake, then the fuel must come from an endogenous source. Adipose tissue reserves are generally sizeable enough to supply fuel through beta-oxidation of fatty acids, leading to the production of KB that are largely produced by the liver (Garber et al., 1974). Ketone bodies can then be transported to the brain across the BBB for use in the production of ATP (Halestrap and Wilson, 2012). As circulating levels of KB become elevated brain usage increases; with capacity for utilization limited by expression of ketolytic enzymes (Morris, 2005). Over time, however, the capacity to compensate with peripheral KB production may diminish without proper exogenous supply through diet or supplementation (Yao et al., 2011). This could lead to a state where the brain becomes dependent on itself as a source of fatty acids and KB.

The myelin insulating neuronal axons in the brain is largely made of various lipids, cholesterol and proteins (Quarles et al., 2006). Thus, it may be a ready source of the fatty acid fuel that may be metabolized into KB for use by the brain. Phospholipase-A2 (PLA2) is an enzyme that catalyzes the cleavage of fatty acids from phospholipids (mainly in cellular membranes) as well as the release of arachidonic acid (AA) and eicosanoid synthesis (Sun et al., 2004; Adibhatla and Hatcher, 2008). When PLA2 is activated in the brain, it may lead to the breakdown of myelin (Adibhatla and Hatcher, 2008), releasing fatty acids for potential use as fuel with ultimate conversion to KB with interaction between astrocytes and neurons. An increased production of ROS, such as hydrogen peroxide, seen in mitochondrial dysfunction also leads to an activation of PLA2 provoking further myelin breakdown (Adibhatla and Hatcher, 2008; Sun et al., 2010; Yao et al., 2011). As the myelin is degraded, white matter changes may become apparent through various neuroimaging modalities and over time may contribute to gross volumetric loss and cognitive changes. White matter abnormalities are a common pathology seen as early as preclinical AD (Burns et al., 2005; Medina et al., 2006). Furthermore, PLA2 has been associated with the pathological response associated with Aβ (Zhu et al., 2006) and has been shown to be increased in the AD brain (Sanchez-Mejia et al., 2008). Work by Sanchez-Mejia et al. (2008) showed that a reduction in PLA2 activation diminished the PLA2-associated neurotoxicity and learning/memory deficits. Thus, the underlying AD-related Aβ accumulation, mitochondrial dysfunction, and bioenergetic shift may each contribute to the activation of PLA2 and ultimately lead to characteristic pathology of the disorder. Yet, it remains to be determined to what extent each of the mediators of PLA2 activation is the primary contributor.

Additional evidence of a bioenergetic shift in AD is the weight changes that are seen in the disorder (White et al., 1998). Individuals prior to AD diagnosis on average tend to weigh more than the general population. Starting with preclinical disease and progression to MCI and Alzheimer's dementia there seems to be a significant weight loss with each stage of decline (White et al., 1998; Johnson et al., 2006). This may be due to a combination of factors, such as decreased appetite, co-morbid depression, and impairments in various cognitive functions (Gillette-Guyonnet et al., 2000). Yet, these weight changes may also relate to the bioenergetic shift in energy metabolism.

Given the current evidence and need to understand AD pathologic processes, we support an updated model for cerebral metabolic changes in AD. The ultimate endpoint of brain energy utilization in AD and many other disorders is hypometabolism, however, a hypermetabolic glucose compensatory response may result from pathology early in disease progression (pre-clinical stage). With increased demand for energy and/or decreasing efficiency of glucose metabolism, alternate fuels (i.e., ketone bodies) may also supplement glucose metabolism. With worsening pathology and significant cell death, global hypometabolism develops. It is likely that these CNS metabolic changes may be provoked by systemic disease. **Figure 1** displays a representation of the metabolic transitions we hypothesize are seen throughout the continuum of sporadic AD.

If a metabolic bioenergetic shift is indeed a feature of AD, several key questions remain to be answered. What causes this shift? Is it an inherent defect in mitochondrial bioenergetics or a result of amyloid, tau, and other AD-related pathology? How do diseases of systemic metabolic dysfunction (insulin

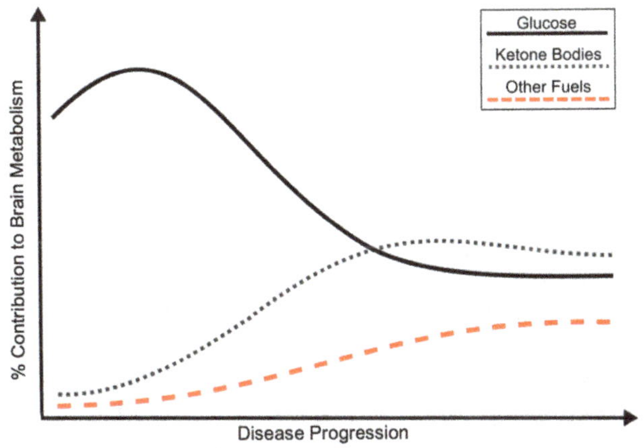

FIGURE 1 | Hypothetical model of the bioenergetic shift in energy metabolism in Alzheimer's disease (AD), as represented by relative contribution of glucose, ketone bodies and other fuels to brain metabolism. Although classically associated with glucose hypometabolism, recent evidence points to an initial glucose hypermetabolic state with potential shift towards use of alternate fuels. Insulin resistance may promote the development of AD through a variety of mechanisms, including a shift in energy metabolism. The bioenergetic shift may also be an independent feature of AD pathology. Black: Glucose metabolism; Gray: Ketone body metabolism; Red: Other fuel metabolism.

resistance, hyperlipidemia, etc.) impact the development of a bioenergetic shift and how does this relate to the susceptibility to develop AD? Further research into the role of metabolic dysfunction and mitochondrial bioenergetics in AD may answer these questions and ultimately fortify our understanding of AD pathogenesis.

Neuroimaging Biomarkers of Bioenergetic Shift in Alzheimer's Disease

Our ability to study the bioenergetic changes in AD is enhanced by newly developed imaging techniques, which may ultimately lead to the identification of a biomarker at the earliest signs of metabolic disturbance in AD and a way to quantify changes secondary to therapeutic intervention.

Although functional imaging of glucose metabolism via FDG PET is commonly used in research and clinical settings, solely visualizing brain glucose metabolism does not provide a comprehensive understanding of the brain's differential use of fuels. In order to appreciate the bioenergetic shift that potentially contributes to the pathogenesis of AD, it is important to study the use of KB, as they are the primary alternate fuel for brain metabolism. Several neuroimaging methods may be utilized for the study of brain KB metabolism, including PET with tracers developed for individual KB and magnetic resonance spectroscopy (MRS; Blomqvist et al., 1995, 2002; Pan et al., 2000; Tremblay et al., 2007, 2008).

Literature regarding the utilization of PET imaging for cerebral alternate energy metabolism is relatively scarce, largely originating from two main laboratories. Work from Blomqvist et al. (1995, 2002) described the use of carbon-11 labeled BHB PET imaging. BHB is one of the KB utilized by the brain and can be readily measured peripherally in the blood (Garber et al., 1974). Studies using this tracer described a BBB transport-dependent uptake of BHB after acute infusion of the KB (Blomqvist et al., 1995, 2002). Findings suggested no significant difference in uptake or utilization of BHB in metabolically healthy subjects and those who had insulin dependent (type 1) diabetes (Blomqvist et al., 2002). An earlier study by the group using the same tracer described BHB utilization increasing linearly with peripheral concentration and showed higher BHB utilization in gray over white matter (Blomqvist et al., 1995). These results were important in establishing a PET technique that may be utilized to visualize differential brain metabolism. Moreover, they provide valuable evidence to how KB utilization changes with peripheral concentration.

More recently, Cunnane and colleagues have developed a carbon-11 labeled radiotracer of AcAc, the other major KB utilized by the brain, for use in PET imaging of brain KB metabolism (Tremblay et al., 2007). Their work describes use of the tracer in rat models of aging and on ketogenic interventions and clinical studies. Results suggest an increased KB uptake in young and aged rats during a ketogenic intervention (Bentourkia et al., 2009; Roy et al., 2012). Importantly elevated cerebral 11C-AcAc uptake corresponds to amount of peripheral KB levels (Bentourkia et al., 2009; Roy et al., 2012). Although the use of an AcAc tracer is exciting and informative, the Cunnane group has implemented a novel dual-tracer PET approach with 11C-AcAc and 18F-FDG at the same imaging session. Several articles in the human population and within rodent models have utilized this dual-tracer technique (Roy et al., 2012; Nugent et al., 2014; Castellano et al., 2015). In a comparison of healthy young (mean age = 26 years) and older adults (mean age = 74 years), both glucose and AcAc metabolism was decreased in older adults relative to the younger cohort (Nugent et al., 2014). A 2015 study has explored cerebral glucose and AcAc metabolism in AD (Castellano et al., 2015). They described a reduction in cerebral glucose metabolism in older adults with mild AD relative to age-matched controls. Interestingly, AcAc did not differ between the groups (Castellano et al., 2015), which may provide a therapeutic outlet for those with AD and related disorders. This dual-tracer technique has the potential to greatly expand our understanding of brain metabolism in healthy vs. pathological conditions, how it is affected in "normal aging" as well as in AD. There is much to be gained from the study of brain KB metabolism, especially when coupled with glucose metabolism. The ability to visualize the bioenergetic shift in energy metabolism may provide further insight into the development of AD and ultimately act as an early biomarker for AD and the ability to determine individuals that may benefit from therapies aimed at providing KB as an alternative source of fuel for therapeutic treatment.

CONCLUSION

In this review, we have discussed the contribution of insulin resistance to the pathogenesis of AD, in particular how insulin resistance may induce a bioenergetic shift in peripheral and CNS energy metabolism, while closing with a review of neuroimaging biomarkers that may be used to identify and better understand the bioenergetic changes seen in AD and potentially response to preventative and therapeutic interventions.

We remain at a time where we have made significant progress in understanding AD without any disease-modifying therapeutics or proven prevention strategies. Yet, we now have the opportunity to explore new areas of research that may expand our knowledgebase and provide a more comprehensive view of AD pathogenesis. One of the most vital areas of need is the study of brain metabolism. Until now we have largely discussed glucose as being the sole player in brain metabolism. In fact, when brain energy is discussed, it is implied that we are referring to glucose metabolism (i.e., cerebral [glucose] metabolism). We take for granted our knowledge that glucose is the primary fuel—that higher uptake is better and that in almost every neurologic and psychiatric condition, glucose metabolism is diminished (Mosconi et al., 2009b; Wallace et al., 2010; Bélanger et al., 2011; Bohnen et al., 2012). Studies describing a state of compensatory or reactive glucose hypermetabolism that precedes significant clinical decline are overshadowed by reports of the hypometabolic state commonly assumed in most neurologic disorders (Bohnen et al., 2012; Borghammer et al., 2012; Cistaro et al., 2012; Lee et al., 2012; Ashraf et al., 2015). Although the cause of this hypermetabolism is not definitively known, it is most likely a compensatory response to injury and initial pathologic processes (Ashraf et al., 2015). If this was an isolated phenomenon, it would be easy to dismiss. However, it has been reported in conditions from Alzheimer's, Parkinson's, Huntington's and ALS, to Down Syndrome, Friedrich's Ataxia and familial Creutzfeldt-Jakob disease in disease-specific patterns (Gilman et al., 1990; Haier et al., 2003; Nagasaka et al., 2011; Borghammer et al., 2012; Cistaro et al., 2012; Lee et al., 2012; Ashraf et al., 2015).

The view of a glucose hypermetabolic state as an early disease event and response to initial pathology is likely a temporary solution to injury with an ultimate decline to decreased glucose utilization. If further evidence supports the occurrence of an initial rise and ultimate decline of cerebral glucose metabolism, then it possible to visualize this shift early (prior to clinical symptomology) and work to prevent the underlying pathology. This primary glucose hypermetabolic shift is likely also supplemented with a increase in utilization of other fuels. With progression of the disease, a potential bioenergetic shift may occur with decreasing reliance on glucose and increased use of alternate energy sources, see **Figure 1**.

Despite the brain's metabolic flexibility, most alternate fuels have been inadequately studied. These are sources of energy that our bodies use on a daily basis. Ketone bodies are an optimal first alternate fuel to study as they have been commonly reported to be the chief alternate source of cerebral energy (Cahill, 2006). Yet, acetate, lactate, pyruvate, amino acids or even glycogen remain largely unstudied (Gonzalez et al., 2005; Boumezbeur et al., 2010; Wallace et al., 2010; Barros, 2013; Cunnane et al., 2016). It is crucial to understand the brain's use of different fuels and how this may change throughout progression of disease. This enables us to appreciate pathophysiology and the body's response to increasing pathology. Moreover, we may be able to characterize "brain metabolic fingerprints" that may be used to offer patients and research participants more personalized therapeutic options if they were to develop a condition impacting brain metabolism. Strategies for prevention and therapeutic approaches may be developed to improve metabolism and clinical function. Importantly, due to the metabolic changes commonly seen in brain disease, any findings from the study of one disorder may have broad application to other neurologic, psychiatric, as well as systemic metabolic conditions.

Studying the brain in any context is truly a new frontier, and we have only recently had the opportunity and tools to study its majesty. By investigating areas such as differential brain energy metabolism, we have the opportunity to greatly advance our understanding of how our brains function in health and disease. Many mysteries and questions remain—and if answered may lead to the successful treatment and prevention of some of the most terrifying diseases of our time.

AUTHOR CONTRIBUTIONS

BJN and SC drafted, revised and approved final version of the manuscript.

FUNDING

This work was supported by National Institutes of Health grants R37-AG10880 (SC), R01-AG027415 (SC) and the Roena B. Kulynych Center for Cognition and Memory Research.

REFERENCES

Abbatecola, A. M., Paolisso, G., Lamponi, M., Bandinelli, S., Lauretani, F., Launer, L., et al. (2004). Insulin resistance and executive dysfunction in older persons. *J. Am. Geriatr. Soc.* 52, 1713–1718. doi: 10.1111/j.1532-5415.2004.52466.x

Abbott, M. A., Wells, D. G., and Fallon, J. R. (1999). The insulin receptor tyrosine kinase substrate p58/53 and the insulin receptor are components of CNS synapses. *J. Neurosci.* 19, 7300–7308.

Adibhatla, R. M., and Hatcher, J. F. (2008). Phospholipase A_2, reactive oxygen species, and lipid peroxidation in CNS pathologies. *BMB Rep.* 41, 560–567. doi: 10.5483/bmbrep.2008.41.8.560

Agrawal, R., Tyagi, E., Shukla, R., and Nath, C. (2011). Insulin receptor signaling in rat hippocampus: a study in STZ (ICV) induced memory deficit model. *Eur. Neuropsychopharmacol.* 21, 261–273. doi: 10.1016/j.euroneuro.2010.11.009

Akash, M. S., Rehman, K., and Chen, S. (2013). Role of inflammatory mechanisms in pathogenesis of type 2 diabetes mellitus. *J. Cell. Biochem.* 114, 525–531. doi: 10.1002/jcb.24402

Akiyama, H., Barger, S., Barnum, S., Bradt, B., Bauer, J., Cole, G. M., et al. (2000). Inflammation and Alzheimer's disease. *Neurobiol. Aging* 21, 383–421. doi: 10.1016/S0197-4580(00)00124-X

Alzheimer's Association. (2015). 2015 Alzheimer's disease facts and figures. *Alzheimers Dement.* 11, 332–384. doi: 10.1016/j.jalz.2015.02.003

Amador-Ortiz, C., Lin, W. L., Ahmed, Z., Personett, D., Davies, P., Duara, R., et al. (2007). TDP-43 immunoreactivity in hippocampal sclerosis and Alzheimer's disease. *Ann. Neurol.* 61, 435–445. doi: 10.1002/ana.21154

Amor, S., Puentes, F., Baker, D., and Van Der Valk, P. (2010). Inflammation in neurodegenerative diseases. *Immunology* 129, 154–169. doi: 10.1111/j.1365-2567.2009.03225.x

Apelt, J., Mehlhorn, G., and Schliebs, R. (1999). Insulin-sensitive GLUT4 glucose transporters are colocalized with GLUT3-expressing cells and demonstrate a chemically distinct neuron-specific localization in rat brain. *J. Neurosci. Res.* 57, 693–705. doi: 10.1002/(sici)1097-4547(19990901)57:5<693::aid-jnr11>3.0.co;2-x

Armstrong, R. A. (2011). The Pathogenesis of Alzheimer's disease: a reevaluation of the "amyloid cascade hypothesis". *Int. J. Alzheimers Dis.* 2011:630865. doi: 10.4061/2011/630865

Ashraf, A., Fan, Z., Brooks, D. J., and Edison, P. (2015). Cortical hypermetabolism in MCI subjects: a compensatory mechanism? *Eur. J. Nucl. Med. Mol. Imaging* 42, 447–458. doi: 10.1007/s00259-014-2919-z

Attwell, D., and Laughlin, S. B. (2001). An energy budget for signaling in the grey matter of the brain. *J. Cereb. Blood Flow Metab.* 21, 1133–1145. doi: 10.1097/00004647-200110000-00001

Authier, F., Posner, B. I., and Bergeron, J. J. (1996). Insulin-degrading enzyme. *Clin. Invest. Med.* 19, 149–160.

Baker, L. D., Cross, D. J., Minoshima, S., Belongia, D., Watson, G. S., and Craft, S. (2011). Insulin resistance and Alzheimer-like reductions in regional cerebral glucose metabolism for cognitively normal adults with prediabetes or early type 2 diabetes. *Arch. Neurol.* 68, 51–57. doi: 10.1001/archneurol.2010.225

Banks, W. A., Jaspan, J. B., Huang, W., and Kastin, A. J. (1997a). Transport of insulin across the blood-brain barrier: saturability at euglycemic doses of insulin. *Peptides* 18, 1423–1429. doi: 10.1016/s0196-9781(97)00231-3

Banks, W. A., Jaspan, J. B., and Kastin, A. J. (1997b). Selective, physiological transport of insulin across the blood-brain barrier: novel demonstration by species-specific radioimmunoassays. *Peptides* 18, 1257–1262. doi: 10.1016/s0196-9781(97)00198-8

Banks, W. A., Owen, J. B., and Erickson, M. A. (2012). Insulin in the brain: There and back again. *Pharmacol. Ther.* 136, 82–93. doi: 10.1016/j.pharmthera.2012.07.006

Barros, L. F. (2013). Metabolic signaling by lactate in the brain. *Trends Neurosci.* 36, 396–404. doi: 10.1016/j.tins.2013.04.002

Baskin, D. G., Figlewicz, D. P., Woods, S. C., Porte, D. Jr., and Dorsa, D. M. (1987). Insulin in the brain. *Annu. Rev. Physiol.* 49, 335–347. doi: 10.1146/annurev.ph.49.030187.002003

Baura, G. D., Foster, D. M., Porte, D. Jr., Kahn, S. E., Bergman, R. N., Cobelli, C., et al. (1993). Saturable transport of insulin from plasma into the central nervous system of dogs *in vivo*. A mechanism for regulated insulin delivery to the brain. *J. Clin. Invest.* 92, 1824–1830. doi: 10.1172/jci116773

Bélanger, M., Allaman, I., and Magistretti, P. J. (2011). Brain energy metabolism: focus on astrocyte-neuron metabolic cooperation. *Cell Metab.* 14, 724–738. doi: 10.1016/j.cmet.2011.08.016

Benedict, C., Hallschmid, M., Hatke, A., Schultes, B., Fehm, H. L., Born, J., et al. (2004). Intranasal insulin improves memory in humans. *Psychoneuroendocrinology* 29, 1326–1334. doi: 10.1016/j.psyneuen.2004.04.003

Benedict, C., Kern, W., Schultes, B., Born, J., and Hallschmid, M. (2008). Differential sensitivity of men and women to anorexigenic and memory-improving effects of intranasal insulin. *J. Clin. Endocrinol. Metab.* 93, 1339–1344. doi: 10.1210/jc.2007-2606

Bentourkia, M., Tremblay, S., Pifferi, F., Rousseau, J., Lecomte, R., and Cunnane, S. (2009). PET study of 11C-acetoacetate kinetics in rat brain during dietary treatments affecting ketosis. *Am. J. Physiol. Endocrinol. Metab.* 296, E796–E801. doi: 10.1152/ajpendo.90644.2008

Berti, V., Murray, J., Davies, M., Spector, N., Tsui, W. H., Li, Y., et al. (2015). Nutrient patterns and brain biomarkers of Alzheimer's disease in cognitively normal individuals. *J. Nutr. Health Aging* 19, 413–423. doi: 10.1007/s12603-014-0534-0

Bezprozvanny, I., and Mattson, M. P. (2008). Neuronal calcium mishandling and the pathogenesis of Alzheimer's disease. *Trends Neurosci.* 31, 454–463. doi: 10.1016/j.tins.2008.06.005

Biessels, G. J., Strachan, M. W., Visseren, F. L., Kappelle, L. J., and Whitmer, R. A. (2014). Dementia and cognitive decline in type 2 diabetes and prediabetic stages: towards targeted interventions. *Lancet Diabetes Endocrinol.* 2, 246–255. doi: 10.1016/s2213-8587(13)70088-3

Bingham, E. M., Hopkins, D., Smith, D., Pernet, A., Hallett, W., Reed, L., et al. (2002). The role of insulin in human brain glucose metabolism: an 18fluoro-deoxyglucose positron emission tomography study. *Diabetes* 51, 3384–3390. doi: 10.2337/diabetes.51.12.3384

Blasko, I., Stampfer-Kountchev, M., Robatscher, P., Veerhuis, R., Eikelenboom, P., and Grubeck-Loebenstein, B. (2004). How chronic inflammation can affect the brain and support the development of Alzheimer's disease in old age: the role of microglia and astrocytes. *Aging Cell* 3, 169–176. doi: 10.1111/j.1474-9728.2004.00101.x

Blass, J. P. (2000). The mitochondrial spiral. An adequate cause of dementia in the Alzheimer's syndrome. *Ann. N Y Acad. Sci.* 924, 170–183. doi: 10.1111/j.1749-6632.2000.tb05576.x

Blass, J. P., and Gibson, G. E. (1991). The role of oxidative abnormalities in the pathophysiology of Alzheimer's disease. *Rev. Neurol. (Paris)* 147, 513–525.

Blázquez, E., Velázquez, E., Hurtado-Carneiro, V., and Ruiz-Albusac, J. M. (2014). Insulin in the brain: its pathophysiological implications for states related with central insulin resistance, type 2 diabetes and Alzheimer's disease. *Front. Endocrinol. (Lausanne)* 5:161. doi: 10.3389/fendo.2014.00161

Blomqvist, G., Alvarsson, M., Grill, V., Von Heijne, G., Ingvar, M., Thorell, J. O., et al. (2002). Effect of acute hyperketonemia on the cerebral uptake of ketone bodies in nondiabetic subjects and IDDM patients. *Am. J. Physiol. Endocrinol. Metab.* 283, E20–E28. doi: 10.1152/ajpendo.00294.2001

Blomqvist, G., Thorell, J. O., Ingvar, M., Grill, V., Widen, L., and Stone-Elander, S. (1995). Use of R-β-[1-11C]hydroxybutyrate in PET studies of regional cerebral uptake of ketone bodies in humans. *Am. J. Physiol.* 269, E948–E959.

Blum-Degen, D., Muller, T., Kuhn, W., Gerlach, M., Przuntek, H., and Riederer, P. (1995). Interleukin-1 β and interleukin-6 are elevated in the cerebrospinal fluid of Alzheimer's and *de novo* Parkinson's disease patients. *Neurosci. Lett.* 202, 17–20. doi: 10.1016/0304-3940(95)12192-7

Bohnen, N. I., Djang, D. S., Herholz, K., Anzai, Y., and Minoshima, S. (2012). Effectiveness and safety of 18F-FDG PET in the evaluation of dementia: a review of the recent literature. *J. Nucl. Med.* 53, 59–71. doi: 10.2967/jnumed.111.096578

Borghammer, P., Hansen, S. B., Eggers, C., Chakravarty, M., Vang, K., Aanerud, J., et al. (2012). Glucose metabolism in small subcortical structures in Parkinson's disease. *Acta Neurol. Scand.* 125, 303–310. doi: 10.1111/j.1600-0404.2011.01556.x

Bosco, D., Fava, A., Plastino, M., Montalcini, T., and Pujia, A. (2011). Possible implications of insulin resistance and glucose metabolism in Alzheimer's disease pathogenesis. *J. Cell. Mol. Med.* 15, 1807–1821. doi: 10.1111/j.1582-4934.2011.01318.x

Boumezbeur, F., Petersen, K. F., Cline, G. W., Mason, G. F., Behar, K. L., Shulman, G. I., et al. (2010). The contribution of blood lactate to brain energy metabolism in humans measured by dynamic 13C nuclear magnetic resonance spectroscopy. *J. Neurosci.* 30, 13983–13991. doi: 10.1523/JNEUROSCI.2040-10.2010

Bowie, C. R., and Harvey, P. D. (2006). Administration and interpretation of the Trail Making Test. *Nat. Protoc.* 1, 2277–2281. doi: 10.1038/nprot.2006.390

Braak, H., Alafuzoff, I., Arzberger, T., Kretzschmar, H., and Del Tredici, K. (2006). Staging of Alzheimer disease-associated neurofibrillary pathology using paraffin sections and immunocytochemistry. *Acta Neuropathol.* 112, 389–404. doi: 10.1007/s00401-006-0127-z

Braak, H., and Braak, E. (1991). Neuropathological stageing of Alzheimer-related changes. *Acta Neuropathol.* 82, 239–259. doi: 10.1007/bf00308809

Brant, A. M., Jess, T. J., Milligan, G., Brown, C. M., and Gould, G. W. (1993). Immunological analysis of glucose transporters expressed in different regions of the rat brain and central nervous system. *Biochem. Biophys. Res. Commun.* 192, 1297–1302. doi: 10.1006/bbrc.1993.1557

Brinton, R. D. (2008a). Estrogen regulation of glucose metabolism and mitochondrial function: therapeutic implications for prevention of Alzheimer's disease. *Adv. Drug Deliv. Rev.* 60, 1504–1511. doi: 10.1016/j.addr.2008.06.003

Brinton, R. D. (2008b). The healthy cell bias of estrogen action: mitochondrial bioenergetics and neurological implications. *Trends Neurosci.* 31, 529–537. doi: 10.1016/j.tins.2008.07.003

Brown, A. M., and Ransom, B. R. (2007). Astrocyte glycogen and brain energy metabolism. *Glia* 55, 1263–1271. doi: 10.1002/glia.20557

Burns, J. M., Church, J. A., Johnson, D. K., Xiong, C., Marcus, D., Fotenos, A. F., et al. (2005). White matter lesions are prevalent but differentially related with cognition in aging and early Alzheimer disease. *Arch. Neurol.* 62, 1870–1876. doi: 10.1001/archneur.62.12.1870

Cahill, G. F. Jr. (2006). Fuel metabolism in starvation. *Annu. Rev. Nutr.* 26, 1–22. doi: 10.1146/annurev.nutr.26.061505.111258

Cai, W., Sakaguchi, M., Kleinridders, A., Gonzalez-Del Pino, G., Dreyfuss, J. M., O'neill, B. T., et al. (2017). Domain-dependent effects of insulin and IGF-1 receptors on signalling and gene expression. *Nat. Commun.* 8:14892. doi: 10.1038/ncomms14892

Cardoso, S. M., Proenca, M. T., Santos, S., Santana, I., and Oliveira, C. R. (2004). Cytochrome c oxidase is decreased in Alzheimer's disease platelets. *Neurobiol. Aging* 25, 105–110. doi: 10.1016/s0197-4580(03)00033-2

Castellano, C. A., Nugent, S., Paquet, N., Tremblay, S., Bocti, C., Lacombe, G., et al. (2015). Lower brain 18F-fluorodeoxyglucose uptake but normal 11C-acetoacetate metabolism in mild Alzheimer's disease dementia. *J. Alzheimers Dis.* 43, 1343–1353. doi: 10.3233/JAD-141074

Chaturvedi, R. K., and Beal, M. F. (2013). Mitochondrial diseases of the brain. *Free Radic. Biol. Medi.ine* 63, 1–29. doi: 10.1016/j.freeradbiomed.2013.03.018

Cheng, G., Huang, C., Deng, H., and Wang, H. (2012). Diabetes as a risk factor for dementia and mild cognitive impairment: a meta-analysis of longitudinal studies. *Intern. Med. J.* 42, 484–491. doi: 10.1111/j.1445-5994.2012.02758.x

Chen, Z., and Zhong, C. (2013). Decoding Alzheimer's disease from perturbed cerebral glucose metabolism: implications for diagnostic and therapeutic strategies. *Prog. Neurobiol.* 108, 21–43. doi: 10.1016/j.pneurobio.2013.06.004

Cholerton, B., Baker, L. D., and Craft, S. (2011). Insulin resistance and pathological brain ageing. *Diabet. Med.* 28, 1463–1475. doi: 10.1111/j.1464-5491.2011.03464.x

Cholerton, B., Baker, L. D., and Craft, S. (2013). Insulin, cognition, and dementia. *Eur. J. Pharmacol.* 719, 170–179. doi: 10.1016/j.ejphar.2013.08.008

Cistaro, A., Valentini, M. C., Chiò, A., Nobili, F., Calvo, A., Moglia, C., et al. (2012). Brain hypermetabolism in amyotrophic lateral sclerosis: a FDG PET study in ALS of spinal and bulbar onset. *Eur. J. Nucl. Med. Mol. Imaging* 39, 251–259. doi: 10.1007/s00259-011-1979-6

Claxton, A., Baker, L. D., Hanson, A., Trittschuh, E. H., Cholerton, B., Morgan, A., et al. (2015). Long-acting intranasal insulin detemir improves cognition for adults with mild cognitive impairment or early-stage Alzheimer's disease dementia. *J. Alzheimers Dis.* 44, 897–906. doi: 10.3233/JAD-141791

Claxton, A., Baker, L. D., Wilkinson, C. W., Trittschuh, E. H., Chapman, D., Watson, G. S., et al. (2013). Sex and ApoE genotype differences in treatment response to two doses of intranasal insulin in adults with mild cognitive impairment or Alzheimer's disease. *J. Alzheimers Dis.* 35, 789–797. doi: 10.3233/JAD-122308

Convit, A., Wolf, O. T., Tarshish, C., and de Leon, M. J. (2003). Reduced glucose tolerance is associated with poor memory performance and hippocampal atrophy among normal elderly. *Proc. Natl. Acad. Sci. U S A* 100, 2019–2022. doi: 10.1073/pnas.0336073100

Cook, D. G., Leverenz, J. B., McMillan, P. J., Kulstad, J. J., Ericksen, S., Roth, R. A., et al. (2003). Reduced hippocampal insulin-degrading enzyme in late-onset Alzheimer's disease is associated with the apolipoprotein E-ϵ4 allele. *Am. J. Pathol.* 162, 313–319. doi: 10.1016/s0002-9440(10)63822-9

Cooper, G. J., Day, A. J., Willis, A. C., Roberts, A. N., Reid, K. B., and Leighton, B. (1989). Amylin and the amylin gene: structure, function and relationship to islet amyloid and to diabetes mellitus. *Biochim. Biophys. Acta* 1014, 247–258. doi: 10.1016/0167-4889(89)90220-6

Correia, S. C., Santos, R. X., Carvalho, C., Cardoso, S., Candeias, E., Santos, M. S., et al. (2012). Insulin signaling, glucose metabolism and mitochondria: major players in Alzheimer's disease and diabetes interrelation. *Brain Res.* 1441, 64–78. doi: 10.1016/j.brainres.2011.12.063

Craft, S. (2007). Insulin resistance and Alzheimer's disease pathogenesis: potential mechanisms and implications for treatment. *Curr. Alzheimer Res.* 4, 147–152. doi: 10.2174/156720507780362137

Craft, S. (2009). The role of metabolic disorders in Alzheimer disease and vascular dementia. *Arch. Neurol.* 66, 300–305. doi: 10.1001/archneurol.2009.27

Craft, S., Asthana, S., Cook, D. G., Baker, L. D., Cherrier, M., Purganan, K., et al. (2003). Insulin dose-response effects on memory and plasma amyloid precursor protein in Alzheimer's disease: interactions with apolipoprotein E genotype. *Psychoneuroendocrinology* 28, 809–822. doi: 10.1016/s0306-4530(02)00087-2

Craft, S., Asthana, S., Newcomer, J. W., Wilkinson, C. W., Matos, I. T., Baker, L. D., et al. (1999). Enhancement of memory in Alzheimer disease with insulin and somatostatin, but not glucose. *Arch. Gen. Psychiatry* 56, 1135–1140. doi: 10.1001/archpsyc.56.12.1135

Craft, S., Baker, L. D., Montine, T. J., Minoshima, S., Watson, G. S., Claxton, A., et al. (2012). Intranasal insulin therapy for alzheimer disease and amnestic mild cognitive impairment: a pilot clinical trial. *Arch. Neurol.* 69, 29–38. doi: 10.1001/archneurol.2011.233

Craft, S., Cholerton, B., and Baker, L. D. (2013). Insulin and Alzheimer's disease: untangling the web. *J. Alzheimers Dis.* 33, S263–S275. doi: 10.3233/JAD-2012-129042

Craft, S., Newcomer, J., Kanne, S., Dagogo-Jack, S., Cryer, P., Sheline, Y., et al. (1996). Memory improvement following induced hyperinsulinemia in Alzheimer's disease. *Neurobiol. Aging* 17, 123–130. doi: 10.1016/0197-4580(95)02002-0

Craft, S., Peskind, E., Schwartz, M. W., Schellenberg, G. D., Raskind, M., and Porte, D. Jr. (1998). Cerebrospinal fluid and plasma insulin levels in Alzheimer's disease: relationship to severity of dementia and apolipoprotein E genotype. *Neurology* 50, 164–168. doi: 10.1212/wnl.50.1.164

Craft, S., and Watson, G. S. (2004). Insulin and neurodegenerative disease: shared and specific mechanisms. *Lancet Neurol.* 3, 169–178. doi: 10.1016/s1474-4422(04)00681-7

Cui, H., Kong, Y., and Zhang, H. (2012). Oxidative stress, mitochondrial dysfunction, and aging. *J. Signal Transduct.* 2012:646354. doi: 10.1155/2012/646354

Cunnane, S. C., Courchesne-Loyer, A., St-Pierre, V., Vandenberghe, C., Pierotti, T., Fortier, M., et al. (2016). Can ketones compensate for deteriorating brain glucose uptake during aging? Implications for the risk and treatment of Alzheimer's disease. *Ann. N Y Acad. Sci.* 1367, 12–20. doi: 10.1111/nyas.12999

Cunnane, S., Nugent, S., Roy, M., Courchesne-Loyer, A., Croteau, E., Tremblay, S., et al. (2011). Brain fuel metabolism, aging and Alzheimer's disease. *Nutrition* 27, 3–20. doi: 10.1016/j.nut.2010.07.021

De Felice, F. G., and Ferreira, S. T. (2014). Inflammation, defective insulin signaling, and mitochondrial dysfunction as common molecular denominators connecting type 2 diabetes to Alzheimer disease. *Diabetes* 63, 2262–2272. doi: 10.2337/db13-1954

De Felice, F. G., and Lourenco, M. V. (2015). Brain metabolic stress and neuroinflammation at the basis of cognitive impairment in Alzheimer's disease. *Front. Aging Neurosci.* 7:94. doi: 10.3389/fnagi.2015.00094

De Felice, F. G., Vieira, M. N., Bomfim, T. R., Decker, H., Velasco, P. T., Lambert, M. P., et al. (2009). Protection of synapses against Alzheimer's-linked toxins: insulin signaling prevents the pathogenic binding of Aβ oligomers. *Proc. Natl. Acad. Sci. U S A* 106, 1971–1976. doi: 10.1073/pnas.0809158106

DeFronzo, R. A. (2010). Insulin resistance, lipotoxicity, type 2 diabetes and atherosclerosis: the missing links. The Claude Bernard Lecture 2009. *Diabetologia* 53, 1270–1287. doi: 10.1007/s00125-010-1684-1

DeFronzo, R. A., Bonadonna, R. C., and Ferrannini, E. (1992). Pathogenesis of NIDDM. A balanced overview. *Diabetes Care* 15, 318–368. doi: 10.2337/diacare.15.3.318

DeFronzo, R. A., and Ferrannini, E. (1991). Insulin resistance. A multifaceted syndrome responsible for NIDDM, obesity, hypertension, dyslipidemia, and atherosclerotic cardiovascular disease. *Diabetes Care* 14, 173–194. doi: 10.2337/diacare.14.3.173

Despa, S., Margulies, K. B., Chen, L., Knowlton, A. A., Havel, P. J., Taegtmeyer, H., et al. (2012). Hyperamylinemia contributes to cardiac dysfunction in obesity and diabetes: a study in humans and rats. *Circ. Res.* 110, 598–608. doi: 10.1161/CIRCRESAHA.111.258285

Devi, L., Alldred, M. J., Ginsberg, S. D., and Ohno, M. (2012). Mechanisms underlying insulin deficiency-induced acceleration of β-amyloidosis in a mouse model of Alzheimer's disease. *PLoS One* 7:e32792. doi: 10.1371/journal.pone.0032792

Devraj, K., Klinger, M. E., Myers, R. L., Mokashi, A., Hawkins, R. A., and Simpson, I. A. (2011). GLUT-1 glucose transporters in the blood-brain barrier: differential phosphorylation. *J. Neurosci. Res.* 89, 1913–1925. doi: 10.1002/jnr.22738

Di Paolo, G., and Kim, T. W. (2011). Linking lipids to Alzheimer's disease: cholesterol and beyond. *Nat. Rev. Neurosci.* 12, 284–296. doi: 10.1038/nrn3012

Ding, F., Yao, J., Rettberg, J. R., Chen, S., and Brinton, R. D. (2013a). Early decline in glucose transport and metabolism precedes shift to ketogenic system in female aging and Alzheimer's mouse brain: implication for bioenergetic intervention. *PLoS One* 8:e79977. doi: 10.1371/journal.pone.0079977

Ding, F., Yao, J., Zhao, L., Mao, Z., Chen, S., and Brinton, R. D. (2013b). Ovariectomy induces a shift in fuel availability and metabolism in the hippocampus of the female transgenic model of familial Alzheimer's. *PLoS One* 8:e59825. doi: 10.1371/journal.pone.0059825

Doody, R. S., Thomas, R. G., Farlow, M., Iwatsubo, T., Vellas, B., Joffe, S., et al. (2014). Phase 3 trials of solanezumab for mild-to-moderate Alzheimer's disease. *N. Engl. J. Med.* 370, 311–321. doi: 10.1056/NEJMoa1312889

Dou, J. T., Chen, M., Dufour, F., Alkon, D. L., and Zhao, W. Q. (2005). Insulin receptor signaling in long-term memory consolidation following spatial learning. *Learn. Mem.* 12, 646–655. doi: 10.1101/lm.88005

Duarte, A. I., Moreira, P. I., and Oliveira, C. R. (2012). Insulin in central nervous system: more than just a peripheral hormone. *J. Aging Res.* 2012:384017. doi: 10.1155/2012/384017

Edland, S. D., Silverman, J. M., Peskind, E. R., Tsuang, D., Wijsman, E., and Morris, J. C. (1996). Increased risk of dementia in mothers of Alzheimer's disease cases: evidence for maternal inheritance. *Neurology* 47, 254–256. doi: 10.1212/WNL.47.1.254

El Messari, S., Leloup, C., Quignon, M., Brisorgueil, M. J., Penicaud, L., and Arluison, M. (1998). Immunocytochemical localization of the insulin-responsive glucose transporter 4 (Glut4) in the rat central nervous system. *J. Comp. Neurol.* 399, 492–512. doi: 10.1002/(sici)1096-9861(19981005)399:4<492::aid-cne4>3.0.co;2-x

Farris, W., Mansourian, S., Chang, Y., Lindsley, L., Eckman, E. A., Frosch, M. P., et al. (2003). Insulin-degrading enzyme regulates the levels of insulin, amyloid β-protein, and the β-amyloid precursor protein intracellular domain *in vivo*. *Proc. Natl. Acad. Sci. U S A* 100, 4162–4167. doi: 10.1073/pnas.0230450100

Festa, A., D'agostino, R. Jr., Howard, G., Mykkänen, L., Tracy, R. P., and Haffner, S. M. (2000). Chronic subclinical inflammation as part of the insulin resistance syndrome: the Insulin Resistance Atherosclerosis Study (IRAS). *Circulation* 102, 42–47. doi: 10.1161/01.cir.102.1.42

Figlewicz, D. P., Szot, P., Israel, P. A., Payne, C., and Dorsa, D. M. (1993). Insulin reduces norepinephrine transporter mRNA *in vivo* in rat locus coeruleus. *Brain Res.* 602, 161–164. doi: 10.1016/0006-8993(93)90258-o

Fratiglioni, L., Ahlbom, A., Viitanen, M., and Winblad, B. (1993). Risk factors for late-onset Alzheimer's disease: a population-based, case-control study. *Ann Neurol* 33, 258–266. doi: 10.1002/ana.410330306

Freiherr, J., Hallschmid, M., Frey, W. H. II, Brunner, Y. F., Chapman, C. D., Holscher, C., et al. (2013). Intranasal insulin as a treatment for Alzheimer's disease: a review of basic research and clinical evidence. *CNS Drugs* 27, 505–514. doi: 10.1007/s40263-013-0076-8

Fukao, T., Song, X. Q., Mitchell, G. A., Yamaguchi, S., Sukegawa, K., Orii, T., et al. (1997). Enzymes of ketone body utilization in human tissues: protein and messenger RNA levels of succinyl-coenzyme A (CoA):3-ketoacid CoA transferase and mitochondrial and cytosolic acetoacetyl-CoA thiolases. *Pediatr. Res.* 42, 498–502. doi: 10.1203/00006450-199710000-00013

Garber, A. J., Menzel, P. H., Boden, G., and Owen, O. E. (1974). Hepatic ketogenesis and gluconeogenesis in humans. *J. Clin. Invest.* 54, 981–989. doi: 10.1172/jci107839

Garwood, C. J., Ratcliffe, L. E., Morgan, S. V., Simpson, J. E., Owens, H., Vazquez-Villaseñor, I., et al. (2015). Insulin and IGF1 signalling pathways in human astrocytes *in vitro* and *in vivo*; characterisation, subcellular localisation and modulation of the receptors. *Mol. Brain* 8:51. doi: 10.1186/s13041-015-0138-6

Gasparini, L., Gouras, G. K., Wang, R., Gross, R. S., Beal, M. F., Greengard, P., et al. (2001). Stimulation of β-amyloid precursor protein trafficking by insulin reduces intraneuronal β-amyloid and requires mitogen-activated protein kinase signaling. *J. Neurosci.* 21, 2561–2570.

Genin, E., Hannequin, D., Wallon, D., Sleegers, K., Hiltunen, M., Combarros, O., et al. (2011). APOE and Alzheimer disease: a major gene with semi-dominant inheritance. *Mol. Psychiatry* 16, 903–907. doi: 10.1038/mp.2011.52

Ghasemi, R., Dargahi, L., Haeri, A., Moosavi, M., Mohamed, Z., and Ahmadiani, A. (2013a). Brain insulin dysregulation: implication for neurological and neuropsychiatric disorders. *Mol. Neurobiol.* 47, 1045–1065. doi: 10.1007/s12035-013-8404-z

Ghasemi, R., Haeri, A., Dargahi, L., Mohamed, Z., and Ahmadiani, A. (2013b). Insulin in the brain: sources, localization and functions. *Mol. Neurobiol.* 47, 145–171. doi: 10.1007/s12035-012-8339-9

Gillette-Guyonnet, S., Nourhashemi, F., Andrieu, S., de Glisezinski, I., Ousset, P. J., Riviere, D., et al. (2000). Weight loss in Alzheimer disease. *Am. J. Clin. Nutr.* 71, 637s–642s.

Gilman, S., Junck, L., Markel, D. S., Koeppe, R. A., and Kluin, K. J. (1990). Cerebral glucose hypermetabolism in Friedreich's ataxia detected with positron emission tomography. *Ann. Neurol.* 28, 750–757. doi: 10.1002/ana.410280605

Goldin, A., Beckman, J. A., Schmidt, A. M., and Creager, M. A. (2006). Advanced glycation end products: sparking the development of diabetic vascular injury. *Circulation* 114, 597–605. doi: 10.1161/circulationaha.106.621854

Gonzalez, S. V., Nguyen, N. H., Rise, F., and Hassel, B. (2005). Brain metabolism of exogenous pyruvate. *J. Neurochem.* 95, 284–293. doi: 10.1111/j.1471-4159.2005.03365.x

Greenwood, C. E., and Winocur, G. (2001). Glucose treatment reduces memory deficits in young adult rats fed high-fat diets. *Neurobiol. Learn. Mem.* 75, 179–189. doi: 10.1006/nlme.2000.3964

Haier, R. J., Alkire, M. T., White, N. S., Uncapher, M. R., Head, E., Lott, I. T., et al. (2003). Temporal cortex hypermetabolism in Down syndrome prior to the onset of dementia. *Neurology* 61, 1673–1679. doi: 10.1212/01.wnl.0000098935.36984.25

Haier, R. J., Head, K., Head, E., and Lott, I. T. (2008). Neuroimaging of individuals with Down's syndrome at-risk for dementia: evidence for possible compensatory events. *Neuroimage* 39, 1324–1332. doi: 10.1016/j.neuroimage.2007.09.064

Haj-ali, V., Mohaddes, G., and Babri, S. H. (2009). Intracerebroventricular insulin improves spatial learning and memory in male Wistar rats. *Behav. Neurosci.* 123, 1309–1314. doi: 10.1037/a0017722

Halestrap, A. P., and Wilson, M. C. (2012). The monocarboxylate transporter family–role and regulation. *IUBMB Life* 64, 109–119. doi: 10.1002/iub.572

Hardy, J. A., and Higgins, G. A. (1992). Alzheimer's disease: the amyloid cascade hypothesis. *Science* 256, 184–185. doi: 10.1126/science.1566067

Hardy, J., and Selkoe, D. J. (2002). The amyloid hypothesis of Alzheimer's disease: progress and problems on the road to therapeutics. *Science* 297, 353–356. doi: 10.1126/science.1072994

Hassing, L. B., Grant, M. D., Hofer, S. M., Pedersen, N. L., Nilsson, S. E., Berg, S., et al. (2004). Type 2 diabetes mellitus contributes to cognitive decline in old age: a longitudinal population-based study. *J. Int. Neuropsychol. Soc.* 10, 599–607. doi: 10.1017/S1355617704104165

Havrankova, J., Roth, J., and Brownstein, M. (1978a). Insulin receptors are widely distributed in the central nervous system of the rat. *Nature* 272, 827–829. doi: 10.1038/272827a0

Havrankova, J., Schmechel, D., Roth, J., and Brownstein, M. (1978b). Identification of insulin in rat brain. *Proc. Natl. Acad. Sci. U S A* 75, 5737–5741. doi: 10.1073/pnas.75.11.5737

Hirvonen, J., Virtanen, K. A., Nummenmaa, L., Hannukainen, J. C., Honka, M. J., Bucci, M., et al. (2011). Effects of insulin on brain glucose metabolism in impaired glucose tolerance. *Diabetes* 60, 443–447. doi: 10.2337/db10-0940

Ho, L., Qin, W., Pompl, P. N., Xiang, Z., Wang, J., Zhao, Z., et al. (2004). Diet-induced insulin resistance promotes amyloidosis in a transgenic mouse model of Alzheimer's disease. *FASEB J.* 18, 902–904. doi: 10.1096/fj.03-0978fje

Houten, S. M., and Wanders, R. J. (2010). A general introduction to the biochemistry of mitochondrial fatty acid β-oxidation. *J. Inherit. Metab. Dis.* 33, 469–477. doi: 10.1007/s10545-010-9061-2

Howard, R., McShane, R., Lindesay, J., Ritchie, C., Baldwin, A., Barber, R., et al. (2012). Donepezil and memantine for moderate-to-severe Alzheimer's disease. *N. Engl. J. Med.* 366, 893–903. doi: 10.1056/NEJMoa1106668

Ito, S., Ohtsuki, S., and Terasaki, T. (2006). Functional characterization of the brain-to-blood efflux clearance of human amyloid-β peptide (1–40) across the rat blood-brain barrier. *Neurosci. Res.* 56, 246–252. doi: 10.1016/j.neures.2006.07.006

Jackson, K., Barisone, G. A., Diaz, E., Jin, L. W., DeCarli, C., and Despa, F. (2013). Amylin deposition in the brain: a second amyloid in Alzheimer disease? *Ann. Neurol.* 74, 517–526. doi: 10.1002/ana.23956

Johnson, D. K., Wilkins, C. H., and Morris, J. C. (2006). Accelerated weight loss may precede diagnosis in Alzheimer disease. *Arch. Neurol.* 63, 1312–1317. doi: 10.1001/archneur.63.9.1312

Johri, A., and Beal, M. F. (2012). Mitochondrial dysfunction in neurodegenerative diseases. *J. Pharmacol. Exp. Ther.* 342, 619–630. doi: 10.1124/jpet.112.192138

Kadish, I., Thibault, O., Blalock, E. M., Chen, K. C., Gant, J. C., Porter, N. M., et al. (2009). Hippocampal and cognitive aging across the lifespan: a bioenergetic shift precedes and increased cholesterol trafficking parallels memory impairment. *J. Neurosci.* 29, 1805–1816. doi: 10.1523/JNEUROSCI.4599-08.2009

Kamagate, A., Qu, S., Perdomo, G., Su, D., Kim, D. H., Slusher, S., et al. (2008). FoxO1 mediates insulin-dependent regulation of hepatic VLDL production in mice. *J. Clin. Invest.* 118, 2347–2364. doi: 10.1172/JCI32914

Karch, C. M., Jeng, A. T., Nowotny, P., Cady, J., Cruchaga, C., and Goate, A. M. (2012). Expression of novel Alzheimer's disease risk genes in control and Alzheimer's disease brains. *PLoS One* 7:e50976. doi: 10.1371/journal.pone.0050976

Katakam, P. V. G., Snipes, J. A., Steed, M. M., and Busija, D. W. (2012). Insulin-induced generation of reactive oxygen species and uncoupling of nitric oxide synthase underlie the cerebrovascular insulin resistance in obese rats. *J. Cereb. Blood Flow Metab.* 32, 792–804. doi: 10.1038/jcbfm.2011.181

Kern, W., Peters, A., Fruehwald-Schultes, B., Deininger, E., Born, J., and Fehm, H. L. (2001). Improving influence of insulin on cognitive functions in humans. *Neuroendocrinology* 74, 270–280. doi: 10.1159/000054694

Kerti, L., Witte, A. V., Winkler, A., Grittner, U., Rujescu, D., and Floel, A. (2013). Higher glucose levels associated with lower memory and reduced hippocampal microstructure. *Neurology* 81, 1746–1752. doi: 10.1212/01.WNL.0000435561.00234.ee

Ketterer, C., Tschritter, O., Preissl, H., Heni, M., Häring, H.-U., and Fritsche, A. (2011). Insulin sensitivity of the human brain. *Diabetes Res. Clin. Pract.* 93, S47–S51. doi: 10.1016/S0168-8227(11)70013-4

Khansari, N., Shakiba, Y., and Mahmoudi, M. (2009). Chronic inflammation and oxidative stress as a major cause of age-related diseases and cancer. *Recent Pat. Inflamm. Allergy Drug Discov.* 3, 73–80. doi: 10.2174/187221309787158371

Kim, J. A., Wei, Y., and Sowers, J. R. (2008). Role of mitochondrial dysfunction in insulin resistance. *Circ. Res.* 102, 401–414. doi: 10.1161/CIRCRESAHA.107.165472

Kleinridders, A. (2016). Deciphering brain insulin receptor and insulin-like growth factor 1 receptor signalling. *J. Neuroendocrinol.* 28:11. doi: 10.1111/jne.12433

Kleinridders, A., Ferris, H. A., Cai, W., and Kahn, C. R. (2014). Insulin action in brain regulates systemic metabolism and brain function. *Diabetes* 63, 2232–2243. doi: 10.2337/db14-0568

Kopf, S. R., and Baratti, C. M. (1999). Effects of posttraining administration of insulin on retention of a habituation response in mice: participation of a central cholinergic mechanism. *Neurobiol. Learn. Mem.* 71, 50–61. doi: 10.1006/nlme.1998.3831

Kubaszek, A., Pihlajamaki, J., Komarovski, V., Lindi, V., Lindström, J., Eriksson, J., et al. (2003). Promoter polymorphisms of the TNF-α (G-308A) and IL-6 (C-174G) genes predict the conversion from impaired glucose tolerance to type 2 diabetes: the Finnish Diabetes Prevention Study. *Diabetes* 52, 1872–1876. doi: 10.2337/diabetes.52.7.1872

Kurochkin, I. V., and Goto, S. (1994). Alzheimer's β-amyloid peptide specifically interacts with and is degraded by insulin degrading enzyme. *FEBS Lett.* 345, 33–37. doi: 10.1016/0014-5793(94)00387-4

Lee, J. (2013). Adipose tissue macrophages in the development of obesity-induced inflammation, insulin resistance and type 2 diabetes. *Arch. Pharm. Res.* 36, 208–222. doi: 10.1007/s12272-013-0023-8

Lee, C. C., Kuo, Y. M., Huang, C. C., and Hsu, K. S. (2009). Insulin rescues amyloid β-induced impairment of hippocampal long-term potentiation. *Neurobiol. Aging* 30, 377–387. doi: 10.1016/j.neurobiolaging.2007.06.014

Lee, S. J., Lee, W. Y., Kim, Y. K., An, Y. S., Cho, J. W., Choi, J. Y., et al. (2012). Apparent relative hypermetabolism of selective brain areas in Huntington disease and importance of reference region for analysis. *Clin. Nucl. Med.* 37, 663–668. doi: 10.1097/rlu.0b013e3182478bf2

Lesnefsky, E. J., Moghaddas, S., Tandler, B., Kerner, J., and Hoppel, C. L. (2001). Mitochondrial dysfunction in cardiac disease: ischemia-reperfusion, aging, and heart failure. *J. Mol. Cell. Cardiol.* 33, 1065–1089. doi: 10.1006/jmcc.2001.1378

Lim, Y. A., Rhein, V., Baysang, G., Meier, F., Poljak, A., Raftery, M. J., et al. (2010). Aβ and human amylin share a common toxicity pathway via mitochondrial dysfunction. *Proteomics* 10, 1621–1633. doi: 10.1002/pmic.200900651

Liu, Y., Liu, F., Grundke-Iqbal, I., Iqbal, K., and Gong, C.-X. (2011). Deficient brain insulin signalling pathway in Alzheimer's disease and diabetes. *J. Pathol.* 225, 54–62. doi: 10.1002/path.2912

Livingstone, C., Lyall, H., and Gould, G. W. (1995). Hypothalamic GLUT 4 expression: a glucose- and insulin-sensing mechanism? *Mol. Cell. Endocrinol.* 107, 67–70. doi: 10.1016/0303-7207(94)03423-q

Lowell, B. B., and Shulman, G. I. (2005). Mitochondrial dysfunction and type 2 diabetes. *Science* 307, 384–387. doi: 10.1126/science.1104343

Lund-Andersen, H. (1979). Transport of glucose from blood to brain. *Physiol. Rev.* 59, 305–352.

Luo, F., Rustay, N. R., Ebert, U., Hradil, V. P., Cole, T. B., Llano, D. A., et al. (2012). Characterization of 7- and 19-month-old Tg2576 mice using multimodal *in vivo* imaging: limitations as a translatable model of Alzheimer's disease. *Neurobiol. Aging* 33, 933–944. doi: 10.1016/j.neurobiolaging.2010.08.005

Lüth, H. J., Ogunlade, V., Kuhla, B., Kientsch-Engel, R., Stahl, P., Webster, J., et al. (2005). Age- and stage-dependent accumulation of advanced glycation end products in intracellular deposits in normal and Alzheimer's disease brains. *Cereb. Cortex* 15, 211–220. doi: 10.1093/cercor/bhh123

Madamanchi, N. R., and Runge, M. S. (2007). Mitochondrial dysfunction in atherosclerosis. *Circ. Res.* 100, 460–473. doi: 10.1161/01.RES.0000258450.44413.96

Maimaiti, S., Frazier, H. N., Anderson, K. L., Ghoweri, A. O., Brewer, L. D., Porter, N. M., et al. (2017). Novel calcium-related targets of insulin in hippocampal neurons. *Neuroscience* 364, 130–142. doi: 10.1016/j.neuroscience.2017.09.019

Mammucari, C., and Rizzuto, R. (2010). Signaling pathways in mitochondrial dysfunction and aging. *Mech. Ageing Dev.* 131, 536–543. doi: 10.1016/j.mad.2010.07.003

McDermott, J. R., and Gibson, A. M. (1997). Degradation of Alzheimer's β-amyloid protein by human and rat brain peptidases: involvement of insulin-degrading enzyme. *Neurochem. Res.* 22, 49–56. doi: 10.1023/A:1027325304203

Medina, D., DeToledo-Morrell, L., Urresta, F., Gabrieli, J. D., Moseley, M., Fleischman, D., et al. (2006). White matter changes in mild cognitive impairment and AD: a diffusion tensor imaging study. *Neurobiol. Aging* 27, 663–672. doi: 10.1016/j.neurobiolaging.2005.03.026

Montgomery, M. K., and Turner, N. (2015). Mitochondrial dysfunction and insulin resistance: an update. *Endocr. Connect.* 4, R1–R15. doi: 10.1530/ec-14-0092

Morris, A. (2005). Cerebral ketone body metabolism. *J. Inherit. Metab. Dis.* 28, 109–121. doi: 10.1007/s10545-005-5518-0

Mosconi, L. (2005). Brain glucose metabolism in the early and specific diagnosis of Alzheimer's disease. FDG-PET studies in MCI and AD. *Eur. J. Nucl. Med. Mol. Imaging* 32, 486–510. doi: 10.1007/s00259-005-1762-7

Mosconi, L., Brys, M., Switalski, R., Mistur, R., Glodzik, L., Pirraglia, E., et al. (2007). Maternal family history of Alzheimer's disease predisposes to reduced brain glucose metabolism. *Proc. Natl. Acad. Sci. U S A* 104, 19067–19072. doi: 10.1073/pnas.0705036104

Mosconi, L., Mistur, R., Switalski, R., Brys, M., Glodzik, L., Rich, K., et al. (2009a). Declining brain glucose metabolism in normal individuals with a maternal history of Alzheimer disease. *Neurology* 72, 513–520. doi: 10.1212/01.wnl.0000333247.51383.43

Mosconi, L., Mistur, R., Switalski, R., Tsui, W. H., Glodzik, L., Li, Y., et al. (2009b). FDG-PET changes in brain glucose metabolism from normal cognition to pathologically verified Alzheimer's disease. *Eur. J. Nucl. Med. Mol. Imaging* 36, 811–822. doi: 10.1007/s00259-008-1039-z

Mosconi, L., Pupi, A., and De Leon, M. J. (2008). Brain glucose hypometabolism and oxidative stress in preclinical Alzheimer's disease. *Ann. N Y Acad. Sci.* 1147, 180–195. doi: 10.1196/annals.1427.007

Muniyappa, R., Montagnani, M., Koh, K. K., and Quon, M. J. (2007). Cardiovascular actions of insulin. *Endocr. Rev.* 28, 463–491. doi: 10.1210/er.2007-0006

Nagasaka, T., Nagasaka, K., Ohta, E., Shindo, K., Takiyama, Y., Shiozawa, Z., et al. (2011). Cerebral hypermetabolism demonstrated by FDG PET in familial Creutzfeldt-Jakob disease. *Clin. Nucl. Med.* 36, 725–727. doi: 10.1097/rlu.0b013e31821a2604

Neumann, K. F., Rojo, L., Navarrete, L. P., Farías, G., Reyes, P., and Maccioni, R. B. (2008). Insulin resistance and Alzheimer's disease: molecular links & clinical implications. *Curr. Alzheimer Res.* 5, 438–447. doi: 10.2174/156720508785908919

Novak, V., Milberg, W., Hao, Y., Munshi, M., Novak, P., Galica, A., et al. (2014). Enhancement of vasoreactivity and cognition by intranasal insulin in type 2 diabetes. *Diabetes Care* 37, 751–759. doi: 10.2337/dc13-1672

Nugent, S., Tremblay, S., Chen, K. W., Ayutyanont, N., Roontiva, A., Castellano, C. A., et al. (2014). Brain glucose and acetoacetate metabolism: a comparison of young and older adults. *Neurobiol. Aging* 35, 1386–1395. doi: 10.1016/j.neurobiolaging.2013.11.027

Oskarsson, M. E., Paulsson, J. F., Schultz, S. W., Ingelsson, M., Westermark, P., and Westermark, G. T. (2015). *In vivo* seeding and cross-seeding of localized amyloidosis: a molecular link between type 2 diabetes and Alzheimer disease. *Am. J. Pathol.* 185, 834–846. doi: 10.1016/j.ajpath.2014.11.016

Pan, J. W., Rothman, T. L., Behar, K. L., Stein, D. T., and Hetherington, H. P. (2000). Human brain β-hydroxybutyrate and lactate increase in fasting-induced ketosis. *J. Cereb. Blood Flow Metab.* 20, 1502–1507. doi: 10.1097/00004647-200010000-00012

Pancani, T., Anderson, K. L., Porter, N. M., and Thibault, O. (2011). Imaging of a glucose analog, calcium and NADH in neurons and astrocytes: dynamic responses to depolarization and sensitivity to pioglitazone. *Cell Calcium* 50, 548–558. doi: 10.1016/j.ceca.2011.09.002

Park, C. R., Seeley, R. J., Craft, S., and Woods, S. C. (2000). Intracerebroventricular insulin enhances memory in a passive-avoidance task. *Physiol. Behav.* 68, 509–514. doi: 10.1016/s0031-9384(99)00220-6

Park, L. C., Zhang, H., Sheu, K. F., Calingasan, N. Y., Kristal, B. S., Lindsay, J. G., et al. (1999). Metabolic impairment induces oxidative stress, compromises inflammatory responses, and inactivates a key mitochondrial enzyme in microglia. *J. Neurochem.* 72, 1948–1958. doi: 10.1046/j.1471-4159.1999.0721948.x

Parker, W. D. Jr., Filley, C. M., and Parks, J. K. (1990). Cytochrome oxidase deficiency in Alzheimer's disease. *Neurology* 40, 1302–1303. doi: 10.1212/WNL.40.8.1302

Pellerin, L., Bouzier-Sore, A. K., Aubert, A., Serres, S., Merle, M., Costalat, R., et al. (2007). Activity-dependent regulation of energy metabolism by astrocytes: an update. *Glia* 55, 1251–1262. doi: 10.1002/glia.20528

Pérez, A., Morelli, L., Cresto, J. C., and Castaño, E. M. (2000). Degradation of soluble amyloid β-peptides 1-40, 1-42, and the Dutch variant 1-40Q by insulin degrading enzyme from Alzheimer disease and control brains. *Neurochem. Res.* 25, 247–255. doi: 10.1023/A:1007527721160

Piroli, G. G., Grillo, C. A., Reznikov, L. R., Adams, S., McEwen, B. S., Charron, M. J., et al. (2007). Corticosterone impairs insulin-stimulated translocation of GLUT4 in the rat hippocampus. *Neuroendocrinology* 85, 71–80. doi: 10.1159/000101694

Poisnel, G., Hérard, A. S., El Tannir El Tayara, N., Bourrin, E., Volk, A., Kober, F., et al. (2012). Increased regional cerebral glucose uptake in an APP/PS1 model of Alzheimer's disease. *Neurobiol. Aging* 33, 1995–2005. doi: 10.1016/j.neurobiolaging.2011.09.026

Pradhan, A. D., Manson, J. E., Rifai, N., Buring, J. E., and Ridker, P. M. (2001). C-reactive protein, interleukin 6 and risk of developing type 2 diabetes mellitus. *JAMA* 286, 327–334. doi: 10.1001/jama.286.3.327

Purdon, A. D., Rosenberger, T. A., Shetty, H. U., and Rapoport, S. I. (2002). Energy consumption by phospholipid metabolism in mammalian brain. *Neurochem. Res.* 27, 1641–1647. doi: 10.1023/A:1021635027211

Qiu, W. Q., Walsh, D. M., Ye, Z., Vekrellis, K., Zhang, J., Podlisny, M. B., et al. (1998). Insulin-degrading enzyme regulates extracellular levels of amyloid β-protein by degradation. *J. Biol. Chem.* 273, 32730–32738. doi: 10.1074/jbc.273.49.32730

Quarles, R. H., Macklin, W. B., and Morell, P. (2006). *Myelin Formation, Structure and Biochemistry.* London: Elsevier.

Ramasamy, R., Vannucci, S. J., Yan, S. S., Herold, K., Yan, S. F., and Schmidt, A. M. (2005). Advanced glycation end products and RAGE: a common thread in aging, diabetes, neurodegeneration, and inflammation. *Glycobiology* 15, 16R–28R. doi: 10.1093/glycob/cwi053

Reagan, L. P., Gorovits, N., Hoskin, E. K., Alves, S. E., Katz, E. B., Grillo, C. A., et al. (2001). Localization and regulation of GLUTx1 glucose transporter in the hippocampus of streptozotocin diabetic rats. *Proc. Natl. Acad. Sci. U S A* 98, 2820–2825. doi: 10.1073/pnas.051629798

Reaven, G. M. (1983). Insulin resistance in noninsulin-dependent diabetes mellitus. Does it exist and can it be measured? *Am. J. Med.* 74, 3–17. doi: 10.1016/0002-9343(83)90650-2

Reaven, G. M. (2003). The insulin resistance syndrome. *Curr. Atheroscler. Rep.* 5, 364–371. doi: 10.1007/s11883-003-0007-0

Reddy, P. H. (2009). Amyloid β, mitochondrial structural and functional dynamics in Alzheimer's disease. *Exp. Neurol.* 218, 286–292. doi: 10.1016/j.expneurol.2009.03.042

Reed, B., Villeneuve, S., Mack, W., DeCarli, C., Chui, H. C., and Jagust, W. (2014). Associations between serum cholesterol levels and cerebral amyloidosis. *JAMA Neurol.* 71, 195–200. doi: 10.1001/jamaneurol.2013.5390

Reger, M. A., Watson, G. S., Frey, W. H., Baker, L. D., Cholerton, B., Keeling, M. L., et al. (2006). Effects of intranasal insulin on cognition in memory-impaired older adults: Modulation by APOE genotype. *Neurobiology of Aging* 27, 451–458. doi: 10.1016/j.neurobiolaging.2005.03.016

Reger, M. A., Watson, G. S., Green, P. S., Baker, L. D., Cholerton, B., Fishel, M. A., et al. (2008). Intranasal insulin administration dose-dependently modulates verbal memory and plasma amyloid-β in memory-impaired older adults. *J. Alzheimers Dis.* 13, 323–331. doi: 10.3233/jad-2008-13309

Reiman, E. M., Caselli, R. J., Yun, L. S., Chen, K., Bandy, D., Minoshima, S., et al. (1996). Preclinical evidence of Alzheimer's disease in persons homozygous for the epsilon 4 allele for apolipoprotein E. *N. Engl. J. Med.* 334, 752–758. doi: 10.1056/nejm199603213341202

Reitz, C. (2013). Dyslipidemia and the risk of Alzheimer's disease. *Curr. Atheroscler. Rep.* 15:307. doi: 10.1007/s11883-012-0307-3

Robinson, P. J., Noronha, J., DeGeorge, J. J., Freed, L. M., Nariai, T., and Rapoport, S. I. (1992). A quantitative method for measuring regional *in vivo* fatty-acid incorporation into and turnover within brain phospholipids: review and critical analysis. *Brain Res. Brain Res. Rev.* 17, 187–214. doi: 10.1016/0165-0173(92)90016-f

Roden, M., Perseghin, G., Petersen, K. F., Hwang, J. H., Cline, G. W., Gerow, K., et al. (1996). The roles of insulin and glucagon in the regulation of hepatic glycogen synthesis and turnover in humans. *J. Clin. Invest.* 97, 642–648. doi: 10.1172/jci118460

Rojas, S., Herance, J. R., Gispert, J. D., Abad, S., Torrent, E., Jiménez, X., et al. (2013). *In vivo* evaluation of amyloid deposition and brain glucose metabolism of 5XFAD mice using positron emission tomography. *Neurobiol. Aging* 34, 1790–1798. doi: 10.1016/j.neurobiolaging.2012.12.027

Roriz-Filho, J. S., Sá-Roriz, T. M., Rosset, I., Camozzato, A. L., Santos, A. C., Chaves, M. L. F., et al. (2009). (Pre)diabetes, brain aging and cognition. *Biochim. Biophys. Acta* 1792, 432–443. doi: 10.1016/j.bbadis.2008.12.003

Roy, M., Nugent, S., Tremblay-Mercier, J., Tremblay, S., Courchesne-Loyer, A., Beaudoin, J.-F., et al. (2012). The ketogenic diet increases brain glucose and ketone uptake in aged rats A dual tracer PET and volumetric MRI study. *Brain Res.* 1488, 14–23. doi: 10.1016/j.brainres.2012.10.008

Ryu, J. K., and McLarnon, J. G. (2009). A leaky blood-brain barrier, fibrinogen infiltration and microglial reactivity in inflamed Alzheimer's disease brain. *J. Cell. Mol. Med.* 13, 2911–2925. doi: 10.1111/j.1582-4934.2008.00434.x

Salloway, S., Sperling, R., Fox, N. C., Blennow, K., Klunk, W., Raskind, M., et al. (2014). Two phase 3 trials of bapineuzumab in mild-to-moderate Alzheimer's disease. *N. Engl. J. Med.* 370, 322–333. doi: 10.1056/NEJMoa1304839

Saltiel, A. R., and Kahn, C. R. (2001). Insulin signalling and the regulation of glucose and lipid metabolism. *Nature* 414, 799–806. doi: 10.1038/414799a

Sanchez-Mejia, R. O., Newman, J. W., Toh, S., Yu, G. Q., Zhou, Y., Halabisky, B., et al. (2008). Phospholipase A2 reduction ameliorates cognitive deficits in a mouse model of Alzheimer's disease. *Nat. Neurosci.* 11, 1311–1318. doi: 10.1038/nn.2213

Sasaki, N., Fukatsu, R., Tsuzuki, K., Hayashi, Y., Yoshida, T., Fujii, N., et al. (1998). Advanced glycation end products in Alzheimer's disease and other neurodegenerative diseases. *Am. J. Pathol.* 153, 1149–1155. doi: 10.1016/S0002-9440(10)65659-3

Savage, D. B., Petersen, K. F., and Shulman, G. I. (2007). Disordered lipid metabolism and the pathogenesis of insulin resistance. *Physiol. Rev.* 87, 507–520. doi: 10.1152/physrev.00024.2006

Scheff, S. W., Price, D. A., Schmitt, F. A., and Mufson, E. J. (2006). Hippocampal synaptic loss in early Alzheimer's disease and mild cognitive impairment. *Neurobiol. Aging* 27, 1372–1384. doi: 10.1016/j.neurobiolaging.2005.09.012

Schiöth, H. B., Craft, S., Brooks, S. J., Frey, W. H. II, and Benedict, C. (2012). Brain insulin signaling and Alzheimer's disease: current evidence and future directions. *Mol. Neurobiol.* 46, 4–10. doi: 10.1007/s12035-011-8229-6

Schneider, L. S., Dagerman, K. S., Higgins, J. P., and McShane, R. (2011a). Lack of evidence for the efficacy of memantine in mild Alzheimer disease. *Arch. Neurol.* 68, 991–998. doi: 10.1001/archneurol.2011.69

Schneider, L. S., Insel, P. S., and Weiner, M. W. (2011b). Treatment with cholinesterase inhibitors and memantine of patients in the Alzheimer's disease neuroimaging initiative. *Arch. Neurol.* 68, 58–66. doi: 10.1001/archneurol.2010.343

Schönfeld, P., and Reiser, G. (2013). Why does brain metabolism not favor burning of fatty acids to provide energy? Reflections on disadvantages of the use of free fatty acids as fuel for brain. *J. Cereb. Blood Flow Metab.* 33, 1493–1499. doi: 10.1038/jcbfm.2013.128

Schulingkamp, R. J., Pagano, T. C., Hung, D., and Raffa, R. B. (2000). Insulin receptors and insulin action in the brain: review and clinical implications. *Neurosci. Biobehav. Rev.* 24, 855–872. doi: 10.1016/s0149-7634(00)00040-3

Schwartz, M., and Baruch, K. (2014). The resolution of neuroinflammation in neurodegeneration: leukocyte recruitment via the choroid plexus. *EMBO J.* 33, 7–22. doi: 10.1002/embj.201386609

Schwartz, M. W., Figlewicz, D. F., Kahn, S. E., Baskin, D. G., Greenwood, M. R., and Porte, D. Jr. (1990). Insulin binding to brain capillaries is reduced in genetically obese, hyperinsulinemic Zucker rats. *Peptides* 11, 467–472. doi: 10.1016/0196-9781(90)90044-6

Selkoe, D. J. (1996). Amyloid β-protein and the genetics of Alzheimer's disease. *J. Biol. Chem.* 271, 18295–18298. doi: 10.1074/jbc.271.31.18295

Selkoe, D. J. (2002). Alzheimer's disease is a synaptic failure. *Science* 298, 789–791. doi: 10.1126/science.1074069

Shah, K., Desilva, S., and Abbruscato, T. (2012). The role of glucose transporters in brain disease: diabetes and Alzheimer's Disease. *Int. J. Mol. Sci.* 13, 12629–12655. doi: 10.3390/ijms131012629

Shulman, G. I., Rothman, D. L., Jue, T., Stein, P., DeFronzo, R. A., and Shulman, R. G. (1990). Quantitation of muscle glycogen synthesis in normal subjects and subjects with non-insulin-dependent diabetes by 13C nuclear magnetic resonance spectroscopy. *N. Engl. J. Med.* 322, 223–228. doi: 10.1056/nejm199001253220403

Sims, N. R., Finegan, J. M., Blass, J. P., Bowen, D. M., and Neary, D. (1987). Mitochondrial function in brain tissue in primary degenerative dementia. *Brain Res.* 436, 30–38. doi: 10.1016/0006-8993(87)91553-8

Singh, R., Barden, A., Mori, T., and Beilin, L. (2001). Advanced glycation end-products: a review. *Diabetologia* 44, 129–146. doi: 10.1007/s001250051591

Skeberdis, V. A., Lan, J., Zheng, X., Zukin, R. S., and Bennett, M. V. (2001). Insulin promotes rapid delivery of N-methyl-D- aspartate receptors to the cell surface by exocytosis. *Proc. Natl. Acad. Sci. U S A* 98, 3561–3566. doi: 10.1073/pnas.051634698

Small, G. W., Ercoli, L. M., Silverman, D. H., Huang, S. C., Komo, S., Bookheimer, S. Y., et al. (2000). Cerebral metabolic and cognitive decline in persons at genetic risk for Alzheimer's disease. *Proc. Natl. Acad. Sci. U S A* 97, 6037–6042. doi: 10.1073/pnas.090106797

Sperling, R. A., Aisen, P. S., Beckett, L. A., Bennett, D. A., Craft, S., Fagan, A. M., et al. (2011). Toward defining the preclinical stages of Alzheimer's disease: recommendations from the National Institute on Aging-Alzheimer's Association workgroups on diagnostic guidelines for Alzheimer's disease. *Alzheimers Dement.* 7, 280–292. doi: 10.1016/j.jalz.2011.03.003

Sridhar, G. R., Lakshmi, G., and Nagamani, G. (2015). Emerging links between type 2 diabetes and Alzheimer's disease. *World J. Diabetes* 6, 744–751. doi: 10.4239/wjd.v6.i5.744

Srikanth, V., Maczurek, A., Phan, T., Steele, M., Westcott, B., Juskiw, D., et al. (2011). Advanced glycation endproducts and their receptor RAGE in Alzheimer's disease. *Neurobiol. Aging* 32, 763–777. doi: 10.1016/j.neurobiolaging.2009.04.016

Srodulski, S., Sharma, S., Bachstetter, A. B., Brelsfoard, J. M., Pascual, C., Xie, X. S., et al. (2014). Neuroinflammation and neurologic deficits in diabetes linked to brain accumulation of amylin. *Mol. Neurodegener.* 9:30. doi: 10.1186/1750-1326-9-30

Starkov, A. A., Fiskum, G., Chinopoulos, C., Lorenzo, B. J., Browne, S. E., Patel, M. S., et al. (2004). Mitochondrial α-ketoglutarate dehydrogenase complex generates reactive oxygen species. *J. Neurosci.* 24, 7779–7788. doi: 10.1523/JNEUROSCI.1899-04.2004

Stockhorst, U., De Fries, D., Steingrueber, H.-J., and Scherbaum, W. A. (2004). Insulin and the CNS: effects on food intake, memory and endocrine parameters and the role of intranasal insulin administration in humans. *Physiol. Behav.* 83, 47–54. doi: 10.1016/j.physbeh.2004.07.022

Strachan, M. W. (2011). R D Lawrence Lecture 2010. The brain as a target organ in Type 2 diabetes: exploring the links with cognitive impairment and dementia. *Diabet. Med.* 28, 141–147. doi: 10.1111/j.1464-5491.2010.03199.x

Stranahan, A. M., Norman, E. D., Lee, K., Cutler, R. G., Telljohann, R. S., Egan, J. M., et al. (2008). Diet-induced insulin resistance impairs hippocampal synaptic plasticity and cognition in middle-aged rats. *Hippocampus* 18, 1085–1088. doi: 10.1002/hipo.20470

Sudoh, S., Frosch, M. P., and Wolf, B. A. (2002). Differential effects of proteases involved in intracellular degradation of amyloid b-protein between detergent-soluble and -insoluble pools in CHO-695 cells. *Biochemistry* 41, 1091–1099. doi: 10.1021/bi011193l

Sun, G. Y., Shelat, P. B., Jensen, M. B., He, Y., Sun, A. Y., and Simonyi, A. (2010). Phospholipases A2 and inflammatory responses in the central nervous system. *Neuromolecular Med.* 12, 133–148. doi: 10.1007/s12017-009-8092-z

Sun, G. Y., Xu, J., Jensen, M. D., and Simonyi, A. (2004). Phospholipase A2 in the central nervous system: implications for neurodegenerative diseases. *J. Lipid Res.* 45, 205–213. doi: 10.1194/jlr.r300016-jlr200

Swardfager, W., Lanctot, K., Rothenburg, L., Wong, A., Cappell, J., and Herrmann, N. (2010). A meta-analysis of cytokines in Alzheimer's disease. *Biol. Psychiatry* 68, 930–941. doi: 10.1016/j.biopsych.2010.06.012

Swerdlow, R. H., Burns, J. M., and Khan, S. M. (2010). The Alzheimer's disease mitochondrial cascade hypothesis. *J. Alzheimers Dis.* 20, S265–S279. doi: 10.3233/JAD-2010-100339

Swerdlow, R. H., and Khan, S. M. (2004). A "mitochondrial cascade hypothesis" for sporadic Alzheimer's disease. *Med. Hypotheses* 63, 8–20. doi: 10.1016/j.mehy.2003.12.045

Szendroedi, J., Phielix, E., and Roden, M. (2011). The role of mitochondria in insulin resistance and type 2 diabetes mellitus. *Nat. Rev. Endocrinol.* 8, 92–103. doi: 10.1038/nrendo.2011.138

Takeda, S., Sato, N., Ikimura, K., Nishino, H., Rakugi, H., and Morishita, R. (2013). Increased blood-brain barrier vulnerability to systemic inflammation in an Alzheimer disease mouse model. *Neurobiol. Aging* 34, 2064–2070. doi: 10.1016/j.neurobiolaging.2013.02.010

Tamaki, C., Ohtsuki, S., and Terasaki, T. (2007). Insulin facilitates the hepatic clearance of plasma amyloid β-peptide (1 40) by intracellular translocation of low-density lipoprotein receptor-related protein 1 (LRP-1) to the plasma membrane in hepatocytes. *Mol. Pharmacol.* 72, 850–855. doi: 10.1124/mol.107.036913

Taylor, R. W., and Turnbull, D. M. (2005). Mitochondrial DNA mutations in human disease. *Nat. Rev. Genet.* 6, 389–402. doi: 10.1038/nrg1606

Tilvis, R. S., Kähönen-Väre, M. H., Jolkkonen, J., Valvanne, J., Pitkala, K. H., and Strandberg, T. E. (2004). Predictors of cognitive decline and mortality of aged people over a 10-year period. *J. Gerontol. A Biol. Sci. Med. Sci.* 59, 268–274. doi: 10.1093/gerona/59.3.m268

Townsend, M., Mehta, T., and Selkoe, D. J. (2007). Soluble Aβ inhibits specific signal transduction cascades common to the insulin receptor pathway. *J. Biol. Chem.* 282, 33305–33312. doi: 10.1074/jbc.M610390200

Tremblay, S., Ouellet, R., Bénard, F., and Cunnane, S. C. (2008). Automated synthesis of 11C-β-hydroxybutyrate by enzymatic conversion of 11C-acetoacetate using β-hydroxybutyrate dehydrogenase. *J. Labelled Comp. Radiopharm.* 51, 242–245. doi: 10.1002/jlcr.1504

Tremblay, S., Ouellet, R., Rodrigue, S., Langlois, R., Bénard, F., and Cunnane, S. C. (2007). Automated synthesis of 11C-acetoacetic acid, a key alternate brain fuel to glucose. *Appl. Radiat. Isot.* 65, 934–940. doi: 10.1016/j.apradiso.2007.03.015

Unger, J. W., Livingston, J. N., and Moss, A. M. (1991). Insulin receptors in the central nervous system: localization, signalling mechanisms and functional aspects. *Prog. Neurobiol.* 36, 343–362. doi: 10.1016/0301-0082(91)90015-s

Unoki, H., Bujo, H., Yamagishi, S., Takeuchi, M., Imaizumi, T., and Saito, Y. (2007). Advanced glycation end products attenuate cellular insulin sensitivity by increasing the generation of intracellular reactive oxygen species in adipocytes. *Diabetes Res. Clin. Pract.* 76, 236–244. doi: 10.1016/j.diabres.2006.09.016

Unoki, H., and Yamagishi, S. (2008). Advanced glycation end products and insulin resistance. *Curr. Pharm. Des.* 14, 987–989. doi: 10.2174/138161208784139747

Vaishnavi, S. N., Vlassenko, A. G., Rundle, M. M., Snyder, A. Z., Mintun, M. A., and Raichle, M. E. (2010). Regional aerobic glycolysis in the human brain. *Proc. Natl. Acad. Sci. U S A* 107, 17757–17762. doi: 10.1073/pnas.1010459107

Vanhanen, M., Koivisto, K., Kuusisto, J., Mykkänen, L., Helkala, E. L., Hänninen, T., et al. (1998). Cognitive function in an elderly population with persistent impaired glucose tolerance. *Diabetes Care* 21, 398–402. doi: 10.2337/diacare.21.3.398

Vlassenko, A. G., Vaishnavi, S. N., Couture, L., Sacco, D., Shannon, B. J., Mach, R. H., et al. (2010). Spatial correlation between brain aerobic glycolysis and amyloid-β (Aβ) deposition. *Proc. Natl. Acad. Sci. U S A* 107, 17763–17767. doi: 10.1073/pnas.1010461107

Wallace, D. C., Fan, W., and Procaccio, V. (2010). Mitochondrial energetics and therapeutics. *Annu. Rev. Pathol.* 5, 297–348. doi: 10.1146/annurev.pathol.4.110807.092314

Wallum, B. J., Taborsky, G. J. Jr., Porte, D. Jr., Figlewicz, D. P., Jacobson, L., Beard, J. C., et al. (1987). Cerebrospinal fluid insulin levels increase during intravenous insulin infusions in man. *J. Clin. Endocrinol. Metab.* 64, 190–194. doi: 10.1210/jcem-64-1-190

Wang, X., Su, B., Lee, H. G., Li, X., Perry, G., Smith, M. A., et al. (2009). Impaired balance of mitochondrial fission and fusion in Alzheimer's disease. *J. Neurosci.* 29, 9090–9103. doi: 10.1523/JNEUROSCI.1357-09.2009

Wang, X., Su, B., Siedlak, S. L., Moreira, P. I., Fujioka, H., Wang, Y., et al. (2008). Amyloid-β overproduction causes abnormal mitochondrial dynamics via differential modulation of mitochondrial fission/fusion proteins. *Proc. Natl. Acad. Sci. U S A* 105, 19318–19323. doi: 10.1073/pnas.0804871105

Watson, G. S., and Craft, S. (2006). Insulin resistance, inflammation, and cognition in Alzheimer's disease: lessons for multiple sclerosis. *J. Neurol. Sci.* 245, 21–33. doi: 10.1016/j.jns.2005.08.017

Wautier, J. L., Zoukourian, C., Chappey, O., Wautier, M. P., Guillausseau, P. J., Cao, R., et al. (1996). Receptor-mediated endothelial cell dysfunction in diabetic vasculopathy. Soluble receptor for advanced glycation end products blocks hyperpermeability in diabetic rats. *J. Clin. Invest.* 97, 238–243. doi: 10.1172/jci118397

Wei, Y. H., and Lee, H. C. (2002). Oxidative stress, mitochondrial DNA mutation, and impairment of antioxidant enzymes in aging. *Exp. Biol. Med. (Maywood)* 227, 671–682. doi: 10.1177/153537020222700901

Werther, G. A., Hogg, A., Oldfield, B. J., Mckinley, M. J., Figdor, R., Allen, A. M., et al. (1987). Localization and characterization of insulin receptors in rat brain and pituitary gland using *in vitro* autoradiography and computerized densitometry. *Endocrinology* 121, 1562–1570. doi: 10.1210/endo-121-4-1562

White, H., Pieper, C., and Schmader, K. (1998). The association of weight change in Alzheimer's disease with severity of disease and mortality: a longitudinal analysis. *J. Am. Geriatr. Soc.* 46, 1223–1227. doi: 10.1111/j.1532-5415.1998.tb04537.x

Whitmer, R. A., Gustafson, D. R., Barrett-Connor, E., Haan, M. N., Gunderson, E. P., and Yaffe, K. (2008). Central obesity and increased risk of dementia more than three decades later. *Neurology* 71, 1057–1064. doi: 10.1212/01.wnl.0000306313.89165.ef

Willette, A. A., Bendlin, B. B., Starks, E. J., Birdsill, A. C., Johnson, S. C., Christian, B. T., et al. (2015a). Association of insulin resistance with cerebral glucose uptake in late middle-aged adults at risk for Alzheimer disease. *JAMA Neurol.* 72, 1013–1020. doi: 10.1001/jamaneurol.2015.0613

Willette, A. A., Modanlo, N., and Kapogiannis, D. (2015b). Insulin resistance predicts medial temporal hypermetabolism in mild cognitive impairment conversion to Alzheimer disease. *Diabetes* 64, 1933–1940. doi: 10.2337/db14-1507

Woods, S. C., Seeley, R. J., Baskin, D. G., and Schwartz, M. W. (2003). Insulin and the blood-brain barrier. *Curr. Pharm. Des.* 9, 795–800. doi: 10.2174/1381612033455323

Wyss-Coray, T., and Rogers, J. (2012). Inflammation in Alzheimer disease-a brief review of the basic science and clinical literature. *Cold Spring Harb. Perspect. Med.* 2:a006346. doi: 10.1101/cshperspect.a006346

Yaffe, K., Blackwell, T., Kanaya, A. M., Davidowitz, N., Barrett-Connor, E., and Krueger, K. (2004). Diabetes, impaired fasting glucose, and development of cognitive impairment in older women. *Neurology* 63, 658–663. doi: 10.1212/01.WNL.0000134666.64593.ba

Yaffe, K., Blackwell, T., Whitmer, R. A., Krueger, K., and Barrett Connor, E. (2006). Glycosylated hemoglobin level and development of mild cognitive impairment or dementia in older women. *J. Nutr. Health Aging* 10, 293–295.

Yamagishi, S., Maeda, S., Matsui, T., Ueda, S., Fukami, K., and Okuda, S. (2012). Role of advanced glycation end products (AGEs) and oxidative stress in vascular complications in diabetes. *Biochim. Biophys. Acta* 1820, 663–671. doi: 10.1016/j.bbagen.2011.03.014

Yao, J., and Brinton, R. D. (2011). Targeting mitochondrial bioenergetics for Alzheimer's prevention and treatment. *Curr. Pharm. Des.* 17, 3474–3479. doi: 10.2174/138161211798072517

Yao, J., and Brinton, R. D. (2012). Estrogen regulation of mitochondrial bioenergetics: implications for prevention of Alzheimer's disease. *Adv. Pharmacol.* 64, 327–371. doi: 10.1016/b978-0-12-394816-8.00010-6

Yao, J., Hamilton, R. T., Cadenas, E., and Brinton, R. D. (2010). Decline in mitochondrial bioenergetics and shift to ketogenic profile in brain during reproductive senescence. *Biochim. Biophys. Acta* 1800, 1121–1126. doi: 10.1016/j.bbagen.2010.06.002

Yao, J., Irwin, R., Chen, S., Hamilton, R., Cadenas, E., and Brinton, R. D. (2012). Ovarian hormone loss induces bioenergetic deficits and mitochondrial β-amyloid. *Neurobiol. Aging* 33, 1507–1521. doi: 10.1016/j.neurobiolaging.2011.03.001

Yao, J., Irwin, R. W., Zhao, L., Nilsen, J., Hamilton, R. T., and Brinton, R. D. (2009). Mitochondrial bioenergetic deficit precedes Alzheimer's pathology in female mouse model of Alzheimer's disease. *Proc. Natl. Acad. Sci. U S A* 106, 14670–14675. doi: 10.1073/pnas.0903563106

Yao, J., Rettberg, J. R., Klosinski, L. P., Cadenas, E., and Brinton, R. D. (2011). Shift in brain metabolism in late onset alzheimer's disease: implications for biomarkers and therapeutic interventions. *Mol. Aspects Med.* 32, 247–257. doi: 10.1016/j.mam.2011.10.005

Yan, L. M., Velkova, A., and Kapurniotu, A. (2014). Molecular characterization of the hetero-assembly of β-amyloid peptide with islet amyloid polypeptide. *Curr. Pharm. Des.* 20, 1182–1191. doi: 10.2174/13816128113199990064

Zhang, Y., Zhou, B., Deng, B., Zhang, F., Wu, J., Wang, Y., et al. (2013). Amyloid-β induces hepatic insulin resistance *in vivo* via JAK2. *Diabetes* 62, 1159–1166. doi: 10.2337/db12-0670

Zhao, W. Q., and Alkon, D. L. (2001). Role of insulin and insulin receptor in learning and memory. *Mol. Cell. Endocrinol.* 177, 125–134. doi: 10.1016/s0303-7207(01)00455-5

Zhao, W.-Q., Chen, H., Quon, M. J., and Alkon, D. L. (2004). Insulin and the insulin receptor in experimental models of learning and memory. *Eur. J. Pharmacol.* 490, 71–81. doi: 10.1016/j.ejphar.2004.02.045

Zhao, W., Chen, H., Xu, H., Moore, E., Meiri, N., Quon, M. J., et al. (1999). Brain insulin receptors and spatial memory. Correlated changes in gene expression, tyrosine phosphorylation, and signaling molecules in the hippocampus of water maze trained rats. *J. Biol. Chem.* 274, 34893–34902. doi: 10.1074/jbc.274.49.34893

Zhu, D., Lai, Y., Shelat, P. B., Hu, C., Sun, G. Y., and Lee, J. C. (2006). Phospholipases A2 mediate amyloid-β peptide-induced mitochondrial dysfunction. *J. Neurosci.* 26, 11111–11119. doi: 10.1523/jneurosci.3505-06.2006

Zhao, N., Liu, C. C., Van Ingelgom, A. J., Martens, Y. A., Linares, C., Knight, J. A., et al. (2017). Apolipoprotein E4 impairs neuronal insulin signaling by trapping insulin receptor in the endosomes. *Neuron* 96, 115.e5–129.e5. doi: 10.1016/j.neuron.2017.09.003

Zhao, L., Teter, B., Morihara, T., Lim, G. P., Ambegaokar, S. S., Ubeda, O. J., et al. (2004). Insulin-degrading enzyme as a downstream target of insulin receptor signaling cascade: implications for Alzheimer's disease intervention. *J. Neurosci.* 24, 11120–11126. doi: 10.1523/JNEUROSCI.2860-04.2004

8

APOE and Alzheimer's Disease: Neuroimaging of Metabolic and Cerebrovascular Dysfunction

*Jason A. Brandon, Brandon C. Farmer, Holden C. Williams and Lance A. Johnson**

Department of Physiology, University of Kentucky, Lexington, KY, United States

***Correspondence:**
Lance A. Johnson
johnson.lance@uky.edu

Apolipoprotein E4 (ApoE4) is the strongest genetic risk factor for late onset Alzheimer's Disease (AD), and is associated with impairments in cerebral metabolism and cerebrovascular function. A substantial body of literature now points to E4 as a driver of multiple impairments seen in AD, including blunted brain insulin signaling, mismanagement of brain cholesterol and fatty acids, reductions in blood brain barrier (BBB) integrity, and decreased cerebral glucose uptake. Various neuroimaging techniques, in particular positron emission topography (PET) and magnetic resonance imaging (MRI), have been instrumental in characterizing these metabolic and vascular deficits associated with this important AD risk factor. In the current mini-review article, we summarize the known effects of *APOE* on cerebral metabolism and cerebrovascular function, with a special emphasis on recent findings via neuroimaging approaches.

Keywords: ApoE, apolipoprotein E, cerebral, metabolism, brain, imaging, neurodegeneration, Alzheimer's Disease (AD)

INTRODUCTION

Apolipoprotein E (ApoE) plays an critical role in the metabolism of lipoproteins and redistribution of cholesterol, and has long been studied in relation to atherosclerosis and cardiovascular disease (Mahley and Rall, 2000; Eichner et al., 2002; Pendse et al., 2009). In the periphery, apoE is primarily produced by the liver, but is also expressed by a number of other tissues (Driscoll and Getz, 1984; Zechner et al., 1991). In the brain, apoE is primarily produced by astrocytes, and it plays a critical role in neuronal maintenance and repair (Xu et al., 1996, 2006; Mahley and Rall, 2000). In humans, there are three major isoforms of apoE: E2, E3 and E4 (Mahley and Rall, 2000). E3 is the major isoform expressed in humans, and the effects of E2 and E4 are typically compared to those of E3 to determine relative risk (Phillips, 2014). Importantly, *APOE* is the strongest genetic risk factor for late onset Alzheimer's Disease (AD), with E4 conferring between a 3- (heterozygous) to 15-fold (homozygous) increase in risk of AD (Farrer et al., 1997; Raber et al., 2004). Conversely, E2 is associated with increased longevity and a decreased risk of AD (Farrer et al., 1997; Garatachea et al., 2014).

Normal synaptic function requires a multitude of energy-intensive processes, and a complex and intricately linked interplay between neurons and supporting glia is necessary to maintain efficient energy metabolism (Belanger et al., 2011). Metabolic dysfunction, as in the case of insulin resistance (IR) and type 2 diabetes, increases the risk of dementia and shares several pathological characteristics with AD, such as inflammation, increases in oxidative stress and vascular dysfunction (Craft, 2009; Walker and Harrison, 2015). Metabolic disorders also increase in incidence with age (Narayan et al., 2006) and a rapidly ageing demographic means the number of individuals suffering from both metabolic disorders and AD is expanding precipitously.

It is now well established that E4 is associated with various impairments in CNS metabolism, most notably decreased cerebral glucose uptake. A substantial body of literature now suggests that

E4 carriage can in itself be viewed as a form of cerebral metabolic dysfunction. In the current mini-review article, we summarize important recent findings related to apoE's role in modulating cerebral metabolism and cerebrovascular function, with a special emphasis on neuroimaging approaches (see **Figure 1**).

APOE, CEREBRAL GLUCOSE METABOLISM, AND PERIPHERAL GLUCOSE REGULATION

^{18}F-Fluorodeoxyglucose positron emission topography (FDG-PET) is commonly used to measure cerebral glucose metabolism. A reduction in cerebral metabolic rate of glucose (CMRglc), as measured by FDG-PET, is now considered one of the hallmarks of AD (Small et al., 2000). FDG-PET is able to differentiate AD from other types of dementia with a high degree of specificity due to specific regional patterns (Laforce and Rabinovici, 2011). Clinical AD symptoms essentially never occur without glucose hypometabolism, and the extent of the metabolic changes are strongly correlated with the severity of clinical symptoms (Grady et al., 1986; Haxby et al., 1990; Blass, 2002). Furthermore, recent evidence suggests that these alterations in glucose metabolism occur very early in the neurodegenerative process (Small et al., 1995; Reiman et al., 1996; de Leon et al., 2001; Mosconi et al., 2008).

Interestingly, a pattern of brain glucose hypometabolism regionally similar to that observed in AD has been described in individuals with E4 in a number of studies over the past two decades (reviewed in more detail here, Wolf et al., 2013). This pattern of decreased cerebral glucose metabolism is observed even in non-demented, cognitively normal E4 carriers (Small et al., 1995, 2000; Reiman et al., 1996, 2001) thereby lending support to this being an inherent biological feature of E4, rather than simply a byproduct of dementia (Reiman et al., 2004). Importantly, these metabolic deficits are present decades in advance of AD onset in E4 individuals—reductions in cerebral glucose utilization are observed in normal E4 individuals as young as their 20–30s (Reiman et al., 2004). This pattern of cerebral glucose hypometabolism in young E4 carriers is considered the earliest brain abnormality described to date in living individuals at risk for AD (Mosconi et al., 2008). Below, we summarize some more recent findings that may shed light on this well-established E4-associated phenomenon, including studies that look beyond FDG-PET imaging.

A recent study by Nielsen et al. (2017) examined how peripheral apoE levels affect cognition, gray matter volume (GMV) and cerebral glucose metabolism in an isoform-dependent manner. They showed that females not only have higher plasma levels of total apoE and apoE4 compared to males, but also see significant increases in the apoE3 isoform with age (Nielsen et al., 2017). In the same study, higher ratios of apoE4/apoE3 were negatively associated with CMRglc and GMV. These results may point toward an important role for peripheral apoE levels in modulating brain health and may offer insight into the higher risk of AD in women, particularly women with E4 (Altmann et al., 2014; Nielsen et al., 2017).

Several recent studies have explored the connection between E4, glucose metabolism and amyloid pathology. For example, by comparing FDG-PET data using β-amyloid as a continuous variable, Carbonell et al. (2016) showed that E4 and β-amyloid have a strong association with glucose hypometabolism during early AD stages. Cognitively normal E4 carriers have increased Aβ deposition, with a nonlinear relationship with age; albeit subtle effects on GMV and glucose metabolism compared to FDG-PET scans of other cognitively normal noncarriers (Gonneaud et al., 2016).

Other groups have recently begun to probe the relationship of peripheral glucose regulation and insulin sensitivity to cerebral metabolism. For example, Foley et al. (2016) showed that in E4 carriers, the degree of glucose dysregulation (measured by fasting blood glucose concentration and HbA1C) correlates with reduced cortical thickness; in fact, those diagnosed with diabetes demonstrated a level of cortical thinning comparable to that of preclinical AD. Additionally, impaired glycemia (defined here as a fasting glucose $\geq$100 mg/dL) and E4 genotype are independent risk factors for cerebral amyloid deposition in cortical regions, but do not appear to have an additive effect (Morris et al., 2016). E4 also confers a greater risk of age-related white matter hyperintensities in diabetics aged 73–76 years and acts as a predictor for progression of white matter hyperintensities (Cox et al., 2017). Finally, post-mortem studies of young adult E4 carriers showed upregulation of several transporters (GLUT1, GLUT3 and MCT2), metabolic enzymes (hexokinase, SCOT and AACS), and mitochondrial complexes I, II, IV, suggestive of inherent apoE-associated alterations in metabolism (Valla et al., 2010; Perkins et al., 2016).

Increasing evidence suggests that cognitive impairment resulting from IR and E4 share common neuropathological features and involve similar changes in metabolism and cerebrovascular function. For instance, the cerebrovascular pathology observed in diabetic patients and in individuals with E4 show significant overlap (Walker and Harrison, 2015) and both IR and E4 have been independently associated with brain glucose hypometabolism and reduced cerebral blood flow (CBF; Thambisetty et al., 2010; Filippini et al., 2011; Pallas and Larson, 1996; Chung et al., 2015). Additionally, these two risk factors appear to interact to impair cognition and drive neurodegeneration (Peila et al., 2002; Dore et al., 2009; Salameh et al., 2016; Johnson et al., 2017a,b). Along these lines, a number of recent studies directly implicate E4 in pathways of insulin signaling (Wolf et al., 2013). For example, in both human apoE mice and postmortem human brain tissue, E4 reduced the expression of insulin signaling proteins such as IRS1 and Akt (Ong et al., 2014; Keeney et al., 2015). In a mouse model of AD, E4 expression accelerated cognitive deficits and exaggerated impairments in insulin signaling (Chan et al., 2015, 2016). Importantly, a recent study by Zhao et al. (2017) showed that E4 directly impairs cerebral insulin signaling in an age-dependent manner, and that peripheral IR and E4 also acted synergistically to impair insulin signaling in the brain. Finally, E4+ individuals do not cognitively benefit from intranasal insulin administration, suggestive of brain IR (Reger et al., 2006; Hanson et al., 2015b). Together, these findings may suggest a metabolic

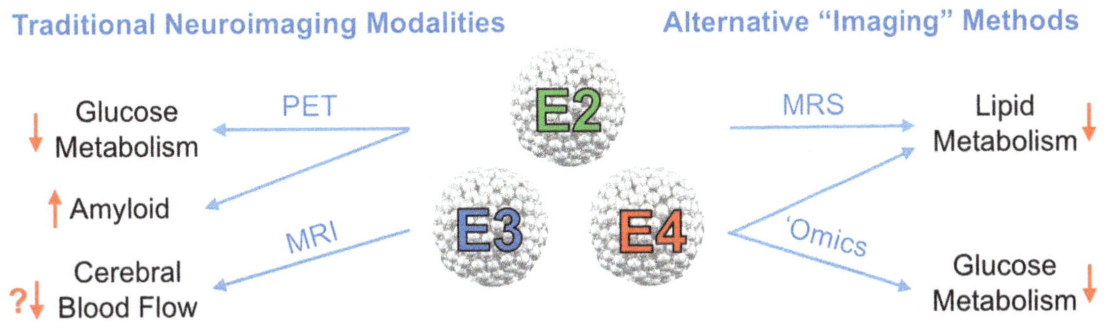

FIGURE 1 | Neuroimaging approaches to study the effects of the Apolipoprotein E (ApoE) isoforms on cerebral metabolism. Left: traditional neuroimaging techniques, in particular positron emission topography (PET) and magnetic resonance imaging (MRI), have been invaluable in characterizing the metabolic and cerebrovascular deficits associated with APOE4, the strongest genetic risk factor for late onset Alzheimer's disease (AD). ^{18}F-Fluorodeoxyglucose positron emission topography (FDG-PET) imaging has consistently shown a pattern of brain glucose hypometabolism in individuals with E4, while amyloid PET imaging shows increased amyloid deposition. Some, but not all, blood oxygen level dependent (BOLD) functional magnetic resonance imaging (fMRI) studies in E4 individuals have shown decreased cerebral blood flow (CBF). Right: other alternative, or non-imaging methods of visualizing vascular and metabolic changes may prove instrumental in elucidating apoE isoform-specific effects on AD risk and progression. Magnetic resonance spectroscopy (MRS), metabolomics and lipidomics studies have implicated E4 in multiple pathways of lipid and glucose metabolism (effects of E4 denoted by red arrows).

dysregulation in early life stages preceding disease onset (Perkins et al., 2016).

APOE AND BRAIN LIPID METABOLISM

ApoE serves as the primary lipid carrier protein in the brain, carrying cholesterol synthesized from astrocytes to neurons in HDL-like lipoprotein particles. These lipid carrying lipoproteins have been shown to interact with Aβ (Sanan et al., 1994). In both transgenic AD mouse models and in post-mortem AD tissue, apoE and its corresponding cholesterol were shown to co-localize with Aβ plaques (Panchal et al., 2010; Lazar et al., 2013). Interestingly, lipid associated E4 has a higher Aβ binding affinity than the delipidated isoforms (Sanan et al., 1994). While this may suggest that cholesterol is involved in E4 driven AD pathology, the mechanism by which apoE-shuttled cholesterol interacts with Aβ is unclear.

In addition to *APOE* associated alterations in brain cholesterol, studies have shown that there is an isoform-dependent usage of fatty acids in both mice and humans. Arbones-Mainar et al. (2016) showed that E4 mice exhibit a metabolic shift toward fatty acid oxidation compared to controls using indirect calorimetry. In humans, it has been reported that E4 individuals β-oxidize uniformly labeled docosahexaenoic acid at higher rates than age- and disease-matched controls (Chouinard-Watkins et al., 2013). E4 expressing mice have also shown to have dysregulated fatty acid synthesis in the entorhinal cortex (Nuriel et al., 2017). Specifically, targeted metabolomics of E4 entorhinal cortices revealed significant changes in multiple glycerolipid and glycerophospholipid species, (Johnson et al., 2017a) as well as seven fatty acid species, (Nuriel et al., 2017) when compared to E3 mice. Thus, in addition to the glucose and insulin impairments described in the previous section, these studies point to a potential lipid mismanagement in E4 carriers which may contribute to AD pathogenesis.

APOE, CEREBRAL BLOOD FLOW AND CEREBRAL AMYLOID ANGIOPATHY

Similar to dynamic vasculature meeting metabolic needs through hyperemic action in skeletal muscle, a related theory has been posited in the brain as so called "neurovascular coupling". These events are the observed increases in CBF to meet hyperactive neuronal activity. Initially thought to be a response to an oxygen deficit, there is now evidence suggesting direct action of various vasoactive agents on the local vasculature to modulate CBF. Neurovascular coupling is the basis for routinely used imaging platforms including functional magnetic resonance imaging (fMRI). The blood oxygen level dependent (BOLD) contrast response represents an fMRI signal comprised of both a blood flow and metabolic component, as each voxel reflects changes in deoxyhemoglobin and CBF.

Some studies suggest that cerebral hypoperfusion precedes, and possibly contributes to, the onset of dementia (Ruitenberg et al., 2005). Because metabolic rate and CBF are coupled, alterations in cerebral metabolism are likely to affect CBF (Koehler et al., 2009). However, it remains unclear whether cerebral hypoperfusion is a driver of cognitive decline, or whether the deficits simply reflect diminished metabolic demand due to aging and/or neurodegeneration. Given the importance of an efficient and responsive vascular system, it has been proposed that the accelerated AD pathogenesis associated with E4 may result from detrimental cerebrovasculature effects (Tai et al., 2016).

It is well established that CBF is decreased in AD patients (Celsis et al., 1997; Roher et al., 2012). However, both increased (Scarmeas et al., 2005; Thambisetty et al., 2010; Filippini et al., 2011) and decreased (Wierenga et al., 2013; Zlatar et al., 2014) CBF has been observed in individuals with E4, with results differing depending on age (Filippini et al., 2011). Reduced CBF in multiple brain regions has been observed in elderly E4 carriers relative to non-carriers (Filippini et al., 2011). Cognitively normal E4 individuals also show sharper age-related declines in regional CBF (Thambisetty et al., 2010) and *APOE* modifies the association between cognitive function and age-related changes in CBF (Wierenga et al., 2013). In addition to these differences in resting CBF, several studies have shown differences in functional activation, as measured by BOLD fMRI, in middle aged and older E4 individuals (Scarmeas et al., 2005). Functional differences in CBF have been noted in individuals as early as their 20s (Scarmeas et al., 2005) suggesting that E4-associated alterations in brain physiology occur early in life—in the absence of gross neuropathological changes and preceding cognitive impairments (Di Battista et al., 2016).

Evidence from studies using human apoE mice also highlight CBF as a potential link between E4 and impaired cognition. For example, Wiesmann et al. (2016) recently used a flow-sensitive MRI technique to show that 18-month old E4 mice have reduced CBF compared to WT mice. Using MRI, Lin et al. (2017) similarly showed that compared to WT mice, E4 mice have reduced CBF. Furthermore, they showed improvements in CBF in E4 mice following treatment with rapamycin, a pleiotropic compound with various metabolic effects, and provided evidence that the blood brain barrier (BBB) is involved in mediating these effects (Lin et al., 2017). Our own group recently showed that both diet-induced IR and E4 decreased cerebral blood volume (CBV) as measured with optical microangiography (Johnson et al., 2017b). We further demonstrated that an oral glucose gavage selectively improved cognitive performance in E4 mice with IR, and that this spike in blood glucose resulted in a significant increase in CBV. Interestingly, our results in this mouse model of human apoE mirrored a recent clinical research study, in which E4 carriers showed acute cognitive benefits from a high glycemic index meal (Hanson et al., 2015a). However, it should be noted that not all studies of CBF or CBV in human apoE mice have been in consensus. For example, a recent study using a steady-state gadolinium-enhanced fMRI technique showed that, compared to E3 mice, aged E4 mice were found to have higher CBV in the hippocampal formations (Nuriel et al., 2017).

BBB dysfunction can lead to impairments in microvascular function, and thus represents a potential pathway leading to neurodegeneration and AD (Zlokovic, 2013). In fact, multiple studies have linked *APOE* genotype with BBB function, with E4 leading to higher BBB permeability, decreased cerebral vascularization, thinner vessel walls and reduced CBF (Bell et al., 2012; Alata et al., 2015). Importantly, these E4-associated vascular defects were observed as early as 2 weeks of age (Bell et al., 2012) well preceding the neuronal and synaptic dysfunction that is observed in these mice in late age.

Apart from its effect on AD risk, E4 has also been independently linked to the development of cerebral amyloid angiopathy (CAA). A majority of AD brains show CAA, which is a result of amyloid deposition within the walls of small vessels in the leptomeninges and brain parenchyma. A recent study from Nielsen et al. (2017) showed increased incidence of CAA in ApoE4 postmortem brain tissues. Interestingly, they also found an association with E2, but this finding is not consistent across other studies (Rannikmae et al., 2014). CAA has been studied in the context of AD mouse models as well. Deletion of murine *APOE* in two mouse models of Aβ deposition resulted in abolishment of Aβ deposits in the brain parenchyma and cerebrovasculature (Holtzman et al., 2000). This deletion also resulted in less CAA-associated microhemorrhage (Fryer et al., 2005). These data demonstrate that apoE facilitates the formation of cerebrovascular plaques, which are pathological hallmarks of CAA. As compliance decreases with increased deposition of insoluble material, it is probable that cerebrovascular amyloid has substantial effects on the hemodynamics of the brain microvasculature. Could deposition of Aβ in the microvascular walls be a primary cause of the decreased CBF in E4 individuals? Questions such as these highlight the need for further studies examining CBF in the context of CAA.

LIMITATIONS OF CEREBRAL METABOLIC IMAGING, ALTERNATIVE "IMAGING" APPROACHES AND FUTURE DIRECTIONS

While they have provided an invaluable knowledge base, each brain imaging technology described above comes with its own set of limitations. Of particular importance in regards to the E4-associated phenomenon of cerebral glucose hypometabolism, are the limitations to biological interpretation of FDG-PET measures. Mainly that CMRglc as determined by FDG-PET is based on blood flow, 2-deoxyglucose (not glucose) transport out of the bloodstream, and phosphorylation of 2DG by the enzyme hexokinase. Thus, the process and its interpretation are restricted to the initial biochemical steps of glycolysis. In theory, the net rate of 2DG uptake is equal to the net rate of the entire glycolytic pathway at steady state (Reivich et al., 1969; Sokoloff et al., 1977; Sokoloff, 1977, 1984; Phelps et al., 1979). However, limited resolution means the cell type(s) responsible remain unknown, and there is no information on whether glucose is eventually converted to ATP in mitochondria, enters the pentose phosphate pathway, is stored as glycogen, or converted to lactate (Mosconi, 2013). Thus, future studies aimed at tracing glucose and other metabolites to their eventual fate will be critical in expanding our understanding of *APOE*'s effects on cerebral metabolism.

Outside of traditional PET- and MRI-based approaches, a few other imaging modalities have been applied to the question of *APOE* influences on cerebral metabolism. For example, magnetic resonance spectroscopy (MRS) has been used by several groups to examine common metabolite concentrations in control and AD individuals of various *APOE* genotypes, as well as human apoE mice. Results have been conflicting, with some groups showing increased choline/creatine and myo-inositol/creatine ratios in E4 carriers (Gomar et al., 2014; Riese et al., 2015) while others showed no *APOE* differences in measured metabolites (Kantarci et al.,

2000; Suri et al., 2017). Finally, Dumanis et al. (2013) used MRS in human apoE mice to show a decrease in production of glutamate and increased levels of glutamine in E4 mice.

New applications of established imaging modalities are also providing novel insight into cerebral metabolism. For example, a recent study by Shokouhi et al. (2017) utilized a novel FDG-PET analysis, the regional FDG time correlation coefficient (rFTC) to sensitively measure longitudinal changes in metabolism in cognitively normal individuals. By capturing within-subject similarities between baseline and follow-up regional radiotracer distributions, they showed that rFTC decline was significantly steeper in E4 carriers compared to noncarriers (Shokouhi et al., 2017). PET can provide measurement of not only CMRglc, but also metabolic rate of oxygen ($CMRO_2$), thereby allowing estimation of glucose metabolism outside of oxidative phosphorylation, or aerobic glycolysis. A series of articles by Raichle and colleagues have shed new light on the importance of cerebral rates of aerobic glycolysis by defining a new measure of aerobic glycolysis, the glycolytic index (GI), and applying this measure to pertinent studies of regional metabolic variability, amyloid deposition, and cognitive activation. Vaishnavi et al. (2010) showed strong regional variations in aerobic glycolysis, with two cortical regions (the default mode network and areas in the frontal and parietal cortex), showing the highest rate. Further, the areas of the normal brain that demonstrate the highest rates of aerobic glycolysis show near complete overlap with areas of the AD brain that preferentially accumulate amyloid, and it has thus been suggested that impairments in aerobic glycolysis may contribute to AD pathophysiology (Vlassenko et al., 2010). Finally, Shannon et al. (2016) combined fMRI and PET to examine the metabolic profile of activated brain areas before and after a task, and demonstrate that aerobic glycolysis is indeed enhanced in areas undergoing learning induced plasticity. Interestingly, declines in cerebral glucose utilization are greater than those in blood flow and oxygen consumption in the early stages of AD (Lying-Tunell et al., 1981; Hoyer et al., 1991; Fukuyama et al., 1994; Blass, 2002). This discrepancy in the initial stages of the disease may suggest that changes in aerobic glycolysis are an influential metabolic feature of early AD, and raises several important questions, including: Do differences in aerobic glycolysis underlie the hypometabolism observed in young E4 carriers?

Finally, other non-imaging methods of "visualizing" metabolic changes may prove instrumental in elucidating *APOE*-driven alterations in cerebral metabolism. For example, two groups have applied metabolomic analyses to brain tissue from human apoE expressing mice (Johnson et al., 2017a; Nuriel et al., 2017). Nuriel et al. (2017) used a mass spectrometry (MS) based metabolomics technique to report an E4-associated downregulation of several fatty acid species and an upregulation of multiple TCA-cycle metabolites, among other changes. Our own recent study applied an integrated 'omics approach to provide insight into the metabolic pathways altered in E4 brains (Johnson et al., 2017a). Combining measures of DNA hydroxymethylation and MS-based metabolomics, we identified novel E4-associated alterations in multiple pathways, most notably purine metabolism, glutamate metabolism, and the pentose phosphate pathway (Johnson et al., 2017a).

SUMMARY

Over the years, the neuropathological characterization of AD has expanded beyond the classic descriptions of amyloid and tau pathology to include metabolic and vascular dysfunction. Advances in brain imaging, most notably PET and MRI, have been invaluable in broadening our understanding of AD pathophysiology. Specifically, the metabolic and cerebrovascular dysfunction described by these studies includes reductions in brain glucose uptake, blunted insulin signaling, alterations in brain lipid metabolism, loss of BBB integrity and deficits in CBF. As reviewed above, many similar alterations have been observed in E4+ individuals, sometimes early in life and often even in the absence of cognitive impairment. Perhaps reflected in the sum of these findings is an inherent inability of E4+ individuals to efficiently regulate cerebral metabolism; although whether it occurs at the level of the BBB or cellular uptake, oxidative phosphorylation, aerobic glycolysis or elsewhere remains unclear. Future studies aimed at expanding the important knowledge base established by PET, MRI and other traditional imaging techniques will be critical in better understanding how E4 drives metabolic dysfunction in AD, and essential in identifying new therapeutic targets to correct these deficiencies in order to delay or prevent AD.

AUTHOR CONTRIBUTIONS

JB, BF, HW and LJ wrote and edited the manuscript. All authors read and approved the final version of the manuscript.

FUNDING

This work was supported by an Institutional Development Award (IDeA) from the National Institute of General Medical Sciences of the National Institutes of Health under Grant No. P20GM103527. The content is solely the responsibility of the authors and does not necessarily represent the official views of the funding sources.

REFERENCES

Alata, W., Ye, Y., St-Amour, I., Vandal, M., and Calon, F. (2015). Human apolipoprotein E ε4 expression impairs cerebral vascularization and blood-brain barrier function in mice. *J. Cereb. Blood Flow Metab.* 35, 86–94. doi: 10.1038/jcbfm.2014.172

Altmann, A., Tian, L., Henderson, V. W., and Greicius, M. D., and Alzheimer's Disease Neuroimaging Initiative Investigators. (2014). Sex modifies the

APOE-related risk of developing Alzheimer disease. *Ann. Neurol.* 75, 563–573. doi: 10.1002/ana.24135

Arbones-Mainar, J. M., Johnson, L. A., Torres-Perez, E., Garcia, A. E., Perez-Diaz, S., Raber, J., et al. (2016). Metabolic shifts toward fatty-acid usage and increased thermogenesis are associated with impaired adipogenesis in mice expressing human APOE4. *Int. J. Obes.* 40, 1574–1581. doi: 10.1038/ijo.2016.93

Belanger, M., Allaman, I., and Magistretti, P. J. (2011). Brain energy metabolism: focus on astrocyte-neuron metabolic cooperation. *Cell Metab.* 14, 724–738. doi: 10.1016/j.cmet.2011.08.016

Bell, R. D., Winkler, E. A., Singh, I., Sagare, A. P., Deane, R., Wu, Z., et al. (2012). Apolipoprotein E controls cerebrovascular integrity via cyclophilin A. *Nature* 485, 512–516. doi: 10.1038/nature11087

Blass, J. P. (2002). Alzheimer's disease and Alzheimer's dementia: distinct but overlapping entities. *Neurobiol. Aging* 23, 1077–1084. doi: 10.1016/s0197-4580(02)00036-2

Carbonell, F., Zijdenbos, A. P., McLaren, D. G., Iturria-Medina, Y., and Bedell, B. J. (2016). Modulation of glucose metabolism and metabolic connectivity by β-amyloid. *J. Cereb. Blood Flow Metab.* 36, 2058–2071. doi: 10.1177/0271678x16654492

Celsis, P., Agniel, A., Cardebat, D., Demonet, J. F., Ousset, P. J., and Puel, M. (1997). Age related cognitive decline: a clinical entity? A longitudinal study of cerebral blood flow and memory performance. *J. Neurol. Neurosurg. Psychiatry* 62, 601–608. doi: 10.1136/jnnp.62.6.601

Chan, E. S., Chen, C., Cole, G. M., and Wong, B. S. (2015). Differential interaction of Apolipoprotein-E isoforms with insulin receptors modulates brain insulin signaling in mutant human amyloid precursor protein transgenic mice. *Sci. Rep.* 5:13842. doi: 10.1038/srep13842

Chan, E. S., Shetty, M. S., Sajikumar, S., Chen, C., Soong, T. W., and Wong, B. S. (2016). ApoE4 expression accelerates hippocampus-dependent cognitive deficits by enhancing Aβ impairment of insulin signaling in an Alzheimer's disease mouse model. *Sci. Rep.* 6:26119. doi: 10.1038/srep26119

Chouinard-Watkins, R., Rioux-Perreault, C., Fortier, M., Tremblay-Mercier, J., Zhang, Y., Lawrence, P., et al. (2013). Disturbance in uniformly 13C-labelled DHA metabolism in elderly human subjects carrying the apoE ε4 allele. *Br. J. Nutr.* 110, 1751–1759. doi: 10.1017/S0007114513001268

Chung, C. C., Pimentel, D., Jor'dan, A. J., Hao, Y., Milberg, W., and Novak, V. (2015). Inflammation-associated declines in cerebral vasoreactivity and cognition in type 2 diabetes. *Neurology* 85, 450–458. doi: 10.1212/WNL.0000000000001820

Cox, S. R., Ritchie, S. J., Dickie, D. A., Pattie, A., Royle, N. A., Corley, J., et al. (2017). Interaction of APOE ε4 and poor glycemic control predicts white matter hyperintensity growth from 73 to 76. *Neurobiol. Aging* 54, 54–58. doi: 10.1016/j.neurobiolaging.2017.02.014

Craft, S. (2009). The role of metabolic disorders in Alzheimer disease and vascular dementia: two roads converged. *Arch. Neurol.* 66, 300–305. doi: 10.1001/archneurol.2009.27

de Leon, M. J., Convit, A., Wolf, O. T., Tarshish, C. Y., DeSanti, S., Rusinek, H., et al. (2001). Prediction of cognitive decline in normal elderly subjects with 2-[^{18}F]fluoro-2-deoxy-D-glucose/poitron-emission tomography (FDG/PET). *Proc. Natl. Acad. Sci. U S A* 98, 10966–10971. doi: 10.1073/pnas.191044198

Di Battista, A. M., Heinsinger, N. M., and Rebeck, G. W. (2016). Alzheimer's disease genetic risk factor APOE-ε4 also affects normal brain function. *Curr. Alzheimer Res.* 13, 1200–1207. doi: 10.2174/1567205013666160401115127

Dore, G. A., Elias, M. F., Robbins, M. A., Elias, P. K., and Nagy, Z. (2009). Presence of the APOE ε4 allele modifies the relationship between type 2 diabetes and cognitive performance: the Maine-Syracuse Study. *Diabetologia* 52, 2551–2560. doi: 10.1007/s00125-009-1497-2

Driscoll, D. M., and Getz, G. S. (1984). Extrahepatic synthesis of apolipoprotein E. *J. Lipid Res.* 25, 1368–1379.

Dumanis, S. B., DiBattista, A. M., Miessau, M., Moussa, C. E., and Rebeck, G. W. (2013). APOE genotype affects the presynaptic compartment of glutamatergic nerve terminals. *J. Neurochem.* 124, 4–14. doi: 10.1111/j.1471-4159.2012.07908.x

Eichner, J. E., Dunn, S. T., Perveen, G., Thompson, D. M., Stewart, K. E., and Stroehla, B. C. (2002). Apolipoprotein E polymorphism and cardiovascular disease: a HuGE review. *Am. J. Epidemiol.* 155, 487–495. doi: 10.1093/aje/155.6.487

Farrer, L. A., Cupples, L. A., Haines, J. L., Hyman, B., Kukull, W. A., Mayeux, R., et al. (1997). Effects of age, sex, and ethnicity on the association between apolipoprotein E genotype and Alzheimer disease. *JAMA* 278, 1349–1356. doi: 10.1001/jama.1997.03550160069041

Filippini, N., Ebmeier, K. P., MacIntosh, B. J., Trachtenberg, A. J., Frisoni, G. B., Wilcock, G. K., et al. (2011). Differential effects of the APOE genotype on brain function across the lifespan. *Neuroimage* 54, 602–610. doi: 10.1016/j.neuroimage.2010.08.009

Foley, J. M., Salat, D. H., Stricker, N. H., McGlinchey, R. E., Milberg, W. P., Grande, L. J., et al. (2016). Glucose dysregulation interacts with APOE-4 to potentiate temporoparietal cortical thinning. *Am. J. Alzheimers Dis. Other Demen.* 31, 76–86. doi: 10.1177/1533317515587084

Fryer, J. D., Simmons, K., Parsadanian, M., Bales, K. R., Paul, S. M., Sullivan, P. M., et al. (2005). Human apolipoprotein E4 alters the amyloid-β 40:42 ratio and promotes the formation of cerebral amyloid angiopathy in an amyloid precursor protein transgenic model. *J. Neurosci.* 25, 2803–2810. doi: 10.1523/JNEUROSCI.5170-04.2005

Fukuyama, H., Ogawa, M., Yamauchi, H., Yamaguchi, S., Kimura, J., Yonekura, Y., et al. (1994). Altered cerebral energy metabolism in Alzheimer's disease: a PET study. *J. Nucl. Med.* 35, 1–6.

Garatachea, N., Emanuele, E., Calero, M., Fuku, N., Arai, Y., Abe, Y., et al. (2014). ApoE gene and exceptional longevity: insights from three independent cohorts. *Exp. Gerontol.* 53, 16–23. doi: 10.1016/j.exger.2014.02.004

Gomar, J. J., Gordon, M. L., Dickinson, D., Kingsley, P. B., Ulug, A. M., Keehlisen, L., et al. (2014). APOE genotype modulates proton magnetic resonance spectroscopy metabolites in the aging brain. *Biol. Psychiatry* 75, 686–692. doi: 10.1016/j.biopsych.2013.05.022

Gonneaud, J., Arenaza-Urquijo, E. M., Fouquet, M., Perrotin, A., Fradin, S., de La Sayette, V., et al. (2016). Relative effect of APOE ε4 on neuroimaging biomarker changes across the lifespan. *Neurology* 87, 1696–1703. doi: 10.1212/WNL.0000000000003234

Grady, C. L., Haxby, J. V., Schlageter, N. L., Berg, G., and Rapoport, S. I. (1986). Stability of metabolic and neuropsychological asymmetries in dementia of the Alzheimer type. *Neurology* 36, 1390–1392. doi: 10.1212/WNL.36.10.1390

Hanson, A. J., Bayer, J. L., Baker, L. D., Cholerton, B., VanFossen, B., Trittschuh, E., et al. (2015a). Differential effects of meal challenges on cognition, metabolism, and biomarkers for apolipoprotein E ε4 carriers and adults with mild cognitive impairment. *J. Alzheimers Dis.* 48, 205–218. doi: 10.3233/JAD-150273

Hanson, A. J., Craft, S., and Banks, W. A. (2015b). The APOE genotype: modification of therapeutic responses in Alzheimer's disease. *Curr. Pharm. Des.* 21, 114–120. doi: 10.2174/1381612820666141020164222

Haxby, J. V., Grady, C. L., Koss, E., Horwitz, B., Heston, L., Schapiro, M., et al. (1990). Longitudinal study of cerebral metabolic asymmetries and associated neuropsychological patterns in early dementia of the Alzheimer type. *Arch. Neurol.* 47, 753–760. doi: 10.1001/archneur.1990.00530070043010

Holtzman, D. M., Fagan, A. M., Mackey, B., Tenkova, T., Sartorius, L., Paul, S. M., et al. (2000). Apolipoprotein E facilitates neuritic and cerebrovascular plaque formation in an Alzheimer's disease model. *Ann. Neurol.* 47, 739–747. doi: 10.1002/1531-8249(200006)47:6<739::aid-ana6>3.3.co;2-#

Hoyer, S., Nitsch, R., and Oesterreich, K. (1991). Predominant abnormality in cerebral glucose utilization in late-onset dementia of the Alzheimer type: a cross-sectional comparison against advanced late-onset and incipient early-onset cases. *J. Neural Transm. Park. Dis. Dement. Sect.* 3, 1–14. doi: 10.1007/bf02251132

Johnson, L. A., Torres, E. R., Impey, S., Stevens, J. F., and Raber, J. (2017a). Apolipoprotein E4 and insulin resistance interact to impair cognition and alter the epigenome and metabolome. *Sci. Rep.* 7:43701. doi: 10.1038/srep43701

Johnson, L. A., Torres, E. R., Weber Boutros, S., Patel, E., Akinyeke, T., Alkayed, N. J., et al. (2017b). Apolipoprotein E4 mediates insulin resistance-associated cerebrovascular dysfunction and the post-prandial response. *J. Cereb. Blood Flow Metab.* doi: 10.1177/0271678x17746186 [Epub ahead of print].

Kantarci, K., Jack, C. R. Jr., Xu, Y. C., Campeau, N. G., O'Brien, P. C., Smith, G. E., et al. (2000). Regional metabolic patterns in mild cognitive impairment and Alzheimer's disease: a 1H MRS study. *Neurology* 55, 210–217. doi: 10.1212/wnl.55.2.210

Keeney, J. T., Ibrahimi, S., and Zhao, L. (2015). Human ApoE isoforms differentially modulate glucose and amyloid metabolic pathways in female brain: evidence of the mechanism of neuroprotection by apoE2 and implications for Alzheimer's disease prevention and early intervention. *J. Alzheimers Dis.* 48, 411–424. doi: 10.3233/JAD-150348

Koehler, R. C., Roman, R. J., and Harder, D. R. (2009). Astrocytes and the regulation of cerebral blood flow. *Trends Neurosci.* 32, 160–169. doi: 10.1016/j.tins.2008.11.005

Laforce, R. Jr., and Rabinovici, G. D. (2011). Amyloid imaging in the differential diagnosis of dementia: review and potential clinical applications. *Alzheimers Res. Ther.* 3:31. doi: 10.1186/alzrt93

Lazar, A. N., Bich, C., Panchal, M., Desbenoit, N., Petit, V. W., Touboul, D., et al. (2013). Time-of-flight secondary ion mass spectrometry (TOF-SIMS) imaging reveals cholesterol overload in the cerebral cortex of Alzheimer disease patients. *Acta Neuropathol.* 125, 133–144. doi: 10.1007/s00401-012-1041-1

Lin, A. L., Jahrling, J. B., Zhang, W., DeRosa, N., Bakshi, V., Romero, P., et al. (2017). Rapamycin rescues vascular, metabolic and learning deficits in apolipoprotein E4 transgenic mice with pre-symptomatic Alzheimer's disease. *J. Cereb. Blood Flow Metab.* 37, 217–226. doi: 10.1177/0271678x15621575

Lying-Tunell, U., Lindblad, B. S., Malmlund, H. O., and Persson, B. (1981). Cerebral blood flow and metabolic rate of oxygen, glucose, lactate, pyruvate, ketone bodies and amino acids. *Acta Neurol. Scand.* 63, 337–350. doi: 10.1111/j.1600-0404.1981.tb00788.x

Mahley, R. W., and Rall, S. C. Jr. (2000). Apolipoprotein E: far more than a lipid transport protein. *Annu. Rev. Genomics Hum. Genet.* 1, 507–537. doi: 10.1146/annurev.genom.1.1.507

Morris, J. K., Vidoni, E. D., Wilkins, H. M., Archer, A. E., Burns, N. C., Karcher, R. T., et al. (2016). Impaired fasting glucose is associated with increased regional cerebral amyloid. *Neurobiol. Aging* 44, 138–142. doi: 10.1016/j.neurobiolaging.2016.04.017

Mosconi, L. (2013). Glucose metabolism in normal aging and Alzheimer's disease: methodological and physiological considerations for PET studies. *Clin. Transl. Imaging* 1, 217–233. doi: 10.1007/s40336-013-0026-y

Mosconi, L., De Santi, S., Li, J., Tsui, W. H., Li, Y., Boppana, M., et al. (2008). Hippocampal hypometabolism predicts cognitive decline from normal aging. *Neurobiol. Aging* 29, 676–692. doi: 10.1016/j.neurobiolaging.2006.12.008

Narayan, K. M., Boyle, J. P., Geiss, L. S., Saaddine, J. B., and Thompson, T. J. (2006). Impact of recent increase in incidence on future diabetes burden: U.S., 2005–2050. *Diabetes Care* 29, 2114–2116. doi: 10.2337/dc06-1136

Nielsen, H. M., Chen, K., Lee, W., Chen, Y., Bauer, R. J. III., Reiman, E., et al. (2017). Peripheral apoE isoform levels in cognitively normal APOE ε3/ε4 individuals are associated with regional gray matter volume and cerebral glucose metabolism. *Alzheimers Res. Ther.* 9:5. doi: 10.1186/s13195-016-0231-9

Nuriel, T., Angulo, S. L., Khan, U., Ashok, A., Chen, Q., Figueroa, H. Y., et al. (2017). Neuronal hyperactivity due to loss of inhibitory tone in APOE4 mice lacking Alzheimer's disease-like pathology. *Nat. Commun.* 8:1464. doi: 10.1038/s41467-017-01444-0

Ong, Q. R., Chan, E. S., Lim, M. L., Cole, G. M., and Wong, B. S. (2014). Reduced phosphorylation of brain insulin receptor substrate and Akt proteins in apolipoprotein-E4 targeted replacement mice. *Sci. Rep.* 4:3754. doi: 10.1038/srep03754

Pallas, F., and Larson, D. F. (1996). Cerebral blood flow in the diabetic patient. *Perfusion* 11, 363–370. doi: 10.1177/026765919601100502

Panchal, M., Loeper, J., Cossec, J. C., Perruchini, C., Lazar, A., Pompon, D., et al. (2010). Enrichment of cholesterol in microdissected Alzheimer's disease senile plaques as assessed by mass spectrometry. *J. Lipid Res.* 51, 598–605. doi: 10.1194/jlr.M001859

Peila, R., Rodriguez, B. L., Launer, L. J., and Honolulu-Asia Aging Study. (2002). Type 2 diabetes, APOE gene, and the risk for dementia and related pathologies: the honolulu-asia aging study. *Diabetes* 51, 1256–1262. doi: 10.2337/diabetes.51.4.1256

Pendse, A. A., Arbones-Mainar, J. M., Johnson, L. A., Altenburg, M. K., and Maeda, N. (2009). Apolipoprotein E knock-out and knock-in mice: atherosclerosis, metabolic syndrome, and beyond. *J. Lipid Res.* 50, S178–S182. doi: 10.1194/jlr.r800070-jlr200

Perkins, M., Wolf, A. B., Chavira, B., Shonebarger, D., Meckel, J. P., Leung, L., et al. (2016). Altered energy metabolism pathways in the posterior cingulate in young adult apolipoprotein E ε4 carriers. *J. Alzheimers Dis.* 53, 95–106. doi: 10.3233/JAD-151205

Phelps, M. E., Huang, S. C., Hoffman, E. J., Selin, C., Sokoloff, L., and Kuhl, D. E. (1979). Tomographic measurement of local cerebral glucose metabolic rate in humans with (F-18)2-fluoro-2-deoxy-D-glucose: validation of method. *Ann. Neurol.* 6, 371–388. doi: 10.1002/ana.410060502

Phillips, M. C. (2014). Apolipoprotein E isoforms and lipoprotein metabolism. *IUBMB Life* 66, 616–623. doi: 10.1002/iub.1314

Raber, J., Huang, Y., and Ashford, J. W. (2004). ApoE genotype accounts for the vast majority of AD risk and AD pathology. *Neurobiol. Aging* 25, 641–650. doi: 10.1016/j.neurobiolaging.2003.12.023

Rannikmae, K., Kalaria, R. N., Greenberg, S. M., Chui, H. C., Schmitt, F. A., Samarasekera, N., et al. (2014). APOE associations with severe CAA-associated vasculopathic changes: collaborative meta-analysis. *J. Neurol. Neurosurg. Psychiatry* 85, 300–305. doi: 10.1136/jnnp-2013-306485

Reger, M. A., Watson, G. S., Frey, W. H. II., Baker, L. D., Cholerton, B., Keeling, M. L., et al. (2006). Effects of intranasal insulin on cognition in memory-impaired older adults: modulation by APOE genotype. *Neurobiol. Aging* 27, 451–458. doi: 10.1016/j.neurobiolaging.2005.03.016

Reiman, E. M., Caselli, R. J., Chen, K., Alexander, G. E., Bandy, D., and Frost, J. (2001). Declining brain activity in cognitively normal apolipoprotein E ε4 heterozygotes: a foundation for using positron emission tomography to efficiently test treatments to prevent Alzheimer's disease. *Proc. Natl. Acad. Sci. U S A* 98, 3334–3339. doi: 10.1073/pnas.061509598

Reiman, E. M., Caselli, R. J., Yun, L. S., Chen, K., Bandy, D., Minoshima, S., et al. (1996). Preclinical evidence of Alzheimer's disease in persons homozygous for the ε4 allele for apolipoprotein E. *N. Engl. J. Med.* 334, 752–758. doi: 10.1056/nejm199603213341202

Reiman, E. M., Chen, K., Alexander, G. E., Caselli, R. J., Bandy, D., Osborne, D., et al. (2004). Functional brain abnormalities in young adults at genetic risk for late-onset Alzheimer's dementia. *Proc. Natl. Acad. Sci. U S A* 101, 284–289. doi: 10.1073/pnas.2635903100

Reivich, M., Jehle, J., Sokoloff, L., and Kety, S. S. (1969). Measurement of regional cerebral blood flow with antipyrine-14C in awake cats. *J. Appl. Physiol.* 27, 296–300. doi: 10.1152/jappl.1969.27.2.296

Riese, F., Gietl, A., Zölch, N., Henning, A., O'Gorman, R., Kalin, A. M., et al. (2015). Posterior cingulate γ-aminobutyric acid and glutamate/glutamine are reduced in amnestic mild cognitive impairment and are unrelated to amyloid deposition and apolipoprotein E genotype. *Neurobiol. Aging* 36, 53–59. doi: 10.1016/j.neurobiolaging.2014.07.030

Roher, A. E., Debbins, J. P., Malek-Ahmadi, M., Chen, K., Pipe, J. G., Maze, S., et al. (2012). Cerebral blood flow in Alzheimer's disease. *Vasc. Health Risk Manag.* 8, 599–611. doi: 10.2147/VHRM.S34874

Ruitenberg, A., den Heijer, T., Bakker, S. L., van Swieten, J. C., Koudstaal, P. J., Hofman, A., et al. (2005). Cerebral hypoperfusion and clinical onset of dementia: the Rotterdam Study. *Ann. Neurol.* 57, 789–794. doi: 10.1002/ana.20493

Salameh, T. S., Rhea, E. M., Banks, W. A., and Hanson, A. J. (2016). Insulin resistance, dyslipidemia, and apolipoprotein E interactions as mechanisms in cognitive impairment and Alzheimer's disease. *Exp. Biol. Med. Maywood* 241, 1676–1683. doi: 10.1177/1535370216660770

Sanan, D. A., Weisgraber, K. H., Russell, S. J., Mahley, R. W., Huang, D., Saunders, A., et al. (1994). Apolipoprotein E associates with β amyloid peptide of Alzheimer's disease to form novel monofibrils. Isoform apoE4 associates more efficiently than apoE3. *J. Clin. Invest.* 94, 860–869. doi: 10.1172/jci117407

Scarmeas, N., Habeck, C. G., Hilton, J., Anderson, K. E., Flynn, J., Park, A., et al. (2005). APOE related alterations in cerebral activation even at college age. *J. Neurol. Neurosurg. Psychiatry* 76, 1440–1444. doi: 10.1136/jnnp.2004.053645

Shannon, B. J., Vaishnavi, S. N., Vlassenko, A. G., Shimony, J. S., Rutlin, J., and Raichle, M. E. (2016). Brain aerobic glycolysis and motor adaptation learning. *Proc. Natl. Acad. Sci. U S A* 113, E3782–E3791. doi: 10.1073/pnas.1604977113

Shokouhi, S., Riddle, W. R., and Kang, H. (2017). A new data analysis approach for measuring longitudinal changes of metabolism in cognitively normal elderly adults. *Clin. Interv. Aging* 12, 2123–2130. doi: 10.2147/CIA.S150859

Small, G. W., Ercoli, L. M., Silverman, D. H., Huang, S. C., Komo, S., Bookheimer, S. Y., et al. (2000). Cerebral metabolic and cognitive decline in persons at genetic risk for Alzheimer's disease. *Proc. Natl. Acad. Sci. U S A* 97, 6037–6042. doi: 10.1073/pnas.090106797

Small, G. W., Mazziotta, J. C., Collins, M. T., Baxter, L. R., Phelps, M. E., Mandelkern, M. A., et al. (1995). Apolipoprotein E type 4 allele and cerebral glucose metabolism in relatives at risk for familial Alzheimer disease. *JAMA* 273, 942–947. doi: 10.1001/jama.1995.03520360056039

Sokoloff, L. (1977). Relation between physiological function and energy metabolism in the central nervous system. *J. Neurochem.* 29, 13–26. doi: 10.1111/j.1471-4159.1977.tb03919.x

Sokoloff, L. (1984). Modeling metabolic processes in the brain *in vivo*. *Ann. Neurol.* 15, S1–S11. doi: 10.1002/ana.410150703

Sokoloff, L., Reivich, M., Kennedy, C., Des Rosiers, M. H., Patlak, C. S., Pettigrew, K. D., et al. (1977). The [^{14}C]deoxyglucose method for the measurement of local cerebral glucose utilization: theory, procedure, and normal values in the conscious and anesthetized albino rat. *J. Neurochem.* 28, 897–916. doi: 10.1111/j.1471-4159.1977.tb10649.x

Suri, S., Emir, U., Stagg, C. J., Near, J., Mekle, R., Schubert, F., et al. (2017). Effect of age and the APOE gene on metabolite concentrations in the posterior cingulate cortex. *Neuroimage* 152, 509–516. doi: 10.1016/j.neuroimage.2017.03.031

Tai, L. M., Thomas, R., Marottoli, F. M., Koster, K. P., Kanekiyo, T., Morris, A. W., et al. (2016). The role of APOE in cerebrovascular dysfunction. *Acta Neuropathol.* 131, 709–723. doi: 10.1007/s00401-016-1547-z

Thambisetty, M., Beason-Held, L., An, Y., Kraut, M. A., and Resnick, S. M. (2010). APOE ε4 genotype and longitudinal changes in cerebral blood flow in normal aging. *Arch. Neurol.* 67, 93–98. doi: 10.1001/archneurol.2009.913

Vaishnavi, S. N., Vlassenko, A. G., Rundle, M. M., Snyder, A. Z., Mintun, M. A., and Raichle, M. E. (2010). Regional aerobic glycolysis in the human brain. *Proc. Natl. Acad. Sci. U S A* 107, 17757–17762. doi: 10.1073/pnas.1010459107

Valla, J., Yaari, R., Wolf, A. B., Kusne, Y., Beach, T. G., Roher, A. E., et al. (2010). Reduced posterior cingulate mitochondrial activity in expired young adult carriers of the APOE ε4 allele, the major late-onset alzheimer's susceptibility gene. *J. Alzheimers Dis.* 22, 307–313. doi: 10.3233/JAD-2010-100129

Vlassenko, A. G., Vaishnavi, S. N., Couture, L., Sacco, D., Shannon, B. J., Mach, R. H., et al. (2010). Spatial correlation between brain aerobic glycolysis and amyloid-β (Aβ) deposition. *Proc. Natl. Acad. Sci. U S A* 107, 17763–17767. doi: 10.1073/pnas.1010461107

Walker, J. M., and Harrison, F. E. (2015). Shared neuropathological characteristics of obesity, type 2 diabetes and Alzheimer's disease: impacts on cognitive decline. *Nutrients* 7, 7332–7357. doi: 10.3390/nu7095341

Wierenga, C. E., Clark, L. R., Dev, S. I., Shin, D. D., Jurick, S. M., Rissman, R. A., et al. (2013). Interaction of age and APOE genotype on cerebral blood flow at rest. *J. Alzheimers Dis.* 34, 921–935. doi: 10.3233/JAD-121897

Wiesmann, M., Zerbi, V., Jansen, D., Haast, R., Lütjohann, D., Broersen, L. M., et al. (2016). A dietary treatment improves cerebral blood flow and brain connectivity in aging apoE4 mice. *Neural Plast.* 2016:6846721. doi: 10.1155/2016/6846721

Wolf, A. B., Caselli, R. J., Reiman, E. M., and Valla, J. (2013). APOE and neuroenergetics: an emerging paradigm in Alzheimer's disease. *Neurobiol. Aging* 34, 1007–1017. doi: 10.1016/j.neurobiolaging.2012.10.011

Xu, Q., Bernardo, A., Walker, D., Kanegawa, T., Mahley, R. W., and Huang, Y. (2006). Profile and regulation of apolipoprotein E (ApoE) expression in the CNS in mice with targeting of green fluorescent protein gene to the ApoE locus. *J. Neurosci.* 26, 4985–4994. doi: 10.1523/JNEUROSCI.5476-05.2006

Xu, P. T., Schmechel, D., Rothrock-Christian, T., Burkhart, D. S., Qiu, H. L., Popko, B., et al. (1996). Human apolipoprotein E2, E3, and E4 isoform-specific transgenic mice: human-like pattern of glial and neuronal immunoreactivity in central nervous system not observed in wild-type mice. *Neurobiol. Dis.* 3, 229–245. doi: 10.1006/nbdi.1996.0023

Zechner, R., Moser, R., Newman, T. C., Fried, S. K., and Breslow, J. L. (1991). Apolipoprotein E gene expression in mouse 3T3-L1 adipocytes and human adipose tissue and its regulation by differentiation and lipid content. *J. Biol. Chem.* 266, 10583–10588.

Zhao, N., Liu, C. C., Van Ingelgom, A. J., Martens, Y. A., Linares, C., Knight, J. A., et al. (2017). Apolipoprotein E4 impairs neuronal insulin signaling by trapping insulin receptor in the endosomes. *Neuron* 96, 115.e5–129.e5. doi: 10.1016/j.neuron.2017.09.003

Zlatar, Z. Z., Wierenga, C. E., Bangen, K. J., Liu, T. T., and Jak, A. J. (2014). Increased hippocampal blood flow in sedentary older adults at genetic risk for Alzheimer's disease. *J. Alzheimers Dis.* 41, 809–817. doi: 10.3233/JAD-132252

Zlokovic, B. V. (2013). Cerebrovascular effects of apolipoprotein E: implications for Alzheimer disease. *JAMA Neurol.* 70, 440–444. doi: 10.1001/jamaneurol.2013.2152

9

Brain–Blood Partition Coefficient and Cerebral Blood Flow in Canines Using Calibrated Short TR Recovery (CaSTRR) Correction Method

*Scott W. Thalman[1,2], David K. Powell[1,3], Margo Ubele[2], Christopher M. Norris[2,4], Elizabeth Head[5,6] and Ai-Ling Lin[1,2,4,7]**

[1] F. Joseph Halcomb III, Department of Biomedical Engineering, University of Kentucky, Lexington, KY, United States, [2] Sanders–Brown Center on Aging, University of Kentucky, Lexington, KY, United States, [3] Magnetic Resonance Imaging and Spectroscopy Center, University of Kentucky, Lexington, KY, United States, [4] Department of Pharmacology and Nutritional Sciences, University of Kentucky, Lexington, KY, United States, [5] Department of Pathology and Laboratory Medicine, University of California, Irvine, Irvine, CA, United States, [6] University of California Irvine Institute for Memory Impairments and Neurological Disorders (UCI MIND), University of California, Irvine, Irvine, CA, United States, [7] Department of Neuroscience, University of Kentucky, Lexington, KY, United States

***Correspondence:**
Ai-Ling Lin
ailing.lin@uky.edu

The brain–blood partition coefficient (BBPC) is necessary for quantifying cerebral blood flow (CBF) when using tracer based techniques like arterial spin labeling (ASL). A recent improvement to traditional MRI measurements of BBPC, called calibrated short TR recovery (CaSTRR), has demonstrated a significant reduction in acquisition time for BBPC maps in mice. In this study CaSTRR is applied to a cohort of healthy canines (n = 17, age = 5.0 – 8.0 years) using a protocol suited for application in humans at 3T. The imaging protocol included CaSTRR for BBPC maps, pseudo-continuous ASL for CBF maps, and high resolution anatomical images. The standard CaSTRR method of normalizing BBPC to gadolinium-doped deuterium oxide phantoms was also compared to normalization using hematocrit (Hct) as a proxy value for blood water content. The results show that CaSTRR is able to produce high quality BBPC maps with a 4 min acquisition time. The BBPC maps demonstrate significantly higher BBPC in gray matter (0.83 ± 0.05 mL/g) than in white matter (0.78 ± 0.04 mL/g, p = 0.006). Maps of CBF acquired with pCASL demonstrate a negative correlation between gray matter perfusion and age (p = 0.003). Voxel-wise correction for BBPC is also shown to improve contrast to noise ratio between gray and white matter in CBF maps. A novel aspect of the study was to show that that BBPC measurements can be calculated based on the known Hct of the blood sample placed in scanner. We found a strong correlation (R^2 = 0.81 in gray matter, R^2 = 0.59 in white matter) established between BBPC maps normalized to the doped phantoms and BBPC maps normalized using Hct. This obviates the need for doped water phantoms which simplifies both the acquisition protocol and the post-processing methods. Together this suggests that CaSTRR represents a feasible, rapid method to account for BBPC variability when quantifying CBF. As canines have been used widely for aging and Alzheimer's disease studies, the CaSTRR method established in the animals may further improve CBF measurements and advance our understanding of cerebrovascular changes in aging and neurodegeneration.

Keywords: cerebral blood flow, brain–blood partition coefficient, calibrated short TR recovery, arterial spin labeling, perfusion, magnetic resonance imaging, canines

INTRODUCTION

When using tracer-based techniques like arterial spin labeling (ASL) to quantify cerebral blood flow (CBF), it is necessary to determine the partition coefficient of the tracer between the perfused tissue and the arterial blood. ASL is a non-invasive, quantitative magnetic resonance imaging (MRI) technique that uses magnetically labeled protons in the water molecules of the blood as the tracer (Williams et al., 1992; Petcharunpaisan et al., 2010; Alsop et al., 2015). So in the case of ASL, the relevant partition coefficient is the brain–blood partition coefficient of water (BBPC) which is the ratio of the solubility of water in brain tissue to the solubility of water in the blood. The BBPC is tissue specific and varies with age, species, pathology, and brain region (Herscovitch and Raichle, 1985; Kudomi et al., 2005; Leithner et al., 2010; Hirata et al., 2011). This means that BBPC should be determined experimentally for each subject.

However, the standard practice in ASL studies is to assume a constant BBPC value of 0.9 mL/g for all regions of the brain regardless of the known variability of this parameter (Herscovitch and Raichle, 1985; Alsop et al., 2015). This assumption is made because the previously published MRI methods to experimentally determine BBPC required prohibitively long acquisition times and ASL studies were generally focused on gray matter perfusion where BBPC variability was assumed to be small (Roberts et al., 1996; Leithner et al., 2010). A recent study in mice at 7T reported an 87% reduction in the acquisition time for BBPC maps using an MRI technique called calibrated short TR recovery (CaSTRR) (Thalman et al., 2019). Like previous methods, CaSTRR determines relative proton density using a series of gradient echo acquisitions with varying repetition times (TR) and then calibrates the proton density map using a set of deuterium doped phantoms which provide an absolute scale of water content. The method is accelerated in CaSTRR by using shorter TR values and using gadolinium doped water phantoms to acquire similar quality BBPC maps in a fraction of the time.

The goal of this study is to apply the CaSTRR technique to a cohort of healthy canines using a protocol suited for application in humans at 3T. To do so we acquired BBPC images using a CaSTRR protocol adapted for use on a 3T human scanner. We then acquired CBF maps using pseudo-continuous ASL (pCASL) to assess the effect of BBPC correction on CBF maps, and high resolution anatomical images using magnetization prepared rapid acquisition gradient echo (MPRAGE) to facilitate segmentation and coregistration. Finally, we compare two methods of normalizing the proton density maps using the doped water phantoms and using blood water content derived from Hct values.

MATERIALS AND METHODS

Animals

All animal experiments were performed in accordance with NIH guidelines and approved by the University of Kentucky Institutional Animal Care and Use Committee (approval number #2017-2680). Middle aged beagles (n = 17, age = 5.0–8.0 years, male = 24%) were acquired as part of a longitudinal study on aging and Alzheimer's disease. The scans in this report represent pretreatment observations, and all animals were healthy at the time of their scans. The animals were anesthetized during the MRI procedure using 3–4 mg/Kg propofol for induction and 1–4% isoflurane mixed with air for maintenance. Respiratory rate, heart rate, body temperature, and blood pressure were monitored and maintained throughout the procedure. Two 5 mL vials of blood were drawn from the jugular vein using ethylenediaminetetraacetate (EDTA) treated vials. One of these was placed in the scanner with the animal according to the CaSTRR protocol, and the other was sent for laboratory analysis including Hct (ANTECH Diagnostics, Louisville, KY, United States).

Scanning Procedure

Magnetic resonance imaging experiments were performed using a 3T Siemens Prisma scanner (Siemens, Erlangen, Germany) at the MRI and Spectroscopy Center at the University of Kentucky. The animal was placed prone with their head resting in a 155 mm diameter, 15 channel transmit/receive birdcage coil commonly used for scanning human knees. The doped water phantoms along with blood sample were centered on the top of the head. The CaSTRR, pCASL, and MPRAGE acquisitions were all acquired in a single scanning session.

Calibrated Short TR Recovery Imaging

For the CaSTRR proton density measurements a series of 2-D image stacks were acquired using a phase-spoiled, fast low-angle shot gradient echo (FLASH-GRE) sequence with varying repetition times (TR = 125, 250, 500, 1000, and 2000 ms) (Thalman et al., 2019). The shortest possible echo time (TE = 1.9 ms) was used to minimize T2* decay. Image matrix parameters were: field of view = 135 × 124 mm, matrix = 96 × 88, in-plane resolution = 1.4 × 1.4 mm, slice thickness = 3 mm, number of slices = 30, flip angle = 90°, acquisition time = 4 min, labeling offset = 12 mm (see **Figure 1A**). A B_1 mapping was done to confirm accuracy and homogeneity of the B_1 field. A simulation with a saline phantom was used to simulate the gradient echo signal over a range of flip angles (see **Supplementary Figure S1**).

A Qualitative proton density map was calculated for each subject in a voxel-wise manner by fitting the signal recovery curve to the mono-exponential equation $S = M_0*[1\text{-}e\hat{}(-TR/T_1)]$ to yield a map of M_0 in arbitrary units. Next a Bayesian bias field correction (**Figure 2**) was applied to the M_0 maps to account for inhomogeneity in the receiver coil profile (Iglesiast et al., 2016). The low spatial frequency bias field was calculated using 4th order polynomials and six Gaussian components. To avoid artificially attenuating the higher signal water phantoms, the blood and water phantoms were excluded when calculating the smooth bias field, and the correction was then applied to the entire volume (see **Figures 1B,C**).

The calculation of M_0 values by voxel-wise exponential regression on the signal recovery curves resulted in a range of M_0 values on an arbitrary scale. Due to the qualitative nature

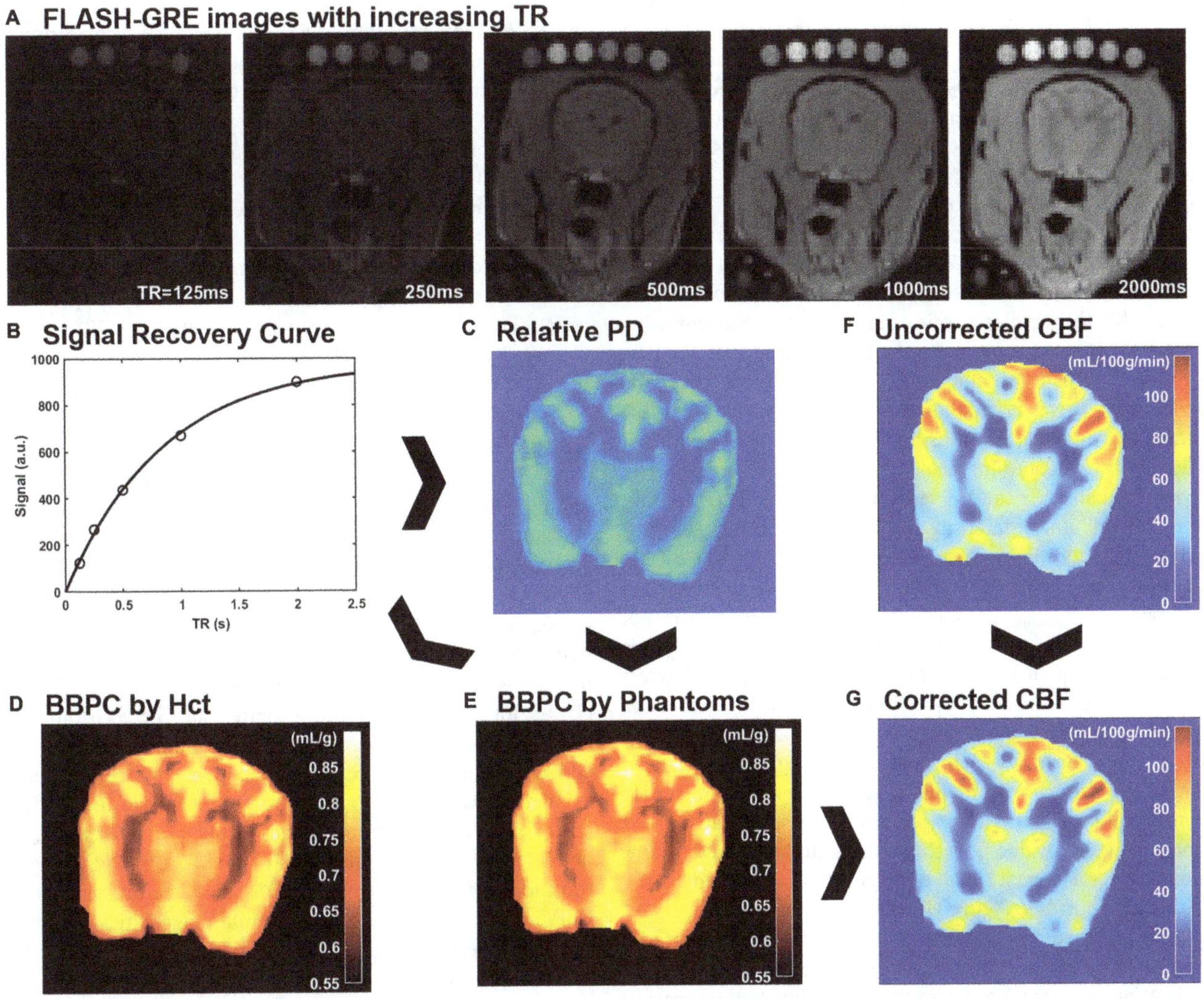

FIGURE 1 | An explanation of CaSTRR and pCASL methods used in this study. CaSTRR utilizes a series of FLASH-GRE acquisitions with varying TR which include a blood sample and gadolinium-doped deuterium samples placed on the head **(A)**. An exponential regression is fit to the signal recovery curve for each voxel **(B)** yielding a map of relative proton density values **(C)**. The relative proton density values are calibrated using either water content estimated from hematocrit (Hct) **(D)** or the scale of water content present in the phantoms **(E)**. Uncorrected CBF maps are derived from pCASL acquisitions **(F)** and are corrected on a voxel-wise basis using the BBPC map normalized to the phantoms to create a corrected map of CBF **(G)**.

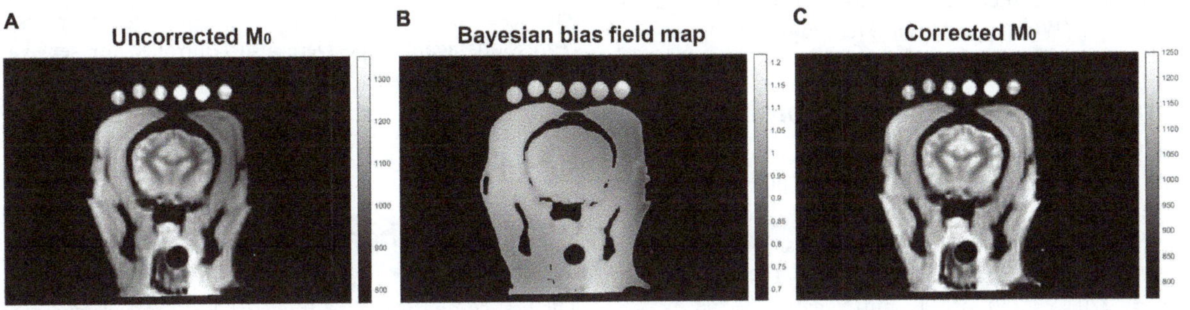

FIGURE 2 | A representative images of M_0 as calculated by exponential regression **(A)**, signal inhomogeneity determined by Bayesian bias field correction **(B)**, and corrected M_0 **(C)**.

of MRI signal measurement, the average value of M_0 in brain tissue varied from subject to subject on this arbitrary scale. Therefore, the M_0 maps were calibrated to absolute water content in two ways. The first follows the previously published CaSTRR technique which uses a series of five phantoms containing mixtures of deuterium oxide and distilled water at 40, 30, 20, 10, and 0% (Thalman et al., 2019). These phantoms were also doped with 0.18 mM gadobutrol (Gadavist, Bayer Healthcare Pharmaceuticals, Whippany, NJ, United States) to reduce the longitudinal relaxation rate (T1) to be similar to the T1 of brain tissue ($\approx$ 1.2 s). Because the deuterium oxide does not produce signal in MRI this creates a scale of known water concentration from 60–100% water. Each voxel in the image can then be normalized to this internal scale to yield a measure of absolute water content. It was noted, however, that in subjects where the arbitrary M_0 values of brain tissue were high, the M_0 values of the doped water phantoms tended to be higher than expected. This meant that while the M_0 value of tissues increased linearly with the overall image intensity, the M_0 values of the phantoms exhibited a quadratic increase over the range of arbitrary M_0 values measured. The result was that the ratio of average $M_{0,tissue}$ to average $M_{0,phantoms}$ used in image normalization was not constant from subject to subject but had a strong negative linear relationship to the phantom signal intensity. To correct for the relationship, linear regression of this ratio against the average M_0 value of the phantoms was used to quantify the quadratic error term for each subject. This negative error term was then subtracted from the blood and tissue M_0 values prior to normalization. Finally, a linear regression was calculated based on the average M_0 value in each phantom and its known water content, and every voxel in the image was normalized to the resultant equation (see **Figure 1E**).

The second method of calibrating M_0 maps utilized the arterial Hct value to determine the absolute water content of the blood sample. Water content was determined according to the equation $WC_{blood} = -0.271^{*}Hct + 0.912$ (Lijnema et al., 1993). The M_0 image was then normalized such that the average water content in the blood sample matched the average value calculated according to hematocrit.

Brain–blood partition coefficient maps were generated for both normalization methods by comparing the measured water content of each voxel in the brain to the average water content of the blood using the equation $BBPC = WC_{brain}/(WC_{blood}{}^{*}1.04\ g/mL)$ (see **Figure 1D**).

Cerebral Blood Flow and Anatomical Imaging

The CBF maps were acquired using a pCASL sequence with a three-dimensional gradient and spin echo (GRASE) readout (Alsop et al., 2015). The acquisition parameters were as follows: TR/TE/TI = 3200/16/1400 ms, field of view = 270 × 250 × 90 mm, matrix = 96 × 88, resolution = 3 × 3 × 3 mm, acquisition time = 6:15 min (see **Figure 1F**).

Because the original CBF maps were created with an assumed BBPC value of 0.9 mL/g, corrected maps were generated by dividing the entire map by this value and then multiplying by the BBPC map in a voxel-wise manner. BBPC correction was performed using the BBPC maps generated using the gadolinium doped water phantoms (see **Figure 1G**).

Contrast to noise ratio (CNR) was calculated according to the equation $CNR = (Mean_{gray} - Mean_{white})/Pooled\ Standard\ Deviation$ (Cohen, 1988).

Anatomical images were acquired using a high resolution T1 weighted magnetization prepared rapid acquisition gradient echo (MPRAGE) sequence as recommended for optimal use with FreeSurfer (MGH, 2009). Scan parameters were: TR/TE = 1690/2.56 ms, flip angle = 12°, field of view = 320 × 320 × 160 mm, matrix = 256 × 256 × 128, resolution = 0.8 × 0.8 × 0.8 mm, acquisition time = 10:49 min.

Image Analysis

All images were coregistered by first resampling the anatomical volumes to match the slice thickness of the CaSTRR and pCASL acquisitions. The CaSTRR and pCASL volumes were then registered to the anatomical using an intensity-based registration algorithm in Matlab (Mathworks, Natick, MA, United States) (Styner et al., 2000). The brain region of interest was extracted manually, and then segmented into gray and white regions of interest using an expectation maximization algorithm with classes for gray matter, white matter, and cerebrospinal fluid (Wells et al., 1996). To avoid partial volume effects, the gray and white matter regions of interest in each slice were eroded by two pixels. Due to image inhomogeneities in the MPRAGE acquisitions in some animals, the segmentation algorithm often failed to adequately segment gray and white matter regions in the most rostral and caudal sections of the brain. While the BBPC maps did not display these inhomogeneities, the regions of interest were not reliable for analysis. For this reason, we chose to include only the centermost 10 slices in our analysis. These regions of interest were then applied to the BBPC and CBF maps. All image analysis was performed in Matlab (Mathworks, Natick, MA, United States).

Statistical Analysis

All statistical analysis was performed in Matlab. Data is expressed as mean ± standard deviation. Gray and white matter comparisons were assessed using three-way analysis of covariance with age, sex, and tissue type as independent variables. Linear regressions against age were also controlled for sex. Values of $p < 0.05$ were considered statistically significant.

RESULTS

BBPC Is Higher in Gray Matter Than in White Matter

The first comparison was drawn on BBPC maps generated using the previously published CaSTRR method of normalizing to the gadolinium doped water phantoms (see **Figure 1E**). The average BBPC in gray matter was 0.83 ± 0.05 mL/g which is 5.6% higher than the BBPC in white matter (0.78 ± 0.04 mL/g, $p = 0.007$)

(see **Figure 3B**). When plotted against age, neither the gray nor the white matter regions of interest demonstrated a significant correlation over the age range studied (gray matter: $p = 0.645$, white matter: $p = 0.483$ (see **Figure 3A**).

Gray Matter CBF Is Negatively Correlated With Age

Next, gray and white matter perfusion were compared in uncorrected CBF maps (see **Figure 1F**) and again in corrected CBF maps (see **Figure 1G**) which used the standard CaSTRR derived BBPC maps for correction (see **Figure 1E**). Gray matter has 45% higher CBF than white matter in the uncorrected CBF maps (CBF_{gray} = 81 ± 12 mL/100g/min, CBF_{white} = 56 ± 12 mL/100 g/min, $p < 0.001$) and 53% higher CBF in the maps corrected for BBPC ($cCBF_{gray}$ = 73 ± 13 mL/100 g/min, $cCBF_{white}$ = 49 ± 11 mL/100 g/min, $p < 0.01$) (see **Figure 4B**). Gray matter demonstrated a significant negative correlation with age with a reduction of 7.5 ± 2.1 mL/100 g/min each year or 9% of the average perfusion (CBF_{gray} = 128 – 7.5 * Age mL/100 g/min, $p = 0.003$). The corrected CBF maps also revealed a reduction of 6.6 ± 2.6 mL/100 g/min/year ($cCBF_{gray}$ = 117 – 6.6 * Age mL/100 g/min, $p = 0.02$), but this relationship was not significantly different in the corrected maps than the uncorrected ($p = 0.81$). While there appears to be a downward trend in white matter perfusion with age, this correlation was not statistically significant in the uncorrected CBF maps ($p = 0.20$) or the corrected maps ($p = 0.33$) (see **Figure 4A**).

BBPC Correction Improved Contrast to Noise Ratio in CBF Maps

Next, the CNR of corrected CBF maps (see **Figure 1G**) was compared to uncorrected CBF maps (see **Figure 1F**). On average BBPC correction improved CNR between gray and white matter regions of the CBF maps by 3.6% (95% confidence interval = 0.6 – 6.5%). The average uncorrected CNR was 0.81 and the average corrected CNR was 0.84.

BBPC Values Generated Using Hematocrit to Estimate Water Content Agree With Those Generated Using Water Phantoms

The final comparison was between maps normalized using the doped water phantoms (see **Figure 1E**) to ones normalized using Hct derived blood water content (see **Figure 1D**), we observed positive correlations between the BBPC values generated using these two methods. The Pearson correlation was $R^2 = 0.81$ for gray matter indicating strong correlation between these measures in this region (see **Figure 5A**). Due to higher variability in the white matter regions the correlation was moderate in white matter ($R^2 = 0.59$) (see **Figure 5C**).

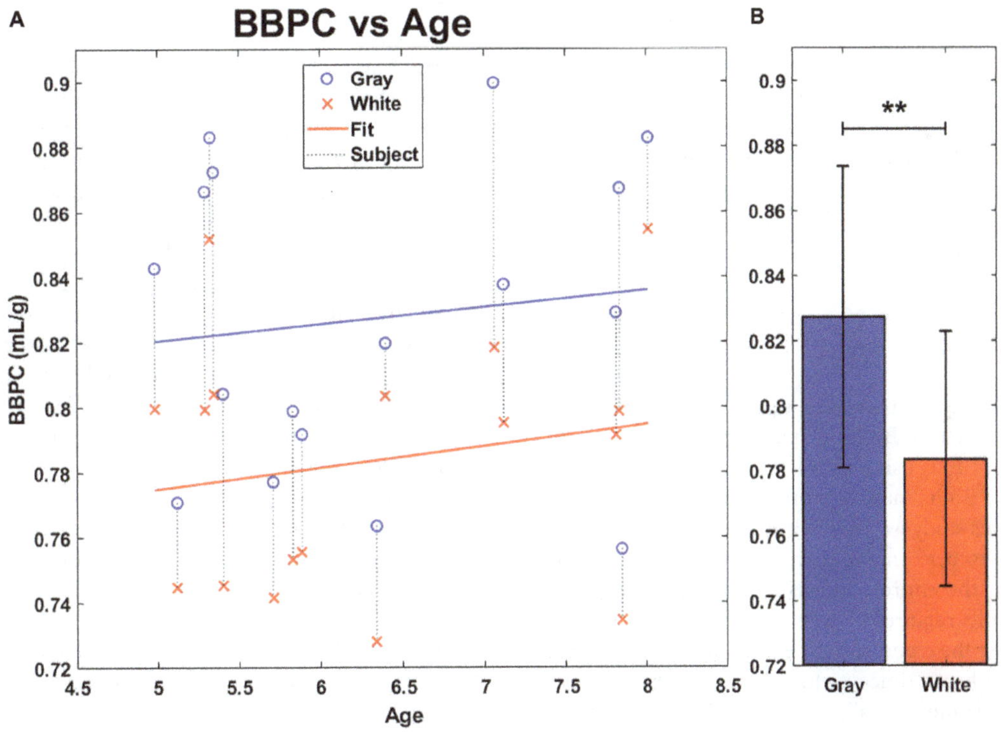

FIGURE 3 | Average BBPC in gray matter (blue) and white matter (red) regions of interest plotted against age **(A)** and as group averages **(B)**. Regions corresponding to the same animal are connected with a vertical dotted line. No significant linear correlation to age was found in either region. Average BBPC in gray matter was which is 5.6% higher than in white matter ($BBPC_{gray}$ = 0.83 ± 0.05 mL/g, $BBPC_{white}$ 0.78 ± 0.04 mL/g, ** indicates p < 0.01, error bars represent 1 standard deviation).

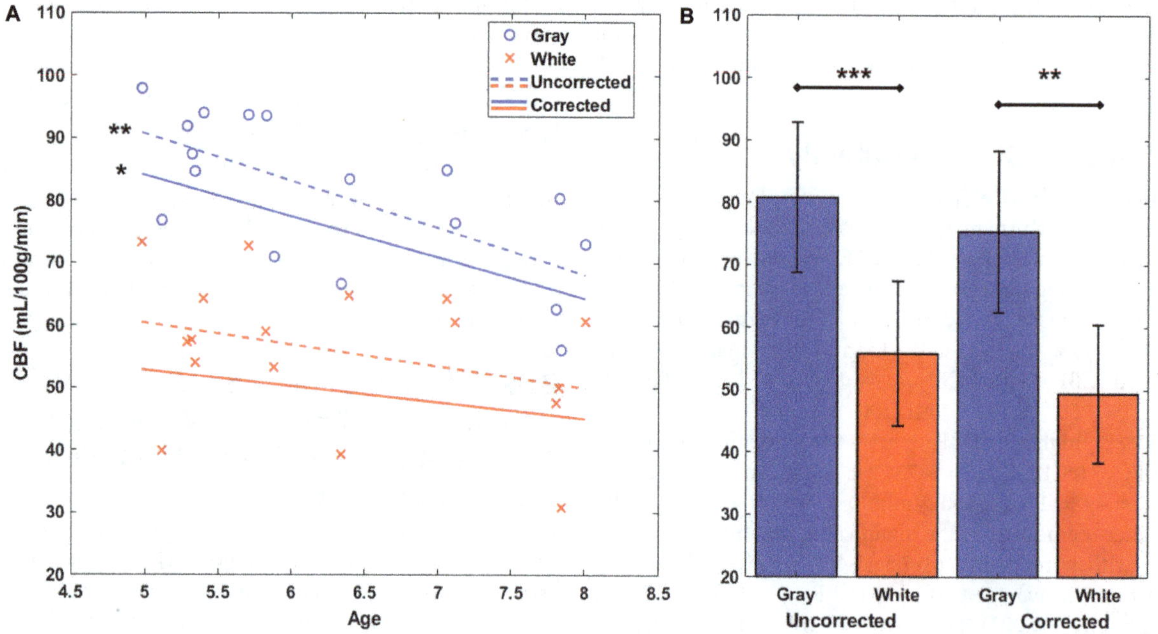

FIGURE 4 | Gray and white matter perfusion plotted against age **(A)**. Plotted points represent uncorrected average CBF for each animal. Gray matter CBF demonstrates a negative linear correlation with age in both uncorrected CBF maps (CBF_{gray} = 128 – 7.5 * Age mL/100 g/min) and maps corrected using measured BBPC ($cCBF_{gray}$ = 117 – 6.6 * Age mL/100 g/min). Linear regression was not significant in the white matter region in either case. When considered as group averages **(B)**, the gray matter has significantly higher CBF in both uncorrected (CBF_{gray} = 81 ± 12 mL/100 g/min, CBF_{white} = 56 ± 12 mL/100 g/min), and corrected maps ($cCBF_{gray}$ = 73 ± 13 mL/100 g/min, $cCBF_{white}$ = 49 ± 11 mL/100 g/min). * indicates $p < 0.05$, ** indicates $p < 0.01$, *** indicates $p < 0.001$, error bars represent 1 standard deviation.

The measured BBPC values were slightly lower in maps normalized to hematocrit, though not statistically different, and Bland-Altman analysis demonstrates no significant bias in either region of interest (see **Figures 5B,D**). Again the BBPC in gray matter was 5.9% higher than in white matter when using Hct to normalize ($BBPC_{gray}$ = 0.81 ± 0.06 mL/g, $BBPC_{white}$ = 0.77 ± 0.05 mL/g, $p = 0.02$).

DISCUSSION

The CaSTRR technique represents a significant improvement in the acquisition speed of BBPC maps. A previously published report measuring BBPC using a 1.5T human scanner acquired a single slice of the BBPC map in approximately 30 min (Roberts et al., 1996). In this study we were able to produce BBPC maps of sufficient quality to perform voxel-wise correction of CBF maps with coverage of the entire brain using a CaSTRR acquisition protocol that only required 4 min of scan time. This is an improvement over the reported CaSTRR technique in mice which required 17 min of scan time due to the much higher resolution requirement of scanning small animals at 7T (Thalman et al., 2019). A 4 min scan time is comparable to the acquisition time of the pCASL technique for CBF. The experiment was also done with commercially available equipment and pulse sequences that are directly applicable for use with a human subject. Furthermore, the CaSTRR scans were performed with the same birdcage receive coil that was used for the pCASL acquisitions. This was not possible when scanning mice at 7T and represents a significant advantage of scanning at lower fields. The greatly reduced scan time and ready availability of equipment and pulse sequences demonstrate that CaSTRR is a feasible approach to correct CBF maps using empirically measured BBPC values instead of assuming a constant value for all tissue types, pathologies, ages, and species. This technique has the potential for rapid translation to use in human studies.

While BBPC has not been previously reported in canines, our reported values of 0.83 ± 0.05 mL/g in gray matter and 0.78 ± 0.04 mL/g in white matter are lower than published reports in humans, non-human primates, and mice (Herscovitch and Raichle, 1985; Kudomi et al., 2005; Leithner et al., 2010). One possible reason for this is the temperature discrepancy between the blood sample and the brain tissue. When measured at room temperature instead of physiologic temperature, the proton density of the blood could be overestimated by as much as 5% causing BBPC to be underestimated by the same amount (Tofts, 2003). The amount of inter-species variability in BBPC values is further evidence for the importance of empirical BBPC correction when quantifying CBF.

The correlation between the two methods of normalization represents a distinct advantage of this study. Our results suggest that the CaSTRR technique can be further simplified by omitting the gadolinium doped water phantoms. One of the difficulties of this study was the non-linear signal increase observed in

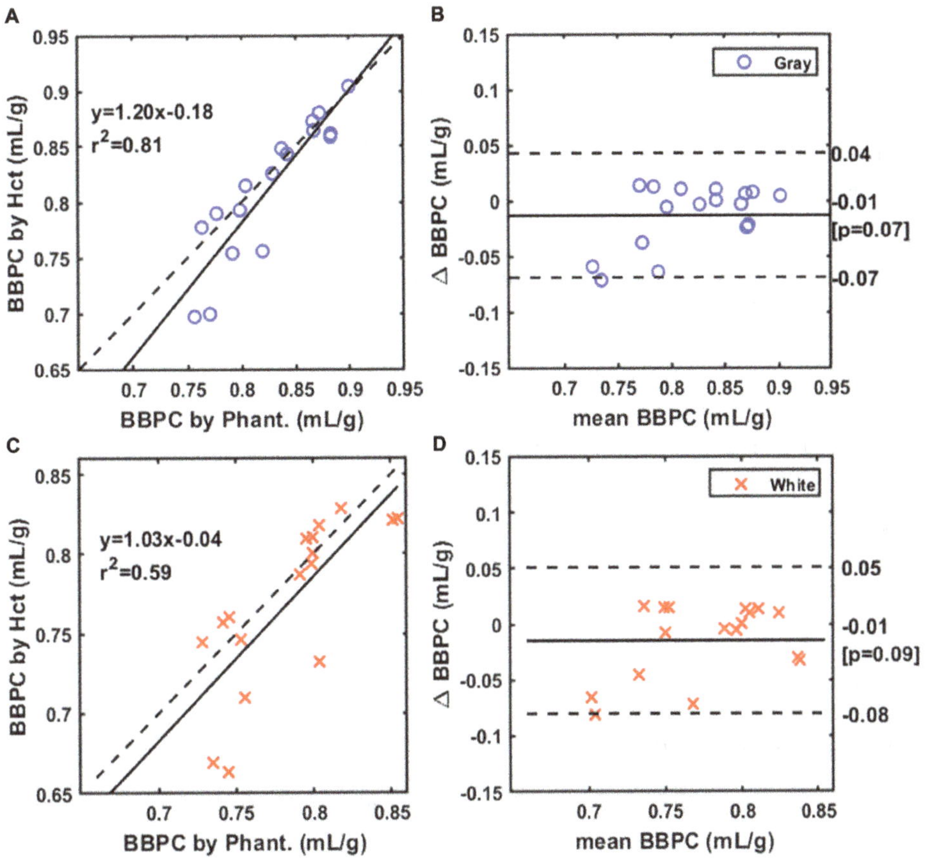

FIGURE 5 | Correlation of BBPC values in maps normalized according to hematocrit (Hct) with values in maps normalized to the gadolinium-doped phantoms. Correlation is very strong for the gray matter BBPC values (R^2 = 0.81) **(A)** and moderately strong for white matter (R^2 = 0.59) **(C)**. Bland-Altman analysis demonstrates no significant bias in either gray **(B)** or white matter values **(D)**.

the water phantoms. This is possibly due to the pre-scan normalization algorithm of the scanner used for this study and/or reduced T2* decay in the water phantoms. These effects would likely be specific to a given scanner and would need to be determined empirically. However, the correlation between BBPC values derived using the water phantoms with those derived using Hct indicate that future studies using CaSTRR could rely solely on the water content determined by the hematocrit. This would also obviate the need for correcting the non-linear signal increases observed in the water phantoms as done in this study.

Another significant advantage of this study is the use of Bayesian bias field correction to account for inhomogeneities in the receiver coil sensitivity profile. The CaSTRR method described in mice assumed a sufficiently homogenous profile in the birdcage receive coil, but observed significant signal loss near the large ear canals of the mouse (Thalman et al., 2019). Other BBPC studies attempted to correct for bias field using a separate measurement on a uniform phantom (Roberts et al., 1996; Leithner et al., 2010), but it is unlikely that the receiver profile would be the same when measuring the non-uniform tissue of a live subject.

Arterial spin labeling has an inherently low signal to noise ratio because it is a subtractive technique. Including an empirical measurement of BBPC to the quantification of CBF will increase noise, as we observed in the greater variance of CBF values in the corrected maps. However, there was an improvement in contrast to noise between areas with significantly different BBPC values despite this addition of noise. This could become important when studying perfusion in models of pathology where the tissue composition is likely to change.

Canines have been widely used for aging and neurodegeneration studies (Martin et al., 2011; Vite and Head, 2014; Triani et al., 2018). There are many examples of pathologies that could affect water balance in the brain. Brain edema caused by ischemia (Rosenberg, 1999), infection (Niemoller and Tauber, 1989), or trauma (Winkler et al., 2016) can cause localized increases in free water and potentially affect the BBPC. Another important field of interest where ASL is commonly used is the study of Alzheimer's disease (AD). The deposition of hydrophobic amyloid-β protein, which is a hallmark of AD pathology, may reduce the BBPC in regions of plaque development (Aleksis et al., 2017). AD occurs in the context of aging and typically causes pronounced brain atrophy

(Bobinski et al., 1999). Both of these could result in reduced brain water content and therefore reduced BBPC. Both brain volume (Duning et al., 2005) and Hct (Jimenez et al., 1999) can also change significantly with a subject's level of hydration. So while our result showed that BBPC correction did not affect the observed relationship between CBF and age between the ages of 5–8 year, it is possible that BBPC correction could improve sensitivity in studies where BBPC is expected to change significantly. In future studies, CaSTRR imaging could be used to study how BBPC changes in canines with pathology and could also be used to account for water balance effects when measuring perfusion.

We acknowledge that in addition to CaSTRR, other efforts have also been made to improve the BBPC measurement, CBF quantification, and gray-white CBF contrast. It has been reported that a uniform, brain-tissue-type-dependent magnetization image could be generated using a sensitivity calibration (Dai et al., 2011). Another study showed that BBPC can be improved by exploiting the partial-volume data to adjust the ratio between BBPC and the proton density-weighted image (Ahlgren et al., 2018). Furthermore, gray-white matter CBF can be enhanced with background suppression methods (van Osch et al., 2009). Here we provide another approach that can quantify BBPC rapidly, and improve CBF quantification and gray-white CBF contrast using Hct calibration.

CONCLUSION

In conclusion, this study demonstrates the feasibility of CaSTRR as a method to correct CBF measurements for regional and inter-subject variability in BBPC. Further, we demonstrated that the correction can be achieved using Hct calibration. The developed CaSTRR method has potential contribution for future translational studies in aging and neurodegeneration.

AUTHOR CONTRIBUTIONS

ST was responsible for the experimental and scanning protocol design, analysis software development, image acquisition, data and statistical analyses, and manuscript preparations. DP contributed to the sequence development, scanning protocol design, technical support, and manuscript editing. MU was responsible for the animal handling, image acquisition, laboratory samples, and manuscript editing. CN and EH contributed to the project design, animal acquisition, data interpretation, and manuscript editing. A-LL was the primary investigator and contributed to the project design, interpretation of the results, and manuscript preparation.

FUNDING

This research was supported by the National Institute of Health (NIH) (Grant Numbers R01AG054459, RF1AG062480, R01AG056998, and T32AG057461). The 7T ClinScan small animal MRI scanner of the University of Kentucky was funded by the S10 NIH Shared Instrumentation Program Grant (Grant Number 1S10RR029541-01).

ACKNOWLEDGMENTS

The authors would like to thank Kathy Boaz, Stephanie Krumholz, and Beverly Meacham for their assistance in animal handling and MRI experiments.

SUPPLEMENTARY MATERIAL

FIGURE S1 | B_1 mapping. The B_1 mapping was aquired using a *Tfl_b1map* sequence with a saline phantom (salinity is the same as mammalian extracellular space). Right image proportional to flip angle, showing maximum flip angle variation of 4% over a 10 cm phantom. The FOV is comparible to beagle's brain, which is approximately 4 cm × 5 cm × 7 cm. **(Left)** The magnitude image. **(Right)** A flip angle map where the intensity is linearly proportional to the flip angle. The examples are shown in two ROIs: 83.8 and 89.5 degrees, respectively.

REFERENCES

Ahlgren, A., Wirestam, R., Knutsson, L., and Petersen, E. T. (2018). Improved calculation of the equilibrium magnetization of arterial blood in arterial spin labeling. *Magn. Reson. Med.* 80, 2223–2231. doi: 10.1002/mrm.27193

Aleksis, R., Oleskovs, F., Jaudzems, K., Pahnke, J., and Biverstal, H. (2017). Structural studies of amyloid-beta peptides: unlocking the mechanism of aggregation and the associated toxicity. *Biochimie* 140, 176–192. doi: 10.1016/j.biochi.2017.07.011

Alsop, D. C., Detre, J. A., Golay, X., Gunther, M., Hendrikse, J., Hernandez-Garcia, L., et al. (2015). Recommended implementation of arterial spin-labeled perfusion MRI for clinical applications: a consensus of the ISMRM perfusion study group and the European consortium for ASL in dementia. *Magn. Reson. Med.* 73, 102–116. doi: 10.1002/mrm.25197

Bobinski, M., De Leon, M. J., Wegiel, J., Desanti, S., Convit, A., Saint Louis, L. A., et al. (1999). The histological validation of post mortem magnetic resonance imaging-determined hippocampal volume in Alzheimer's disease. *Neuroscience* 95, 721–725. doi: 10.1016/s0306-4522(99)00476-5

Cohen, J. (1988). *Statistical Power Analysis for the Behavioral Sciences.* Hillsdale, NJ: Lawrence Erlbaum Associates.

Dai, W., Robson, P. M., Shankaranarayanan, A., and Alsop, D. C. (2011). Sensitivity calibration with a uniform magnetization image to improve arterial spin labeling perfusion quantification. *Magn. Reson. Med.* 66, 1590–1600. doi: 10.1002/mrm.22954

Duning, T., Kloska, S., Steinstrater, O., Kugel, H., Heindel, W., and Knecht, S. (2005). Dehydration confounds the assessment of brain atrophy. *Neurology* 64, 548–550. doi: 10.1212/01.wnl.0000150542.16969.cc

Herscovitch, P., and Raichle, M. E. (1985). What is the correct value for the brain-blood partition coefficient for water? *J. Cereb. Blood Flow Metab.* 5, 65–69. doi: 10.1038/jcbfm.1985.9

Hirata, K., Hattori, N., Katoh, C., Shiga, T., Kuroda, S., Kubo, N., et al. (2011). Regional partition coefficient of water in patients with cerebrovascular disease and its effect on rCBF assessment. *Nucl. Med. Commun.* 32, 63–70. doi: 10.1097/MNM.0b013e3283412106

Iglesiast, J. E., Paz-Alonso, P., Lerma-Usabiaga, G., Insausti, R., Miller, K., and Caballero-Gaudes, C. (2016). "Simultaneous Bayesian correction of slab boundary artifacts and bias field for high resolution ex vivo MRI," in *Proceedings of the 13th International Symposium on Biomedical Imaging (ISBI)*, (Piscataway, NJ: IEEE), 1384–1387.

Jimenez, C., Melin, B., Koulmann, N., Allevard, A. M., Launay, J. C., and Savourey, G. (1999). Plasma volume changes during and after acute variations of body hydration level in humans. *Eur. J. Appl. Physiol. Occup. Physiol.* 80, 1–8. doi: 10.1007/s004210050550

Kudomi, N., Hayashi, T., Teramoto, N., Watabe, H., Kawachi, N., Ohta, Y., et al. (2005). Rapid quantitative measurement of CMRO(2) and CBF by dual administration of (15)O-labeled oxygen and water during a single PET scan-a validation study and error analysis in anesthetized monkeys. *J. Cereb. Blood Flow Metab.* 25, 1209–1224. doi: 10.1038/sj.jcbfm.9600118

Leithner, C., Muller, S., Fuchtemeier, M., Lindauer, U., Dirnagl, U., and Royl, G. (2010). Determination of the brain-blood partition coefficient for water in mice using MRI. *J. Cereb. Blood Flow Metab.* 30, 1821–1824. doi: 10.1038/jcbfm.2010.160

Lijnema, T. H., Huizenga, J. R., Jager, J., Mackor, A. J., and Gips, C. H. (1993). Gravimetric determination of the water concentration in whole blood, plasma and erythrocytes and correlations with hematological and clinicochemical parameters. *Clin. Chim. Acta* 214, 129–138. doi: 10.1016/0009-8981(93)90105-d

Martin, S. B., Dowling, A. L., and Head, E. (2011). Therapeutic interventions targeting beta amyloid pathogenesis in an aging dog model. *Curr. Neuropharmacol.* 9, 651–661. doi: 10.2174/157015911798376217

MGH, (2009). *FreeSurfer Suggested Morphometry Protocols.* Available at: http://surfer.nmr.mgh.harvard.edu/fswiki/FreeSurferWiki?action=AttachFile&do=get&target=FreeSurfer_Suggested_Morphometry_Protocols.pdf (accessed April 29, 2019).

Niemoller, U. M., and Tauber, M. G. (1989). Brain edema and increased intracranial pressure in the pathophysiology of bacterial meningitis. *Eur. J. Clin. Microbiol. Infect. Dis.* 8, 109–117. doi: 10.1007/bf01963892

Petcharunpaisan, S., Ramalho, J., and Castillo, M. (2010). Arterial spin labeling in neuroimaging. *World J. Radiol.* 2, 384–398. doi: 10.4329/wjr.v2.i10.384

Roberts, D. A., Rizi, R., Lenkinski, R. E., and Leigh, J. S. Jr. (1996). Magnetic resonance imaging of the brain: blood partition coefficient for water: application to spin-tagging measurement of perfusion. *J. Magn. Reson. Imaging* 6, 363–366. doi: 10.1002/jmri.1880060217

Rosenberg, G. A. (1999). Ischemic brain edema. *Prog. Cardiovasc. Dis.* 42, 209–216.

Styner, M., Brechbuhler, C., Szckely, G., and Gerig, G. (2000). Parametric estimate of intensity inhomogeneities applied to MRI. *IEEE Trans. Med. Imaging* 19, 153–165. doi: 10.1109/42.845174

Thalman, S. W., Powell, D. K., and Lin, A. L. (2019). Novel calibrated short TR recovery (CaSTRR) method for brain-blood partition coefficient correction enhances gray-white matter contrast in blood flow measurements in mice. *Front. Neurosci.* 13:308. doi: 10.3389/fnins.2019.00308

Tofts, P. S. (ed.) (2003). "PD: Proton Density of Tissue Water," in *Quantitative MRI of the Brain*, (Chichester: John Wiley).

Triani, F., Tramutola, A., Di Domenico, F., Sharma, N., Butterfield, D. A., Head, E., et al. (2018). Biliverdin reductase-A impairment links brain insulin resistance with increased Abeta production in an animal model of aging: implications for Alzheimer disease. *Biochim. Biophys. Acta Mol. Basis Dis.* 1864, 3181–3194. doi: 10.1016/j.bbadis.2018.07.005

van Osch, M. J., Teeuwisse, W. M., Van Walderveen, M. A., Hendrikse, J., Kies, D. A., and Van Buchem, M. A. (2009). Can arterial spin labeling detect white matter perfusion signal? *Magn. Reson. Med.* 62, 165–173. doi: 10.1002/mrm.22002

Vite, C. H., and Head, E. (2014). Aging in the canine and feline brain. *Vet. Clin. North Am. Small Anim. Pract.* 44, 1113–1129. doi: 10.1016/j.cvsm.2014.07.008

Wells, W. M., Grimson, W. E. L., Kikinis, R., and Jolesz, F. A. (1996). Adaptive segmentation of MRI data. *IEEE Trans. Med. Imaging* 15, 429–442. doi: 10.1109/42.511747

Williams, D. S., Detre, J. A., Leigh, J. S., and Koretsky, A. P. (1992). Magnetic resonance imaging of perfusion using spin inversion of arterial water. *Proc. Natl Acad. Sci. U.S.A.* 89, 212–216.

Winkler, E. A., Minter, D., Yue, J. K., and Manley, G. T. (2016). Cerebral edema in traumatic brain injury: pathophysiology and prospective therapeutic targets. *Neurosurg. Clin. N. Am.* 27, 473–488. doi: 10.1016/j.nec.2016.05.008

10

In vivo Brainstem Imaging in Alzheimer's Disease: Potential for Biomarker Development

David J. Braun[1] and Linda J. Van Eldik[1,2,3]*

[1] Sanders-Brown Center on Aging, University of Kentucky, Lexington, KY, United States, [2] Spinal Cord and Brain Injury Research Center, University of Kentucky, Lexington, KY, United States, [3] Department of Neuroscience, University of Kentucky, Lexington, KY, United States

***Correspondence:**
Linda J. Van Eldik
linda.vaneldik@uky.edu

The dearth of effective treatments for Alzheimer's disease (AD) is one of the largest public health issues worldwide, costing hundreds of billions of dollars per year. From a therapeutic standpoint, research efforts to date have met with strikingly little clinical success. One major issue is that trials begin after substantial pathological change has occurred, and it is increasingly clear that the most effective treatment regimens will need to be administered earlier in the disease process. In order to identify individuals within the long preclinical phase of AD who are likely to progress to dementia, improvements are required in biomarker development. One potential area of research that might prove fruitful in this regard is the *in vivo* detection of brainstem pathology. The brainstem is known to undergo pathological changes very early and progressively in AD. With an updated and harmonized AD research framework, and emerging advances in neuroimaging technology, the potential to leverage knowledge of brainstem pathology into biomarkers for AD will be discussed.

Keywords: Alzheimer's disease, brainstem, neuroimaging, imaging, *in vivo*, locus coeruleus, raphe nucleus, biomarker

INTRODUCTION

Dementia is a global public health crisis, affecting around 47 million people worldwide and projected to nearly triple by 2050 as the global population increases in average age (World Health Organization, 2017). Alzheimer's disease (AD) is the most common cause of aging-related dementia, accounting for 60–80% of cases (Alzheimer's Association, 2017). Even a relatively small reduction or delay in AD incidence therefore has the potential to dramatically reduce dementia burden (Barnes and Yaffe, 2011). Unfortunately, current AD treatments are only moderately and transiently effective, and many promising treatments have fallen short in late-stage clinical trials (Mehta et al., 2017). One major obstacle is the need for refined early-stage biomarkers that can reliably predict who within the AD spectrum will develop dementia. The brainstem has long been recognized as a site with early and significant susceptibility to AD-type neuropathological change (Mann, 1983), but it has been difficult to access this region *in vivo*. Advances in non-invasive neuroimaging techniques are beginning to allow antemortem assessment of this crucial region, thereby opening the possibility of using early brainstem changes as AD biomarkers. This might extend the window in which preclinical AD is detectable or, in conjunction with other biomarkers, better define those patients most likely to experience cognitive dysfunction in the future. This concept will be discussed in light of the current AD research framework and recent neuroimaging advances.

ALZHEIMER'S DISEASE PATHOLOGY AND DIAGNOSTIC CRITERIA

The essential neuropathologic features of AD consist of extracellular deposits of amyloid beta peptide (Aβ), and intracellular accumulations of modified tau protein called neurofibrillary tangles (NFTs). These pathologies are accompanied by neuronal injury and neurodegeneration, leading to progressive cognitive impairment and culminating in dementia. An updated clinical staging of AD was defined in 2011 by a joint workgroup of the National Institute on Aging and the Alzheimer's Association (NIA-AA) (Albert et al., 2011; McKhann et al., 2011; Sperling et al., 2011; Montine et al., 2012). Associated with this, the NIA-AA published neuropathologic guidelines to score AD-associated neuropathology as well as assess commonly appearing comorbid pathologies (Montine et al., 2012). Importantly, the 2011 guidelines also formalized the use of imaging and cerebrospinal fluid (CSF) biomarkers to define "preclinical AD," wherein an individual has abnormal AD-type pathological changes and no or only subtle cognitive/behavioral symptoms. Validated *in vivo* markers for AD-type neuropathologic change include CSF levels of $A\beta_{42}$ and phosphorylated tau, increased positron emission tomography (PET) ligand binding for amyloid or tau within the cortex, glucose hypometabolism as measured by fluorodeoxyglucose PET (FDG-PET), and brain atrophy as measured by structural magnetic resonance imaging (MRI) (Tan et al., 2014). This biomarker-defined preclinical AD framework is particularly useful as the preclinical phase can extend more than a decade before the onset of clinically defined symptoms (Quiroz et al., 2018), and therefore represents a promising window for therapeutic intervention.

The disparity between reference to AD as a clinical syndrome versus a neuropathologic phenomenon has led to some confusion, however. For example, around 30% of patients clinically diagnosed with AD do not have significant AD neuropathology at autopsy and a similar proportion of cognitively unimpaired patients do (Davis et al., 1999; Neuropathology Group, 2001). In an attempt to harmonize definitions and clarify research efforts, the NIA-AA recently released an updated 2018 framework, building upon the 2011 biomarker-based approach in defining preclinical AD (Jack et al., 2018; Khachaturian et al., 2018; Knopman et al., 2018; Silverberg et al., 2018). This new system categorizes all patients by the presence or absence of biomarker-based pathology in three categories to generate an "ATN" profile: A for amyloid, T for tau, and N for neurodegeneration. Additionally, there is a cognitive staging scheme of cognitively unimpaired, mild cognitive impairment (MCI), or dementia overlaid on the ATN biomarker profiles (**Table 1**). An individual must have biomarker group A pathology (reduced CSF $A\beta_{42}$, increased amyloid PET, etc.) to be placed on the AD spectrum, irrespective of cognitive or other pathological changes. The framework is flexible in that it can incorporate new ATN biomarkers as they become validated, or entirely new biomarker categories. As will be discussed below, neuropathological data indicate that neuroimaging-accessible changes within the brainstem may be useful additions to the T or N biomarker groupings.

BRAINSTEM CHANGES IN AD

Although considerable focus in the AD field has been placed on pathological changes in cortical, hippocampal, and basal forebrain regions, brainstem pathology has also been described since at least the 1930s (Hannah, 1936). The brainstem is a small and complex region, serving as a major relay center and signal integrator for the central nervous system (CNS). Rostro-caudally it is comprised of the midbrain, pons, and medulla, together containing the majority of neurons belonging to several widely projecting monoaminergic modulatory systems. These monoamine transmitters include serotonin (5-HT) and the catecholamines dopamine and noradrenaline (NA), the dysfunction of which have been well-described in AD (Trillo et al., 2013; Šimić et al., 2017). Early and severe AD-associated changes occur in the major brainstem serotonergic and noradrenergic nuclei, the dorsal raphe nucleus (DRN) and locus coeruleus (LC), respectively, a brief summary of which is provided below. For more in depth reading, several comprehensive reviews have been published (Szabadi, 2013; Trillo et al., 2013; Giorgi et al., 2017; Šimić et al., 2017).

The Dorsal Raphe Nucleus

The DRN is one of a cluster of serotonergic nuclei, located near the midline in the dorsal midbrain and pons. It contains the majority of brainstem serotonergic neurons and is comprised of about 235,000 neurons in the adult human brain, roughly 70% of which produce 5-HT. The DRN sends ascending projections to regions such as the cortex, hippocampus, and striatum, as well as descending projections to the lower brainstem and spinal cord (Šimić et al., 2017). The serotonergic neurons of the DRN undergo substantial cell loss in AD (Lyness et al., 2003), and tangle pathology occurs early in the disease process (Rüb et al., 2000; Grinberg et al., 2009; Braak et al., 2011; Ehrenberg et al., 2017). Dysfunction in the serotonergic system has been strongly implicated in the behavioral and psychological symptoms of dementia (BPSD), such as agitation, aggression, hallucinations, and depression (Lanctôt et al., 2001). In particular, depressive symptoms later in life appear to be a feature of preclinical neurodegenerative changes, even before the onset of cognitive decline (Donovan et al., 2015; Singh-Manoux et al., 2017). Similarly, the DRN (along with the LC) is heavily involved in regulation of the sleep/wake cycle and cognitively normal individuals meeting criteria for preclinical AD have measurably worse sleep quality versus controls (Ju et al., 2013).

The Locus Coeruleus

The LC is a long and narrow nucleus in the brainstem pons, averaging about 14.5 mm long and up to about 2.5 mm

TABLE 1 | Overview of NIA-AA ATN biomarker scores and cognitive staging.

Cognitive stage	A	T	N	Description of ATN profile and cognitive stage
Cognitively unimpaired (CU)	−	−	−	Normal AD biomarkers, CU
	+	−	−	Preclinical Alzheimer's pathologic change, CU
	+	+	−	Preclinical AD
	+	+	+	
	+	−	+	Alzheimer's and concomitant non-Alzheimer's pathologic change, CU
	−	+	−	Non-Alzheimer's pathologic change, CU
	−	−	+	
	−	+	+	
Mild cognitive impairment (MCI)	−	−	−	Normal AD biomarkers, MCI
	+	−	−	Alzheimer's pathologic change with MCI
	+	+	−	AD with MCI (prodromal AD)
	+	+	+	
	+	−	+	Alzheimer's and concomitant non-Alzheimer's pathologic change, MCI
	−	+	−	Non-Alzheimer's pathologic change with MCI
	−	−	+	
	−	+	+	
Dementia (DM)	−	−	−	Normal AD biomarkers, MCI
	+	−	−	Alzheimer's pathologic change with dementia
	+	+	−	AD with dementia
	+	+	+	
	+	−	+	Alzheimer's and concomitant non-Alzheimer's pathologic change, DM
	−	+	−	Non-Alzheimer's pathologic change with dementia
	−	−	+	
	−	+	+	

Only those with A biomarkers (A+) are considered to be on the AD pathological spectrum. Biomarkers for A (amyloid) include CSF $A\beta_{42}$ and amyloid PET. Biomarkers for T (tau) include CSF p-tau and tau PET. Biomarkers for N (neurodegeneration) include CSF total tau, structural changes detectable by MRI (i.e., atrophy), and FDG-PET. Neuroimaging-detectable brainstem changes might inform the T or N categories, or potentially comprise a separate category in future iterations of the NIA-AA research framework.

thick (Fernandes et al., 2012). It extends caudally along the cerebral aqueduct from the level of the inferior colliculus, ending ventrolateral to the floor of the fourth ventricle. It consists of only about 20 to 30,000 neurons per side in the healthy adult (German et al., 1988; Baker et al., 1989). Despite its small size, the LC provides the majority of central noradrenergic innervation via extensive projections throughout the CNS and it plays important roles across behavioral, cognitive, and physiological domains. It has also been implicated in early BPSD changes (Matthews et al., 2002) and tangle pathology in the LC occurs early and progressively throughout the disease process, even prior to tangle pathology within the DRN (Ehrenberg et al., 2017). Interestingly, the first detectable tau pathology within the brain is in the LC, appearing even in cognitively normal young individuals (Braak et al., 2011), and it has been speculated that LC damage and noradrenergic dysfunction might potentiate pathology in target regions such as cortex and hippocampus (Heneka et al., 2010; Braun et al., 2014; Feinstein et al., 2016). The LC undergoes severe topographic degeneration in AD, such that areas containing neurons reciprocally connected to hippocampal and cortical forebrain regions are selectively lost (Marcyniuk et al., 1986; Lyness et al., 2003; Zarow et al., 2003; Theofilas et al., 2017), and LC degeneration correlates with cognitive dysfunction (Grudzien et al., 2007). It is important to note here that the distinct but common condition known as primary age-related tauopathy (PART) also manifests with early LC tau pathology (Nelson et al., 2016). AD-related LC tau pathology by definition refers only to that co-occurring with amyloid biomarker changes (*e.g.*, reduced CSF $A\beta_{42}$, increased cortical amyloid PET).

Although the DRN and LC are quite small, the pathology within them occurs early, progressively, and severely, increasing the likelihood of neuroimaging-based detection in the preclinical phase of disease. How this might practically be achieved is the topic of the following section.

NEUROIMAGING THE BRAINSTEM

Of the non-invasive imaging modalities available, MRI and PET are those most commonly used in AD research (**Table 2**). MRI is primarily used to rule out other causes of dementia (e.g., stroke) and assess brain structural alterations informative of neurodegenerative change (Kehoe et al., 2014). It can also measure functional parameters relevant to AD pathology such as tissue perfusion (Wolk and Detre, 2012) or blood brain barrier (BBB) integrity (Raja et al., 2017); however, these methods have yet to be validated for biomarker use. PET in the AD context is employed primarily for assessment of levels of Aβ or tau, and to measure brain glucose hypometabolism with FDG-PET (Bao et al., 2017; Rice and Bisdas, 2017; Villemagne et al., 2018). These measurements are taken in relevant cortical and hippocampal regions, due in part to logistical considerations that have limited the use of these modalities for brainstem evaluation. The brainstem is a small structure with substantial anatomical complexity, requiring high resolution to visualize its component structures, and there is little endogenous contrast to enable the easy separation of nuclei. Additionally, significant physiological noise is present from cardiorespiratory systems, making fine-grained measurements difficult even with higher resolution systems (for review see Sclocco et al., 2017). Nonetheless, refined techniques are increasing the sensitivity of brainstem measurement, and a recent MRI study successfully identified reductions in dorsal midbrain volume in AD patients, corresponding to the location of the raphe nuclei (Lee et al., 2015). The increasing adoption of ultra-high-field (UHF) magnets for MRI (Deistung et al., 2013) and the High-Resolution Research Tomograph (HRRT) for PET (Schain et al., 2013), along with improved analytical methods (Iglesias et al., 2015), are enhancing the accessibility of these small brainstem regions to neuroimaging.

Neuroimaging the DRN

The imaging of individual brainstem raphe nuclei poses some challenges (Kranz et al., 2012). However, it has primarily been achieved with the use of PET radioligands specific for 5-HT receptors or the 5-HT transporter (Kranz et al., 2012; Paterson et al., 2013; Schain et al., 2013; Kumar and Mann, 2014; Zhang et al., 2017). There are only two studies directly assessing the DRN *in vivo* in AD spectrum changes, both using functional MRI (fMRI). In one, reduced default mode network connectivity of the DRN was found in patients with AD, distinctive from changes observed in dementia with Lewy bodies (Zhou et al., 2010). A combined PET and fMRI study found reduced 5-HT transporter in the DRN of patients with MCI versus controls, associated with reduced functional connectivity between the hippocampus and DRN (Barrett et al., 2017). In addition, neuroimaging alterations in DRN are observable in patients with anxiety (Lanzenberger et al., 2007; Lee et al., 2011; Johnston et al., 2015; Pillai et al., 2018) and major depressive disorder (Lee et al., 2011; Johnston et al., 2015; Pillai et al., 2018), indicating that such changes might also be detectable in patients with BPSD due to AD. Interestingly, one group has successfully used a fusion PET/MRI system with both HRRT PET and UHF MRI (7T) for brainstem serotonergic imaging (Cho et al., 2007). With this system, all 5 individual raphe nuclei have been visualized using UHF MRI and FDG-PET or ^{11}C-DASB PET (a radioligand for the 5-HT transporter) (Son et al., 2014). This raises the immediate possibility of testing the hypothesis that neurodegenerative biomarker changes may be observable in the DRN in early stages of AD. Whether such a system might also be able to detect other pathology (e.g., tau PET) in the DRN remains to be seen, but such a study would be well worth the effort. A major caveat is that the current cost and rarity of such systems limit their use; however, they are likely to become more common with time (Nensa et al., 2014), especially in light of demonstrated utility in dementia research (Dukart et al., 2011). Specific funding to equip Alzheimer's Disease Research Centers with such systems would rapidly expand their use and facilitate research in this domain.

Neuroimaging the LC

The biosynthesis of catecholamines in humans is associated with the production of neuromelanin, putatively a mechanism to reduce oxidative damage (Zecca et al., 2008). The noradrenergic LC is no exception, with neuromelanin levels increasing with age and then starting to decline around the seventh decade of life (Mann and Yates, 1974). Conveniently, neuromelanin has paramagnetic properties that allow regions with a high neuromelanin content to be directly imaged with T1-weighted or magnetization transfer weighted MRI scans on widely used 3T magnets (Sasaki et al., 2006, 2008). This neuromelanin-sensitive MRI (NM-MRI) allows for reliable mapping of the human LC (Keren et al., 2009, 2015; Tona et al., 2017). Although this property is increasingly being exploited, only two studies have applied this approach to AD patients *in vivo*. In one study, a non-significant reduction in neuromelanin signal versus controls was found, however, only 6 AD patients were included in the study (Miyoshi et al., 2013). A subsequent larger study of 22 AD, 38 MCI, and 26 controls reported

TABLE 2 | Validated and potential neuroimaging-based biomarkers for AD-relevant pathology.

	Pathology	Imaging technique/sequence
Validated AD neuroimaging biomarkers[1]	Amyloid (A)	Amyloid PET
	Tau (T)	Tau PET
	Hypometabolism (N)	FDG-PET
	Atrophy (N)	Structural MRI
Potential AD neuroimaging biomarkers	Perfusion	Arterial spin labeling, contrast-enhanced MRI
	BBB integrity	Contrast-enhanced MRI
	Vascular reactivity	Blood-oxygen-level-dependent MRI
	Functional connectivity	Blood-oxygen-level-dependent MRI
	Neurotransmitter dysfunction	Neuromelanin-sensitive MRI, MRS, PET
	White matter disruption	Diffusion tensor imaging
	Neuroinflammation	MRS, translocator protein PET*
	Synaptic dysfunction	Synaptic vesicle glycoprotein 2A PET*

*Included are pathologies that have been reported in AD and techniques used to image them in vivo. The techniques listed have also been successfully applied to the brainstem in the published literature in various contexts, with the exception of the newer PET indicators of neuroinflammation and synaptic dysfunction, marked by *. MRS, magnetic resonance spectroscopy. [1]Validated AD neuroimaging biomarkers are those described in the recently updated NIA-AA research framework (Jack et al., 2018).*

significantly reduced LC neuromelanin signal in both MCI and AD patients as compared with controls, with no difference between MCI or AD groups (Takahashi et al., 2015). This latter finding indicates that neuronal loss might occur relatively early in these patients, even before clinically detectable cognitive impairment. Interestingly, a study of healthy individuals showed that the LC neuromelanin signal positively correlates with established proxies of neural reserve such as years of education (Clewett et al., 2016), a finding in line with other data that implicate the LC as a physiological substrate of cognitive reserve (Robertson, 2013; Wilson et al., 2013). Further, another recent study found that reduced LC neuromelanin signal was associated with poorer memory even in healthy older adults, particularly for emotionally negative events (Hämmerer et al., 2018). Such findings raise the possibility that LC neuromelanin signal may have prognostic value for older individuals in preclinical stages of AD, well before cognitive impairment.

In addition to NM-MRI, there have been studies examining LC functional connectivity in healthy and clinical populations. These studies have primarily focused on psychiatric symptoms, showing that LC functional connectivity with certain limbic regions is increased in patients with generalized anxiety disorder (Meeten et al., 2016), post-traumatic stress disorder (Steuwe et al., 2015), or those at high risk for schizophrenia (Anticevic et al., 2014). Whether such changes are also present in AD patients with BPSD has yet to be determined. Additionally, PET radioligands have been developed that bind the noradrenaline transporter (NET) (Stehouwer and Goodman, 2009; Adhikarla et al., 2016) and various adrenoceptor subtypes (Lehto et al., 2015; Phan et al., 2017). These have even been combined with NM-MRI, in a study demonstrating a correlation between LC neuromelanin signal and NET binding in certain LC projection areas in Parkinson's disease (Sommerauer et al., 2018). Although various studies have found that NET density is decreased within the LC of the AD brain (Tejani-Butt et al., 1993; Szot et al., 2000; Gulyás et al., 2010), this has yet to be reported in AD patients *in vivo*.

SUMMARY

Thanks to recent advances in neuroimaging technologies, particularly UHF MRI, HRRT PET, and hybrid PET/MRI systems, the capacity to measure AD-associated brainstem pathology *in vivo* has reached a point where we can begin to assess its utility. Given the neuropathological findings described above, it is reasonable to expect alterations in these regions in at least a subset of patients with preclinical AD or even preclinical Alzheimer's pathologic change (**Table 1**). One of the first questions to address is whether neuroimaging-detectable LC or DRN pathology, either alone or in some combination with other markers, can help predict which patients on the AD spectrum will go on to develop AD dementia. The LC in particular seems promising in light of the aforementioned evidence indicating its early loss in size (Theofilas et al., 2017) and its potential role as a substrate of cognitive reserve (Wilson et al., 2013; Clewett et al., 2016; Hämmerer et al., 2018). Additionally, the technology to assess its integrity *in vivo* is already in increasingly widespread use. Indeed, a recent systematic review of LC NM-MRI studies by Liu et al. (2017) identified areas where this technique can be improved, particularly in terms of standardization of LC signal measurements and methods of sub-regional analysis. This latter aspect may be especially useful given the topographic specificity of LC degeneration in AD. Additionally, the advent of new PET radioligands for synaptic dysfunction and neuroinflammatory change (Bao et al., 2017; **Table 2**) opens new possibilities. Neuroinflammation in particular is increasingly appreciated for its significant role in the early etiology of AD, and various MRS-detectable metabolites have historically been taken as indicators of neuroinflammatory changes (Quarantelli, 2015). More recently, progress has been made in PET imaging of translocator protein (TSPO) as a biomarker of activated microglia and astrocytes (Kreisl et al., 2018).

Despite the promise, there is much to be studied before such strategies might be employed in the clinic. The aforementioned studies have been small in both size and number, and they need to be expanded and replicated. A more fundamental question of whether brainstem neuroimaging is likely to provide benefit above and beyond other biomarkers remains and, while it is too early to say, we believe that the potential is worth investigating as technological advancements allow it. Finally, whether or not neuroimaging within the LC or DRN becomes useful clinically, the techniques outlined here afford an opportunity to advance our understanding not only of AD pathological progression, but other neurodegenerative diseases as well.

AUTHOR CONTRIBUTIONS

DB wrote the manuscript. All authors conceived, revised, and approved the final manuscript.

FUNDING

This work was supported in part by the Weston Brain Institute and National Institutes of Health (F32-AG058456).

REFERENCES

Adhikarla, V., Zeng, F., Votaw, J., Goodman, M., and Nye, J. (2016). Compartmental modeling of [11C]MENET binding to the norepinephrine transporter in the healthy human brain. *Nucl. Med. Biol.* 43, 318–323. doi: 10.1016/j.nucmedbio.2016.02.008

Albert, M., DeKosky, S., Dickson, D., Dubois, B., Feldman, H., Fox, N., et al. (2011). The diagnosis of mild cognitive impairment due to Alzheimer's disease: recommendations from the National Institute on Aging-Alzheimer's association workgroups on diagnostic guidelines for Alzheimer's disease. *Alzheimers Dement.* 7, 270–279. doi: 10.1016/j.jalz.2011.03.008

Alzheimer's Association (2017). Alzheimer's disease facts and figures. *Alzheimers Dement.* 13, 325–373. doi: 10.1016/j.jalz.2017.02.001

Anticevic, A., Tang, Y., Cho, Y., Repovs, G., Cole, M., Savic, A., et al. (2014). Amygdala connectivity differs among chronic, early course, and individuals at risk for developing schizophrenia. *Schizophr. Bull.* 40, 1105–1116. doi: 10.1093/schbul/sbt165

Baker, K. G., Törk, I., Hornung, J. P., and Halasz, P. (1989). The human locus coeruleus complex: an immunohistochemical and three dimensional reconstruction study. *Exp. Brain Res.* 77, 257–270. doi: 10.1007/BF00274983

Bao, W., Jia, H., Finnema, S., Cai, Z., Carson, R., and Huang, Y. (2017). PET Imaging for early detection of Alzheimer's disease. *PET Clin.* 12, 329–350. doi: 10.1016/j.cpet.2017.03.001

Barnes, D., and Yaffe, K. (2011). The projected effect of risk factor reduction on Alzheimer's disease prevalence. *Lancet Neurol.* 10, 819–828. doi: 10.1016/S1474-4422(11)70072-2

Barrett, F., Workman, C., Sair, H., Savonenko, A., Kraut, M., Sodums, D., et al. (2017). Association between serotonin denervation and resting-state functional connectivity in mild cognitive impairment. *Hum. Brain Mapp.* 38, 3391–3401. doi: 10.1002/hbm.23595

Braak, H., Thal, D. R., Ghebremedhin, E., and Del Tredici, K. (2011). Stages of the pathologic process in Alzheimer disease: age categories from 1 to 100 years. *J. Neuropathol. Exp. Neurol.* 70, 960–969. doi: 10.1097/NEN.0b013e318232a379

Braun, D., Madrigal, J. L., and Feinstein, D. L. (2014). Noradrenergic regulation of glial activation: molecular mechanisms and therapeutic implications. *Curr. Neuropharmacol.* 12, 342–352. doi: 10.2174/1570159X12666140828220938

Cho, Z., Son, Y., Kim, H., Kim, K., Oh, S., Han, J., et al. (2007). A hybrid PET-MRI: an integrated molecular-genetic imaging system with HRRT-PET and 7.0-T MRI. *Int. J. Imaging Syst. Technol.* 17, 252–265. doi: 10.1002/ima.20119

Clewett, D., Lee, T.-H., Greening, S., Ponzio, A., Margalit, E., and Mather, M. (2016). Neuromelanin marks the spot: identifying a locus coeruleus biomarker of cognitive reserve in healthy aging. *Neurobiol. Aging* 37, 117–126. doi: 10.1016/j.neurobiolaging.2015.09.019

Davis, D. G., Schmitt, F. A., Wekstein, D. R., and Markesbery, W. R. (1999). Alzheimer neuropathologic alterations in aged cognitively normal subjects. *J. Neuropathol. Exp. Neurol.* 58, 376–388. doi: 10.1097/00005072-199904000-00008

Deistung, A., Schäfer, A., Schweser, F., Biedermann, U., Güllmar, D., Trampel, R., et al. (2013). High-resolution MR imaging of the human brainstem *In vivo* at 7 Tesla. *Front. Hum. Neurosci.* 7:710. doi: 10.3389/fnhum.2013.00710

Donovan, N., Hsu, D., Dagley, A., Schultz, A., Amariglio, R., Mormino, E., et al. (2015). Depressive symptoms and biomarkers of Alzheimer's Disease in cognitively normal older adults. *J. Alzheimers Dis.* 46, 63–73. doi: 10.3233/JAD-142940

Dukart, J., Mueller, K., Horstmann, A., Barthel, H., Möller, H. E., Villringer, A., et al. (2011). Combined evaluation of FDG-PET and MRI improves detection and differentiation of dementia. *PLoS One* 6:e18111. doi: 10.1371/journal.pone.0018111

Ehrenberg, A. J., Nguy, A. K., Theofilas, P., Dunlop, S., Suemoto, C. K., Lorenzo Alho, A. T., et al. (2017). Quantifying the accretion of hyperphosphorylated tau in the locus coeruleus and dorsal raphe nucleus: the pathological building blocks of early Alzheimer's disease. *Neuropathol. Appl. Neurobiol.* 43, 393–408. doi: 10.1111/nan.12387

Feinstein, D., Kalinin, S., and Braun, D. (2016). Causes, consequences, and cures for neuroinflammation mediated via the locus coeruleus: noradrenergic signaling system. *J. Neurochem.* 139, 154–178. doi: 10.1111/jnc.13447

Fernandes, P., Regala, J., Correia, F., and Gonçalves-Ferreira, A. J. (2012). The human locus coeruleus 3-D stereotactic anatomy. *Surg. Radiol. Anat.* 34, 879–885. doi: 10.1007/s00276-012-0979-y

German, D. C., Walker, B. S., Manaye, K., Smith, W. K., Woodward, D. J., and North, A. J. (1988). The human locus coeruleus: computer reconstruction of cellular distribution. *J. Neurosci.* 8, 1776–1788. doi: 10.1523/JNEUROSCI.08-05-01776.1988

Giorgi, F., Ryskalin, L., Ruffoli, R., Biagioni, F., Limanaqi, F., Ferrucci, M., et al. (2017). The neuroanatomy of the reticular nucleus locus coeruleus in Alzheimer's Disease. *Front. Neuroanat.* 11:80. doi: 10.3389/fnana.2017.00080

Grinberg, L., Rüb, U., Ferretti, R., Nitrini, R., Farfel, J., Polichiso, L., et al. (2009). The dorsal raphe nucleus shows phospho-tau neurofibrillary changes before the transentorhinal region in Alzheimer's disease. A precocious onset?. *Neuropathol. Appl. Neurobiol.* 35, 406–416. doi: 10.1111/j.1365-2990.2009.00997.x

Grudzien, A., Shaw, P., Weintraub, S., Bigio, E., Mash, D., and Mesulam, M. (2007). Locus coeruleus neurofibrillary degeneration in aging, mild cognitive impairment and early Alzheimer's disease. *Neurobiol. Aging* 28, 327–335. doi: 10.1016/j.neurobiolaging.2006.02.007

Gulyás, B., Brockschnieder, D., Nag, S., Pavlova, E., Kása, P., Beliczai, Z., et al. (2010). The norepinephrine transporter (NET) radioligand (S,S)-[18F]FMeNER-D2 shows significant decreases in NET density in the human brain in Alzheimer's disease: a post-mortem autoradiographic study. *Neurochem. Int.* 56, 789–798. doi: 10.1016/j.neuint.2010.03.001

Hämmerer, D., Callaghan, M., Hopkins, A., Kosciessa, J., Betts, M., Cardenas-Blanco, A., et al. (2018). Locus coeruleus integrity in old age is selectively related to memories linked with salient negative events. *Proc. Nat. Acad. Sci. U.S.A.* 115, 2228–2233. doi: 10.1073/pnas.1712268115

Hannah, J. A. (1936). A case of Alzheimer's disease with neuropathological findings. *Can. Med. Assoc. J.* 35, 361–366.

Heneka, M. T., Nadrigny, F., Regen, T., Martinez-Hernandez, A., Dumitrescu-Ozimek, L., Terwel, D., et al. (2010). Locus ceruleus controls Alzheimer's disease pathology by modulating microglial functions through norepinephrine. *Proc. Natl. Acad. Sci. U.S.A.* 107, 6058–6063. doi: 10.1073/pnas.0909586107

Iglesias, J., Leemput, K., Bhatt, P., Casillas, C., Dutt, S., Schuff, N., et al. (2015). Bayesian segmentation of brainstem structures in MRI. *Neuroimage* 113, 184–195. doi: 10.1016/j.neuroimage.2015.02.065

Jack, C., Bennett, D., Blennow, K., Carrillo, M., Dunn, B., Haeberlein, S., et al. (2018). NIA-AA research framework: toward a biological definition of Alzheimer's disease. *Alzheimers Dement.* 14, 535–562. doi: 10.1016/j.jalz.2018.02.018

Johnston, B., Tolomeo, S., Gradin, V., Christmas, D., Matthews, K., and Steele, D. (2015). Failure of hippocampal deactivation during loss events in treatment-resistant depression. *Brain* 138, 2766–2776. doi: 10.1093/brain/awv177

Ju, Y.-E., McLeland, J., Toedebusch, C., Xiong, C., Fagan, A., Duntley, S., et al. (2013). Sleep quality and preclinical Alzheimer Disease. *JAMA Neurol.* 70, 587–593. doi: 10.1001/jamaneurol.2013.2334

Kehoe, E., McNulty, J., Mullins, P., and Bokde, A. (2014). Advances in MRI biomarkers for the diagnosis of Alzheimer's disease. *Biomark. Med.* 8, 1151–1169. doi: 10.2217/bmm.14.42

Keren, N., Lozar, C., Harris, K., Morgan, P., and Eckert, M. (2009). In vivo mapping of the human locus coeruleus. *Neuroimage* 47, 1261–1267. doi: 10.1016/j.neuroimage.2009.06.012

Keren, N., Taheri, S., Vazey, E., Morgan, P., Granholm, A.-C., Aston-Jones, G., et al. (2015). Histologic validation of locus coeruleus MRI contrast in post-mortem tissue. *Neuroimage* 113, 235–245. doi: 10.1016/j.neuroimage.2015.03.020

Khachaturian, A., Hayden, K., Mielke, M., Tang, Y., Lutz, M., Gustafson, D., et al. (2018). Future prospects and challenges for Alzheimer's disease drug development in the era of the NIA-AA research framework. *Alzheimers Dement.* 14, 532–534. doi: 10.1016/j.jalz.2018.03.003

Knopman, D., Haeberlein, S., Carrillo, M., Hendrix, J., Kerchner, G., Margolin, R., et al. (2018). The national institute on aging and the Alzheimer's association research framework for Alzheimer's disease: perspectives from the research roundtable. *Alzheimers Dement.* 14, 563–575. doi: 10.1016/j.jalz.2018.03.002

Kranz, G., Hahn, A., Savli, M., and Lanzenberger, R. (2012). Challenges in the differentiation of midbrain raphe nuclei in neuroimaging research. *Proc. Natl. Acad. Sci. U.S.A.* 109, E2000–E2000. doi: 10.1073/pnas.1206247109

Kreisl, W. C., Henter, I. D., and Innis, R. B. (2018). Imaging translocator protein as a biomarker of neuroinflammation in dementia. *Adv. Pharmacol.* 82, 163–185. doi: 10.1016/bs.apha.2017.08.004

Kumar, J. S., and Mann, J. J. (2014). PET tracers for serotonin receptors and their applications. *Cent. Nerv. Syst. Agents Med. Chem.* 14, 96–112. doi: 10.2174/1871524914666141030124316

Lanctôt, K. L., Herrmann, N., and Mazzotta, P. (2001). Role of serotonin in the behavioral and psychological symptoms of dementia. *J. Neuropsychiatry Clin. Neurosci.* 13, 5–21. doi: 10.1176/jnp.13.1.5

Lanzenberger, R., Mitterhauser, M., Spindelegger, C., Wadsak, W., Klein, N., Mien, L.-K., et al. (2007). Reduced serotonin-1a receptor binding in social anxiety disorder. *Biol. Psychiatry* 61, 1081–1089. doi: 10.1016/j.biopsych.2006.05.022

Lee, H.-Y., Tae, W., Yoon, H.-K., Lee, B.-T., Paik, J.-W., Son, K.-R., et al. (2011). Demonstration of decreased gray matter concentration in the midbrain encompassing the dorsal raphe nucleus and the limbic subcortical regions in major depressive disorder: an optimized voxel-based morphometry study. *J. Affect. Disord.* 133, 128–136. doi: 10.1016/j.jad.2011.04.006

Lee, J., Ryan, J., Andreescu, C., Aizenstein, H., and Lim, H. (2015). Brainstem morphological changes in Alzheimer's disease. *Neuroreport* 26, 411–415. doi: 10.1097/WNR.0000000000000362

Lehto, J., Johansson, J., Vuorilehto, L., Luoto, P., Arponen, E., Scheinin, H., et al. (2015). Sensitivity of [11C]ORM-13070 to increased extracellular noradrenaline in the CNS – a PET study in human subjects. *Psychopharmacology* 232, 4169–4178. doi: 10.1007/s00213-015-3941-y

Liu, K., Marijatta, F., Hämmerer, D., Acosta-Cabronero, J., Düzel, E., and Howard, R. (2017). Magnetic resonance imaging of the human locus coeruleus: a systematic review. *Neurosci. Biobehav. Rev.* 83, 325–355. doi: 10.1016/j.neubiorev.2017.10.023

Lyness, S. A., Zarow, C., and Chui, H. C. (2003). Neuron loss in key cholinergic and aminergic nuclei in Alzheimer disease: a meta-analysis. *Neurobiol. Aging* 24, 1–23. doi: 10.1016/S0197-4580(02)00057-X

Mann, D. M. (1983). The locus coeruleus and its possible role in ageing and degenerative disease of the human central nervous system. *Mech. Ageing Dev.* 23, 73–94. doi: 10.1016/0047-6374(83)90100-8

Mann, D. M., and Yates, P. O. (1974). Lipoprotein pigments-their relationship to ageing in the human nervous system. II. The melanin content of pigmented nerve cells. *Brain* 97, 489–498. doi: 10.1093/brain/97.1.489

Marcyniuk, B., Mann, D. M. A., and Yates, P. O. (1986). Loss of nerve cells from locus coeruleus in Alzheimer's disease is topographically arranged. *Neurosci. Lett.* 64, 247–252. doi: 10.1016/0304-3940(86)90336-8

Matthews, K., Chen, C., Esiri, M., Keene, J., Minger, S., and Francis, P. (2002). Noradrenergic changes, aggressive behavior, and cognition in patients with dementia. *Biol. Psychiatry* 51, 407–416. doi: 10.1016/S0006-3223(01)01235-5

McKhann, G., Knopman, D., Chertkow, H., Hyman, B., Jack, C., Kawas, C., et al. (2011). The diagnosis of dementia due to Alzheimer's disease: recommendations from the National Institute on Aging-Alzheimer's Association workgroups on diagnostic guidelines for Alzheimer's disease. *Alzheimers Dement.* 7, 263–269. doi: 10.1016/j.jalz.2011.03.005

Meeten, F., Davey, G., Makovac, E., Watson, D., Garfinkel, S., Critchley, H., et al. (2016). Goal directed worry rules are associated with distinct patterns of amygdala functional connectivity and vagal modulation during perseverative cognition. *Front. Hum. Neurosci.* 10:553. doi: 10.3389/fnhum.2016.00553

Mehta, D., Jackson, R., Paul, G., Shi, J., and Sabbagh, M. (2017). Why do trials for Alzheimer's disease drugs keep failing? A discontinued drug perspective for 2010-2015. *Expert Opin. Inv. Drug* 26, 735–739. doi: 10.1080/13543784.2017.1323868

Miyoshi, F., Ogawa, T., Kitao, S., Kitayama, M., Shinohara, Y., Takasugi, M., et al. (2013). Evaluation of parkinson disease and Alzheimer Disease with the use of neuromelanin MR imaging and 123i-metaiodobenzylguanidine scintigraphy. *Am. J. Neuroradiol.* 34, 2113–2118. doi: 10.3174/ajnr.A3567

Montine, T., Phelps, C., Beach, T., Bigio, E., Cairns, N., Dickson, D., et al. (2012). National Institute on Aging–Alzheimer's Association guidelines for the neuropathologic assessment of Alzheimer's disease: a practical approach. *Acta Neuropath.* 123, 1–11. doi: 10.1007/s00401-011-0910-3

Nelson, P., Trojanowski, J., Abner, E., Al-Janabi, O., Jicha, G., Schmitt, F., et al. (2016). "New Old Pathologies": AD, part, and cerebral age-related TDP-43 with sclerosis (CARTS). *J. Neuropathol. Exp. Neurol.* 75, 482–498. doi: 10.1093/jnen/nlw033

Nensa, F., Beiderwellen, K., Heusch, P., and Wetter, A. (2014). Clinical applications of PET/MRI: current status and future perspectives. *Diagn. Interv. Radiol.* 20, 438–447. doi: 10.5152/dir.2014.14008

Neuropathology Group (2001). Pathological correlates of late-onset dementia in a multicentre, community-based population in England and Wales. neuropathology group of the medical research council cognitive function and ageing study (MRC CFAS). *Lancet* 357, 169–175.

Paterson, L., Kornum, B., Nutt, D., Pike, V., and Knudsen, G. (2013). 5-HT radioligands for human brain imaging with PET and SPECT. *Med. Res. Rev.* 33, 54–111. doi: 10.1002/med.20245

Phan, J.-A. A., Landau, A. M., Jakobsen, S., Wong, D. F., and Gjedde, A. (2017). Radioligand binding analysis of α 2 adrenoceptors with [11C]yohimbine in brain in vivo: extended inhibition plot correction for plasma protein binding. *Sci. Rep.* 7:15979. doi: 10.1038/s41598-017-16020-1

Pillai, R., Zhang, M., Yang, J., Mann, J., Oquendo, M., Parsey, R., et al. (2018). Molecular connectivity disruptions in males with major depressive disorder. *J. Cereb. Blood Flow Metab.* doi: 10.1177/0271678X18764053 [Epub ahead of print].

Quarantelli, M. (2015). MRI/MRS in neuroinflammation: methodology and applications. *Clin. Transl. Imaging* 3, 475–489. doi: 10.1007/s40336-015-0142-y

Quiroz, Y., Sperling, R., Norton, D., Baena, A., Arboleda-Velasquez, J., Cosio, D., et al. (2018). Association between amyloid and tau accumulation in young adults with autosomal dominant Alzheimer Disease. *JAMA Neurol.* 75, 548–556. doi: 10.1001/jamaneurol.2017.4907

Raja, R., Rosenberg, G., and Caprihan, A. (2017). MRI measurements of blood-brain barrier function in dementia: a review of recent studies. *Neuropharmacology* 134, 259–271. doi: 10.1016/j.neuropharm.2017.10.034

Rice, L., and Bisdas, S. (2017). The diagnostic value of FDG and amyloid PET in Alzheimer's disease-A systematic review. *Eur. J. Radiol.* 94, 16–24. doi: 10.1016/j.ejrad.2017.07.014

Robertson, I. (2013). A noradrenergic theory of cognitive reserve: implications for Alzheimer's disease. *Neurobiol. Aging* 34, 298–308. doi: 10.1016/j.neurobiolaging.2015.09.019

Rüb, U., Tredici, K., Del Schultz, C., Thal, D. R., Braak, E., and Braak, H. (2000). The evolution of Alzheimer's disease-related cytoskeletal pathology in the human raphe nuclei. *Neuropathol. Appl. Neurobiol.* 26, 553–567. doi: 10.1046/j.0305-1846.2000.00291.x

Sasaki, M., Shibata, E., Tohyama, K., Kudo, K., Endoh, J., Otsuka, K., et al. (2008). Monoamine neurons in the human brain stem: anatomy, magnetic resonance imaging findings, and clinical implications. *Neuroreport* 19:1649. doi: 10.1097/WNR.0b013e328315a637

Sasaki, M., Shibata, E., Tohyama, K., Takahashi, J., Otsuka, K., Tsuchiya, K., et al. (2006). Neuromelanin magnetic resonance imaging of locus ceruleus and substantia nigra in Parkinson's disease. *Neuroreport* 17:1215. doi: 10.1097/01.wnr.0000227984.84927.a7

Schain, M., Tóth, M., Cselényi, Z., Arakawa, R., Halldin, C., Farde, L., et al. (2013). Improved mapping and quantification of serotonin transporter availability in the human brainstem with the HRRT. *Eur. J. Nucl. Med. Mol. Imaging* 40, 228–237. doi: 10.1007/s00259-012-2260-3

Sclocco, R., Beissner, F., Bianciardi, M., Polimeni, J., and Napadow, V. (2017). Challenges and opportunities for brainstem neuroimaging with ultrahigh field MRI. *Neuroimage* 168, 412–426. doi: 10.1016/j.neuroimage.2017.02.052

Silverberg, N., Elliott, C., Ryan, L., Masliah, E., and Hodes, R. (2018). NIA commentary on the NIA-AA research framework: towards a biological definition of Alzheimer's disease. *Alzheimers Dement.* 14, 576–578. doi: 10.1016/j.jalz.2018.03.004

Šimić, G., Babić Leko, M., Wray, S., Harrington, C. R., Delalle, I., Jovanov-Milošević, N., et al. (2017). Monoaminergic neuropathology in Alzheimer's disease. *Prog. Neurobiol.* 151, 101–138. doi: 10.1016/j.pneurobio.2016.04.001

Singh-Manoux, A., Dugravot, A., Fournier, A., Abell, J., Ebmeier, K., Kivimäki, M., et al. (2017). Trajectories of depressive symptoms before diagnosis of dementia: a 28-year follow-up study. *JAMA Psychiatry* 74, 712–718. doi: 10.1001/jamapsychiatry.2017.0660

Sommerauer, M., Fedorova, T. D., Hansen, A. K., Knudsen, K., Otto, M., Jeppesen, J., et al. (2018). Evaluation of the noradrenergic system in Parkinson's disease: an 11C-MeNER PET and neuromelanin MRI study. *Brain* 141, 496–504. doi: 10.1093/brain/awx348

Son, Y.-D., Cho, Z.-H., Choi, E.-J., Kim, J.-H., Kim, H.-K., Lee, S.-Y., et al. (2014). Individually differentiated serotonergic raphe nuclei measured with brain PET/MR imaging. *Radiology* 272, 541–548. doi: 10.1148/radiol.14131547

Sperling, R., Aisen, P., Beckett, L., Bennett, D., Craft, S., Fagan, A., et al. (2011). Toward defining the preclinical stages of Alzheimer's disease: recommendations from the National Institute on Aging-Alzheimer's Association workgroups on diagnostic guidelines for Alzheimer's disease. *Alzheimers Dement.* 7, 280–292. doi: 10.1016/j.jalz.2011.03.003

Stehouwer, J., and Goodman, M. (2009). Fluorine-18 radiolabeled PET tracers for imaging monoamine transporters: dopamine, serotonin, and norepinephrine. *Pet Clin.* 4, 101–128. doi: 10.1016/j.cpet.2009.05.006

Steuwe, C., Daniels, J., Frewen, P., Densmore, M., Theberge, J., and Lanius, R. (2015). Effect of direct eye contact in women with PTSD related to interpersonal trauma: psychophysiological interaction analysis of connectivity of an innate alarm system. *Psychiatry Res. Neuroimaging* 232, 162–167. doi: 10.1016/j.pscychresns.2015.02.010

Szabadi, E. (2013). Functional neuroanatomy of the central noradrenergic system. *J. Psychopharmacol.* 27, 659–693. doi: 10.1177/0269881113490326

Szot, P., Leverenz, J., Peskind, E., Kiyasu, E., Rohde, K., Miller, M., et al. (2000). Tyrosine hydroxylase and norepinephrine transporter mRNA expression in the locus coeruleus in Alzheimer's disease. *Mol. Brain Res.* 84, 135–140. doi: 10.1016/S0169-328X(00)00168-6

Takahashi, J., Shibata, T., Sasaki, M., Kudo, M., Yanezawa, H., Obara, S., et al. (2015). Detection of changes in the locus coeruleus in patients with mild cognitive impairment and Alzheimer's disease: high-resolution fast spin-echo T1-weighted imaging. *Geriatr. Gerontol. Int.* 15, 334–340. doi: 10.1111/ggi.12280

Tan, C.-C. C., Yu, J.-T. T., and Tan, L. (2014). Biomarkers for preclinical Alzheimer's disease. *J. Alzheimers Dis.* 42, 1051–1069. doi: 10.3233/JAD-140843

Tejani-Butt, S., Yang, J., and Zaffar, H. (1993). Norepinephrine transporter sites are decreased in the locus coeruleus in Alzheimer's disease. *Brain Res.* 631, 147–150. doi: 10.1016/0006-8993(93)91201-3

Theofilas, P., Ehrenberg, A., Dunlop, S., Alho, A., Nguy, A., Leite, R., et al. (2017). Locus coeruleus volume and cell population changes during Alzheimer's disease progression: a stereological study in human postmortem brains with potential implication for early-stage biomarker discovery. *Alzheimers Dement.* 13, 236–246. doi: 10.1016/j.jalz.2016.06.2362

Tona, K.-D., Keuken, M., Rover, M., de Lakke, E., Forstmann, B., Nieuwenhuis, S., et al. (2017). In vivo visualization of the locus coeruleus in humans: quantifying the test-retest reliability. *Brain Struct. Funct.* 222, 4203–4217. doi: 10.1007/s00429-017-1464-5

Trillo, L., Das, D., Hsieh, W., Medina, B., Moghadam, S., Lin, B., et al. (2013). Ascending monoaminergic systems alterations in Alzheimer's disease. Translating basic science into clinical care. *Neurosci. Biobehav. Rev.* 37, 1363–1379. doi: 10.1016/j.neubiorev.2013.05.008

Villemagne, V., Doré, V., Burnham, S., Masters, C., and Rowe, C. (2018). Imaging tau and amyloid-β proteinopathies in Alzheimer disease and other conditions. *Nat. Rev. Neurol.* 14, 225. doi: 10.1038/nrneurol.2018.9

Wilson, R., Nag, S., Boyle, P., Hizel, L., Yu, L., Buchman, A., et al. (2013). Neural reserve, neuronal density in the locus ceruleus, and cognitive decline. *Neurology* 80, 1202–1208. doi: 10.1212/WNL.0b013e3182897103

Wolk, D., and Detre, J. (2012). Arterial spin labeling MRI: an emerging biomarker for Alzheimer's disease and other neurodegenerative conditions. *Curr. Opin. Neurol.* 25, 421–428. doi: 10.1097/WCO.0b013e328354ff0a

World Health Organization (2017). *Global Action Plan on the Public Health Response to Dementia 2017–2025.* Geneva: World Health Organization.

Zarow, C., Lyness, S., Mortimer, J., and Chui, H. (2003). Neuronal loss is greater in the locus coeruleus than nucleus basalis and substantia nigra in Alzheimer and Parkinson diseases. *Arch. Neurol.* 60, 337–341. doi: 10.1001/archneur.60.3.337

Zecca, L., Casella, L., Albertini, A., Bellei, C., Zucca, F. A., Engelen, M., et al. (2008). Neuromelanin can protect against iron-mediated oxidative damage in system modeling iron overload of brain aging and Parkinson's disease. *J. Neurochem.* 106, 1866–1875. doi: 10.1111/j.1471-4159.2008.05541.x

Zhang, X., Yang, Z., Lu, G., Yang, G., and Zhang, L. (2017). PET/MR imaging: new frontier in alzheimer's disease and other dementias. *Front. Mol. Neurosci.* 10:343. doi: 10.3389/fnmol.2017.00343

Zhou, J., Greicius, M., Gennatas, E., Growdon, M., Jang, J., Rabinovici, G., et al. (2010). Divergent network connectivity changes in behavioural variant frontotemporal dementia and Alzheimer's disease. *Brain* 133, 1352–1367. doi: 10.1093/brain/awq075

11

Reduced Regional Cerebral Blood Flow Relates to Poorer Cognition in Older Adults With Type 2 Diabetes

Katherine J. Bangen[1,2], Madeleine L. Werhane[2,3], Alexandra J. Weigand[1,2], Emily C. Edmonds[1,2], Lisa Delano-Wood[4,2], Kelsey R. Thomas[2,4], Daniel A. Nation[5], Nicole D. Evangelista[1], Alexandra L. Clark[2,3], Thomas T. Liu[6] and Mark W. Bondi[2,4]*

[1] Research Service, VA San Diego Healthcare System, San Diego, CA, United States, [2] Department of Psychiatry, University of California, San Diego, San Diego, CA, United States, [3] Department of Psychology, San Diego State University, San Diego, CA, United States, [4] Psychology Service, VA San Diego Healthcare System, San Diego, CA, United States, [5] Department of Psychology, University of Southern California, Los Angeles, CA, United States, [6] Department of Radiology and Bioengineering, University of California, San Diego, San Diego, CA, United States

***Correspondence:**
Katherine J. Bangen
kbangen@ucsd.edu

Type 2 diabetes mellitus (T2DM) increases risk for dementia, including Alzheimer's disease (AD). Many previous studies of brain changes underlying cognitive impairment in T2DM have applied conventional structural magnetic resonance imaging (MRI) to detect macrostructural changes associated with cerebrovascular disease such as white matter hyperintensities or infarcts. However, such pathology likely reflects end-stage manifestations of chronic decrements in cerebral blood flow (CBF). MRI techniques that measure CBF may (1) elucidate mechanisms that precede irreversible parenchymal damage and (2) serve as a marker of risk for cognitive decline. CBF measured with arterial spin labeling (ASL) MRI may be a useful marker of perfusion deficits in T2DM and related conditions. We examined associations among T2DM, CBF, and cognition in a sample of 49 well-characterized nondemented older adults. Along with a standard T1-weighted scan, a pseudocontinuous ASL sequence optimized for older adults (by increasing post-labeling delays to allow more time for the blood to reach brain tissue) was obtained on a 3T GE scanner to measure regional CBF in FreeSurfer derived regions of interest. Participants also completed a neuropsychological assessment. Results showed no significant differences between individuals with and without T2DM in terms of cortical thickness or regional brain volume. However, adjusting for age, sex, comorbid vascular risk factors, and reference CBF (postcentral gyrus) older adults with T2DM demonstrated reduced CBF in the hippocampus, and inferior temporal, inferior parietal, and frontal cortices. Lower CBF was associated with poorer memory and executive function/processing speed. When adjusting for diabetes, the significant associations between lower regional CBF and poorer executive function/processing speed remained. Results demonstrate that CBF is reduced in older adults with T2DM, and suggest that CBF alterations likely precede volumetric changes. Notably, relative to nondiabetic control participants, those with T2DM showed lower CBF in predilection sites for AD pathology (medial temporal lobe and inferior parietal regions). Findings augment recent research suggesting that perfusion deficits may underlie cognitive decrements frequently observed among older adults with T2DM. Results also suggest that CBF measured with ASL MRI may reflect an early and important marker of risk of cognitive impairment in T2DM and related conditions.

Keywords: aging, diabetes, vascular risk, arterial spin labeling, cerebral blood flow, neuropsychology, memory, Alzheimer's disease

INTRODUCTION

Type 2 diabetes mellitus (T2DM) is a chronic, highly disabling metabolic disorder that is growing in prevalence at an alarming rate. In 2015, it was estimated that 30.3 million Americans (1 in 10) had either diagnosed or undiagnosed diabetes, the vast majority of whom (90–95%) had T2DM (Prevention, 2017). This is particularly concerning, given that T2DM has been linked to an increased risk for developing mild cognitive impairment (MCI) and dementia including Alzheimer's disease (AD) (Luchsinger et al., 2001; Arvanitakis et al., 2004; Luchsinger et al., 2007; Vagelatos and Eslick, 2013) - conditions that are associated with high health care costs, reduced quality of life, and loss of independence in late adulthood. Even among nondemented older adults, studies have observed increased rates of subtle cognitive impairment and accelerated cognitive decline in individuals with T2DM compared to their nondiabetic counterparts, suggesting that cognitive impairment may be a chronic long-term complication of T2DM (Geijselaers et al., 2015). In T2DM, vascular dysfunction has long been considered the underlying cause of the multi-organ complications of the disease. Cerebrovascular dysfunction, thus, seems to be a possible mechanism by which poor cognitive outcomes occur in diabetes. Indeed, neuropathologic studies have linked T2DM to increased incidence of cerebral infarcts (Peila et al., 2002; Arvanitakis et al., 2006; Sarwar et al., 2010). Furthermore, insulin resistance, hyperglycemia, and inflammation - all which represent defining deleterious metabolic states that occur in diabetes - have been linked to cerebrovascular dysfunction (Brownlee, 2005; Zhou et al., 2014; Chung et al., 2015).

Most previous studies of brain changes underlying cognitive decrements in T2DM have applied conventional structural magnetic resonance imaging (MRI) to detect macrostructural changes associated with cerebral gray matter (GM) atrophy and markers of cerebrovascular disease (CVD) lesions such as white matter hyperintensities (WMH), which are thought to reflect small vessel disease. Many structural neuroimaging studies have shown *in vivo* cerebral atrophy in T2DM that has been linked to poorer cognitive performance across domains including memory, executive functioning, and processing speed (Tiehuis et al., 2009; Hayashi et al., 2011; Moran et al., 2013; Zhang et al., 2014). Results from several of these studies indicate that regional atrophy patterns in T2DM resemble those seen in preclinical AD, with hippocampal atrophy identified as the earliest and most prominent neurodegenerative change (Moran et al., 2013). However, these structural brain changes in T2DM likely reflect end-stage manifestations of chronic decrements in cerebrovascular functioning. Advanced functional MRI techniques that measure cerebral blood flow (CBF) may elucidate the mechanisms that precede the development of irreversible parenchymal damage and serve as an early indicator of impending cognitive decline in at-risk populations.

Arterial spin labeling (ASL) is a non-invasive MRI technique that measures CBF alterations. ASL studies of AD demonstrate similar patterns of regional perfusion compared to studies using fluorodeoxyglucose positron emission tomography (FDG-PET) and single photon emission computed tomography (SPECT) (Chen et al., 2011; Takahashi et al., 2014). ASL techniques have advantages over PET and SPECT, however, related to the nature of the tracer (i.e., magnetically labeled arterial water) (Detre and Alsop, 1999). That is, ASL employs a non-invasive, endogenous tracer rather than an intravenously administered contrast agent. The rapid decay time of the magnetized water molecules (on the order of seconds), moreover, allows for relatively brief scan times (5–10 min) that can provide dynamic CBF estimates with high temporal resolution (Johnson et al., 2005). These advantages, combined with its ability to quantitatively measure cerebral perfusion (in milliliters per 100 g of tissue per minute), make ASL an ideal technique for research and clinical settings (Telischak et al., 2015) designed to monitor neural and vascular changes in healthy older adults (Bangen et al., 2009) and clinical populations (Johnson et al., 2005; Xu et al., 2007; Bangen et al., 2012; Binnewijzend et al., 2013).

There are few publications examining cerebral perfusion and its associations with cognition in individuals with T2DM, and findings across these limited studies are contradictory. In one of the earliest studies, Dandona et al. (1978) measured global CBF by the 133-Xe inhalation method in 59 individuals with T2DM and 28 controls encompassing a wide range of ages. They reported age-related perfusion reductions that were similar in those with and without T2DM. Previous studies employing SPECT have reported that diabetic patients exhibit decreased CBF (Wakisaka et al., 1990; Nagamachi et al., 1994; Sabri et al., 2000) and that these CBF reductions are associated with poorer cognitive performance (Xia et al., 2015). Although the extant literature still remains relatively limited, a handful of studies have attempted to employ ASL to assess associations among diabetes status, CBF, and cognitive functioning. Consistent with the PET and SPECT literature, several studies have reported regional cerebral hypoperfusion in individuals with diabetes (Last et al., 2007; Xia et al., 2015; Cui et al., 2017; Dai et al., 2017), although some studies have reported no such differences between individuals with and without diabetes (Launer et al., 2015; Rusinek et al., 2015). Those studies that do report significant differences, however, have most consistently observed associations between diabetes status and hypoperfusion in posterior cortical regions (e.g., parietal regions) (Last et al., 2007; Xia et al., 2015; Cui et al., 2017; Dai et al., 2017), although some reports document hypoperfusion in frontal, temporal, and limbic regions as well (Xia et al., 2015; Cui et al., 2017; Dai et al., 2017). With respect to cognitive functioning in T2DM, the ASL literature is even further limited. While the available evidence suggests that alterations to CBF in certain regions are associated with poorer cognitive functioning in individuals with T2DM (Novak et al., 2014; Xia et al., 2015; Cui et al., 2017; Dai et al., 2017), these data are extremely limited given the very few published studies to date, and the findings are mixed with respect to the affected cognitive domains.

Although there is mounting evidence to suggest an association between T2DM, CBF, and cognition, prior studies lack the robust methodology needed to reliably assess these associations. Many studies do not specifically explore these associations in an older adult population, despite this population being at an elevated risk for both T2DM and dementia. Moreover, those that do target an older sample employ ASL methods that are not optimized for imaging CBF in older adults, which is problematic considering that this population has expected increases in transport time from the labeling position to the tissue (i.e., longer arterial transit time) relative to younger adults and therefore the post-labeling delay should be adjusted accordingly so that the CBF estimation will not be biased by incomplete delivery of the labeled bolus prior to image acquisition (Alsop et al., 2015). Finally, most studies include relatively limited neuropsychological assessment. Thus, the present study sought to extend the literature by examining the associations among T2DM, CBF, and cognition in a sample of well-characterized nondemented older adults who underwent pseudo-continuous ASL imaging optimized for older adult populations and comprehensive neuropsychological assessment.

MATERIALS AND METHODS

Participants

Forty-nine independently living, nondemented older adults were recruited from ongoing aging studies at the University of California, San Diego (UCSD) and the San Diego VA Healthcare System. Potential participants were excluded if they were younger than 60 years of age; had a history of Type 1 diabetes; had dementia identified by medical, neurological, and neuropsychological examinations; or had a history of stroke or neurologic disease (e.g., Parkinson's disease, multiple sclerosis), head injury with cognitive sequelae, or major psychiatric disorder; or for whom MRI was contraindicated (e.g., individuals with a pacemaker). Of the 49 participants, 11 had T2DM, and 38 were nondiabetic control participants.

Ethics Statement

All participants provided written informed consent prior to enrollment, and data were collected in accordance with ethical standards for research. The UCSD and VA San Diego Healthcare System Institutional Review Boards approved the research protocol.

Clinical and Neuropsychological Assessment

All participants underwent a semi-structured clinical interview assessing medical and psychiatric history; assessment of instrumental activities of daily living; physical examination with brachial artery blood pressure measurement using an automated blood pressure cuff; comprehensive neuropsychological testing; and brain MRI. Participants were classified as having diabetes based on self-report during clinical interview and review of available medical records. Of the 11 participants with T2DM, 10 were being treated with antidiabetic medications (9 with oral glucose lowering agents only and 1 with insulin only).

Presence of additional vascular risk factors included in the Framingham stroke risk profile (FSRP) (D'Agostino et al., 1994) was determined by self-report, medical chart review, and physical examination. These vascular risk factors included: (1) hypertension (defined as systolic blood pressure $\geq$140 mm Hg, diastolic blood pressure $\geq$90 mm Hg, or use of antihypertensive medications); (2) history of cardiovascular disease [e.g., coronary artery disease (myocardial infarction, angina pectoris, coronary insufficiency), intermittent claudication, cardiac failure]; (3) atrial fibrillation; and (4) current cigarette smoking. To characterize the aggregate vascular risk burden of our sample, we also calculated a modified FSRP for each participant (D'Agostino et al., 1994) omitting diabetes. Pulse pressure – a proxy for arterial stiffness – was also calculated (as systolic minus diastolic blood pressure), given that T2DM is associated with arterial stiffening (Winer and Sowers, 2003; Tomiyama et al., 2005). Arterial stiffening is also an AD risk factor that relates to AD cerebrospinal fluid (CSF) biomarkers and cerebrovascular functioning (Nation et al., 2015, 2016b; Werhane et al., 2018) including reduced CBF (Yan et al., 2016).

Global cognition was assessed by the dementia rating scale (DRS) (Mattis, 1988). Episodic memory was assessed by the California Verbal Learning Test-Second Edition (CVLT-II) (Delis et al., 2000) long delay free recall, and delayed recall of the Logical Memory and Visual Reproduction subtests of the Wechsler memory scale – revised (WMS-R) (Wechsler, 1987). Executive function/processing speed was assessed using Trail Making Test, Parts A and B. For each of the five cognitive scores, each participant's raw score was converted to a z-score based on the mean and standard deviation of the entire sample (n = 49). Domain composite scores are the mean of z-scores measured within that domain. In addition, executive function/processing speed composite scores were multiplied by −1 so that positive z-scores represented better performance for all scores. Of note, one participant with T2DM was missing CVLT-II data; one nondiabetic control participant was missing WMS-R Logical Memory data; and one T2DM participant was missing WMS-R Visual Reproduction data. For these three participants who were each missing data for one memory measure, their memory composite score was calculated as the mean of their two existing memory scores. In addition, two T2DM participants were missing both Trail Making Test variables and, therefore, these individuals were not included in the analyses involving the executive function/processing speed composite.

MRI Data Acquisition

Magnetic resonance imaging data were acquired on one of two identical GE Discovery MR 750 3T whole body systems using an 8-channel receive-only head coil (General Electric Medical Systems, Milwaukee, WI, United States) at the UCSD Keck Center for functional MRI. During scanning, participants are provided with ear plugs and MRI-safe noise reduction headphones and instructed to stay still. The scanner room is dark and there is no visual stimulation. Participants are not given instructions to keep their eyes open or closed. A T1-weighted anatomical scan was acquired using a Fast Spoiled Gradient Recall (3DFSPGR) sequence with the following parameters: 172.1 mm contiguous sagittal slices, field of view (FOV) = 25 cm, repetition time (TR) = 8 ms, echo time (TE) = 3.1 ms, flip angle = 12, inversion time (TI) = 600 ms, 256 × 192 matrix, bandwidth = 31.25 kHZ, frequency direction = S–I, NEX = 1, scan time = 8 min, and 13 s.

Resting CBF was acquired using a 2D pseudocontinuous ASL (PCASL) sequence optimized for older adult populations, which increases post-labeling delays to allow more time for the blood to reach brain tissue with the following parameters: TR = 4,500 ms, TE = 3.2 ms, FOV = 24 cm, labeling duration = 1,800 ms, post-labeling delay = 2,000 ms, 24.6 mm slices, with a single shot spiral acquisition and a total scan time of 4:18 min plus a 30 s calibration scan. In addition, a spiral scan with the inversion pulses turned off was acquired to obtain an estimate of the magnetization of CSF. The CSF signal from this scan was used to estimate the equilibrium magnetization of blood, which was used to convert the perfusion signal into calibrated CBF units (i.e., millimeters of blood per 100 g of tissue per minute) (Chalela et al., 2000). A minimum contrast scan was also acquired to adjust for coil inhomogeneities during the CBF quantification step (Wang et al., 2005). Finally, a field map scan was also acquired and used for off-line field map correction to help correct distortion and signal dropout, particularly in the frontal and medial temporal lobes.

MRI Data Processing

MRI data were processed using Analysis of Functional NeuroImages (AFNI) (Cox, 1996), FMRIB Software Library (FSL) (Smith et al., 2004), FreeSurfer, and locally created Matlab scripts.

T1-Weighted Anatomical Images

T1-weighted anatomical images were processed using FreeSurfer 5.1 software. Briefly, images underwent skull stripping, B1 bias field correction, GM–WM segmentation, reconstruction of cortical surface models, and parcellation and labeling of regions on the cortical surface as well as segmentation and labeling of subcortical brain structures (Dale et al., 1999; Fischl et al., 2002). FreeSurfer output (gray–white boundary surface, pial surface, cortical parcellation, and subcortical segmentation) was visually inspected and, when necessary, manual edits were performed to ensure proper region of interest (ROI) segmentation and GM and WM differentiation.

ASL Images

Each participant's raw ASL data (perfusion, CSF, and mincon data), field map, and anatomical data were uploaded for processing to the Cerebral Blood Flow Biomedical Informatics Research Network (CBFBIRN[1]) (Shin et al., 2013) established at the UCSD Center for Functional Magnetic Resonance Imaging). Field map and motion correction; skull-stripping; and tissue segmentation using FSL's Automated Segmentation Tool (FAST) algorithm to define CSF, GM, and WM tissue were completed. The high-resolution T1-weighted image and partial volume segmentations were then registered to ASL space, and partial volume segmentations were down-sampled to the resolution of the ASL data. To correct the CBF measures for partial volume effects and ensure that CBF values were not influenced by known decreased perfusion in WM or increased volume of CSF (Parkes et al., 2004), we utilized the method described by Johnson et al. (2005). These calculations assume that CSF has 0 CBF and that CBF in GM is 2.5 times higher than that in WM. To compute partial volume corrected CBF signal intensities, the following formula was used: CBFcorr = CBFuncorr/(GM + 0.4 × WM) where CBFcorr and CBFuncorr are corrected and uncorrected CBF values, respectively, and GM and WM are the partial volume fractions of GM and WM, respectively. The CBFcorr data was blurred to 4.0 mm full-width at half maximum. Each participant's quantified CBF map (in units of mL/100 g tissue/min) was downloaded to a local server and a threshold was applied that removed values outside of the expected physiological range of CBF (<10 or >150) (Bangen et al., 2014).

FreeSurfer was used to generate anatomical ROIs for the CBF data as well cortical thickness and volume data for these ROIs to be compared between the T2DM and nondiabetic control groups. We examined left and right hemisphere for the following five *a priori* ROIs: (1) hippocampus, (2) inferior temporal cortex, (3) inferior parietal cortex, (4) rostral middle frontal gyrus, and (5) medial orbitofrontal cortex. These ROIs were selected because they have been implicated in cerebrovascular dysfunction in MCI and AD (Du et al., 2002; Nation et al., 2013, 2016a). Many of these regions have been implicated in T2DM in the few existing studies of ASL CBF in this population (Last et al., 2007; Xia et al., 2015; Cui et al., 2017; Dai et al., 2017). The regional GM CBF values (corrected for partial volume effects) from the Desikan et al. (2006) atlas were extracted for each of the ROIs for each hemisphere. See **Figure 1** for a depiction of the *a priori* ROIs used in the primary analyses. In addition, to adjust for individual variation in CBF, postcentral gyrus CBF was used as a reference region and included as a covariate in statistical analyses comparing groups on CBF in the ROIs. This region was selected due to its relative sparing in AD (Thompson et al., 2003) and T2DM-related brain atrophy (Moran et al., 2013; Zhang et al., 2014) as well as its use as a control region in our prior studies of CBF in older adults at increased risk for AD (Bangen et al., 2017).

[1]cbfbirn.ucsd.edu

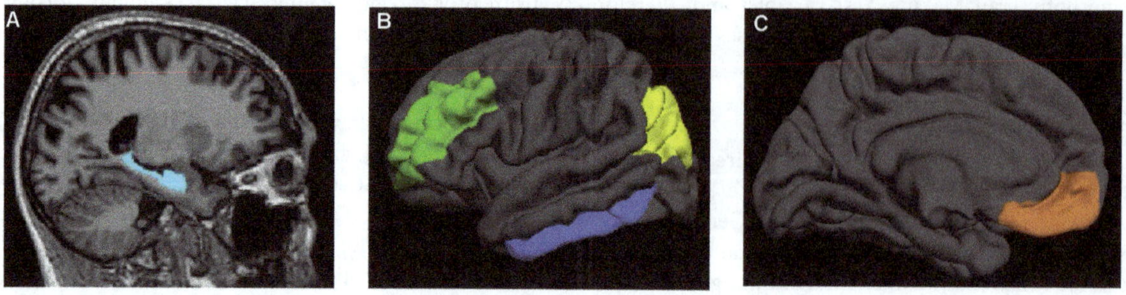

FIGURE 1 | Regions of interest. **(A)** hippocampus; **(B)** rostral middle frontal gyrus (in *green*), inferior temporal cortex (in *blue*), and inferior parietal cortex (in *yellow*); **(C)** medial orbitofrontal cortex (in *orange*).

FreeSurfer-derived intracranial volume was used as a covariate in analyses comparing groups on regional brain volume.

In addition, groups were also compared on FreeSurfer-derived volumes of WM signal abnormalities (WMSAs). WMSAs on MRI refer to regions in the WM that appear hyperintense on T2 fluid-attenuated inversion recovery (FLAIR) but hypointense on T1-weighted images. WMSAs are often observed in aging and conditions including diabetes and are usually thought to reflect small vessel CVD resulting from microvascular hypoperfusion (Garde et al., 2000; O'Sullivan et al., 2002; Brickman et al., 2015; Shen et al., 2017). The FreeSurfer automated segmentation pipeline subdivides brain tissue into regions of GM, WM, and hypointense regions within the WM using a combination of segmentation and a set of anatomical priors (Fischl and Dale, 2000; Fischl et al., 2002). Total volume of WM hypointensities was extracted from FreeSurfer output.

Statistical Analyses

Analysis of variance (ANOVA) and chi-square tests were used to compare those with and without T2DM on demographic and clinical characteristics of interest. Multiple analysis of covariance (MANCOVA) models were used to determine CBF and structural brain differences between T2DM and nondiabetic control participants. The MANCOVA compared CBF in the selected ROIs adjusting for age, sex, modified FSRP (omitting diabetes), and reference CBF (postcentral gyrus). The modified FSRP was used as a covariate in an effort to determine whether any potential groups differences in CBF were related to T2DM rather than possible comorbid vascular risk factors/conditions. This composite measure to assess vascular risk (rather than individuals vascular risk factors) was used to maximize the sample size to independent variable ratio in our analyses. MANCOVAs were also used to determine whether there were group differences in brain structure (i.e., cortical thickness or volume) that might influence CBF findings, particularly given that some previous studies have reported that atrophy may largely explain lower CBF in T2DM (Sabri et al., 2000). One MANCOVA compared cortical thickness in 4 of the 5 ROIs (inferior parietal cortex, inferior parietal cortex, rostral middle frontal gyrus, and medial orbitofrontal cortex) adjusting for age, sex, and modified FSRP. A second MANCOVA compared volume of hippocampus and WM hypointensities adjusting for age, sex, modified FSRP, and intracranial volume. All *a priori* ROIs were entered into the MANCOVAs simultaneously.

Pearson's product-moment correlations examined the associations between cognition and CBF across the entire sample (i.e., collapsed across T2DM and nondiabetic control participants). To minimize comparisons, we examined associations only for those unilateral ROIs that showed significant group differences in CBF. For each significant ROI, we correlated regional CBF with performance in cognitive domains subserved by that region. Specifically, we examined the associations of the memory composite score and CBF in the hippocampus and inferior temporal cortex. In addition, we examined the associations of the executive function/processing speed composite with CBF in the inferior parietal cortex and rostral middle frontal gyrus.

Sensitivity analyses were performed to determine whether results from the primary analyses may have been influenced by potential sex-related CBF differences and/or the presence of comorbid vascular risk factors associated with T2DM (e.g., hypertension). First, we compared men and women (regardless of T2DM status) on mean CBF for regions where differences were observed between the T2DM and nondiabetic control groups. Second, we ran t-test analyses to compare a subset of the sample consisting of nondiabetic control participants ($n = 11$) and T2DM ($n = 11$) participants who were matched so that the two groups did not significantly differ in terms of demographic or covariate variables. Significance levels of 0.05 were used for all analyses. All statistical analyses were conducted using the Statistical Package for the Social Sciences (SPSS) version 24 (SPSS IBM, New York, United States).

Finally, in order to address potential inflation of type I error resulting from multiple comparisons, we applied the Benjamini–Hochberg procedure (Benjamini and Hochberg, 1995). We assessed results when the false discovery rate (FDR) was controlled at 0.05 and 0.10.

RESULTS

Participant Characteristics

Participant demographics and clinical characteristics are presented in **Table 1**. In comparison to the nondiabetic control

TABLE 1 | Demographic and neuropsychological characteristics by T2DM status.

	Nondiabetic (n = 38)	T2DM (n = 11)	F or χ^2	p	Effect size
Demographics*					
Age, years	73.6 (5.9)	72.3 (2.8)	0.49	0.486	$\eta_p^2 = 0.010$
Education, years	17.0 (1.7)	16.6 (2.4)	0.24	0.627	$\eta_p^2 = 0.005$
Sex, M:F	13:25	8:3	5.17	0.023	$\varphi_c = 0.325$
FSRP (%)**	10.1 (7.9)	13.4 (7.8)	1.47	0.232	$\eta_p^2 = 0.030$
Pulse pressure, mmHg	50.5 (11.2)	56.2 (16.1)	1.86	0.179	$\eta_p^2 = 0.038$
Current smoker (%)	5.3	9.1	0.22	0.641	$\varphi_c = 0.067$
History of cardiovascular disease (%)	5.3	9.1	0.22	0.641	$\varphi_c = 0.067$
History of hypertension (%)	52.6	100.0	8.24	0.004	$\varphi_c = 0.410$
History of atrial fibrillation (%)	10.5	9.1	0.02	0.890	$\varphi_c = 0.020$
GDS	3.6 (3.9)	6.1 (3.7)	3.31	0.075	$\eta_p^2 = 0.069$
Cognitive measures* **					
Mean (SD)					
Global cognition (DRS total score)	140.5 (3.4)	138.3 (4.5)	0.94	0.338	$\eta_p^2 = 0.021$
Memory composite	0.18 (0.8)	−0.78 (0.9)	5.80	0.020	$\eta_p^2 = 0.117$
Executive function/processing speed composite	0.20 (0.7)	−0.83 (1.1)	11.72	0.001	$\eta_p^2 = 0.218$

T2DM, type 2 diabetes mellitus; SD, standard deviation; FSRP, Framingham stroke risk profile (D'Agostino et al., 1994); GDS, geriatric depression scale; DRS, Mattis dementia rating scale (Mattis, 1988).

**Data are mean and standard deviation in parentheses unless otherwise noted.*

***Modified FSRP omitting diabetes.*

****DRS total score is a raw score (maximum possible score = 144); memory and executive function/processing speed composite scores are z scores. Results for the group comparisons on DRS and memory and executive function/processing speed composite scores are from analysis of covariance (ANCOVA) models adjusted for age, sex, and education.*

group, the T2DM group had a greater proportion of men relative to women and a greater proportion of individuals with a history of hypertension relative to those with no history of hypertension. There were no significant group differences with respect to mean age, education, aggregate vascular risk (i.e., modified FSRP omitting diabetes), pulse pressure, current smoking status, history of cardiovascular disease, history of atrial fibrillation, and depression. There were no significant group differences in global cognition as assessed by DRS total score. In contrast, those with T2DM performed significantly worse on the memory composite score and the executive function/processing speed composite score.

Regional CBF by T2DM

Group means and differences in CBF for *a priori* ROIs are shown in **Figure 2**. MANCOVA adjusting for age, sex, aggregate vascular risk (i.e., modified FSRP omitting diabetes), and reference CBF (postcentral gyrus) revealed significant effects of T2DM on regional CBF. Specifically, compared to nondiabetic control participants, individuals with T2DM exhibited lower CBF in left hippocampus [$F(1,43) = 5.45$, $p = 0.024$, $\eta_p^2 = 0.113$], right hippocampus [$F(1,43) = 8.81$, $p = 0.005$, $\eta_p^2 = 0.170$], right inferior parietal cortex [$F(1,43) = 11.78$, $p = 0.001$, $\eta_p^2 = 0.215$], right inferior temporal cortex [$F(1,43) = 8.00$, $p = 0.007$, $\eta_p^2 = 0.157$], and right rostral middle frontal gyrus [$F(1,43) = 9.38$, $p = 0.004$, $\eta_p^2 = 0.179$]. Statistical significance of all results described above was retained using a 0.05 FDR.

In contrast, there were no significant group differences for left inferior parietal cortex [$F(1,43) = 0.01$, $p = 0.906$, $\eta_p^2 < 0.001$], left inferior temporal cortex [$F(1,43) = 2.01$, $p = 0.163$, $\eta_p^2 = 0.045$], left medial orbitofrontal cortex [$F(1,43) = 0.16$, $p = 0.690$, $\eta_p^2 = 0.004$], right medial orbitofrontal cortex [$F(1,43) = 0.02$, $p = 0.903$, $\eta_p^2 < 0.001$], or left rostral middle frontal gyrus [$F(1,43) = 1.88$, $p = 0.178$, $\eta_p^2 = 0.042$]. Also, as expected, we confirmed that there were no group differences in terms of postcentral gyrus reference CBF [$F(1,47) = 0.78$, $p = 0.382$, $\eta_p^2 = 0.016$].

Regional Cortical Thickness and Volume by T2DM

Multiple analysis of covariance models adjusting for age, sex, and aggregate vascular risk (i.e., modified FSRP omitting diabetes) (and intracranial volume for analyses with hippocampal volume and WM hypointensities as the dependent variable) examined differences in cortical thickness or volume for the *a priori* ROIs used in the CBF analyses as well as for WM hypointensities. These models revealed no significant group differences in terms of cortical thickness of the right or left inferior parietal cortices [left: ($F(1,44) = 0.58$, $p = 0.452$, $\eta_p^2 = 0.013$); right: ($F(1,44) = 0.50$, $p = 0.502$, $\eta_p^2 = 0.010$)], inferior temporal cortices [left: ($F(1,44) = 0.27$, $p = 0.607$, $\eta_p^2 = 0.006$); right: ($F(1,44) = 0.17$, $p = 0.687$, $\eta_p^2 = 0.004$)], medial orbitofrontal cortices [left: ($F(1,44) = 0.003$, $p = 0.955$, $\eta_p^2 < 0.001$); right: ($F(1,44) = 0.37$, $p = 0.545$, $\eta_p^2 = 0.008$)], or rostral middle frontal gyri [left: ($F(1,44) = 1.44$, $p = 0.237$, $\eta_p^2 = 0.032$); right: ($F(1,44) = 0.94$, $p = 0.337$, $\eta_p^2 = 0.021$)]. Similarly, there were

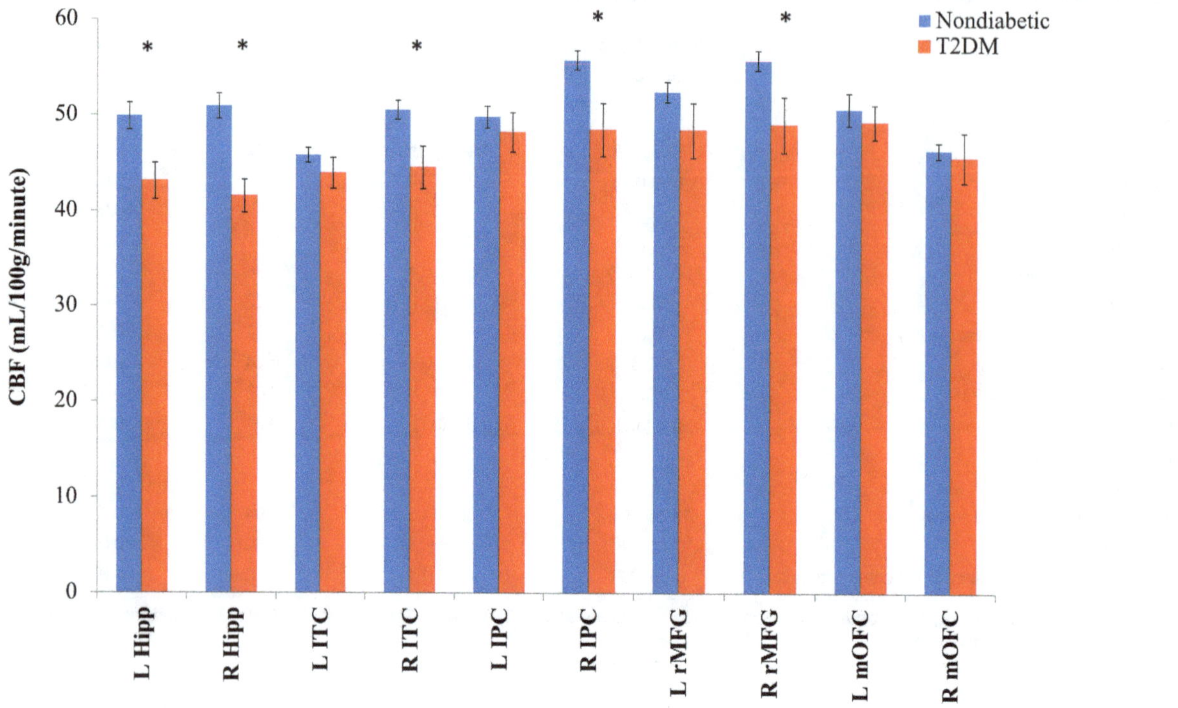

FIGURE 2 | Mean regional CBF for T2DM and nondiabetic control groups. CBF, cerebral blood flow; L, left; R, right; hipp, hippocampus; ITC, inferior temporal cortex; IPC, inferior parietal cortex; rMFG, rostral middle frontal gyrus; mOFC, medial orbitofrontal cortex. $^{*}p < 0.05$. Error bars represent ± 1 standard error.

no significant differences between those with T2DM and the nondiabetic control participants in left or right hippocampal volume [left: ($F(1,43) = 1.32$, $p = 0.258$, $\eta_p^2 = 0.030$); right: ($F(1,43) = 2.06$, $p = 0.158$, $\eta_p^2 = 0.046$)] or volume of WM hypointensities [$F(1,43) = 0.83$, $p = 0.367$, $\eta_p^2 = 0.019$].

Associations Between Regional CBF and Cognition

Correlation analyses were used to examine associations between CBF (in regions for which group differences were found by T2DM status) and cognitive abilities subserved by those particular regions. That is, analyses were performed relating bilateral hippocampal and right inferior temporal CBF to memory and right inferior parietal and right rostral middle frontal CBF to executive function/processing speed. Associations were examined both unadjusted and controlling for diabetes status (present versus absent).

Collapsed across the entire sample, there were significant associations between lower regional CBF and poorer cognitive performance (see **Figure 3** for selected associations for memory and executive function/processing speed with regional CBF). Lower hippocampal and inferior temporal cortex CBF was associated with poorer memory performance. Significant CBF-memory correlations were found for both left hippocampal CBF ($r = 0.31$, $p = 0.016$) and right hippocampal CBF ($r = 0.25$, $p = 0.044$). In contrast, lower right inferior temporal CBF was not significantly associated with poorer memory performance ($r = 0.07$, $p = 0.310$). Significant associations were maintained when FDR was limited to 0.10. In contrast, the association with memory and left hippocampal CBF but not right hippocampal CBF remained significant when FDR was limited to 0.05.

When partial correlations adjusted for diabetes status were performed, the associations between regional CBF and memory were attenuated and no longer statistically significant (left hippocampus: $r = 0.15$, $p = 0.168$; right hippocampus: $r = 0.02$, $p = 0.458$; right inferior temporal gyrus: $r = -0.10$, $p = 0.253$).

Lower CBF in right inferior parietal cortex and rostral middle frontal gyrus was associated with poorer performance on measures of executive function/processing speed (right inferior parietal cortex: $r = 0.36$, $p = 0.007$; right rostral middle frontal gyrus: $r = 0.34$, $p = 0.009$). These significant associations were maintained when FDR was limited to 0.05.

When partial correlation analyses were performed adjusting for diabetes status, the associations between regional CBF and executive function/processing speed were somewhat attenuated although they remained statistically significant for both the right inferior parietal cortex ($r = 0.26$, $p = 0.043$) and right rostral middle frontal gyrus ($r = 0.29$, $p = 0.028$).

Sensitivity Analyses

Given the higher proportion of men in the T2DM group, we performed sensitivity analyses to examine the potential role of sex on CBF in our sample. Similar to our primary analyses examining CBF by T2DM status, we ran MANCOVA models adjusting for age, aggregate vascular risk (i.e., modified FSRP omitting

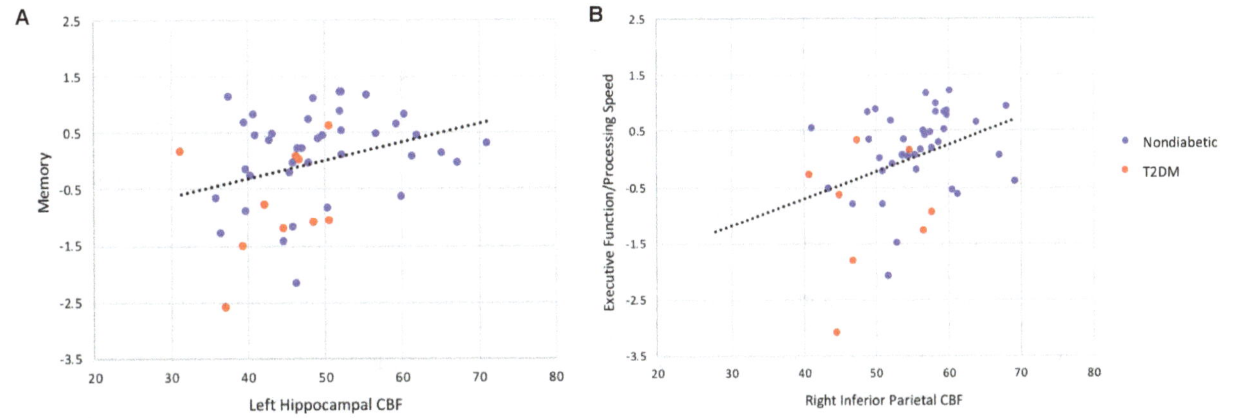

FIGURE 3 | Scatterplots of correlations between cognitive composite scores (z-scores) and regional cerebral blood flow (in units of milliliters per 100 g of tissue per minute). **(A)** Depicts the correlation between memory performance and left hippocampal CBF and **(B)** the correlation between executive function/processing speed and inferior parietal CBF (all p's < 0.05). These significant associations were maintained controlling the FDR at 0.05. When partial correlation analyses were performed adjusting for diabetes status, the association between executive function/processing speed and regional CBF remained statistically significant ($p < 0.05$) whereas the association between memory and regional CBF was no longer significant.

diabetes), and reference CBF (postcentral gyrus) to assess sex-related differences in CBF for those regions where group differences were observed between the nondiabetic controls and T2DM participants. The MANCOVA models revealed no significant differences between men and women across any of these ROIs [left hippocampus: ($F(1,44) = 0.04$, $p = 0.848$, $\eta_p^2 = 0.001$); right hippocampus: ($F(1,44) = 0.54$, $p = 0.465$, $\eta_p^2 = 0.012$); right inferior parietal: ($F(1,44) = 1.62$, $p = 0.210$, $\eta_p^2 = 0.035$); right inferior temporal: ($F(1,44) = 0.75$, $p = 0.393$, $\eta_p^2 = 0.017$); right rostral middle frontal: ($F(1,44) = 0.57$, $p = 0.454$, $\eta_p^2 = 0.013$)].

In addition, we also performed t-test analyses to compare a subset of the sample consisting of nondiabetic control ($n = 11$) and T2DM ($n = 11$) participants who were matched so that the two groups did not significantly differ in terms of demographic or covariate variables including age; sex; aggregate vascular risk; pulse pressure, systolic blood pressure, or diastolic blood pressure; history of cardiovascular disease or atrial fibrillation; or depression (i.e., GDS score). In this matched subsample, findings for group differences in CBF remained statistically and qualitatively similar to the results from analyses including the entire sample. That is, when the T2DM and nondiabetic control groups were equivalent in terms of sex distribution and vascular risk covariates, the T2DM participants showed reduced CBF in left hippocampus ($t = 3.29$, $p = 0.004$, Cohen's $d = 1.40$), right hippocampus ($t = 4.10$, $p = 0.001$, Cohen's $d = 1.75$), right inferior parietal cortex ($t = 2.68$, $p = 0.014$, Cohen's $d = 1.14$), right inferior temporal cortex ($t = 2.90$, $p = 0.009$, Cohen's $d = 1.24$), and right rostral middle frontal gyrus ($t = 2.85$, $p = 0.104$, Cohen's $d = 1.21$). Similar to the primary analyses including the entire sample, there were no significant group differences in any of the other *a priori* ROIs (left inferior parietal cortex: $t = 0.95$, $p = 0.352$, Cohen's $d = 0.41$; left inferior temporal cortex: $t = 1.63$, $p = 0.118$, Cohen's $d = 0.70$; left medial orbitofrontal cortex $t = 1.21$, $p = 0.240$, Cohen's $d = 0.52$; right medial orbitofrontal cortex: $t = 0.75$, $p = 0.462$, Cohen's $d = 0.32$; left rostral middle frontal cortex: $t = 1.74$, $p = 0.097$, Cohen's $d = 0.74$).

DISCUSSION

Our results demonstrate that CBF is reduced in nondemented older adults with T2DM independent of age, sex, and related vascular risk factors. We did not find significant differences between those with and without T2DM in terms of brain structure (cortical thickness or brain volume in regions of interest), suggesting that CBF alterations occur independent of cerebral atrophy and may precede structural changes that have been identified in previous studies. T2DM-related reductions in CBF were pronounced in known predilection sites for AD pathology as well as regions implicated in cerebrovascular dysfunction in early AD (hippocampus, inferior parietal cortex, inferior temporal cortex, and middle frontal regions). Moreover, among older adults both with and without T2DM, lower CBF was associated with poorer cognitive performance in memory and executive/processing speed domains. These findings were somewhat attenuated when analyses were adjusted for diabetes status although associations between regional CBF and executive function/processing speed remained significant in adjusted analyses. Findings add to a growing body of research suggesting that perfusion deficits may underlie cognitive decrements frequently observed among older adults with T2DM. Results also suggest that CBF measured with ASL MRI may reflect an early and important marker of risk of cognitive decline in T2DM and related conditions particularly given that the mean level of performance on cognitive measures in our sample was within the normal range and not objectively impaired.

Several previous studies have examined the association of T2DM and CBF using techniques including PET, SPECT, and ASL, although findings across studies have been mixed. Many studies have reported reduced CBF in T2DM (Last et al., 2007;

Xia et al., 2015; Cui et al., 2017; Dai et al., 2017), although some other studies have reported no differences between individuals with and without T2DM (Tiehuis et al., 2008; Launer et al., 2015; Rusinek et al., 2015). As noted by Dai et al. (2017), studies reporting no alterations in CBF in T2DM relative to nondiabetic control participants typically examined large ROIs such as whole brain GM or large cortical regions. Importantly, previous studies are limited in their ability to reliably detect CBF reductions in the context of T2DM as they typically did not consider the effects of additional vascular risk factors such as hypertension (Dai et al., 2017) or elevated pulse pressure, which commonly co-occur with T2DM, or brain atrophy, which in some instances appears to fully account for decreased CBF (Sabri et al., 2000). Furthermore, few studies have utilized a PCASL sequence and implemented an ASL protocol optimized for use in older adults.

Despite previous findings linking T2DM and elevated blood glucose to cognitive impairment and AD, there are few studies investigating the neuropathologic mechanisms underlying these associations. Although autopsy-based studies have shown that T2DM is linked to cerebral infarcts (Peila et al., 2002; Arvanitakis et al., 2006; Sarwar et al., 2010), its association with AD neuropathology itself (i.e., β-amyloid plaques, Aβ and neurofibrillary tangles, NFT) remains unclear. (Peila et al., 2002; Beeri et al., 2005; Arvanitakis et al., 2006; Ahtiluoto et al., 2010; Malek-Ahmadi et al., 2013). However, some evidence suggests a role for deficiencies in brain insulin in the pathogenesis of AD and have proposed that AD may be "type 3 diabetes" (Steen et al., 2005). In our previous work, we found that midlife elevated blood glucose is predictive of more severe AD pathology (i.e., higher medial temporal lobe NFT pathology) in late life. This work suggests that elevated blood glucose - even many years before death and even among nondiabetic individuals - may have detrimental effects on the brain that ultimately contribute to the development of AD pathology and subsequent cognitive decline (Bangen et al., 2016). The present findings provide additional evidence for the influence of T2DM on changes in AD-vulnerable regions, and they suggest that cerebrovascular dysfunction may underlie the predilection of AD pathology in these regions.

We found lower CBF in T2DM in *a priori* ROIs including medial temporal lobe, parietal, and frontal regions. This pattern is similar to that seen in AD and vascular disease. Medial temporal regions are susceptible to early pathologic and neurodegenerative changes in AD, and alterations in CBF represent a potential mechanism through which these changes may occur. Indeed, many of the regions implicated in the current study, including inferior parietal cortices, are key components of the default mode network, which contributes to episodic memory and executive functioning and has been implicated in preclinical AD (Hampel, 2013). Lifetime cerebral metabolism associated with default mode network activity may predispose these regions to AD-related pathologic changes including Aβ accumulation and may also disrupt connections with the medial temporal lobe, resulting in impaired cognitive function (Buckner et al., 2005). Further, WM lesion pathology in the parietal lobe has been implicated as an early biomarker of AD, and as a marker of small-vessel disease, these lesions may reflect later-stage consequences of chronic hypoperfusion in this region (Lee et al., 2016).

The present findings corroborate previous studies demonstrating hypoperfusion in T2DM in the absence of brain volume differences, suggesting that perfusion alterations are independent of cerebral atrophy (Xia et al., 2015; Jansen et al., 2016). Previous studies have shown that functional changes precede structural changes in the context of AD (Devous, 2002) and T2DM (Musen et al., 2012). Given this, MRI techniques such as ASL have great potential as a non-invasive method for detecting early and/or subtle functional brain changes in asymptomatic individuals. Advanced MRI techniques that measure early physiological changes including alterations in CBF may elucidate the mechanisms that precede the development of irreversible parenchymal/structural damage and serve as a marker of risk for cognitive decline.

Indeed, mounting evidence suggests that ASL CBF represents a useful biomarker in at-risk individuals given that this technique can reliably differentiate those at risk from control participants (Fleisher et al., 2009; Bangen et al., 2012; Wierenga et al., 2012). Furthermore, longitudinal studies have shown that ASL CBF indices predict cognitive decline in older adults with normal cognition (Xekardaki et al., 2015) as well as progression from normal cognition to MCI (Beason-Held et al., 2013), and MCI to AD (Chao et al., 2010). Previous work has shown that CBF alterations are independent of changes in volume and were detectable several years prior to the development of cognitive impairment (Beason-Held et al., 2013). Our current findings emphasize the important link between CBF and cognition, and they provide further support for CBF as a useful marker of vascular risk and correlate of cognitive functioning in nondemented older adults. Furthermore, a recent study showed that there was an increase in perfusion and improvements in cognitive performance after insulin administration in individuals with T2DM which was greater than in the nondiabetic control group, and these insulin-induced changes were associated with vasodilation in the middle cerebral artery territory, suggesting involvement of a vascular mechanism (Novak et al., 2014). Although findings have been mixed, overall it appears that reduced CBF seems to be an early change independent of brain structural changes and may be a viable intervention target for preventing cognitive decline in T2DM. Dissemination of methods capable of detecting cerebrovascular dysfunction prior to the manifestation of these frank lesions would represent a major advancement in early detection and expansion of treatment opportunities to prevent or delay cognitive impairment in these individuals.

Taken together, our findings show an important relationship between cerebral perfusion and memory and executive function in the context of T2DM. Results further highlight the potential value in examining ASL CBF as a sensitive vascular marker in aging, metabolic and vascular conditions, and dementia risk. Strengths of this work include a well-characterized sample, comprehensive neuropsychological assessment, and use of an ASL protocol optimized for use in older adults. However, there are important limitations of this study worth noting. First, our sample size of participants with T2DM is small and thus results should be considered preliminary. Data on glycemic control was not available (e.g., hemoglobin A1c) and therefore not included in our analyses, which should be addressed in future studies. In addition, our sample was predominantly white, generally medically healthy, and relatively well-educated, which may affect generalizability of the findings. Future studies should include larger sample sizes and longitudinal follow-up spanning middle age to older age in order to better understand how changes in CBF may evolve over time and how they influence the development of later-stage structural and pathologic changes that have previously been associated with T2DM. Finally, the nondiabetic control group included a higher proportion of women relative to the T2DM group. Although women have been shown to have higher CBF, some evidence suggests that this difference is diminished with advancing age and that, by the sixth decade, men and women show similar CBF rates (Gur et al., 1987; Gur and Gur, 1990). The mean age of the present sample was approximately 73 (range = 68–88). We performed sensitivity analyses to examine the potential role of sex on CBF in our sample and found that sex was not significantly associated with regional CBF. We performed a second set of sensitivity analyses in a subset of our sample including nondiabetic control participants and those with T2DM who were matched on distribution of sex, pulse pressure and blood pressure, and other important demographic and vascular risk variables. Findings were qualitatively and statistically similar to those from the primary analyses including the entire sample. Nonetheless, future work should aim to replicate our findings in a larger sample with groups matched on sex distribution.

Despite these limitations, our findings, if replicated, may have important research and clinical implications. Indeed, our results show that reduced CBF may be an early marker of incipient change independent of brain structural changes, and it may be a viable intervention target for preventing cognitive decline in T2DM. Dissemination of methods capable of detecting cerebrovascular dysfunction prior to the manifestation of these frank lesions would represent a major advancement in early detection and expansion of treatment opportunities to prevent or delay cognitive impairment in these individuals. For example, pharmacological and behavioral interventions, such as physical exercise, may influence the regulation of CBF and, ultimately, the prevention of cognitive decline in T2DM and related conditions. T2DM is a growing condition that has been linked to the development of substantial cognitive and brain changes, and there is therefore a pressing public health need to identify early biomarkers of cognitive decline in T2DM and related conditions as well as potentially modifiable mechanisms underlying these changes. Such research will help facilitate the development and optimization of targeted interventions to reduce dementia risk while improving the health and functioning of individuals with T2DM and other groups at risk for cognitive decline.

AUTHOR CONTRIBUTIONS

KB designed the study, analyzed and interpreted the data, and wrote and revised the manuscript. MW wrote and revised the manuscript. AW, NE, and AC created figures and revised the manuscript for important intellectual content. EE, LD-W, KT, DN, TL, and MB interpreted the data and revised the manuscript for important intellectual content. All authors approved the submitted version of the manuscript and agree to be accountable for all aspects of the work.

FUNDING

This work was supported by VA Clinical Science Research & Development (Career Development Award-2 1IK2CX000938 to KB and 1IK2CX001415 to EE), the Alzheimer's Association (AARG-18-566254 to KB, AARG-17-500358 to EE, and AARF-17-528918 to KT), and NIH (K24 AG026431 to MB; R01 AG049810 to MB, EE, and LD-W).

REFERENCES

Ahtiluoto, S., Polvikoski, T., Peltonen, M., Solomon, A., Tuomilehto, J., Winblad, B., et al. (2010). Diabetes, Alzheimer disease, and vascular dementia: a population-based neuropathologic study. *Neurology* 75, 1195–1202. doi: 10.1212/WNL.0b013e3181f4d7f8

Alsop, D. C., Detre, J. A., Golay, X., Gunther, M., Hendrikse, J., Hernandez-Garcia, L., et al. (2015). Recommended implementation of arterial spin-labeled perfusion MRI for clinical applications: a consensus of the ISMRM perfusion study group and the European consortium for ASL in dementia. *Magn. Reson. Med.* 73, 102–116. doi: 10.1002/mrm.25197

Arvanitakis, Z., Schneider, J. A., Wilson, R. S., Li, Y., Arnold, S. E., Wang, Z., et al. (2006). Diabetes is related to cerebral infarction but not to AD pathology in older persons. *Neurology* 67, 1960–1965. doi: 10.1212/01.wnl.0000247053.45483.4e

Arvanitakis, Z., Wilson, R. S., Bienias, J. L., Evans, D. A., and Bennett, D. A. (2004). Diabetes mellitus and risk of Alzheimer disease and decline in cognitive function. *Arch. Neurol.* 61, 661–666. doi: 10.1001/archneur.61.5.661

Bangen, K. J., Clark, A. L., Edmonds, E. C., Evangelista, N. D., Werhane, M. L., Thomas, K. R., et al. (2017). Cerebral blood flow and amyloid-beta interact to affect memory performance in cognitively normal older adults. *Front. Aging Neurosci.* 9:181. doi: 10.3389/fnagi.2017.00181

Bangen, K. J., Himali, J. J., Beiser, A. S., Nation, D. A., Libon, D. J., Fox, C. S., et al. (2016). Interaction between midlife blood glucose and apoe genotype predicts later alzheimer's disease pathology. *J. Alzheimers. Dis.* 53, 1553–1562. doi: 10.3233/jad-160163

Bangen, K. J., Nation, D. A., Clark, L. R., Harmell, A. L., Wierenga, C. E., Dev, S. I., et al. (2014). Interactive effects of vascular risk burden and advanced age on cerebral blood flow. *Front. Aging Neurosci.* 6:159. doi: 10.3389/fnagi.2014.00159

Bangen, K. J., Restom, K., Liu, T. T., Jak, A. J., Wierenga, C. E., Salmon, D. P., et al. (2009). Differential age effects on cerebral blood flow and BOLD response to encoding: associations with cognition and stroke risk. *Neurobiol. Aging* 30, 1276–1287. doi: 10.1016/j.neurobiolaging.2007.11.012

Bangen, K. J., Restom, K., Liu, T. T., Wierenga, C. E., Jak, A. J., Salmon, D. P., et al. (2012). Assessment of Alzheimer's Disease risk with functional magnetic resonance imaging: an arterial spin labeling study. *J. Alzheimers Dis.* 31(Suppl. 3), S59–S74. doi: 10.3233/jad-2012-120292

Beason-Held, L. L., Goh, J. O., An, Y., Kraut, M. A., O'Brien, R. J., Ferrucci, L., et al. (2013). Changes in brain function occur years before the onset of cognitive impairment. *J. Neurosci.* 33, 18008–18014. doi: 10.1523/jneurosci.1402-13.2013

Beeri, M. S., Silverman, J. M., Davis, K. L., Marin, D., Grossman, H. Z., Schmeidler, J., et al. (2005). Type 2 diabetes is negatively associated with Alzheimer's disease neuropathology. *J. Gerontol. A Biol. Sci. Med. Sci.* 60, 471–475.

Benjamini, Y., and Hochberg, Y. (1995). Controlling the false discovery rate: a practical and powerful approach to multiple testing. *J. R. Stat. Soc. Ser. B* 57, 289–300.

Binnewijzend, M. A., Kuijer, J. P., Benedictus, M. R., van der Flier, W. M., Wink, A. M., Wattjes, M. P., et al. (2013). Cerebral blood flow measured with 3D pseudocontinuous arterial spin-labeling MR imaging in Alzheimer disease and mild cognitive impairment: a marker for disease severity. *Radiology* 267, 221–230. doi: 10.1148/radiol.12120928

Brickman, A. M., Guzman, V. A., Gonzalez-Castellon, M., Razlighi, Q., Gu, Y., Narkhede, A., et al. (2015). Cerebral autoregulation, beta amyloid, and white matter hyperintensities are interrelated. *Neurosci. Lett.* 592, 54–58. doi: 10.1016/j.neulet.2015.03.005

Brownlee, M. (2005). The pathobiology of diabetic complications: a unifying mechanism. *Diabetes Metab. Res. Rev.* 54, 1615–1625.

Buckner, R. L., Snyder, A. Z., Shannon, B. J., LaRossa, G., Sachs, R., Fotenos, A. F., et al. (2005). Molecular, structural, and functional characterization of Alzheimer's disease: evidence for a relationship between default activity, amyloid, and memory. *J. Neurosci.* 25, 7709–7717. doi: 10.1523/jneurosci.2177-05.2005

Chalela, J. A., Alsop, D. C., Gonzalez-Atavales, J. B., Maldjian, J. A., Kasner, S. E., and Detre, J. A. (2000). Magnetic resonance perfusion imaging in acute ischemic stroke using continuous arterial spin labeling. *Stroke* 31, 680–687.

Chao, L. L., Buckley, S. T., Kornak, J., Schuff, N., Madison, C., Yaffe, K., et al. (2010). ASL perfusion MRI predicts cognitive decline and conversion from MCI to dementia. *Alzheimer Dis. Assoc. Disord.* 24, 19–27. doi: 10.1097/WAD.0b013e3181b4f736

Chen, Y., Wolk, D. A., Reddin, J. S., Korczykowski, M., Martinez, P. M., Musiek, E. S., et al. (2011). Voxel-level comparison of arterial spin-labeled perfusion MRI and FDG-PET in Alzheimer disease. *Neurology* 77, 1977–1985. doi: 10.1212/WNL.0b013e31823a0ef7

Chung, C. C., Pimentel, D., Jor'dan, A. J., Hao, Y., Milberg, W., and Novak, V. (2015). Inflammation-associated declines in cerebral vasoreactivity and cognition in type 2 diabetes. *Neurology* 85, 450–458. doi: 10.1212/wnl.0000000000001820

Cox, R. W. (1996). AFNI: software for analysis and visualization of functional magnetic resonance neuroimages. *Comput. Biomed. Res.* 29, 162–173.

Cui, Y., Liang, X., Gu, H., Hu, Y., Zhao, Z., Yang, X. Y., et al. (2017). Cerebral perfusion alterations in type 2 diabetes and its relation to insulin resistance and cognitive dysfunction. *Brain Imaging Behav.* 11, 1248–1257. doi: 10.1007/s11682-016-9583-9

D'Agostino, R. B., Wolf, P. A., Belanger, A. J., and Kannel, W. B. (1994). Stroke risk profile: adjustment for antihypertensive medication. The Framingham Study. *Stroke* 25, 40–43.

Dai, W., Duan, W., Alfaro, F. J., Gavrieli, A., Kourtelidis, F., and Novak, V. (2017). The resting perfusion pattern associates with functional decline in type 2 diabetes. *Neurobiol. Aging* 60, 192–202. doi: 10.1016/j.neurobiolaging.2017.09.004

Dale, A. M., Fischl, B., and Sereno, M. I. (1999). Cortical surface-based analysis. I. segmentation and surface reconstruction. *Neuroimage* 9, 179–194. doi: 10.1006/nimg.1998.0395

Dandona, P., James, I. M., Newbury, P. A., Woollard, M. L., and Beckett, A. G. (1978). Cerebral blood flow in diabetes mellitus: evidence of abnormal cerebrovascular reactivity. *Br. Med. J.* 2, 325–326.

Delis, D. C., Kramer, J., Kaplan, E., and Ober, B. A. (2000). *The California Verbal Learning Test,* 2nd Edn. New York, NY: Psychological Corporation.

Desikan, R. S., Ségonne, F., Fischl, B., Quinn, B. T., Dickerson, B. C., Blacker, D., et al. (2006). An automated labeling system for subdividing the human cerebral cortex on MRI scans into gyral based regions of interest. *Neuroimage* 31, 968–980. doi: 10.1016/j.neuroimage.2006.01.021

Detre, J. A., and Alsop, D. C. (1999). Perfusion magnetic resonance imaging with continuous arterial spin labeling: methods and clinical applications in the central nervous system. *Eur. J. Radiol.* 30, 115–124.

Devous, M. D. (2002). Functional brain imaging in the dementias: role in early detection, differential diagnosis, and longitudinal studies. *Eur. J. Nucl. Med. Mol. Imaging* 29, 1685–1696. doi: 10.1007/s00259-002-0967-2

Du, A. T., Schuff, N., Laakso, M. P., Zhu, X. P., Jagust, W. J., Yaffe, K., et al. (2002). Effects of subcortical ischemic vascular dementia and AD on entorhinal cortex and hippocampus. *Neurology* 58, 1635–1641.

Fischl, B., and Dale, A. M. (2000). Measuring the thickness of the human cerebral cortex from magnetic resonance images. *Proc. Natl. Acad. Sci. U.S.A.* 97, 11050–11055. doi: 10.1073/pnas.200033797

Fischl, B., Salat, D. H., Busa, E., Albert, M., Dieterich, M., Haselgrove, C., et al. (2002). Whole brain segmentation: automated labeling of neuroanatomical structures in the human brain. *Neuron* 33, 341–355.

Fleisher, A. S., Podraza, K. M., Bangen, K. J., Taylor, C., Sherzai, A., Sidhar, K., et al. (2009). Cerebral perfusion and oxygenation differences in Alzheimer's disease risk. *Neurobiol. Aging* 30, 1737–1748. doi: 10.1016/j.neurobiolaging.2008.01.012

Garde, E., Mortensen, E. L., Krabbe, K., Rostrup, E., and Larsson, H. B. (2000). Relation between age-related decline in intelligence and cerebral white-matter hyperintensities in healthy octogenarians: a longitudinal study. *Lancet* 356, 628–634. doi: 10.1016/s0140-6736(00)02604-0

Geijselaers, S. L. C., Sep, S. J. S., Stehouwer, C. D. A., and Biessels, G. J. (2015). Glucose regulation, cognition, and brain MRI in type 2 diabetes: a systematic review. *Lancet Diabetes Endocrinol.* 3, 75–89. doi: 10.1016/s2213-8587(14)70148-2

Gur, R. C., Gur, R. E., Obrist, W. D., Skolnick, B. E., and Reivich, M. (1987). Age and regional cerebral blood flow at rest and during cognitive activity. *Arch. Gen. Psychiatry* 44, 617–621.

Gur, R. E., and Gur, R. C. (1990). Gender differences in regional cerebral blood flow. *Schizophr. Bull.* 16, 247–254.

Hampel, H. (2013). Amyloid-beta and cognition in aging and Alzheimer's disease: molecular and neurophysiological mechanisms. *J. Alzheimers Dis.* 33(Suppl. 1), S79–S86. doi: 10.3233/jad-2012-129003

Hayashi, K., Kurioka, S., Yamaguchi, T., Morita, M., Kanazawa, I., Takase, H., et al. (2011). Association of cognitive dysfunction with hippocampal atrophy in elderly Japanese people with type 2 diabetes. *Diabetes Res. Clin. Pract.* 94, 180–185. doi: 10.1016/j.diabres.2011.07.002

Jansen, J. F., van Bussel, F. C., van de Haar, H. J., van Osch, M. J., Hofman, P. A., van Boxtel, M. P., et al. (2016). Cerebral blood flow, blood supply, and cognition in type 2 diabetes mellitus. *Sci. Rep.* 6:10. doi: 10.1038/s41598-016-0003-6

Johnson, N. A., Jahng, G. H., Weiner, M. W., Miller, B. L., Chui, H. C., Jagust, W. J., et al. (2005). Pattern of cerebral hypoperfusion in Alzheimer disease and mild cognitive impairment measured with arterial spin-labeling MR imaging: initial experience. *Radiology* 234, 851–859. doi: 10.1148/radiol.2343040197

Last, D., Alsop, D. C., Abduljalil, A. M., Marquis, R. P., de Bazelaire, C., Hu, K., et al. (2007). Global and regional effects of type 2 diabetes on brain tissue volumes and cerebral vasoreactivity. *Diabetes Care* 30, 1193–1199. doi: 10.2337/dc06-2052

Launer, L. J., Lewis, C. E., Schreiner, P. J., Sidney, S., Battapady, H., Jacobs, D. R., et al. (2015). Vascular factors and multiple measures of early brain health: CARDIA brain MRI study. *PLoS One* 10:e0122138. doi: 10.1371/journal.pone.0122138

Lee, S., Viqar, F., Zimmerman, M. E., Narkhede, A., Tosto, G., Benzinger, T. L., et al. (2016). White matter hyperintensities are a core feature of Alzheimer's disease: evidence from the dominantly inherited Alzheimer network. *Ann. Neurol.* 79, 929–939. doi: 10.1002/ana.24647

Luchsinger, J. A., Reitz, C., Patel, B., Tang, M. X., Manly, J. J., and Mayeux, R. (2007). Relation of diabetes to mild cognitive impairment. *Arch. Neurol.* 64, 570–575. doi: 10.1001/archneur.64.4.570

Luchsinger, J. A., Tang, M. X., Stern, Y., Shea, S., and Mayeux, R. (2001). Diabetes mellitus and risk of Alzheimer's disease and dementia with stroke in a multiethnic cohort. *Am. J. Epidemiol.* 154, 635–641.

Malek-Ahmadi, M., Beach, T., Obradov, A., Sue, L., Belden, C., Davis, K., et al. (2013). Increased Alzheimer's disease neuropathology is associated with type 2 diabetes and ApoE epsilon.4 carrier status. *Curr. Alzheimer Res.* 10, 654–659.

Mattis, S. (1988). *Dementia Rating Scale: Professional Manual.* Odessa, FL: Psychological Assessment Resources.

Moran, C., Phan, T. G., Chen, J., Blizzard, L., Beare, R., Venn, A., et al. (2013). Brain atrophy in type 2 diabetes: regional distribution and influence on cognition. *Diabetes Care* 36, 4036–4042. doi: 10.2337/dc13-0143

Musen, G., Jacobson, A. M., Bolo, N. R., Simonson, D. C., Shenton, M. E., McCartney, R. L., et al. (2012). Resting-state brain functional connectivity is altered in type 2 diabetes. *Diabetes Metab. Res. Rev.* 61, 2375–2379. doi: 10.2337/db11-1669

Nagamachi, S., Nishikawa, T., Ono, S., Ageta, M., Matsuo, T., Jinnouchi, S., et al. (1994). Regional cerebral blood flow in diabetic patients: evaluation by N-isopropyl-123I-IMP with SPECT. *Nucl. Med. Commun.* 15, 455–460.

Nation, D. A., Edmonds, E. C., Bangen, K. J., Delano-Wood, L., Scanlon, B. K., Han, S. D., et al. (2015). Pulse pressure in relation to tau-mediated neurodegeneration, cerebral amyloidosis, and progression to dementia in very old adults. *JAMA Neurol.* 72, 546–553. doi: 10.1001/jamaneurol.2014.4477

Nation, D. A., Ho, J., and Yew, B. (2016a). Older adults taking At1-receptor blockers exhibit reduced cerebral amyloid retention. *J. Alzheimers. Dis.* 50, 779–789. doi: 10.3233/jad-150487

Nation, D. A., Preis, S. R., Beiser, A., Bangen, K. J., Delano-Wood, L., Lamar, M., et al. (2016b). Pulse pressure is associated with early brain atrophy and cognitive decline: modifying effects of APOE-epsilon4. *Alzheimer Dis. Assoc. Disord.* 30, 210–215. doi: 10.1097/wad.0000000000000127

Nation, D. A., Wierenga, C. E., Clark, L. R., Dev, S. I., Stricker, N. H., Jak, A. J., et al. (2013). Cortical and subcortical cerebrovascular resistance index in mild cognitive impairment and Alzheimer's disease. *J. Alzheimers Dis.* 36, 689–698. doi: 10.3233/jad-130086

Novak, V., Milberg, W., Hao, Y., Munshi, M., Novak, P., Galica, A., et al. (2014). Enhancement of vasoreactivity and cognition by intranasal insulin in type 2 diabetes. *Diabetes Care* 37, 751–759. doi: 10.2337/dc13-1672

O'Sullivan, M., Lythgoe, D. J., Pereira, A. C., Summers, P. E., Jarosz, J. M., Williams, S. C., et al. (2002). Patterns of cerebral blood flow reduction in patients with ischemic leukoaraiosis. *Neurology* 59, 321–326.

Parkes, L. M., Rashid, W., Chard, D. T., and Tofts, P. S. (2004). Normal cerebral perfusion measurements using arterial spin labeling: reproducibility, stability, and age and gender effects. *Magn. Reson. Med.* 51, 736–743. doi: 10.1002/mrm.20023

Peila, R., Rodriguez, B. L., and Launer, L. J. (2002). Type 2 diabetes, APOE gene, and the risk for dementia and related pathologies: the honolulu-asia aging study. *Diabetes Metab. Res. Rev.* 51, 1256–1262.

Prevention (2017). *National Diabetes Statistics Report, 2017.* Atlanta: US Department of Health and Human Services.

Rusinek, H., Ha, J., Yau, P. L., Storey, P., Tirsi, A., Tsui, W. H., et al. (2015). Cerebral perfusion in insulin resistance and type 2 diabetes. *J. Cereb. Blood Flow Metab.* 35, 95–102. doi: 10.1038/jcbfm.2014.173

Sabri, O., Hellwig, D., Schreckenberger, M., Schneider, R., Kaiser, H. J., Wagenknecht, G., et al. (2000). Influence of diabetes mellitus on regional cerebral glucose metabolism and regional cerebral blood flow. *Nucl. Med. Commun.* 21, 19–29.

Sarwar, N., Aspelund, T., Eiriksdottir, G., Gobin, R., Seshasai, S. R., Forouhi, N. G., et al. (2010). Markers of dysglycaemia and risk of coronary heart disease in people without diabetes: reykjavik prospective study and systematic review. *PLoS Med.* 7:e1000278. doi: 10.1371/journal.pmed.1000278

Shen, Y., Zhao, B., Yan, L., Jann, K., Wang, G., Wang, J., et al. (2017). Cerebral hemodynamic and white matter changes of type 2 diabetes revealed by multi-ti arterial spin labeling and double inversion recovery sequence. *Front. Neurol.* 8:717. doi: 10.3389/fneur.2017.00717

Shin, D. D., Ozyurt, I. B., and Liu, T. T. (2013). The cerebral blood flow biomedical informatics research network (CBFBIRN) database and analysis pipeline for arterial spin labeling MRI data. *Front. Neuroinform.* 7:21. doi: 10.3389/fninf.2013.00021

Smith, S. M., Jenkinson, M., Woolrich, M. W., Beckmann, C. F., Behrens, T. E., Johansen-Berg, H., et al. (2004). Advances in functional and structural MR image analysis and implementation as FSL. *Neuroimage* 23(Suppl. 1), S208–S219. doi: 10.1016/j.neuroimage.2004.07.051

Steen, E., Terry, B. M., Rivera, E. J., Cannon, J. L., Neely, T. R., Tavares, R., et al. (2005). Impaired insulin and insulin-like growth factor expression and signaling mechanisms in Alzheimer's disease–is this type 3 diabetes? *J. Alzheimers Dis.* 7, 63–80.

Takahashi, H., Ishii, K., Hosokawa, C., Hyodo, T., Kashiwagi, N., Matsuki, M., et al. (2014). Clinical application of 3D arterial spin-labeled brain perfusion imaging for Alzheimer disease: comparison with brain perfusion SPECT. *AJNR Am. J. Neuroradiol.* 35, 906–911. doi: 10.3174/ajnr.A3780

Telischak, N. A., Detre, J. A., and Zaharchuk, G. (2015). Arterial spin labeling MRI: clinical applications in the brain. *J. Magn. Reson. Imaging* 41, 1165–1180. doi: 10.1002/jmri.24751

Thompson, P. M., Hayashi, K. M., de Zubicaray, G., Janke, A. L., Rose, S. E., Semple, J., et al. (2003). Dynamics of gray matter loss in Alzheimer's disease. *J. Neurosci.* 23, 994–1005.

Tiehuis, A. M., Mali, W. P., van Raamt, A. F., Visseren, F. L., Biessels, G. J., van Zandvoort, M. J., et al. (2009). Cognitive dysfunction and its clinical and radiological determinants in patients with symptomatic arterial disease and diabetes. *J. Neurol. Sci.* 283, 170–174. doi: 10.1016/j.jns.2009.02.337

Tiehuis, A. M., Vincken, K. L., van den Berg, E., Hendrikse, J., Manschot, S. M., Mali, W. P., et al. (2008). Cerebral perfusion in relation to cognitive function and type 2 diabetes. *Diabetologia* 51, 1321–1326. doi: 10.1007/s00125-008-1041-9

Tomiyama, H., Koji, Y., Yambe, M., Motobe, K., Shiina, K., Gulnisa, Z., et al. (2005). Elevated C-reactive protein augments increased arterial stiffness in subjects with the metabolic syndrome. *Hypertension* 45, 997–1003. doi: 10.1161/01.HYP.0000165018.63523.8a

Vagelatos, N. T., and Eslick, G. D. (2013). Type 2 diabetes as a risk factor for Alzheimer's Disease: the confounders, interactions, and neuropathology associated with this relationship. *Epidemiol. Rev.* 35, 152–160. doi: 10.1093/epirev/mxs012

Wakisaka, M., Nagamachi, S., Inoue, K., Morotomi, Y., Nunoi, K., and Fujishima, M. (1990). Reduced regional cerebral blood flow in aged noninsulin-dependent diabetic patients with no history of cerebrovascular disease: evaluation by N-isopropyl-123I-p-iodoamphetamine with single-photon emission computed tomography. *J. Diabet. Complications* 4, 170–174.

Wang, J., Qiu, M., and Constable, R. T. (2005). In vivo method for correcting transmit/receive nonuniformities with phased array coils. *Magn. Reson. Med.* 53, 666–674. doi: 10.1002/mrm.20377

Wechsler, D. (1987). *Wechsler Memory Scale – Revised.* New York, NY: The Psychological Corporation.

Werhane, M. L., Thomas, K. R., Edmonds, E. C., Bangen, K. J., Tran, M., Clark, A. L., et al. (2018). Differential effect of apoe varepsilon4 status and elevated pulse pressure on functional decline in cognitively normal older adults. *J. Alzheimers Dis.* 62, 1567–1578. doi: 10.3233/jad-170918

Wierenga, C. E., Dev, S. I., Shin, D. D., Clark, L. R., Bangen, K. J., Jak, A. J., et al. (2012). Effect of mild cognitive impairment and APOE genotype on resting cerebral blood flow and its association with cognition. *J. Cereb. Blood Flow Metab.* 32, 1589–1599. doi: 10.1038/jcbfm.2012.58

Winer, N., and Sowers, J. R. (2003). Vascular compliance in diabetes. *Curr. Diab. Rep.* 3, 230–234.

Xekardaki, A., Rodriguez, C., Montandon, M. L., Toma, S., Tombeur, E., Herrmann, F. R., et al. (2015). Arterial spin labeling may contribute to the prediction of cognitive deterioration in healthy elderly individuals. *Radiology* 274, 490–499. doi: 10.1148/radiol.14140680

Xia, W., Rao, H., Spaeth, A. M., Huang, R., Tian, S., Cai, R., et al. (2015). Blood pressure is associated with cerebral blood flow alterations in patients with T2DM as revealed by perfusion functional MRI. *Medicine* 94:e2231. doi: 10.1097/md.0000000000002231

Xu, G., Antuono, P. G., Jones, J., Xu, Y., Wu, G., Ward, D., et al. (2007). Perfusion fMRI detects deficits in regional CBF during memory-encoding tasks in MCI subjects. *Neurology* 69, 1650–1656. doi: 10.1212/01.wnl.0000296941.06685.22

Yan, L., Liu, C. Y., Smith, R. X., Jog, M., Langham, M., Krasileva, K., et al. (2016). Assessing intracranial vascular compliance using dynamic arterial spin labeling. *Neuroimage* 124(Pt A), 433–441. doi: 10.1016/j.neuroimage.2015.09.008

Zhang, Y., Zhang, X., Zhang, J., Liu, C., Yuan, Q., Yin, X., et al. (2014). Gray matter volume abnormalities in type 2 diabetes mellitus with and without mild cognitive impairment. *Neurosci. Lett.* 562, 1–6. doi: 10.1016/j.neulet.2014.01.006

Zhou, H., Zhang, X., and Lu, J. (2014). Progress on diabetic cerebrovascular diseases. *Bosn. J. Basic Med. Sci.* 14, 185–190. doi: 10.17305/bjbms.2014.4.203

12

Preventing P-gp Ubiquitination Lowers Aβ Brain Levels in an Alzheimer's Disease Mouse Model

Anika M. S. Hartz[1,2]*, *Yu Zhong*[1], *Andrew N. Shen*[1], *Erin L. Abner*[1] *and Björn Bauer*[3]

[1]*Sanders-Brown Center on Aging, University of Kentucky, Lexington, KY, United States,* [2]*Department of Pharmacology and Nutritional Sciences, University of Kentucky, Lexington, KY, United States,* [3]*Department of Pharmaceutical Sciences, College of Pharmacy, University of Kentucky, Lexington, KY, United States*

Correspondence:
Anika M. S. Hartz
anika.hartz@uky.edu

One characteristic of Alzheimer's disease (AD) is excessive accumulation of amyloid-β (Aβ) in the brain. Aβ brain accumulation is, in part, due to a reduction in Aβ clearance from the brain across the blood-brain barrier. One key element that contributes to Aβ brain clearance is P-glycoprotein (P-gp) that transports Aβ from brain to blood. In AD, P-gp protein expression and transport activity levels are significantly reduced, which impairs Aβ brain clearance. The mechanism responsible for reduced P-gp expression and activity levels is poorly understood. We recently demonstrated that $A\beta_{40}$ triggers P-gp degradation through the ubiquitin-proteasome pathway. Consistent with these data, we show here that ubiquitinated P-gp levels in brain capillaries isolated from brain samples of AD patients are increased compared to capillaries isolated from brain tissue of cognitive normal individuals. We extended this line of research to *in vivo* studies using transgenic human amyloid precursor protein (hAPP)-overexpressing mice (Tg2576) that were treated with PYR41, a cell-permeable, irreversible inhibitor of the ubiquitin-activating enzyme E1. Our data show that inhibiting P-gp ubiquitination protects the transporter from degradation, and immunoprecipitation experiments confirmed that PYR41 prevented P-gp ubiquitination. We further found that PYR41 treatment prevented reduction of P-gp protein expression and transport activity levels and substantially lowered Aβ brain levels in hAPP mice. Together, our findings provide *in vivo* proof that the ubiquitin-proteasome system mediates reduction of blood-brain barrier P-gp in AD and that inhibiting P-gp ubiquitination prevents P-gp degradation and lowers Aβ brain levels. Thus, targeting the ubiquitin-proteasome system may provide a novel therapeutic approach to protect blood-brain barrier P-gp from degradation in AD and other Aβ-based pathologies.

Keywords: blood-brain barrier, P-glycoprotein, Alzheimer's disease, brain capillaries, amyloid beta, ubiquitin-proteasome system, ubiquitin, proteasome

INTRODUCTION

Accumulation of amyloid-β (Aβ) in the brain is a neuropathological hallmark of Alzheimer's disease (AD; Hardy and Selkoe, 2002). Increasing evidence suggests that Aβ brain accumulation is due to impaired Aβ clearance from the brain (Zlokovic, 2005; Mawuenyega et al., 2010; Wang et al., 2016). Several studies indicate a role for the blood-brain barrier efflux transporter P-glycoprotein (P-gp) in clearing Aβ from brain to blood: (1) P-gp transports Aβ *in vitro* (Lam et al., 2001; Kuhnke et al., 2007; Hartz et al., 2010); (2) in mice lacking P-gp, Aβ clearance is decreased while Aβ brain levels are increased (Cirrito et al., 2005; Yuede et al., 2016); (3) P-gp expression and transport activity are reduced at the blood-brain barrier of several AD mouse models (Hartz et al., 2010; Mehta et al., 2013; Park et al., 2014); and (4) treating human amyloid precursor protein (hAPP) mice with the PXR activator pregnenolone-16-carbonitrile (PCN) induces P-gp expression and activity, which restores Aβ transport and reduces Aβ brain levels (Hartz et al., 2010). (5) Results of multiple studies from different laboratories show that P-gp protein expression levels at the human blood-brain barrier are significantly reduced in AD patients (Wijesuriya et al., 2010; Jeynes and Provias, 2011; Carrano et al., 2014; Chiu et al., 2015). Consistent with reduced P-gp protein expression levels, results of recent PET imaging studies indicate compromised P-gp transport activity in AD patients compared to age-matched cognitive healthy individuals (van Assema et al., 2012; Deo et al., 2014). Thus, existing studies support the conclusion that blood-brain barrier P-gp is reduced in AD, however, more insights into the mechanism that triggers this phenomenon are needed to prevent P-gp loss in AD and improve Aβ brain clearance.

In this regard, we recently reported that exposing isolated rat brain capillaries to $A\beta_{40}$ at concentrations similar to those found in AD patients reduced P-gp protein expression and transport activity levels in a time- and concentration-dependent manner (Hartz et al., 2016). We showed that $A\beta_{40}$ triggers ubiquitination, internalization, and proteasomal degradation of P-gp in isolated rat brain capillaries *ex vivo* (Akkaya et al., 2015; Hartz et al., 2016). Collectively, these results indicate that blood-brain barrier P-gp is part of an Aβ clearance system and that P-gp expression and transport activity levels are reduced in AD, suggesting a link between high Aβ levels and reduced brain capillary P-gp levels in AD pathology.

In the present study, we show that P-gp protein expression and transport activity levels are reduced and that P-gp protein is highly ubiquitinated in isolated human brain capillaries from AD patients compared to P-gp in brain capillaries isolated from age-matched cognitive normal individuals. We extended our previous *ex vivo* findings to *in vivo* studies with hAPP mice by blocking P-gp ubiquitination in hAPP mice, which is the initial step of protein degradation mediated by the ubiquitin-proteasome system. We used transgenic hAPP-overexpressing mice (Tg2576) to test the hypothesis that preventing P-gp reduction results in a reduction of Aβ brain levels. We show here that inhibiting P-gp ubiquitination *in vivo* with PYR41, a cell-permeable, irreversible inhibitor of the ubiquitin-activating enzyme E1, prevents P-gp reduction at the blood-brain barrier and significantly lowers Aβ brain levels *in vivo*.

Together, our findings suggest that targeting the ubiquitin-proteasome system by inhibiting ubiquitination protects brain capillary P-gp and thereby lowers Aβ brain levels.

MATERIALS AND METHODS

Experimental Design and Statistical Analysis

Sample size (animal numbers, number of brain capillaries, number of human tissue samples) for individual experiments were based on power analyses of preliminary data and previously published data (Hartz et al., 2010, 2016, 2017), and are given in the corresponding figure legends. Number of repetitions are stated in the results section and the figure legends.

Results are presented as mean ± SEM. One-way analysis of variance (ANOVA) was used to assess differences in group means. Pre-planned pairwise *post hoc* tests were carried out when the overall F test was significant, and the Bonferroni correction was used to control the type 1 error rate. Statistical significance was set at $\alpha = 0.05$. Data were analyzed using GraphPad Prism® statistical software (version 7.00; RRID:SCR_002798).

Animals

All animal experiments were approved by the University of Kentucky Institutional Animal Care and Use Committee (Protocol #2014-1233; PI: AMS Hartz) and carried out in accordance with AAALAC regulations, the US Department of Agriculture Animal Welfare Act, and the Guide for the Care and Use of Laboratory Animals of the NIH.

Male transgenic hAPP-overexpressing mice (Tg2576 strain; 129S6.Cg-Tg(APPSWE)2576Kha; RRID:IMSR_TAC:2789; $n = 45$) and corresponding male wild type (WT) mice ($n = 15$; RRID:IMSR_TAC:2789) were purchased from Taconic Farms (Germantown, NY, USA). On arrival, mice were 8-week old with an average body weight of 27.1 ± 2.6 *g* (SD) for WT mice and 29.9 ± 2.9 *g* (SD) for hAPP mice. Animals were single-housed in an AALAC-accredited temperature- and humidity-controlled vivarium (23°C, 60%–65% relative humidity, 14:10 light-dark cycle) in cages connected to an EcoFlo Allentown ventilation system (Allentown Inc., Allentown, NJ, USA). Animals had *ad libitum* access to tap water and standard rodent feed (Harlan Teklad Chow 2918, Harlan Laboratories Inc., Indianapolis, IN, USA) and were allowed to habituate to the vivarium for at least 2 weeks after arrival before the start of experiments.

Human Brain Tissue Samples

Human brain tissue samples (inferior parietal lobule) were obtained from the UK-ADC tissue bank (IRB #B15-2602-M). Case inclusion criteria for this study were enrollment in the UK-ADC longitudinal autopsy cohort (Nelson et al., 2007), a post-mortem interval ≤4 h, and a final consensus diagnosis determined by a group of UK-ADC neuropathologists, neuropsychologists, and neurologists. Cases were classified into two groups: Group (1) cognitive normal ($n = 3$; a classification of "normal" denotes a consensus diagnosis of normal cognition and CERAD rating of "criteria not met") and Group (2) AD patients ($n = 3$; Mirra et al., 1991). All brain tissue samples were from female individuals, whose average age at death was 85.5 ± 9.2 years (group 1, cognitive normal, post-mortem interval: 1.5 h ± 0.3 h, Braak stage score: 1 ± 0) and 86.5 ± 9.2 years (group 2, AD, post-mortem interval: 3.5 h ± 0.7 h, Braak stage score: 5.5 ± 0.7).

Chemicals

Antibodies against β-actin (ab8226; RRID:AB_306371), human Aβ40 (ab12265; RRID:AB_298985), human Aβ42 (ab12267; RRID:AB_298987), LRP (ab92544; RRID:AB_2234877), RAGE (ab3611; RRID:AB_303947), APP (ab11118; RRID:AB_442855) and 20S proteasome (ab109530; RRID:AB_10860339; antibody raised against a synthetic peptide within the human proteasome 20S C2 unit (amino acids: 250–350; C terminal)), as well as cyclosporine A (CSA; ab120114) were purchased from Abcam (Cambridge, MA, USA). Modified Dulbecco's phosphate buffered saline (DPBS; with 0.9 mM Ca^{2+} and 0.5 mM Mg^{2+}) was purchased from HyClone (Logan, UT, USA). Complete™ protease inhibitor was purchased from Roche (Mannheim, Germany). C219 antibody against P-gp was purchased from ThermoFisher (MA126528; RRID:AB_795165; Waltham, MA, USA). Fluorescein-hAβ_{42} [fluorescein-A$\beta_{(1-42)}$] was purchased from rPeptide (Bogart, GA, USA). [N- (4-nitrobenzofurazan-7-yl)-D-Lys8]-cyclosporine A (NBD-CSA) was custom-synthesized by R. Wenger (Basel, Switzerland; Wenger, 1986). PSC833 was a kind gift from Novartis (Basel, Switzerland). PYR41, CelLytic™ M, Ficoll® PM 400, bovine serum albumin and all other chemicals were purchased at the highest grade from Sigma-Aldrich (St. Louis, MO, USA).

PYR41 Dosing

Table 1 shows the dosing regimen for this *in vivo* study. Mice were dosed as follows: Group 1: WT mice (n = 15) received *i.p.* vehicle every third day and *p.o.* vehicle on both days between *i.p.* vehicle injections. Group 2: hAPP mice (n = 15) also received *i.p.* vehicle every third day and *p.o.* vehicle on both days between *i.p.* vehicle injections. Group 3: hAPP-PYR41 mice (n = 15) were dosed every third day with 2 mg/kg PYR41 by *i.p.* injection and received *p.o.* vehicle on days between PYR41 treatment. Group 4: hAPP-PYR41/CSA mice (n = 15) were dosed every third day with 2 mg/kg PYR41 by *i.p.* injection and received 25 mg/kg CSA via oral gavage on both days between doses of PYR41.

Blood Collection

Blood samples were collected by facial vein bleeding 24 h prior to the start of the first dose to obtain control values. Twenty-four hours after the last dose, mice were euthanized by CO_2 inhalation, decapitated and trunk blood was collected in heparinized blood collection tubes. Plasma was obtained by centrifugation at 5000× g for 15 min at 4°C and stored at −80°C until further analysis.

Brain Capillary Isolation

Brain capillaries were isolated using a modified method previously described elsewhere (Hartz et al., 2012). Briefly, mice were euthanized with CO_2 followed by decapitation. Brains were removed, cleaned, dissected and homogenized in DPBS containing Ca^{2+}/Mg^{2+} and supplemented with 5 mM D-glucose

TABLE 1 | PYR41 dosing regimen.

Group	Day of treatment													
	1	2	3	4	5	6	7	8	9	10	11	12	13	14
WT	Vehicle (ip)	Vehicle (po)	Vehicle (po)	Vehicle (ip)	Vehicle (po)	Vehicle (po)	Vehicle (ip)	Vehicle (po)	Vehicle (po)	Vehicle (ip)	Vehicle (po)	Vehicle (po)	Vehicle (ip)	Vehicle (po)
hAPP	Vehicle (ip)	Vehicle (po)	Vehicle (po)	Vehicle (ip)	Vehicle (po)	Vehicle (po)	Vehicle (ip)	Vehicle (po)	Vehicle (po)	Vehicle (ip)	Vehicle (po)	Vehicle (po)	Vehicle (ip)	Vehicle (po)
hAPP-PYR41	**PYR41 (ip)**	Vehicle (po)	Vehicle (po)	**PYR41 (ip)**	Vehicle (po)	Vehicle (po)	**PYR41 (ip)**	Vehicle (po)	Vehicle (po)	**PYR41 (ip)**	Vehicle (po)	Vehicle (po)	**PYR41 (ip)**	Vehicle (po)
hAPP-PYR41/CSA	**PYR41 (ip)**	CSA (po)	CSA (po)	**PYR41 (ip)**	CSA (po)	CSA (po)	**PYR41 (ip)**	CSA (po)	CSA (po)	**PYR41 (ip)**	CSA (po)	CSA (po)	**PYR41 (ip)**	CSA (po)

The present dosing regimen was based on a 2-week preliminary dosing study with CD-1 mice (data not shown). WT and hAPP mice were treated according to the following dosing scheme over the course of 14 days: WT and hAPP mice were given vehicle p.o. by oral gavage or by i.p. injection once every 3 days. hAPP-PYR41 mice received 2 mg/kg PYR41 by i.p. injection once every 3 days and vehicle p.o. by oral gavage on all other days. hAPP-PYR41/CSA mice received 2 mg/kg PYR41 by i.p. injection once every 3 days and 25 mg/kg CSA p.o. by oral gavage on all other days.

and 1 mM sodium pyruvate. Ficoll® PM 400 was added to the homogenized brains (final concentration 15%) and the homogenate was centrifuged (5800 *g*, 20 min, 4°C). After centrifugation, the capillary-enriched pellet was collected and resuspended in 1% BSA-DPBS. The capillary suspension was first passed through a 300 μm nylon mesh and then passed over a glass bead column using 1% BSA-DPBS. Capillaries adhering to the glass beads were washed off and collected by agitation in 1% BSA-DPBS. After centrifugation (1500 *g*, 3 min, 4°C), the capillary pellet was washed three times with DPBS (no BSA), collected, and used for experiments or crude membrane isolation.

Brain Capillary Crude Membrane Isolation

Brain capillary crude membranes were isolated as previously described (Hartz et al., 2012). Freshly isolated brain capillaries were homogenized in lysis buffer (CelLytic™ M, Sigma-Aldrich, St. Louis, MO, USA) containing Complete™ protease inhibitor. Homogenates were centrifuged to separate the membrane fraction from organelles and debris (10,000 *g*, 15 min, 4°C), and the resulting membrane-containing supernatant was centrifuged to pellet capillary crude membranes (100,000 *g*, 90 min, 4°C). The resulting pellet containing brain capillary crude membranes was resuspended and stored at −80°C.

Aβ Immunostaining of Brain Capillaries

Aβ immunostaining of mouse brain capillaries was performed as previously described (Hartz et al., 2010). Briefly, isolated mouse brain capillaries were fixed with 3% paraformaldehyde/0.25% glutaraldehyde for 30 min at room temperature. After washing with PBS, capillaries were permeabilized with 0.5% Triton X-100 for 30 min and washed with PBS. Capillaries were blocked with 1% BSA/DPBS for 60 min and incubated overnight at 4°C with a 1:250 (4 μg/ml) dilution of rabbit polyclonal antibody to human Aβ1–40 (hAβ40; ab12265, Abcam, Cambridge, MA, USA; RRID:AB_298985) or rabbit polyclonal to human Aβ1–42 antibody (hAβ42; ab12267; Abcam, Cambridge, MA, USA; RRID:AB_298987). Capillaries were washed with 1% BSA/PBS and incubated with Alexa-Fluor 488-conjugated goat anti-rabbit IgG (1:1000, 1 μg/ml; Invitrogen, Carlsbad, CA, USA; RRID:AB_2576217) for 1 h at 37°C. Nuclei were counterstained with 1 μg/ml 4,6-diamidino-2-phenylindole (DAPI; MilliporeSigma, Burlington, MA, USA; RRID:SCR_014366). Aβ immunofluorescence was visualized with confocal microscopy (Leica TCS SP5 confocal microscope, 63× water objective, NA 1.2, Leica Instruments, Wetzlar, Germany).

From each treatment group, confocal images of seven capillaries were acquired. Aβ membrane immunofluorescence for each capillary was quantitated with ImageJ software v1.48 as previously described (Hartz et al., 2010). A 10 × 10 grid was superimposed on each image, and fluorescence measurements of capillary membranes were taken between intersecting grid lines. Fluorescence intensity for each capillary was the mean of three measurements per capillary.

Aβ ELISA

Human Aβ40 and Aβ42 levels were quantitated in plasma and brain samples by ELISA (KHB3482 (Sensitivity: <6 pg/ml) and KHB3442 (Sensitivity: <10 pg/ml) from Invitrogen, Camarillo, CA, USA) according to the manufacturer's protocol.

Plasma Samples

Blood samples were collected from control, PYR41 and PYR41/CSA-treated hAPP transgenic mice. Plasma was obtained from blood samples by centrifugation at 5000 *g* for 5 min at 4°C, and then diluted with standard diluent buffer provided with the ELISA kit. To determine hAβ40 levels, samples were diluted 1:50; to determine hAβ42 levels, samples were diluted 1:4.

Brain Samples

To determine brain hAβ40 and hAβ42 levels, brain tissue samples were homogenized in guanidine Tris-HCl buffer (5 M, pH 8) to extract Aβ. To determine hAβ40 levels, samples were diluted 1:20 in DPBS buffer containing 5% BSA and 0.03% Tween-20; to determine hAβ42 levels, samples were diluted 1:5. Diluted samples were centrifuged at 16,000 *g* for 20 min at 4°C; the supernatant was used for ELISA analysis.

Absorbance was measured at 450 nm using a Synergy™ H1 Hybrid Multi-Mode Reader (BioTek, Winooski, VT, USA). A standard curve was plotted using Gen5™ software v2.07 to determine the concentration of hAβ40 and hAβ42 in plasma and brain samples; values at 450 nm were corrected for background absorbance; four parameter logistic ELISA curve fitting was selected.

Western Blotting

Protein expression levels from various tissues were determined by Western blotting as described previously (Hartz et al., 2010, 2016). Protein concentration of brain capillary crude membranes was measured with the Bradford assay. Western blots were performed by using the Invitrogen NuPage® Bis-Tris electrophoresis and blotting system. After protein electrophoresis and transfer, blotting membranes were blocked and incubated overnight with the primary antibody as indicated. Membranes were washed and incubated for 1 h with horseradish peroxidase-conjugated ImmunoPure secondary IgG antibody (1:5000, 0.15 μg/ml; Thermo Fisher Scientific, Waltham, MA, USA). Proteins were detected with SuperSignal West Pico Chemoluminescent Substrate (Thermo Fisher Scientific, Waltham, MA, USA). Protein bands were visualized and recorded with a Bio-Rad ChemiDoc XRS+ gel documentation system (Bio-Rad Laboratories, Hercules, CA, USA). Image Lab 5.0 software from Bio-Rad Laboratories (RRID:SCR_014210) was used for densitometric analyses of band intensities and digital molecular weight analyses; the molecular weight marker was RPN800E (GE Healthcare, Chalfont St. Giles, Buckinghamshire, UK). Linear adjustments of contrast and brightness were applied to entire Western blot images. None of the Western blots shown were modified by nonlinear adjustments.

Immunoprecipitation

Immunoprecipitation was carried out as previously reported (Hartz et al., 2016). Briefly, brain capillaries were homogenized in lysis buffer (CelLytic™ M, Sigma-Aldrich, St. Louis, MO, USA) containing Complete™ protease inhibitor. Samples were centrifuged to separate cellular membranes from organelles and debris (10,000 *g*, 15 min, and 4°C). Protein concentration of the supernatants was determined by Bradford assay.

Anti-P-gp antibody (C219, EMD Millipore, Billerica, MA, USA) was coupled with Pierce Protein A/G Plus Agarose (Thermo Fisher Scientific, Waltham, MA, USA) beads overnight at 4°C in TBST (20 mM Tris (pH 8.0), 170 mM NaCl, 0.05% Tween 20) supplemented with 1% BSA. The immune complex was added to the cell lysate and incubated for 3 h at 4°C. Beads were washed with lysis buffer (10 mM Tris (pH 7.5), 2 mM EDTA, 100 mM NaCl, 1% NP-40, 50 mM NaF, 1 mM Na_3VO_4) containing Complete™ protease inhibitor. For ubiquitin immunoprecipitations, the Pierce™ Ubiquitin Enrichment Kit (#89899; Thermo Fisher Scientific, Waltham, MA, USA) was used according to the manufacturer's protocol. Immunoprecipitated proteins were eluted from agarose beads (IP: P-gp) or the ubiquitin affinity resin (IP: ubiquitin) with NuPAGE LDS sample buffer and heated at 70°C for 10 min. IP samples were resolved by SDS-PAGE and analyzed by Western blotting as described above.

Simple Western Assay

Human brain capillary membrane samples were mixed with Wes™ sample buffer and analyzed with a Simple Western assay designed for the Wes™ instrument by ProteinSimple as previously described (San Jose, CA, USA; Hartz et al., 2016). All steps of the Wes™ Master Kit assay were performed according to the manufacturer's protocol. Briefly, glass microcapillaries were loaded with stacking and separation matrices followed by sample loading. During capillary electrophoresis, proteins were separated by size and then immobilized to the capillary wall. P-gp and β-actin were identified with primary antibodies against P-gp (1:100, 3 μg/ml, C219, MA126528, ThermoFisher, Waltham, MA, USA; RRID:AB_795165) and β-actin (1:150, 5 μg/ml, ab8226, Abcam, Cambridge, MA, USA; RRID:AB_306371), respectively, followed by immunodetection using Wes™ Master Kit HRP conjugated anti-mouse secondary antibody and chemiluminescent substrate. Using Compass V. 2.6.5 software, electropherograms were generated for each sample and each protein (P-gp and β-actin). The area under the curve (AUC), which represents the signal intensity of the chemiluminescent reaction was analyzed for P-gp and β-actin. Values given for P-gp protein expression were normalized to β-actin.

P-gp Transport Assay

To determine P-gp transport activity, freshly isolated brain capillaries from WT and hAPP mice were incubated for 1 h at room temperature with the fluorescent P-gp-specific substrate NBD-CSA (2 μM in PBS buffer; Hartz et al., 2004, 2008, 2010). To assess P-gp-mediated Aβ transport, isolated brain capillaries were incubated for 1 h at room temperature with 5 μM fluorescein-hAβ42 in DPBS buffer (Hartz et al., 2010). For each treatment, images of 10 capillaries were acquired by confocal microscopy using the 488 nm line of an argon laser (Leica Instruments, Wetzlar, Germany) of a Leica TCS SP5 confocal microscope with a 63× 1.2 NA water immersion objective. Images were analyzed by quantitating NBD-CSA fluorescence in the capillary lumen using Image J v.1.48v (Wayne Rasband, NIH, USA; RRID:SCR_003070). Specific, luminal NBD-CSA fluorescence was taken as the difference between total luminal fluorescence and fluorescence in the presence of the P-gp-specific inhibitor PSC833 (5 μM; Hartz et al., 2004, 2008, 2010).

RESULTS

P-gp Ubiquitination Levels Are Increased in Brain Capillaries From AD Patients

Several studies have provided evidence showing that P-gp expression levels at the blood-brain barrier are reduced in AD patients compared to control individuals (Wijesuriya et al., 2010; Jeynes and Provias, 2011; Carrano et al., 2014; Chiu et al., 2015). To assess P-gp protein expression in human brain capillaries, we utilized a recently established protocol to isolate brain capillaries from fresh human frontal cortex tissue (Hartz et al., 2017). **Figure 1** shows representative confocal images of a brain capillary isolated from brain tissue of a cognitive-normal individual (CNI) immunostained for P-gp (**Figure 1A**). The negative control (no primary antibody) shows no signal for P-gp (**Figures 1B,B1**: green channel; **B2**: blue channel; **B3**: overlay of green and blue channel; **B4**: transmitted light channel).

We utilized the Simple Western™ assay to quantitate P-gp protein levels in isolated human brain capillaries. This novel assay allows protein quantitation at 10-fold higher sensitivity and better reproducibility compared to Western blotting (Hartz et al., 2017). The assay is based on automated microcapillary electrophoresis; data robustness was tested at the NIH (Chen et al., 2015). **Figure 1C** shows that a band for P-gp was detected in membrane samples of brain capillaries isolated from CNI patients that was between the 180 kDa and 230 kDa bands of the molecular weight marker. Consistent with previous studies (Wijesuriya et al., 2010; Jeynes and Provias, 2011; Carrano et al., 2014; Chiu et al., 2015), we found that P-gp protein levels in brain capillary samples from AD patients were significantly lower compared to brain capillaries from cognitive normal individuals (CNI; **Figure 1C**); β-actin served as loading control. **Figure 1D** shows the electropherogram of the P-gp microcapillary electrophoresis. Analysis of this electropherogram revealed that the P-gp band peaked at 199.8 ± 2.5 kDa; the peak for β-actin was detected at 49.7 ± 2.6 kDa. The bandwidth for P-gp was 24.8 ± 1.9 kDa and ranged from 187.4 kDa to 212.2 kDa; the bandwidth for β-actin was 9.3 ± 1.2 kDa and ranged from 45.1 kDa to 54.35 kDa. In these electropherograms, each AUC is proportional to the amount of protein, allowing comparisons of P-gp levels between CNI and AD patients. Utilizing this method, we found that P-gp protein levels in capillaries isolated from brain tissue of AD patients are 37%

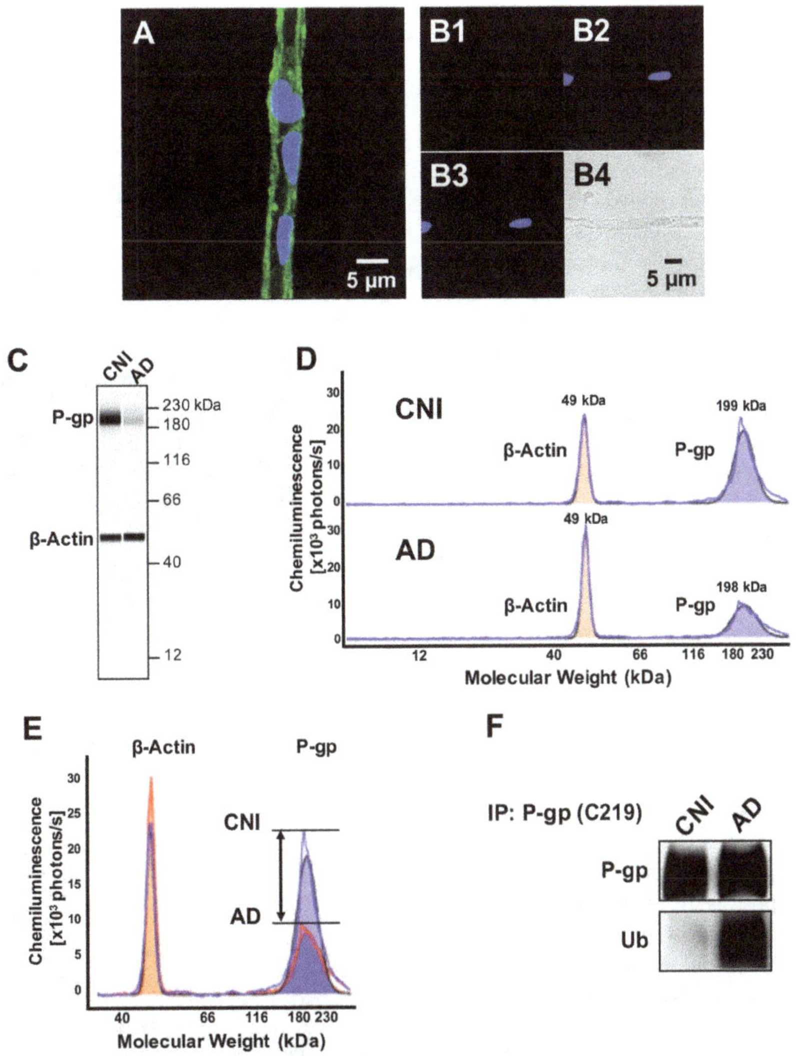

FIGURE 1 | P-glycoprotein (P-gp) protein expression levels are decreased and P-gp ubiquitination levels are increased in brain capillaries from Alzheimer's disease (AD) patients. **(A)** Representative image of a P-gp-immunostained (green) brain capillary isolated from brain tissue of a cognitive normal individual (CNI); nuclei were counterstained with DAPI (blue). **(B)** Negative control (no primary antibody): **(B1**; green channel); **(B2**; blue channel); **(B3**; overlay of green and blue channel) and **(B4**; transmitted light channel). **(C)** Representative WES^{TM} image and **(D)** electropherogram showing reduced P-gp (blue shaded area) protein expression levels in brain capillaries isolated from human brain tissue (frontal cortex) of AD patients (n = 3) vs. CNIs (n = 3). **(E)** Overlay of electropherograms displayed in **(D)** show a reduction in the area under the curve (AUC) that represents P-gp protein expression levels (blue shaded area) in brain capillaries from AD patients (red line) relative to CNI (blue line). In contrast, β-actin levels (orange shaded area) in brain capillaries from AD patients (red line) and CNI (blue line) were the same. **(F)** Western blot showing that ubiquitin levels in P-gp-immunoprecipitates are increased in capillaries from AD patients compared to those from CNI.

lower compared to P-gp protein levels in capillaries isolated from brain samples of CNI (AUC P-gp AD 349670 vs. AUC Pgp CNI 557147 photons × kDa/s). **Figure 1E** shows an overlay of the electropherograms in **Figure 1D**. This overlay shows the difference in peak heights and the areas under the curve (AUC) that represent total protein amount for P-gp and β-actin, respectively, which is a more accurate approach to quantitate protein amount than optical density measurements (O'Neill et al., 2006).

To determine ubiquitinated P-gp levels, we performed immunoprecipitation experiments with brain capillaries from brain tissue of CNI and AD patients and observed that ubiquitination of P-gp was 2.8-fold higher in brain capillaries from patients with AD compared to CNI (n = 3; p = 0.05, **Figure 1F**; Supplementary Figures S1A,B). This indicates that blood-brain barrier P-gp is highly ubiquitinated in patients with AD.

PYR41 Prevents Reduction of P-gp Expression and Activity Levels in hAPP Mice

Ubiquitination of a target protein is carried out by three enzymes. First, ubiquitin is activated by the ubiquitin-activating enzyme

E1. In the second step, ubiquitin is transferred onto the target protein by the conjugating enzyme E2. This ubiquitin transfer is completed in a third step by the ubiquitin ligase E3 resulting in ubiquitination of the target protein.

PYR41 is an E1 ubiquitin-activating enzyme-specific inhibitor that shows little activity on E2 and E3. PYR41 irreversibly blocks ubiquitination, thereby preventing ubiquitin-mediated proteasomal degradation *in vitro* and *in vivo* (Yang et al., 2007; Guan and Ricciardi, 2012). We used PYR41 to test the hypothesis that blocking ubiquitination protects blood-brain barrier P-gp from degradation in transgenic hAPP mice *in vivo*. We dosed young, 8-week old hAPP mice with 2 mg/kg PYR41 i.p. once every 3 days for 14 days (**Table 1**). An additional group of mice received PYR41 in combination with the P-gp inhibitor cyclosporin A (CSA; 25 mg/kg, p.o.) on days between dosing PYR41 alone. These PYR41/CSA-treated mice serve as control group for P-gp transport activity and are used to account for PYR41-treatment effects that depend on P-gp transport activity. WT and hAPP control mice received vehicle. Treatment of hAPP mice with PYR41 restored P-gp protein expression levels in brain capillary membranes to levels observed in vehicle-treated WT mice (**Figure 2A**). We also observed this effect in PYR41/CSA-treated animals. Optical density measurements of P-gp (n = 3, normalized to β-actin) given as percent of WT control mice (SEM, p-value) are: hAPP: 46 ± 10.5% (t = 3.52, p = 0.022; ANOVA *post hoc* test); hAPP-PYR41: 106 ± 11.8% (t = 0.39, p = 0.72; ANOVA *post hoc* test), and hAPP-PYR41/CSA: 106 ± 10.4% (t = 0.39, p = 0.70; ANOVA *post hoc* test).

Next, we determined P-gp transport activity in isolated brain capillaries by using a transport assay we previously described (Hartz et al., 2008, 2010, 2016, 2017). In this assay, freshly isolated brain capillaries are incubated with the fluorescent P-gp substrate NBD-cyclosporin A (NBD-CSA, 2 μM) for 1 h to steady state. Capillaries are then imaged with a confocal microscope followed by quantitative image analysis of NBD-CSA fluorescence in the capillary lumen. In brain capillaries with lower P-gp transport activity compared to control capillaries, less NBD-CSA is transported into the capillary lumen, resulting in lower luminal NBD-CSA fluorescence. Thus, the level of luminal NBD-CSA fluorescence is a measure for P-gp transport activity.

Figure 2B shows representative confocal images of brain capillaries isolated from WT mice, hAPP mice, hAPP mice treated with PYR41 and hAPP mice treated with PYR41/CSA that were exposed to NBD-CSA. Compared to capillaries from WT mice, luminal NBD-CSA fluorescence was decreased in capillaries from hAPP mice and PYR41/CSA-treated hAPP mice, indicating reduced P-gp transport activity levels. In contrast, PYR41 treatment maintained luminal NBD-CSA fluorescence in capillaries from hAPP mice at control levels. Data from confocal image analysis indicate that specific luminal NBD-CSA fluorescence in the lumens of brain capillaries from hAPP mice was reduced by 72% (t = 15.1, p < 0.0001; ANOVA *post hoc* test) relative to WT mice (**Figure 2C**). In contrast, luminal NBD-CSA fluorescence levels in brain capillaries from PYR41-treated hAPP mice were similar to levels measured in capillaries

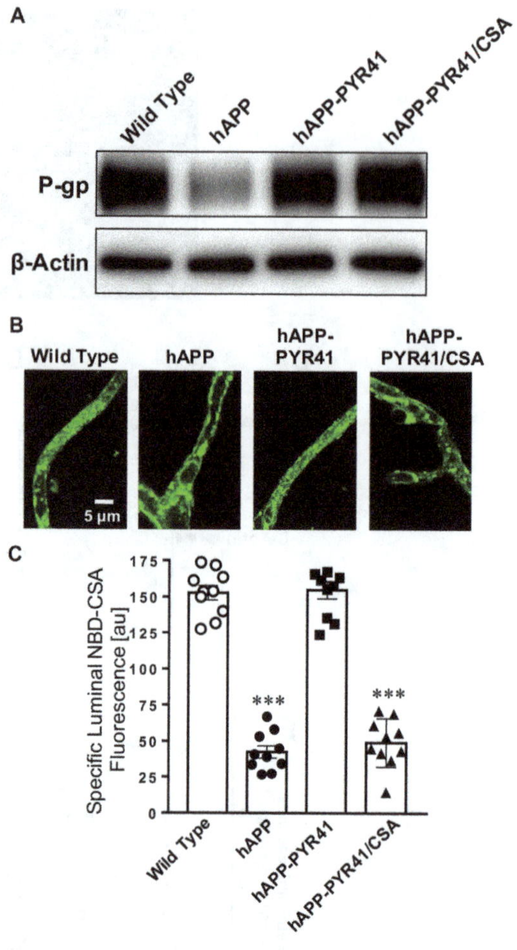

FIGURE 2 | PYR41 prevents reduction of P-gp protein expression and transport activity in human amyloid precursor protein (hAPP) mice. **(A)** Western blot showing that PYR41 treatment restored P-gp protein expression levels in hAPP mice compared to vehicle-treated wild type (WT) mice; β-actin was used as protein loading control. **(B)** Representative confocal images of brain capillaries isolated from WT, hAPP, hAPP-PYR41 and hAPP-PYR41/CSA mice after a 1 h incubation (steady state) with the fluorescent, P-gp-specific substrate NBD-CSA (2 μM). **(C)** Data from ImageJ analysis of confocal images in **(B)** show that luminal NBD-CSA fluorescence was significantly reduced in brain capillaries from hAPP and hAPP-PYR41/CSA mice relative to brain capillaries from WT and hAPP-PYR41 mice. Specific NBD-CSA fluorescence is the difference between total luminal fluorescence and fluorescence in the presence of the P-gp-specific inhibitor PSC833, representing transport activity that is specific to P-gp. Data are mean ± SEM (n = 10 capillaries per treatment group); arbitrary fluorescence units (scale 0–255). Statistics: ***p < 0.001 analysis of variance (ANOVA), significantly lower than WT control group.

from WT mice (t = 0.3, p = 0.81; ANOVA *post hoc* test). In brain capillaries from PYR41-treated hAPP mice that also received CSA to control for P-gp transport activity luminal NBD-CSA fluorescence was reduced by 68% relative to WT mice; this reduction is comparable to that seen in vehicle-treated hAPP mice (t = 13.0, p < 0.0001; ANOVA *post hoc* test).

We repeated this experiment using fluorescein-hAβ_{42} (FL-hAβ_{42}) to test the ability of P-gp to transport Aβ into the lumen of brain capillaries. **Figure 3A** shows representative images of isolated brain capillaries incubated to steady state for 1 h with 5 μM FL-hAβ_{42}. Image analysis shows that luminal FL-hAβ_{42} fluorescence was reduced to 32.6 ± 9.2% (t = 6.4, p < 0.0001; ANOVA *post hoc* test) in capillaries from hAPP mice relative to capillaries from WT mice (**Figure 3B**). Luminal FL-hAβ_{42} fluorescence levels in brain capillaries isolated from PYR41-treated hAPP mice was comparable to fluorescence levels observed in capillaries from WT mice (t = 0.6, p = 0.54; ANOVA *post hoc* test). In contrast, FL-hAβ_{42} fluorescence levels in capillary lumens from PYR41/CSA-treated control mice were significantly reduced (t = 6.87, p < 0.0001; ANOVA *post hoc* test), which was comparable to luminal fluorescence levels in brain capillary lumens of untreated hAPP mice.

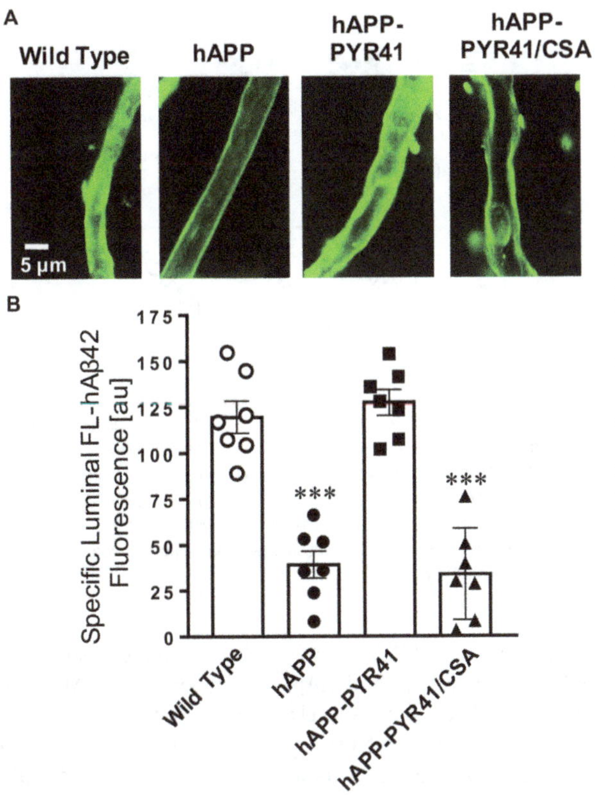

FIGURE 3 | PYR41 treatment restores P-gp-mediated hAβ_{42} transport in hAPP mice. **(A)** Representative confocal images of isolated brain capillaries from WT, hAPP, hAPP-PYR41 and hAPP-PYR41/CSA mice after a 1 h incubation with 5 μM FL-hAβ_{42}. **(B)** Data from ImageJ analysis of confocal images in **(A)** show that luminal FL-hAβ_{42} levels were significantly reduced in brain capillaries from hAPP and hAPP-PYR41/CSA mice relative to brain capillaries from WT and hAPP-PYR41 mice. In contrast, luminal FL-hAβ_{42} fluorescence levels in brain capillaries from PYR41-treated hAPP mice are comparable to those in isolated brain capillaries from WT mice indicating that PYR41-treatment restored P-gp transport activity. Specific FL-hAβ_{42} fluorescence is the difference between total luminal fluorescence and fluorescence in the presence of the P-gp-specific inhibitor PSC833, representing FL-hAβ_{42} transport into the lumen of brain capillaries that is specific to P-gp. Data are mean ± SEM (n = 7 capillaries per treatment group); arbitrary fluorescence units (scale 0–255). Statistics: ***p < 0.001 (ANOVA), significantly lower than WT control group.

Together, the data in **Figures 2, 3** demonstrate that PYR41 treatment of young hAPP mice attenuated reduction of both P-gp protein expression and transport activity levels. This suggests that PYR41 prevented P-gp degradation through the ubiquitin-proteasome system.

PYR41 Treatment of hAPP Mice Prevents P-gp Ubiquitination *in Vivo*

PYR41 is a cell-permeable, specific and irreversible inhibitor of the ubiquitin-activating enzyme E1, which is responsible for mediating the first step of ubiquitination of proteins that are proteasome targets. Thus, PYR41 inhibits ubiquitination of proteins, thereby preventing their degradation by the ubiquitin-proteasome system. To determine the effect of PYR41 treatment on the ubiquitination status of P-gp at the blood-brain barrier, we performed immunoprecipitation experiments with isolated brain capillaries from PYR41-treated and untreated hAPP mice. The Western blot in **Figure 4A** shows that immunoprecipitated P-gp protein levels were similar in brain capillaries from hAPP mice and hAPP mice treated with PYR41 and PYR41/CSA. We observed high levels of ubiquitinated P-gp in isolated capillaries from hAPP mice. In contrast, brain capillaries isolated from PYR-41 and PYR41/CSA-treated hAPP mice had no detectable levels of ubiquitinated P-gp. These data indicate that PYR41 treatment was effective to prevent ubiquitination of P-gp in brain capillaries.

The Western blot in **Figure 4B** shows protein expression levels of P-gp and other proteins involved in Aβ production or transport, as well as signaling molecules associated with P-gp reduction. Data from isolated brain capillaries from hAPP mice showed a reduction in P-gp protein expression levels relative to P-gp levels in WT mice, an effect that was blocked with PYR41 and PYR41/CSA treatment. Importantly, PYR41 and PYR41/CSA treatment did not alter protein expression levels of other proteins associated with Aβ production (hAPP), Aβ clearance (LRP1), Aβ transport (RAGE), or the degradation of P-gp (Nedd-4, 20S Proteasome).

Together, these data demonstrate that PYR41 treatment prevented P-gp ubiquitination in capillaries isolated from hAPP mice but did not affect other proteins involved in Aβ production or transport.

PYR41 Treatment of hAPP Mice Lowers Aβ Levels

In a next step, we determined the consequences of PYR41 treatment on Aβ levels in plasma, capillary membranes, and brain tissue. We measured hAβ_{40} and hAβ_{42} levels in plasma by ELISA and found no difference in hAβ_{40} and hAβ_{42} plasma levels among PYR41-treated, PYR41/CSA-treated, and untreated hAPP mice (**Figures 5A,B**). Samples from WT mice were not included since WT mice do not express human Aβ.

We also immunostained isolated brain capillaries for hAβ_{40} and hAβ_{42} to determine capillary-associated Aβ levels. Brain capillaries isolated from vehicle-treated hAPP mice stained positive for both Aβ peptides (**Figures 6A,B**). PYR41-treatment decreased membrane-associated immunofluorescence of hAβ_{40}

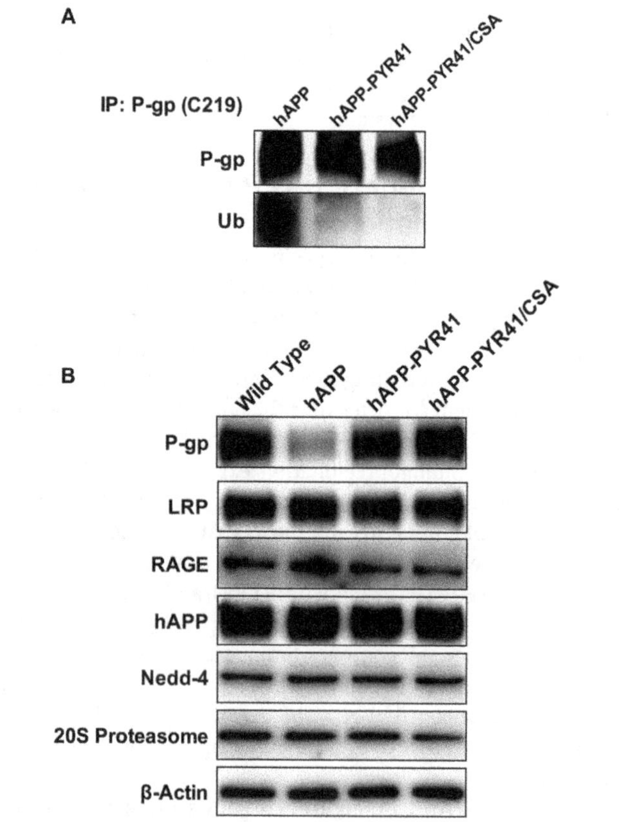

FIGURE 4 | PYR41 prevents P-gp ubiquitination in hAPP mice. **(A)** Western blot showing that treating hAPP mice with PYR41 reduces ubiquitin levels in P-gp-immunoprecipitates from isolated brain capillaries. P-gp was immunoprecipitated in capillary samples isolated from hAPP, hAPP-PYR41 and hAPP-PYR41/CSA mice, and examined for P-gp and ubiquitin levels by Western blotting (brain capillaries isolated from pooled tissue; $n = 15$ mice per treatment group). **(B)** Western blot showing that PYR41 and PYR41/CSA treatment of mice had only an effect on P-gp protein expression levels, whereas levels of LRP, RAGE, hAPP, Nedd-4 and the 20S proteasome were not affected in isolated brain capillaries (pooled tissue; $n = 15$ mice per treatment group).

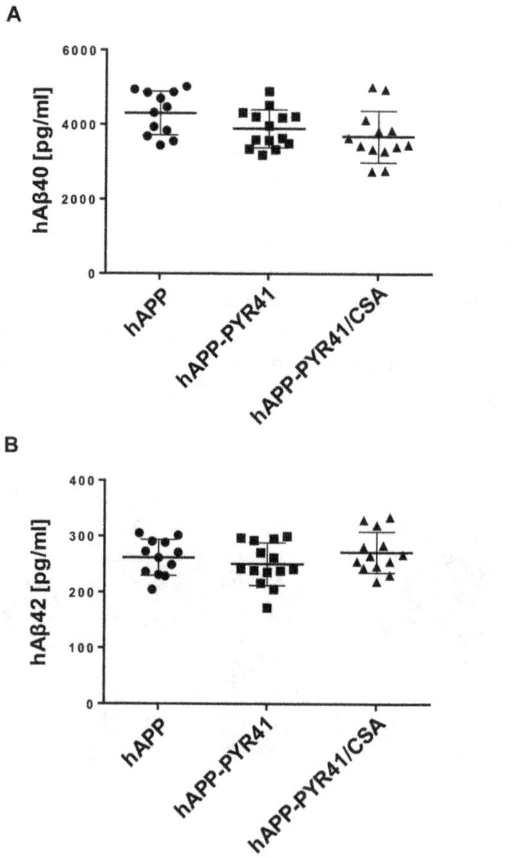

FIGURE 5 | PYR41 treatment has no effect on Aβ plasma levels. **(A)** $hA\beta_{40}$ levels (pg/ml) in plasma samples from hAPP mice treated with vehicle, PYR41, or PYR41/CSA determined by ELISA. Data are given for each animal (hAPP: $n = 12$; hAPP-PYR41: $n = 14$; hAPP-PYR41/CSA: $n = 13$). **(B)** $hA\beta_{42}$ plasma levels (pg/ml) in samples from hAPP mice treated with vehicle ($n = 12$), PYR41 ($n = 14$), or PYR41/CSA ($n = 13$). Statistics: ANOVA; Data between groups are not significantly different.

by 16 ± 5.2% ($t = 8.9$, $p < 0.0001$; ANOVA *post hoc* test) and that of $hA\beta_{42}$ by 20 ± 2.2% ($t = 3.1$, $p = 0.0094$; ANOVA *post hoc* test) relative to untreated hAPP mice. However, this effect was not observed in Aβ-immunostained brain capillaries from PYR41/CSA-treated hAPP mice, indicating that inhibiting P-gp transport activity with CSA blocks the reduction in Aβ levels in brain capillaries.

Finally, data from Western blot analyses showed a significant reduction of $hA\beta_{40}$ and $hA\beta_{42}$ protein levels in brain tissue samples of PYR41-treated hAPP mice relative to untreated hAPP mice (**Figure 7A**). This was not the case in brain tissue from PYR41-treated mice that also received CSA to control for P-gp transport activity. Optical density measurements of Western blots revealed that PYR41 treatment reduced brain $hA\beta_{40}$ levels by 42 ± 6.8% ($t = 6.3$, $p < 0.003$; df = 4, *t*-test) and $hA\beta_{42}$ levels by 47 ± 4.5% ($t = 10.5$, $p < 0.0004$; df = 4, *t*-test) compared to vehicle-treated hAPP mice. Consistent with our Western blot results, data from ELISA analysis of brain samples also showed a reduction in $hA\beta_{40}$ and $hA\beta_{42}$ brain levels in hAPP mice treated with PYR41. $hA\beta_{40}$ levels were reduced by 53.3 ± 0.51% ($t = 11.4$, $p = 0.0005$; ANOVA *post hoc* test) and $hA\beta_{42}$ levels were reduced by 33.3 ± 0.08% ($t = 4.9$, $p = 0.018$; ANOVA *post hoc* test), respectively (**Figures 7B,C**). Together these data indicate that PYR41 treatment prevents P-gp degradation, which results in a reduction in $hA\beta_{40}$ and $hA\beta_{42}$ brain levels in hAPP mice.

In summary, our data indicate that blocking P-gp ubiquitination prevents P-gp degradation, which ultimately leads to a reduction in Aβ brain levels. Thus, targeting the ubiquitin-proteasome system early in AD could be a therapeutic strategy to protect brain capillary P-gp and thereby lower Aβ brain levels.

DISCUSSION

We recently reported that P-gp protein expression and transport activity levels are significantly reduced at the blood-brain barrier

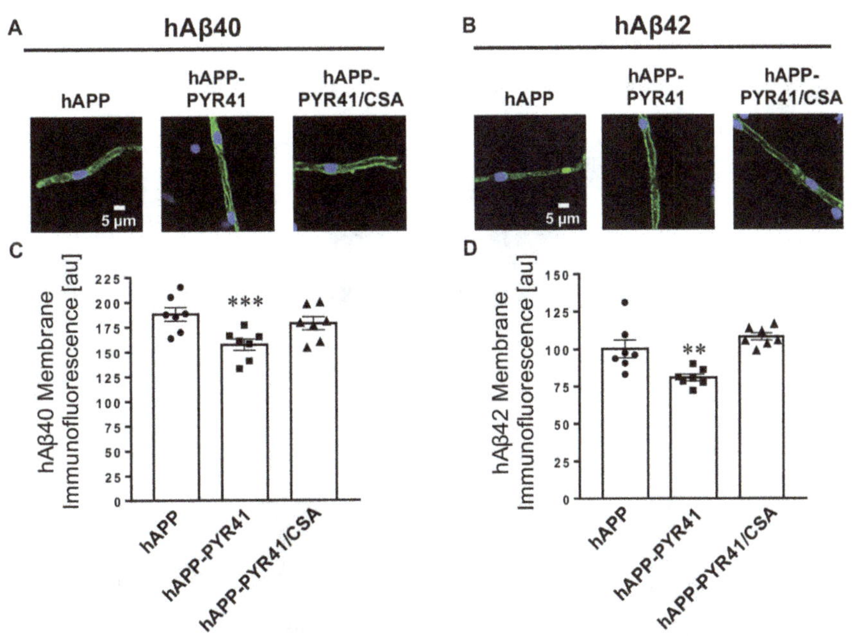

FIGURE 6 | PYR41 treatment reduces Aβ levels in brain capillary membranes. Representative confocal images of **(A)** $hA\beta_{40}$-immunostained and **(B)** $hA\beta_{42}$-immunostained brain capillaries isolated from vehicle-, PYR41- and PYR41/CSA-treated hAPP mice. Data from image analysis with ImageJ show that **(C)** $hA\beta_{40}$ and **(D)** $hA\beta_{42}$ membrane immunofluorescence is lower in capillaries isolated from PYR41-treated hAPP compared to control hAPP mice and mice that received PYR41/CSA. Data are mean ± SEM ($n = 7$ brain capillaries per treatment group); shown are arbitrary fluorescence units (scale 0–255). Statistics: $^{**}p < 0.01$ (ANOVA), $^{***}p < 0.001$ (ANOVA) significantly lower than hAPP vehicle-treated mice.

in young, 12-week old hAPP mice that do not display cognitive deficits yet (Hartz et al., 2010). We also demonstrated that $A\beta_{40}$ triggers reduction of P-gp expression and activity levels by activating the ubiquitin-proteasome system which leads to degradation of the transporter (Akkaya et al., 2015; Hartz et al., 2016). One consequence of reduced P-gp levels is impaired Aβ clearance from brain to blood across the blood-brain barrier (Hartz et al., 2010). The present study extends our previous *ex vivo* findings to an *in vivo* therapeutic strategy designed to prevent loss of P-gp by targeting the ubiquitin-proteasome system.

Here, we report that P-gp protein expression levels are reduced and P-gp ubiquitination levels are increased in isolated capillaries from AD patients relative to CNIs (**Figure 1**). Further, we show that treatment of 8–12-week old hAPP mice with PYR41, a specific and irreversible inhibitor of ubiquitin-activating enzyme E1, prevented degradation of P-gp in brain capillaries from hAPP mice (**Figure 2**). P-gp transport activity levels in PYR41-treated hAPP mice were comparable to those in control WT mice, and P-gp-mediated $A\beta_{40}$ transport activity was also fully restored to control levels in brain capillaries isolated from PYR41-treated hAPP mice (**Figure 3**). We found that PYR41 treatment reduced levels of ubiquitinated P-gp in brain capillaries from hAPP mice, indicating successful inhibition of E1 function *in vivo* (**Figure 4A**). Other proteins involved in Aβ production and/or transport were not affected by PYR41 treatment (**Figure 4B**). While our data suggest that PYR41 treatment prevented P-gp ubiquitination in brain capillaries isolated from hAPP mice without affecting proteins involved in Aβ production or transport (**Figure 4B**), we cannot fully exclude that PYR41 had no effect on other proteins that could also be involved in Aβ brain accumulation. PYR41 treatment did not affect Aβ plasma levels in hAPP mice, but slightly reduced $hA\beta_{40}$ and $hA\beta_{42}$ levels in brain capillaries (**Figures 5**, **6**). PYR41 treatment did, however, significantly reduce hAβ brain levels in PYR41-treated hAPP mice compared to vehicle- and PYR41/CSA-treated hAPP control mice (**Figure 7**).

Together, we provide *in vivo* evidence that inhibiting the ubiquitin-proteasome system blocks the reduction of P-gp levels and lowers Aβ brain levels in an AD mouse model. In the following sections we discuss different aspects of our study and put our findings in context with existing reports.

The Ubiquitin-Proteasome System Is Involved in P-gp Regulation

The ubiquitin-proteasome system is responsible for degradation of proteins, and therefore, essential for proteostasis (Ciechanover, 1994; Ciechanover and Kwon, 2015). The first step in protein degradation by the ubiquitin-proteasome system is ubiquitination of the target protein that is to be degraded. In a four-step process, a cascade of ubiquitin-activating, -conjugating, -ligating and -elongating enzymes (E1–E4) mediate the conjugation of ubiquitin to an amino group of the target protein. After addition of a polyubiquitin chain on the target protein, the now ubiquitinated membrane

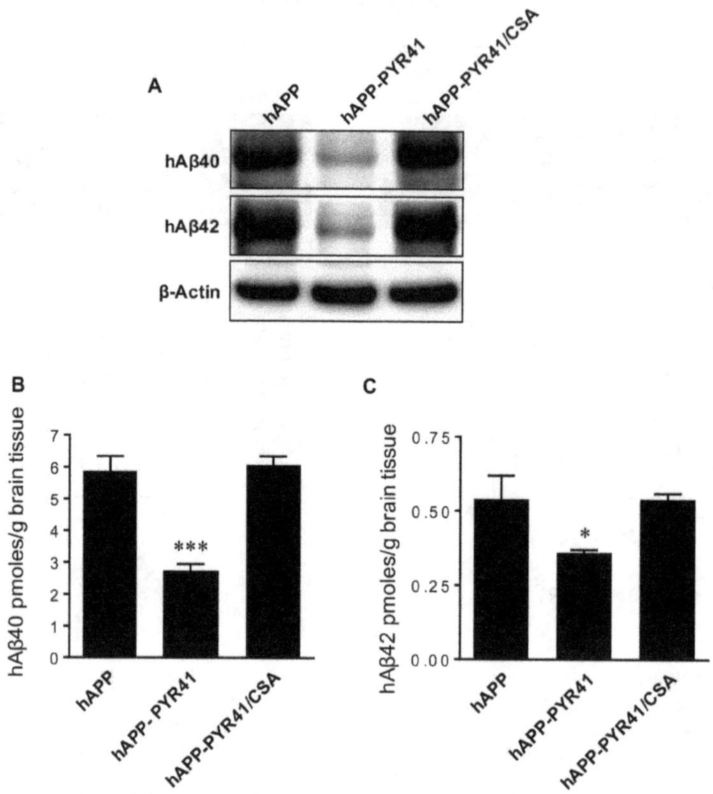

FIGURE 7 | PYR41 treatment reduces Aβ brain levels in hAPP mice. **(A)** Western blots showing PYR41 treatment reduced $hA\beta_{40}$ and $hA\beta_{42}$ protein expression levels in total brain tissue in hAPP mice compared to vehicle-treated WT mice or hAPP mice treated with PYR41/CSA; β-actin was used as protein loading control. ELISA analysis of brain tissue revealed that PYR41 significantly reduced protein levels of **(B)** $hA\beta_{40}$ by 53.3 ± 0.51% and **(C)** $hA\beta_{42}$ by 33.3 ± 0.08%. Data are mean ± SEM (pooled tissue from 15 mice per treatment group). Statistics: $^*p < 0.05$ and $^{***}p < 0.001$ (ANOVA), significantly lower than hAPP vehicle-treated mice.

protein is internalized, recognized by the 26S proteasome complex and is then degraded in an ATP-driven process. The way proteins are ubiquitinated is complex and multifaceted. Some proteins are tagged with one ubiquitin molecule in a process referred to as monoubiquitination. Other proteins undergo multi-monoubiquitination during which different amino acid residues of the same target protein receive each one ubiquitin molecule. In contrast, polyubiquitination describes a process during which several ubiquitin molecules are added to one target protein resulting in linear or branched polyubiquitinated chains with different topologies. Mono- and polyubiquitination affects proteins in many ways: it can affect protein activity, promote or prevent protein interactions, alter protein cellular location or signal protein degradation via the proteasome.

Our previous work and the present study show that blood-brain barrier P-gp protein expression levels, and thus, P-gp transport activity levels, are regulated by the ubiquitin-proteasome system (Akkaya et al., 2015; Hartz et al., 2016). Our findings suggest that increased proteasomal degradation of P-gp is responsible for reduced P-gp expression and activity levels in AD. Our work is consistent with findings from other groups showing that the ubiquitin-proteasome system regulates localization, protein expression, and transport function of human P-gp (Loo and Clarke, 1998; Zhang et al., 2004). Katayama et al. (2013) demonstrated in the human colorectal cancer cell lines HCT-15 and SW620 that FBXO15, a subunit of the ubiquitin E3 ligase, is a negative regulator of P-gp protein expression. Data from immunoprecipitation experiments indicated that FBXO15 binds to P-gp and enhances ubiquitination of the transporter. FBXO15 knockdown led to increased P-gp expression and transport activity in both cancer cell lines. In the same study, Katayama et al. (2013) also demonstrated that the ubiquitin E3 ligase complex SCFFbx15 recognizes P-gp as a substrate and brings the transporter in contact with the ubiquitin-conjugating enzyme Ube2r1, which ubiquitinates P-gp. More recently, Katayama et al. (2016) showed that inactivating MAPK signaling with small-molecule inhibitors leads to increased Ube2r1 expression levels, which, in turn, promotes P-gp degradation through the proteasome. Ravindranath et al. (2015) showed that the ubiquitin E3-ligase FBXO21 also catalyzes P-gp ubiquitination, thereby targeting it for subsequent proteasomal degradation. In addition, Rao et al. (2006) showed that the E3 ubiquitin ligase, RING finger protein 2 (RNF2), interacts with the linker region of human P-gp and the authors demonstrated that co-expression of RNF2 and P-gp results in decreased ATPase activity and proteolytic protection of the transporter in Sf9 insect cells. Together, data from various groups suggest that P-gp expression and transport activity are regulated by the ubiquitin-proteasome system.

Our previously published work indicates that $A\beta_{40}$ triggers P-gp ubiquitination, resulting in internalization and proteasomal degradation of the transporter (Hartz et al., 2016). Further, we have demonstrated that P-gp may be a substrate for the ubiquitin E3-ligase Nedd-4 (Akkaya et al., 2015). In the present study, we expand this line of research by inhibiting P-gp ubiquitination with the ubiquitin-activating enzyme E1 inhibitor PYR41 in a mouse AD model *in vivo* and show that blocking P-gp ubiquitination prevents loss of P-gp and lowers Aβ brain levels.

In addition to P-gp, other proteins are also thought to facilitate Aβ transport across the blood-brain barrier such as the low-density lipoprotein receptor-related protein (LRP; Deane et al., 2008; Storck et al., 2016). Similar to P-gp, LRP levels were reduced in brain capillaries from various AD mouse models and in post-mortem brain tissue from AD patients (Donahue et al., 2006; Silverberg et al., 2010). Like P-gp, degradation of LRP is mediated by the proteasome, however, LRP degradation appears to be independent from ubiquitination. In this regard, Melman et al. (2002) have demonstrated that tyrosine and di-leucine motifs within the LRP cytoplasmic tail mediate rapid endocytosis followed by proteasomal degradation, a process that does not require ubiquitination. Deane et al. (2004) showed that Aβ enhanced LRP proteasomal degradation in brain capillaries of 6–9-month old hAPP mice with cognitive impairment. The low LRP levels and the behavior deficits in these mice are consistent with reduced LRP levels in Aβ-accumulating mice and patients with AD and familial cerebrovascular β-amyloidosis (Deane et al., 2004). These findings suggest that reduced expression and activity levels of P-gp and LRP in brain capillaries, which contributes to Aβ pathology, result from similar augmentations of the ubiquitin-proteasome system, where P-gp is affected by enhanced ubiquitination and LRP is affected by enhanced direct proteasomal degradation.

The Ubiquitin-Proteasome System in Alzheimer's Disease

Protein misfolding, protein mishandling and deficits in protein quality control often drive neurodegenerative disease pathology (Urushitani et al., 2002; Kabashi et al., 2004; Ross and Pickart, 2004). These abnormal processes can lead to accumulation of Aβ in the brain and intraneuronal aggregation of hyper-phosphorylated tau protein, both of which are hallmarks of AD (Oddo, 2008; Riederer et al., 2011; Morawe et al., 2012; Hong et al., 2014; Gentier and van Leeuwen, 2015; Gadhave et al., 2016). Numerous studies reported that the activity of the ubiquitin-proteasome system is reduced in AD. For example, data from post-mortem studies of patients with late-stage AD showed accumulation of ubiquitin in both plaques and tangles and increased levels of a variety of ubiquinated proteins (Perry et al., 1987; Keck et al., 2003). One explanation for this finding is a dysfunctional ubiquitin-proteasome system, where ubiquitinated proteins accumulate in the tissue but are not further degraded by the proteasome. Indeed, Keller et al. (2000) observed a significant decrease in proteasome activity in the hippocampus, parahippocampal gyrus, middle temporal gyri, and inferior parietal lobule of patients with AD compared to cognitive normal individuals. Moreover, in AD, the proteolytic activity of the 26S proteasome appears to be impaired, resulting in oxidation and downregulation of ubiquitin C-terminal hydrolase 1 (UCH1), which is responsible for ubiquitin turnover (Almeida et al., 2006). Further, mutant ubiquitin, UBB^{+1}, is a hallmark of various neurodegenerative diseases. Elevated UBB^{+1} levels in the brain directly inhibit proteasome activity, which is thought to lead to Aβ accumulation and hyper-phosphorylated tau, and thus, constitutes a risk factor for AD (Lindsten et al., 2002; van Leeuwen et al., 2006; Shabek et al., 2009; Dennissen et al., 2010; Ciechanover and Kwon, 2015). Collectively, growing evidence suggests that a dysfunctional ubiquitin-proteasome system contributes to AD pathology. However, little is known about the mechanisms that drive irregular activity of the complex ubiquitin-proteasome system, what brain regions and brain cell types are affected is not fully understood, and during which disease stages these changes occur is unclear. In contrast to brain tissue, our previous reports and the present study indicate that in the brain capillaries of the blood-brain barrier, the ubiquitin-proteasome system is overly active, leading to ubiquitination and degradation of membrane proteins such as P-gp (Akkaya et al., 2015; Hartz et al., 2016). The discrepancy between impaired proteasome activity in brain tissue and increased proteasome activity in brain capillary endothelial cells could be due to tissue-specific differences of the 20S proteasome. This explanation is supported by multiple reports showing that enzymes of the ubiquitin pathway (E1–4) are expressed in a tissue-specific manner and that alterations in ubiquitin ligase activity, proteasome subunit composition, and proteasome-interacting proteins are tissue-specific and adapt to functional needs in their respective tissues (Patel and Majetschak, 2007; Mayor and Peng, 2012; Kniepert and Groettrup, 2014; Ortega and Lucas, 2014).

In addition to tissue-specific differences, it is possible that proteasome activity changes with age, and thus, could be time- or even context-dependent. Current studies in our laboratory are aimed at determining levels of ubiquitination and 20S proteasome activity in hAPP mice at different ages.

The Ubiquitin-Proteasome System as a Therapeutic Target

Collectively, our previous and present findings suggest that the ubiquitin-proteasome system is involved in reducing P-gp protein expression and transport activity levels in AD. Based on data from our studies, preventing P-gp loss by targeting the ubiquitin-proteasome pathway could potentially serve as therapeutic strategy to protect P-gp from degradation, reduce Aβ brain accumulation, and slow AD progression. While targeting ubiquitination may represent a new therapeutic strategy, developing drugs that target the ubiquitin activating, conjugating, ligating and elongating enzymes E1–E4 remains a challenge. These enzymes do not have a well-defined catalytic pocket, which makes the design of specific small molecule inhibitors difficult (Nalepa et al., 2006). Further, ubiquitination is a complex process that depends on dynamic protein-protein interactions that are difficult to disrupt with small molecules. In addition, as the name indicates, ubiquitination is a ubiquitous process present in all cells of the body, and thus, selectively targeting one tissue and not others is challenging. Consequently, FDA-approved drugs that specifically and selectively block ubiquitination are currently not available.

A different therapeutic option could be to target the proteasome itself. Currently, two FDA-approved small-molecule 20S proteasome inhibitors are on the market for cancer therapy: bortezomib (Velcade®) and carfilxomib (Krypolis®). Both drugs show efficacy in multiple myeloma with manageable pharmacokinetic properties and a relatively low side effect profile. Since the 20S proteasome subunit is the proteolytic core of the multi-subunit 26S proteasome proteolytic complex, both inhibitors—bortezomib and carfilxomib—also affect the activity of the entire 26S proteasome complex. While targeting the proteasome is an option, two points need more reflection. First, the potential inverse relationship between dysfunction of the ubiquitin-proteasome system in the brain relative to the blood-brain barrier must be taken into consideration. Inhibiting the 20S proteasome may be particularly beneficial in the early stages of AD to prevent P-gp loss and facilitate Aβ clearance. However, 20S proteasome inhibition may be detrimental in later AD stages when the ubiquitin-proteasome system is greatly impaired in the brain. Second, 20S proteasome inhibition is only feasible and can only be fully taken advantage of when AD is diagnosed early. While significant efforts have been made to identify biomarkers and develop novel imaging techniques that allow early AD diagnosis, no tools are currently available in the clinic and early AD diagnosis, prior to the appearance of behavioral symptoms, remains a formidable challenge.

In summary, in the present *in vivo* study we show that preventing ubiquitination of P-gp at the blood-brain barrier protects the transporter from degradation, which substantially lowers Aβ brain levels in an AD mouse model. These data suggest a novel therapeutic avenue that helps protect P-gp by limiting Aβ-induced P-gp degradation for improved Aβ clearance across the blood-brain barrier in AD.

AUTHOR CONTRIBUTIONS

AH and BB contributed to the major design, acquisition, analysis and interpretation of data for the work and wrote and revised the manuscript. YZ carried out ELISAs and experiments with isolated human capillaries. AS contributed to Western blot data analysis and drafted parts of the manuscript. EA provided all statistical analyses. All authors were involved in drafting and revising the work for important intellectual content. All authors approved the final version and agreed to be accountable for all aspects of the work in ensuring that questions related to the accuracy or integrity of any part of the work are appropriately investigated and resolved.

FUNDING

This project was supported by Grant No. 2R01AG039621 from the National Institute on Aging (to AH). The content is solely the responsibility of the authors and does not necessarily represent the official views of the National Institute on Aging or the National Institutes of Health.

ACKNOWLEDGMENTS

We thank the members of the Hartz and Bauer laboratories for proofreading the manuscript.

REFERENCES

Akkaya, B. G., Zolnerciks, J. K., Ritchie, T. K., Bauer, B., Hartz, A. M., Sullivan, J. A., et al. (2015). The multidrug resistance pump ABCB1 is a substrate for the ubiquitin ligase NEDD4-1. *Mol. Membr. Biol.* 32, 39–45. doi: 10.3109/09687688.2015.1023378

Almeida, C. G., Takahashi, R. H., and Gouras, G. K. (2006). β-Amyloid accumulation impairs multivesicular body sorting by inhibiting the ubiquitin-proteasome system. *J. Neurosci.* 26, 4277–4288. doi: 10.1523/JNEUROSCI.5078-05.2006

Carrano, A., Snkhchyan, H., Kooij, G., van der Pol, S., van Horssen, J., Veerhuis, R., et al. (2014). ATP-binding cassette transporters P-glycoprotein and breast cancer related protein are reduced in capillary cerebral amyloid angiopathy. *Neurobiol. Aging* 35, 565–575. doi: 10.1016/j.neurobiolaging.2013.09.015

Chen, J.-Q., Wakefield, L. M., and Goldstein, D. J. (2015). Capillary nano-immunoassays: advancing quantitative proteomics analysis, biomarker assessment and molecular diagnostics. *J. Transl. Med.* 13:182. doi: 10.1186/s12967-015-0537-6

Chiu, C., Miller, M. C., Monahan, R., Osgood, D. P., Stopa, E. G., and Silverberg, G. D. (2015). P-glycoprotein expression and amyloid accumulation in human aging and Alzheimer's disease: preliminary observations. *Neurobiol. Aging* 36, 2475–2482. doi: 10.1016/j.neurobiolaging.2015.05.020

Ciechanover, A. (1994). The ubiquitin-proteasome proteolytic pathway. *Cell* 79, 13–21. doi: 10.1016/0092-8674(94)90396-4

Ciechanover, A., and Kwon, Y. T. (2015). Degradation of misfolded proteins in neurodegenerative diseases: therapeutic targets and strategies. *Exp. Mol. Med.* 47:e147. doi: 10.1038/emm.2014.117

Cirrito, J. R., Deane, R., Fagan, A. M., Spinner, M. L., Parsadanian, M., Finn, M. B., et al. (2005). P-glycoprotein deficiency at the blood-brain barrier increases amyloid-β deposition in an Alzheimer disease mouse model. *J. Clin. Invest.* 115, 3285–3290. doi: 10.1172/JCI25247

Deane, R., Sagare, A., Hamm, K., Parisi, M., Lane, S., Finn, M. B., et al. (2008). apoE isoform-specific disruption of amyloid β peptide clearance from mouse brain. *J. Clin. Invest.* 118, 4002–4013. doi: 10.1172/JCI36663

Deane, R., Wu, Z., Sagare, A., Davis, J., Du Yan, S., Hamm, K., et al. (2004). LRP/amyloid β-peptide interaction mediates differential brain efflux of Aβ isoforms. *Neuron* 43, 333–344. doi: 10.1016/j.neuron.2004.07.017

Dennissen, F., Kholod, N., Steinbusch, H., and Van Leeuwen, F. (2010). Misframed proteins and neurodegeneration: a novel view on Alzheimer's and Parkinson's diseases. *Neurodegener. Dis.* 7, 76–79. doi: 10.1159/000285510

Deo, A. K., Borson, S., Link, J. M., Domino, K., Eary, J. F., Ke, B., et al. (2014). Activity of P-glycoprotein, a β-amyloid transporter at the blood-brain barrier, is compromised in patients with mild Alzheimer disease. *J. Nucl. Med.* 55, 1106–1111. doi: 10.2967/jnumed.113.130161

Donahue, J. E., Flaherty, S. L., Johanson, C. E., Duncan, J. A., Silverberg, G. D., Miller, M. C., et al. (2006). RAGE, LRP-1 and amyloid-β protein in Alzheimer's disease. *Acta Neuropathol.* 112, 405–415. doi: 10.1007/s00401-006-0115-3

Gadhave, K., Bolshette, N., Ahire, A., Pardeshi, R., Thakur, K., Trandafir, C., et al. (2016). The ubiquitin proteasomal system: a potential target for the management of Alzheimer's disease. *J. Cell. Mol. Med.* 20, 1392–1407. doi: 10.1111/jcmm.12817

Gentier, R. J., and van Leeuwen, F. W. (2015). Misframed ubiquitin and impaired protein quality control: an early event in Alzheimer's disease. *Front. Mol. Neurosci.* 8:47. doi: 10.3389/fnmol.2015.00047

Guan, H., and Ricciardi, R. P. (2012). Transformation by E1A oncoprotein involves ubiquitin-mediated proteolysis of the neuronal and tumor repressor REST in the nucleus. *J. Virol.* 86, 5594–5602. doi: 10.1128/JVI.06811-11

Hardy, J., and Selkoe, D. J. (2002). The amyloid hypothesis of Alzheimer's disease: progress and problems on the road to therapeutics. *Science* 297, 353–356. doi: 10.1126/science.1072994

Hartz, A. M., Bauer, B., Block, M. L., Hong, J. S., and Miller, D. S. (2008). Diesel exhaust particles induce oxidative stress, proinflammatory signaling and P-glycoprotein up-regulation at the blood-brain barrier. *FASEB J.* 22, 2723–2733. doi: 10.1096/fj.08-106997

Hartz, A. M., Bauer, B., Fricker, G., and Miller, D. S. (2004). Rapid regulation of P-glycoprotein at the blood-brain barrier by endothelin-1. *Mol. Pharmacol.* 66, 387–394. doi: 10.1124/mol.104.001503

Hartz, A. M., Bauer, B., Soldner, E. L., Wolf, A., Boy, S., Backhaus, R., et al. (2012). Amyloid-β contributes to blood-brain barrier leakage in transgenic human amyloid precursor protein mice and in humans with cerebral amyloid angiopathy. *Stroke* 43, 514–523. doi: 10.1161/STROKEAHA.111.627562

Hartz, A. M., Miller, D. S., and Bauer, B. (2010). Restoring blood-brain barrier P-glycoprotein reduces brain amyloid-β in a mouse model of Alzheimer's disease. *Mol. Pharmacol.* 77, 715–723. doi: 10.1124/mol.109.061754

Hartz, A. M., Pekcec, A., Soldner, E. L., Zhong, Y., Schlichtiger, J., and Bauer, B. (2017). P-gp protein expression and transport activity in rodent seizure models and human epilepsy. *Mol. Pharm.* 14, 999–1011. doi: 10.1021/acs.molpharmaceut.6b00770

Hartz, A. M., Zhong, Y., Wolf, A., LeVine, H., III, Miller, D. S., and Bauer, B. (2016). Aβ40 reduces P-glycoprotein at the blood-brain barrier through the ubiquitin-proteasome pathway. *J. Neurosci.* 36, 1930–1941. doi: 10.1523/JNEUROSCI.0350-15.2016

Hong, L., Huang, H.-C., and Jiang, Z.-F. (2014). Relationship between amyloid-β and the ubiquitin-proteasome system in Alzheimer's disease. *Neurol. Res.* 36, 276–282. doi: 10.1179/1743132813Y.0000000288

Jeynes, B., and Provias, J. (2011). The case for blood-brain barrier dysfunction in the pathogenesis of Alzheimer's disease. *J. Neurosci. Res.* 89, 22–28. doi: 10.1002/jnr.22527

Kabashi, E., Agar, J. N., Taylor, D. M., Minotti, S., and Durham, H. D. (2004). Focal dysfunction of the proteasome: a pathogenic factor in a mouse model of amyotrophic lateral sclerosis. *J. Neurochem.* 89, 1325–1335. doi: 10.1111/j.1471-4159.2004.02453.x

Katayama, K., Fujiwara, C., Noguchi, K., and Sugimoto, Y. (2016). RSK1 protects P-glycoprotein/ABCB1 against ubiquitin-proteasomal degradation by downregulating the ubiquitin-conjugating enzyme E2 R1. *Sci. Rep.* 6:36134. doi: 10.1038/srep36134

Katayama, K., Noguchi, K., and Sugimoto, Y. (2013). FBXO15 regulates P-glycoprotein/ABCB1 expression through the ubiquitin-proteasome pathway in cancer cells. *Cancer Sci.* 104, 694–702. doi: 10.1111/cas.12145

Keck, S., Nitsch, R., Grune, T., and Ullrich, O. (2003). Proteasome inhibition by paired helical filament-tau in brains of patients with Alzheimer's disease. *J. Neurochem.* 85, 115–122. doi: 10.1046/j.1471-4159.2003.01642.x

Keller, J. N., Hanni, K. B., and Markesbery, W. R. (2000). Impaired proteasome function in Alzheimer's disease. *J. Neurochem.* 75, 436–439. doi: 10.1046/j.1471-4159.2000.0750436.x

Kniepert, A., and Groettrup, M. (2014). The unique functions of tissue-specific proteasomes. *Trends Biochem. Sci.* 39, 17–24. doi: 10.1016/j.tibs.2013.10.004

Kuhnke, D., Jedlitschky, G., Grube, M., Krohn, M., Jucker, M., Mosyagin, I., et al. (2007). MDR1-P-glycoprotein (ABCB1) mediates transport of Alzheimer's amyloid-β peptides–implications for the mechanisms of A β clearance at the blood-brain barrier. *Brain Pathol.* 17, 347–353. doi: 10.1111/j.1750-3639.2007.00075.x

Lam, F. C., Liu, R. H., Lu, P. H., Shapiro, A. B., Renoir, J. M., Sharom, F. J., et al. (2001). β-Amyloid efflux mediated by p-glycoprotein. *J. Neurochem.* 76, 1121–1128. doi: 10.1046/j.1471-4159.2001.00113.x

Lindsten, K., de Vrij, F. M., Verhoef, L. G., Fischer, D. F., van Leeuwen, F. W., Hol, E. M., et al. (2002). Mutant ubiquitin found in neurodegenerative disorders is a ubiquitin fusion degradation substrate that blocks proteasomal degradation. *J. Cell Biol.* 157, 417–427. doi: 10.1083/jcb.200111034

Loo, T. W., and Clarke, D. M. (1998). Quality control by proteases in the endoplasmic reticulum removal of a protease-sensitive site enhances expression of human P-glycoprotein. *J. Biol. Chem.* 273, 32373–32376. doi: 10.1074/jbc.273.49.32373

Mawuenyega, K. G., Sigurdson, W., Ovod, V., Munsell, L., Kasten, T., Morris, J. C., et al. (2010). Decreased clearance of CNS β-amyloid in Alzheimer's disease. *Science* 330, 1774–1774. doi: 10.1126/science.1197623

Mayor, U., and Peng, J. (2012). Deciphering tissue-specific ubiquitylation by mass spectrometry. *Methods Mol. Biol.* 832, 65–80. doi: 10.1007/978-1-61779-474-2_3

Mehta, D. C., Short, J. L., and Nicolazzo, J. A. (2013). Altered brain uptake of therapeutics in a triple transgenic mouse model of Alzheimer's disease. *Pharm. Res.* 30, 2868–2879. doi: 10.1007/s11095-013-1116-2

Melman, L., Geuze, H. J., Li, Y., McCormick, L. M., Van Kerkhof, P., Strous, G. J., et al. (2002). Proteasome regulates the delivery of LDL receptor-related protein into the degradation pathway. *Mol. Biol. Cell* 13, 3325–3335. doi: 10.1091/mbc.e02-03-0152

Mirra, S. S., Heyman, A., McKeel, D., Sumi, S., Crain, B. J., Brownlee, L., et al. (1991). The consortium to establish a registry for Alzheimer's disease (CERAD) part II. Standardization of the neuropathologic assessment of Alzheimer's disease. *Neurology* 41:479. doi: 10.1212/wnl.41.4.479

Morawe, T., Hiebel, C., Kern, A., and Behl, C. (2012). Protein homeostasis, aging and Alzheimer's disease. *Mol. Neurobiol.* 46, 41–54. doi: 10.1007/s12035-012-8246-0

Nalepa, G., Rolfe, M., and Harper, J. W. (2006). Drug discovery in the ubiquitin-proteasome system. *Nat. Rev. Drug Discov.* 5, 596–613. doi: 10.1038/nrd2056

Nelson, P. T., Jicha, G. A., Schmitt, F. A., Liu, H., Davis, D. G., Mendiondo, M. S., et al. (2007). Clinicopathologic correlations in a large Alzheimer disease center autopsy cohort: neuritic plaques and neurofibrillary tangles "do count" when staging disease severity. *J. Neuropathol. Exp. Neurol.* 66, 1136–1146. doi: 10.1097/nen.0b013e31815c5efb

Oddo, S. (2008). The ubiquitin-proteasome system in Alzheimer's disease. *J. Cell. Mol. Med.* 12, 363–373. doi: 10.1111/j.1582-4934.2008.00276.x

O'Neill, R. A., Bhamidipati, A., Bi, X., Deb-Basu, D., Cahill, L., Ferrante, J., et al. (2006). Isoelectric focusing technology quantifies protein signaling in 25 cells. *Proc. Natl. Acad. Sci. U S A* 103, 16153–16158. doi: 10.1073/pnas.0607973103

Ortega, Z., and Lucas, J. J. (2014). Ubiquitin-proteasome system involvement in Huntington's disease. *Front. Mol. Neurosci.* 7:77. doi: 10.3389/fnmol.2014.00077

Park, R., Kook, S., Park, J., and Mook-Jung, I. (2014). Aβ1–42 reduces P-glycoprotein in the blood-brain barrier through RAGE-NF-κB signaling. *Cell Death Dis.* 5:e1299. doi: 10.1038/cddis.2014.258

Patel, M. B., and Majetschak, M. (2007). Distribution and interrelationship of ubiquitin proteasome pathway component activities and ubiquitin pools in various porcine tissues. *Physiol. Res.* 56, 341–350.

Perry, G., Friedman, R., Shaw, G., and Chau, V. (1987). Ubiquitin is detected in neurofibrillary tangles and senile plaque neurites of Alzheimer disease brains. *Proc. Natl. Acad. Sci. U S A* 84, 3033–3036. doi: 10.1073/pnas.84.9.3033

Rao, P. S., Mallya, K. B., Srivenugopal, K. S., Balaji, K., and Rao, U. S. (2006). RNF2 interacts with the linker region of the human P-glycoprotein. *Int. J. Oncol.* 29, 1413–1419.

Ravindranath, A. K., Kaur, S., Wernyj, R. P., Kumaran, M. N., Miletti-Gonzalez, K. E., Chan, R., et al. (2015). CD44 promotes multi-drug resistance by protecting P-glycoprotein from FBXO21-mediated ubiquitination. *Oncotarget* 6, 26308–26321. doi: 10.18632/oncotarget.4763

Riederer, B. M., Leuba, G., Vernay, A., and Riederer, I. M. (2011). The role of the ubiquitin proteasome system in Alzheimer's disease. *Exp. Biol. Med.* 236, 268–276. doi: 10.1258/ebm.2010.010327

Ross, C. A., and Pickart, C. M. (2004). The ubiquitin-proteasome pathway in Parkinson's disease and other neurodegenerative diseases. *Trends Cell Biol.* 14, 703–711. doi: 10.1016/j.tcb.2004.10.006

Shabek, N., Herman-Bachinsky, Y., and Ciechanover, A. (2009). Ubiquitin degradation with its substrate, or as a monomer in a ubiquitination-independent mode, provides clues to proteasome regulation. *Proc. Natl. Acad. Sci. U S A* 106, 11907–11912. doi: 10.1073/pnas.0905746106

Silverberg, G. D., Messier, A. A., Miller, M. C., Machan, J. T., Majmudar, S. S., Stopa, E. G., et al. (2010). Amyloid efflux transporter expression at the blood-brain barrier declines in normal aging. *J. Neuropathol. Exp. Neurol.* 69, 1034–1043. doi: 10.1097/NEN.0b013e3181f46e25

Storck, S. E., Meister, S., Nahrath, J., Meißner, J. N., Schubert, N., Di Spiezio, A., et al. (2016). Endothelial LRP1 transports amyloid-β_{1-42} across the blood-brain barrier. *J. Clin. Invest.* 126, 123–136. doi: 10.1172/JCI81108

Urushitani, M., Kurisu, J., Tsukita, K., and Takahashi, R. (2002). Proteasomal inhibition by misfolded mutant superoxide dismutase 1 induces selective motor neuron death in familial amyotrophic lateral sclerosis. *J. Neurochem.* 83, 1030–1042. doi: 10.1046/j.1471-4159.2002.01211.x

van Assema, D. M., Lubberink, M., Bauer, M., van der Flier, W. M., Schuit, R. C., Windhorst, A. D., et al. (2012). Blood-brain barrier P-glycoprotein function in Alzheimer's disease. *Brain* 135, 181–189. doi: 10.1093/brain/awr298

van Leeuwen, F., van Tijn, P., Sonnemans, M., Hobo, B., Mann, D., Van Broeckhoven, C., et al. (2006). Frameshift proteins in autosomal dominant forms of Alzheimer disease and other tauopathies. *Neurology* 66, S86–S92. doi: 10.1212/01.wnl.0000193882.46003.6d

Wang, W., Bodles-Brakhop, A. M., and Barger, S. W. (2016). A role for P-glycoprotein in clearance of alzheimer amyloid β-peptide from the brain. *Curr. Alzheimer Res.* 13, 615–620. doi: 10.2174/1567205013666160314151012

Wenger, R. M. (1986). Cyclosporine and analogues—isolation and synthesis—mechanism of action and structural requirements for pharmacological activity. *Fortschr. Chem. Org. Naturst.* 50, 123–168. doi: 10.1007/978-3-7091-8888-0_4

Wijesuriya, H. C., Bullock, J. Y., Faull, R. L., Hladky, S. B., and Barrand, M. A. (2010). ABC efflux transporters in brain vasculature of Alzheimer's subjects. *Brain Res.* 1358, 228–238. doi: 10.1016/j.brainres.2010.08.034

Yang, Y., Kitagaki, J., Dai, R.-M., Tsai, Y. C., Lorick, K. L., Ludwig, R. L., et al. (2007). Inhibitors of ubiquitin-activating enzyme (E1), a new class of potential cancer therapeutics. *Cancer Res.* 67, 9472–9481. doi: 10.1158/0008-5472.CAN-07-0568

Yuede, C. M., Lee, H., Restivo, J. L., Davis, T. A., Hettinger, J. C., Wallace, C. E., et al. (2016). Rapid *in vivo* measurement of β-amyloid reveals biphasic clearance kinetics in an Alzheimer's mouse model. *J. Exp. Med.* 213, 677–685. doi: 10.1084/jem.20151428

Zhang, Z., Wu, J.-Y., Hait, W. N., and Yang, J.-M. (2004). Regulation of the stability of P-glycoprotein by ubiquitination. *Mol. Pharmacol.* 66, 395–403. doi: 10.1124/mol.104.001966

Zlokovic, B. V. (2005). Neurovascular mechanisms of Alzheimer's neurodegeneration. *Trends Neurosci.* 28, 202–208. doi: 10.1016/j.tins.2005.02.001

13

Hyperhomocysteinemia as a Risk Factor for Vascular Contributions to Cognitive Impairment and Dementia

*Brittani R. Price, Donna M. Wilcock and Erica M. Weekman**

Department of Physiology, Sanders-Brown Center on Aging, University of Kentucky, Lexington, KY, United States

Correspondence:
Erica M. Weekman
emweek2@uky.edu

Behind only Alzheimer's disease, vascular contributions to cognitive impairment and dementia (VCID) is the second most common cause of dementia, affecting roughly 10–40% of dementia patients. While there is no cure for VCID, several risk factors for VCID, such as diabetes, hypertension, and stroke, have been identified. Elevated plasma levels of homocysteine, termed hyperhomocysteinemia (HHcy), are a major, yet underrecognized, risk factor for VCID. B vitamin deficiency, which is the most common cause of HHcy, is common in the elderly. With B vitamin supplementation being a relatively safe and inexpensive therapeutic, the treatment of HHcy-induced VCID would seem straightforward; however, preclinical and clinical data shows it is not. Clinical trials using B vitamin supplementation have shown conflicting results about the benefits of lowering homocysteine and issues have arisen over proper study design within the trials. Studies using cell culture and animal models have proposed several mechanisms for homocysteine-induced cognitive decline, providing other targets for therapeutics. For this review, we will focus on HHcy as a risk factor for VCID, specifically, the different mechanisms proposed for homocysteine-induced cognitive decline and the clinical trials aimed at lowering plasma homocysteine.

Keywords: hyperhomocysteinemia, vascular cognitive impairment and dementia, B vitamins, homocysteine, dementia

INTRODUCTION

Vascular contributions to cognitive impairment and dementia (VCID) are defined as the conditions arising from vascular brain injuries that induce significant changes to memory, thinking, and behavior. It is the leading cause of dementia behind only Alzheimer's disease (AD); however, there is increasing awareness of the co-morbidity of VCID and AD (Bowler et al., 1998; Zekry et al., 2002; Langa et al., 2004; Jellinger and Attems, 2010). Roughly 60% of AD patients have VCID, and it is thought that vascular injuries act as an extra "hit" to the brain that lowers the threshold for cognitive impairment in persons with AD pathology (Schneider and Bennett, 2010; Vemuri and Knopman, 2016). Also, it is suggested that patients with both AD pathology and VCID have a shorter time to dementia and their rate of cognitive decline is faster (Schneider and Bennett, 2010; Vemuri and Knopman, 2016). Recent studies have also shown that vascular injury precedes AD pathologies, highlighting a role for the vasculature in AD progression (Canobbio et al., 2015; Janota et al., 2016).

While there is no cure for VCID, several studies have identified risk factors that can be modified to reduce risk of developing VCID. A major, yet underrecognized, modifiable risk factor for VCID is hyperhomocysteinemia (HHcy). Defined as elevated plasma levels of homocysteine, a non-protein forming amino acid, HHcy has been identified as a risk factor for cardiovascular disease, stroke, VCID, and AD (Graham et al., 1997; Bostom et al., 1999; Eikelboom et al., 1999; Beydoun et al., 2014). Studies have shown that serum homocysteine levels are inversely related to cognitive function in patients with dementia and elevated levels are more common among VCID patients than among AD patients (Miller et al., 2002; Clarke et al., 2003). Elevated plasma homocysteine is also associated with hippocampal atrophy, white matter lesions, and lacunar infarcts (Vermeer et al., 2002; Firbank et al., 2010). In the clinic, it is clear that HHcy plays a role in VCID; however, the mechanisms of homocysteine-induced cognitive impairment and the clinical implications of reducing homocysteine remain unclear. This review paper will focus on proposed mechanisms of homocysteine in the brain, and the clinical trials aimed at lowering homocysteine levels.

HOMOCYSTEINE METABOLISM

Homocysteine is produced in all cells and involved in the metabolism of cysteine and methionine (Selhub, 1999). Normal levels of homocysteine range between 5 and 15 μmol/L. Levels between 15 and 30 μmol/L are considered mild, levels at 30–100 μmol/L are moderate and levels above 100 μmol/L are considered severe HHcy. During normal metabolism, ATP activates methionine to form *S*-adenosylmethionine (SAM). SAM is a methyl donor to several different receptors and forms *S*-adenosylhomocysteine (SAH) as a by-product of this methyl reaction. SAH can then be hydrolyzed to form homocysteine. Homocysteine can also go through two different re-methylation processes to form methionine again. In one pathway, folate is reduced to tetrahydrofolate which is then converted to 5, 10-methylenetetrahydrofolate. Methylenetetrahydrofolate reductase (MTHFR) reduces 5, 10-methylenetetrahydrofate to 5-methyltetrahydrofolate. Finally, 5-methyltetrahydrofolate and the essential cofactor vitamin B12 add a methyl group to homocysteine to form methionine again. In an alternative pathway, betaine–homocysteine *S*-methyltransferase (BHMT) uses betaine synthesized from choline as a methyl group to convert homocysteine back to methionine.

Homocysteine can also go through a transsulfuration pathway to form cysteine. Serine can be enzymatically added to homocysteine by cystathionine beta synthase (CBS) and vitamin B6 to form cystathionine (Locasale, 2013). Cystathionine can then be cleaved by cystathionine gamma lyase (CGL) to form cysteine. While cysteine can be converted back to cystathionine, cystathionine cannot be converted to homocysteine again. The homocysteine metabolic pathway is shown in **Figure 1**.

MECHANISMS OF HOMOCYSTEINE-INDUCED COGNITIVE IMPAIRMENT

Posttranslational Modification of Proteins

As mentioned above, homocysteine is produced in all cells; however, its conversion to cysteine or back to methionine does not. The brain lacks both CGL and BHMT, making it dependent on the folate cycle for re-methylation of homocysteine to methionine (Sunden et al., 1997). While this makes the brain especially vulnerable to raised levels of homocysteine, the mechanisms of homocysteine toxicity in the brain remain unclear, with several different mechanisms proposed. Some studies suggest the post-translational modification of proteins by homocysteine, termed homocysteinylation, contributes to its toxicity, especially since the degree of homocysteinylation is proportional to increased level of plasma homocysteine (Jakubowski, 1999; Jakubowski et al., 2000; Perla-Kajan et al., 2007). In the presence of adenosine triphosphate, methionyl-tRNA synthase catalyzes the conversion of homocysteine to homocysteine-thiolactone, which has been shown to homocysteinylate proteins and alter their functions. Specifically, homocysteine thiolactone acts as a Na/K ATPase inhibitor in the hippocampus and cortex of rat brain cells, thus changing the membrane potential of neurons (Rasic-Markovic et al., 2009).

Oxidative Stress

Other studies suggest homocysteine induces cellular damage via oxidative stress. As mentioned above, during normal homocysteine metabolism, cysteine is produced. Cysteine is a precursor for glutathione, which is a tripeptide that ultimately reduces reactive oxygen species. Without homocysteine conversion to cysteine, either due to CBS mutations or a diet lacking in vitamin B6, glutathione levels decrease, leading to increased reactive oxygen species and ultimately oxidative stress. Homocysteine metabolism is also regulated by the redox potential in a cell since several enzymes involved in its metabolism are regulated by the oxidative status (Zou and Banerjee, 2005). In one instance, the activity of methionine synthase is lowered when reactive oxygen species are high (Zou and Banerjee, 2005). Studies have also shown an increase in neurodegeneration due to homocysteine-related oxidative stress. In cultured embryonic cortical neurons and differentiated SH-SY-5Y human neuroblastoma cells grown in folate free media, there was an increase in cytosolic calcium, reactive oxygen species, and apoptosis (Ho et al., 2003). A significant increase in homocysteine was also found and inhibiting formation of homocysteine prevented the increase in reactive oxygen species. The increase in reactive oxygen species due to HHcy also alters smooth muscle function and promotes proliferation of smooth muscles cells (Welch and Loscalzo, 1998). Homocysteine has also been shown to inhibit endothelial nitric oxide synthase (eNOS) activity in cultured aortic endothelial cells from adult mice (Jiang et al., 2005) and humans (Jiang et al., 2005). In a genetic mouse model of HHcy where the CBS gene is absent, homozygote knockout mice show reduced eNOS activity compared to wildtype mice (Jiang et al., 2005). While the decreased activity of eNOS can affect oxidative stress, it also inhibits endothelial-dependent vasodilation. Taken together with the changes in vascular smooth muscle cells, these data provide further insight into how homocysteine is a risk factor for VCID.

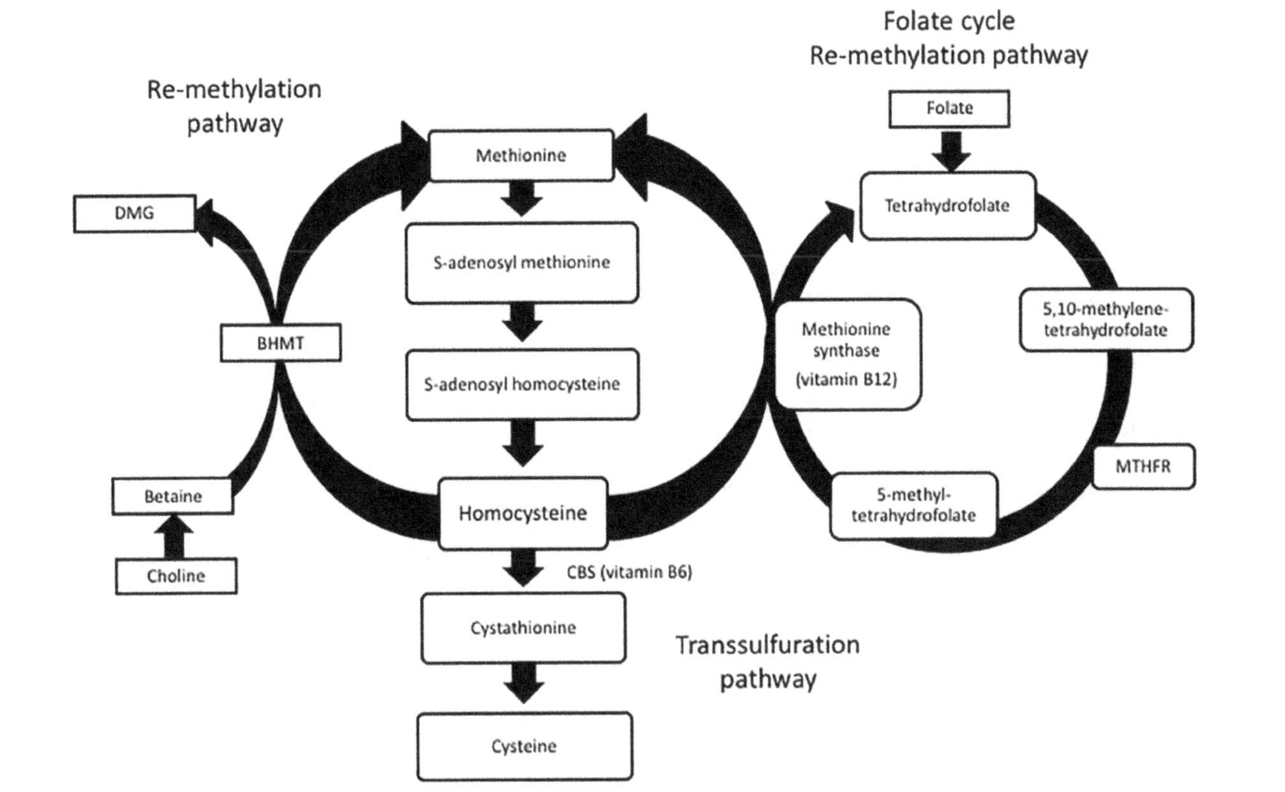

FIGURE 1 | Homocysteine metabolism: homocysteine is converted to methionine or cysteine via remethylation or transsulfuration pathways. Dimethylglycine (DMG), betaine-homocysteine *S*-methyltransferase (BHMT), methylenetetrahydrofolate reductase (MTHFR).

AMPA and NMDA Receptors

Another proposed mechanism for homocysteine neurodegeneration involves homocysteine's role as an agonist for AMPA (both metabotropic and ionotropic) and NMDA receptors. Homocysteic acid, an oxidative product of homocysteine that is released in response to excitatory stimulation, acts an excitatory neurotransmitter by activating the NMDA receptor (Cuenod et al., 1990). Activation of both AMPA and NMDA receptors leads to increased intracellular calcium, which in turn leads to activation of several kinases (Robert et al., 2005). Overstimulation of these receptors due to HHcy can then lead to increased free radicals and caspases, which leads to apoptosis (Mattson and Shea, 2003) and neurodegeneration. Using an NMDA antagonist can block the neurotoxic effects of homocysteic acid in the brain (Olney et al., 1987).

Cerebrovascular

The study of animal models has also lent insight into the mechanisms of homocysteine toxicity and its role in VCID. Several animal models have shown that high plasma levels of homocysteine are sufficient to cause cognitive deficits and vascular adverse events in the brain. Induction of HHcy in an animal model can be achieved via genetic manipulation or diet. Genetic manipulation of either CBS or MTHFR can produce mouse models of HHcy. In humans, deficiencies in CBS result in elevated plasma levels of homocysteine and thrombosis and are the most common cause of hereditary HHcy. $CBS^{\pm}$ heterozygote mice have a 50% lower CBS activity compared to wildtype mice and develop mild HHcy (Watanabe et al., 1995). These mice show endothelial damage, thickened cerebral arteriolar walls, mild hypertension, and blood–brain barrier dysfunction (Baumbach et al., 2002; Weiss et al., 2003; Kamath et al., 2006). In humans, there are several polymorphisms in MTHFR that produce HHcy and neurological conditions such as a progressive demyelinating neuropathy and cognitive impairment (Clayton et al., 1986; Hyland et al., 1988; Surtees et al., 1991). Chen et al. (2001) deleted the MTHFR gene to create a mouse model of HHcy that exhibits motor and gait abnormalities within 5 weeks after birth. $MTHFR^{-/-}$ homozygotes also present with some loss of function in cerebral vessels and abnormal lipid deposition in the aorta and disruption of the laminar structure of the cerebellum with no obvious changes in the cortex or cerebrum (Neves et al., 2004).

Unlike MTHFR and CBS knockout mice, dietary induction of HHcy allows for age related HHcy to be studied. Dietary induction of HHcy in mice and rats can be achieved through a reduction in the essential cofactors needed for homocysteine conversion (folate, vitamins B6, and B12) or enrichment in methionine, which increases the conversion of methionine to homocysteine. A combination of these diets or even a diet of increased homocysteine can also be used to induce HHcy. Troen et al. (2008) showed that feeding mice a B vitamin deficient diet resulted in cognitive impairment on the Morris water maze and rarefaction of brain capillaries. In another animal model, 6-month-old Sprague–Dawley rats were placed on a diet deficient in folate for 8 weeks. By the end of the 8 weeks, the rats on the folate deficient diet had increased homocysteine levels, ultrastructural changes to cerebral capillaries, endothelial damage, swelling of pericytes, basement membrane thickening, and fibrosis (Kim et al., 2002). Cognitive impairments, decreased acetylcholine in the brain and microhemorrhages were seen in rats that were fed a diet high in homocysteine for 5 or 15 months (Pirchl et al., 2010).

Our lab has also recently developed a model of VCID by inducing HHcy in order to investigate the mechanisms of homocysteine-induced cognitive impairment. We placed 3-month-old C57BL6 mice on a combination diet that is deficient in folate and vitamins B6 and B12 and enriched in methionine (Sudduth et al., 2013) for 3 months. At the end of the 3 months, plasma homocysteine levels reached moderate levels in the mice on the homocysteine diet (82.93 ± 3.561 μmol/L compared to 5.89 ± 0.385 μmol/L in the control mice). When tested on the radial arm water maze for behavioral deficits, these mice exhibited significant cognitive impairments in spatial memory. Prussian blue staining and magnetic resonance imaging showed microhemorrhages were the main cerebrovascular pathology induced by the HHcy diet. The mice on the HHcy diet also had an increase in several pro-inflammatory cytokines along with an increase in matrix metalloproteinase 9 (MMP9) activity. MMP9 has been shown to degrade tight junctions, leading to microhemorrhages and dystroglycans, and the pro-inflammatory cytokines, tumor necrosis factor alpha (TNFα), and interleukin 1 beta (IL-1β), stimulate its transcription (Galis et al., 1994; Vecil et al., 2000; Michaluk et al., 2007; Candelario-Jalil et al., 2011; Klein and Bischoff, 2011). Previous studies have also shown homocysteine can induce MMP9 release from mouse cerebral microvessel endothelial cells (Shastry and Tyagi, 2004). Based on this data, another possible mechanism for homocysteine-induced cognitive impairment could be the pro-inflammatory mediated increase in MMP9 leading to tight junction degradation, microhemorrhages, and, finally, cognitive impairment.

Astrocytes

In addition to the pathologies listed above, we have also shown that astrocytic end-feet are disrupted in the mice on the HHcy diet (Sudduth et al., 2017). In the brain, astrocytes make up 50% of the cells and their processes, termed astrocytic end-feet, sheath arterioles, and capillaries. The main function of astrocytic end-feet is to maintain ionic and osmotic homeostasis in the brain (Simard and Nedergaard, 2004). To do this, astrocytes have aquaporin four water channels and several potassium channels located at their end-feet. In our mice on the HHcy diet, we found a significant decrease in these channels, as well as other structural markers located at the end-foot. These decreases in the end-foot channels occur after 10 weeks on the HHcy diet. Cognitive deficits and microhemorrhages are also seen starting at 10 weeks on diet. Interestingly, increases in the pro-inflammatory cytokines, TNFα, and IL-1 β, occur after only 6 weeks on diet. We had also previously shown that MMP9 was significantly increased in mice on the HHcy diet (Sudduth et al., 2013). Taken together, we hypothesize that another mechanism of homocysteine-induced cognitive impairment involves the inflammatory-MMP9 pathway. In our hypothesis, homocysteine increases TNFα and IL-1β expression, which in turn activates MMP9, which degrades dystroglycans, a key structural component that anchors the astrocytic end-foot to the basal lamina of the vessels. This disruption of the astrocytic end-foot leads to impaired ionic and osmotic buffering and eventual cognitive impairment.

While several mechanisms of homocysteine-induced cognitive impairment and neurodegeneration have been proposed and discussed here, it is unlikely that homocysteine acts through only one of these mechanisms. Homocysteine may act through several, if not all of these mechanisms. It is also unclear whether the high levels of homocysteine or the lack of B vitamins is the main cause behind the cognitive impairment seen in hyperhomocysteinemic patients. Discussed next are the clinical implications of HHcy and the potential therapeutics tested in clinical trials to lower homocysteine levels and improve cognition.

HYPERHOMOCYSTEINEMIA IN THE CLINICAL SETTING

Extensive clinical data support the role of HHcy as a risk factor for VCID. Given that normal and abnormal values are set by individual clinical laboratories, mild-moderate HHcy is loosely defined by clinical standards (Moll and Varga, 2015). However, plasma homocysteine concentrations ranging from 15 and 100 μmol/L are uniformly considered to be indicative of clinically relevant HHcy. Gibson et al. (1964) reported vascular anomalies in patients with homocystinuria (elevated concentration of homocysteine in both plasma and urine), and McCully (1969) introduced his homocysteine hypothesis which connected HHcy with an increased risk of atherosclerosis (Abraham and Cho, 2010). To date, HHcy continues to serve as a widely recognized risk factor for coronary artery disease (CAD), peripheral vascular disease, myocardial infarction (MI), and cerebrovascular disease (CVD; Maron and Loscalzo, 2009). Of particular importance here is the association between HHcy and CVD. CVD can manifest as a stroke, white matter disease, cerebral large vessel disease (atherosclerosis), and cerebral small vessel disease (arteriosclerosis), all of which can independently induce cognitive impairment ranging from subtle deficits to frank dementia (Troen et al., 2008; Maron and Loscalzo, 2009; Hainsworth et al., 2016). Furthermore, HHcy has been associated with hippocampal and white matter atrophy in older subjects with mild hypertension, as well as an increased rate of hippocampal atrophy and cognitive decline in elderly patients (Clarke et al., 1998; Firbank et al., 2010). As suggested by the variety of cellular actions of homocysteine described above, there is no shortage of candidate mechanisms by which HHcy induces cognitive impairment despite known etiologies.

Hyperhomocysteinemia vs. Homocystinuria

Both genetic mutations and dietary vitamin deficiencies can affect homocysteine levels resulting in HHcy. Several polymorphisms (notably C677T and A1298C) have been identified in the MTHFR gene in humans, which can induce severe HHcy (>100 μmol/L, termed homocystinuria) by limiting conversion of homocysteine back to methionine (Moll and Varga, 2015; Hainsworth et al., 2016). While rare, these polymorphisms induce progressive demyelinating neuropathy and cognitive impairment (Clayton et al., 1986; Hyland et al., 1988; Surtees et al., 1991). That being said, deficiencies in CBS, the rate-limiting enzyme of the aforementioned transsulfuration pathway, are the most common cause of homocystinuria and may result in thrombosis and low levels of cysteine (Sacharow et al., 1993). In contrast to HHcy, homocystinuria is a rare autosomal recessive metabolic disorder characterized by severely elevated plasma homocysteine and subsequently elevated urine homocysteine concentrations. Patients suffering homocystinuria present with developmental delay, osteoporosis, ocular abnormalities, thromoemobolic disease, and severe premature atherosclerosis (Poloni et al., 2018). Given that less marked elevations in plasma homocysteine (i.e., HHcy) are much more common, homocystinuria will not be further discussed in this review. Less marked elevations in plasma homocysteine, referred to as HHcy, may be attributed to factors such as smoking, aging, renal failure, and low dietary levels of folate and vitamins B6 and B12 (Hainsworth et al., 2016).

Prevalence of B Vitamin Deficiency

As suggested, clinical mild–moderate HHcy is common, especially in elderly patients, with the majority of cases resulting from insufficient B vitamin status (Joosten et al., 1993; Troen et al., 2008). The association of B vitamin status and normal central nervous system function dates back to 1849 when Addison reported on the "wandering mind" of patients with pernicious anemia (Smith and Refsum, 2016). Reports of insufficient B vitamin status with concomitant induction of HHcy trace back to a landmark report by the Framingham Heart Study in 1993. A cohort of 1041 elderly participants (418 men, 623 women) between the ages of 67 and 96 showed that plasma homocysteine becomes elevated due to dietary deficiencies in B6 and folic acid and decreased absorption of B12 (Selhub, 2006; McCully, 2007):

According to the Framingham report, daily intake of 3 mg vitamin B6 and 400 μg of folic acid are required to prevent elevations in plasma homocysteine concentration (Selhub, 2006; McCully, 2007). In support of these amounts of dietary B vitamins, the Nurses' Health Study revealed that similar levels of dietary B6 and folic acid prevent mortality and morbidity from heart disease (Rimm et al., 1998; McCully, 2007). In the United States, mandatory fortification of grains with folic acid was authorized in 1996 and fully implemented in 1998 (Crider et al., 2011). Prior to fortification of grain products, intakes of B6 and folic acid were well below the recommended quantities (McCully, 2007). By contrast, with the exception of those partaking in a vegan diet, vitamin B12 intake is typically adequate. However, in those >65 years of age lack of gastric acidity, decreased intrinsic factor synthesis by gastric mucosal cells, and history or presence of *H. pylori* infection may contribute to inadequate B12 absorption (McCully, 2007). Not to mention, the aging process itself is associated with decreased ability to absorb B vitamins, which can lead to a gradually rising plasma homocysteine concentration (estimated at 1 μmol/L/decade) (McCully, 2007). Literature now suggests between 5 and 30% of the general population, and 25% of those with vascular diseases, to be affected by HHcy (Selhub, 2006; Peng et al., 2015; Yeh et al., 2016). Granted, because blood homocysteine panels are generally ordered only when patients experience a MI or stroke without traditional risk factors, the aforementioned prevalence of HHcy in the general population is likely skewed and possibly underestimated.

HHcy, B Vitamin Status, and Cognition

Regardless, public significance of HHcy in the elderly population should not be ignored given that it is easily treatable with B vitamin fortification and serves as a modifiable risk factor for development of cognitive decline, dementia, and AD. A number of early cross-sectional studies relating HHcy or insufficient B vitamin status to cognitive impairment led to generation of the hypotheses suggesting a causal link. In effort to address whether the hypothesis that HHcy induces cognitive impairment is correct, a number of clinical trials have assessed B vitamin refortification with cognitive endpoints. These vitamin refortification trials are outlined in **Table 1**. Additionally, several meta-analyses of these intervention trials have been conducted (Wald et al., 2010; Ford and Almeida, 2012; Clarke et al., 2014). Upon review, the general consensus suggests that homocysteine-lowering by B vitamin refortification has no significant effect on individual or global cognitive domains despite three trials (FACIT, WAFACS, VITACOG) supporting a beneficial effect. However, when interpreting the results of these trials one needs to consider the fact that many were compromised by the challenges of performing a cognitive clinical trial (cohort age, B vitamin status of said cohort, trial duration, statistical power, etc.).

Limitations of Clinical Trials

As suggested, a number of factors related to trial design and implementation must be considered. First and foremost, the hypothesis being tested should be considered. Assuming the hypothesis is that homocysteine-lowering supplementation with B vitamins slows and/or prevents cognitive decline, those randomized to the placebo arm of the trial must exhibit cognitive decline. As reviewed in **Table 1**, as well as the aforementioned meta-analyses, the majority of trials conducted fail to report significant cognitive decline in those randomized to the placebo arm. Meaning these trials are limited to showing only that B vitamin treatment does not worsen cognition. Additionally, the age range of trial participants must be considered. Referring to the hypothesis above, if cognition is a study measure the age of the participants should reflect the timeframe in which cognitive decline and dementia occur. Duration of the intervention must also be considered given that elderly individuals exhibiting

TABLE 1 | B vitamin clinical trials.

Reference	Sample size	Mean participant age (years)	Selection criteria	Intervention	Duration of intervention (years)	Cognitive domains assessed	Additional Study Endpoints	Study Conclusion	Study Limitations
Lewerin et al., 2005	*n* = 209; 126 intervention, 69 placebo	76	Community-dwelling men and women	Placebo vs. 500 μg B12, 800 μg folic acid, 3 mg B6	0.3	Short-term memory, long-term memory, perceptual speed, verbal ability, spatial ability, inductive reasoning	Plasma [Hcy], postural-locomotor-manual (PLM) test	Despite normalization of plasma [Hcy], B vitamin supplementation did not improve cognitive performance.	No reported, significant decline in cognition observed in participants randomized to the placebo arm.
Eussen et al., 2006	*n* = 195; 65 intervention, 65 placebo	82–83	Patients with suspected, mild B12 deficiency	Placebo vs. 1000 μg B12 vs. 1000 μg B12, 400 μg folic acid	0.5	Attention, construction, sensorimotor speed, short-term memory, executive function	Plasma [Hcy]	Supplementation with B12 alone or in combination with folic acid does not improve cognitive performance.	No reported, significant decline in cognition observed in participants randomized to the placebo arm.
Stott et al., 2005	*n* = 185; 23–24/group	72–76	Patients with ischemic vascular disease	Placebo vs. 400 μg B12, 2.5 mg folic acid, 25 mg B6, 25 mg B2 (alone and in various combinations)	1	TICS-M, Information processing	Plasma [Hcy]	Despite normalization of plasma [Hcy], B vitamin supplementation did not improve cognitive performance.	No reported, significant decline in cognition observed in participants randomized to the placebo arm.
VISP Trial Toole et al., 2004	*n* = 3680; 1853 low-dose intervention, 1827 high-dose intervention	66	Patients with history of non-disabling cerebral infarction	Low-dose: 6 μg B12, 20 μg folic acid, 0.2 mg B6 vs. high-dose: 400 μg B12, 2.5 mg folic acid, 25 mg B6	1.8	MMSE	Plasma [Hcy], recurrent cerebral infarction, CHD, death	Despite normalization of plasma [Hcy] in both the low-dose and high-dose intervention groups, supplementation did not improve cognitive performance.	No reported, significant decline in cognition observed in participants randomized to the low-dose intervention.
VITACOG trial Smith et al., 2010; de Jager et al., 2012	*n* = 168; 85 intervention, 83 placebo	76–77	Patients > 70 years with evident MCI (MCI = TICS–M 17–29/30)	Placebo vs. oral TrioBe Plus® containing 0.8 mg folic acid, 0.5 mg B12, 20 mg B6	2	Episodic memory, semantic memory, global cognition (MMSE)	Plamsa [Hcy], Rate of brain atrophy	Sevenfold less regional atrophy in intervention group vs. placebo group. However, this effect was significant only in those with elevated Hcy above the median (i.e., >11.3 μmol.L). Individuals with baseline plasma Hcy above the median, cognitive decline was prevented across all domains assessed.	VITACOG was not powered to detect any effect of plasma [Hcy] on cognition.

(Continued)

TABLE 1 | Continued

Reference	Sample size	Mean participant age (years)	Selection criteria	Intervention	Duration of intervention (years)	Cognitive domains assessed	Additional Study Endpoints	Study Conclusion	Study Limitations
McMahon et al., 2006	n = 253; 127 intervention, 126 placebo	73–74	Patients with plasma [Hcy] > 13 μmol/L but normal creatinine concentrations	Placebo vs. 500 μg B12, 1000 μg folic acid, 10 mg B6	2.2	Short-term memory, Learning capacity, Verbal fluency, Semantic fluency, Information processing, Reasoning ability	Plasma [Hcy], Plasma [creatinine]	Despite normalization of plasma [Hcy], B vitamin supplementation did not improve cognitive performance. In fact, information processing speed was improved in those randomized to the placebo arm.	No reported, significant decline in cognition observed in participants randomized to the placebo arm.
FACIT Trial Durga et al., 2007	n = 818; 405 intervention, 413 placebo	60	Patients with plasma [Hcy] > 13 and <26 μmol/L	Placebo vs. 800 μg folic acid	3	Memory, Sensorimotor speed, Complex speed, Information processing, Verbal fluency	N/A	Folic acid supplementation improved subdomains of cognitive function that typically decline with age.	N/A
Vitatops Trial Study Group, 2010	*n* = 8164; 4089 intervention, 4075 placebo	62–63	Patients with recent stroke or TIA	Placebo vs. 0.5 mg B12, 2 mg folic acid, 25 mg B6	3.2	MMSE	Plasma [Hcy], stroke, MI, vascular death	Despite normalization of plasma [Hcy], B vitamin supplementation did not improve global cognitive performance.	Baseline cognitive scores not provided.
NORVIT Trial Bonaa et al., 2006	*n* = 3749; 937 folic acid, B12, B6, 935 folic acid and B12, 934 plus B6, 943 placebo	62–63	Patients ages 30–85 years exhibiting acute MI 7 days before randomization.	Placebo vs. 40 mg B6 vs. 0.8 mg folic acid, 0.4 mg B12 vs. 0.8 mg folic acid, 0.4 mg B12, 40 mg B16 (latter referred to as “combination therapy)	3.3	None	Death, MI, unstable angina pectoris requiring hospitalization, coronary revascularization with percutaneous coronary intervention or coronary artery bypass grafting, and stroke	Despite normalization of plasma [Hcy], B vitamin supplementation did not reduce the risk of recurrent CVD following acute MI. A harmful effect from combined B vitamin supplementation was suggested.	Cognition was not assessed.
SU.FOL.OM3 Trial Andreeva et al., 2011	*n* = 1748; 884 intervention, 864 control (no supplementation)	61	Patients with vascular disease	Placebo vs. 20 μg B12, 560 μg CH3-THF, 3 mg B6 ± 600 mg 2:1 ratio of eicosapentaenoic and docosahexaenoic acid	4.5	TICS-M	Plasma [Hcy]	Despite normalization of plasma [Hcy], B vitamin supplementation did not improve global cognitive performance. However, a possible effect of B vitamin supplementation on cognitive function in those with history of stroke was noted.	Baseline cognitive scores not provided.

(Continued)

TABLE 1 | Continued

Reference	Sample size	Mean participant age (years)	Selection criteria	Intervention	Duration of intervention (years)	Cognitive domains assessed	Additional Study Endpoints	Study Conclusion	Study Limitations
HOPE-2 Trial Lonn et al., 2006	n = 5522; 2758 intervention, 2764 placebo	69	Patients with history of vascular disease or with history of diabetes and atherosclerosis	Placebo vs. 1 mg B12, 2.5 mg folic acid, 50 mg B6	4.8	MMSE	Plasma [Hcy], death resulting from CVD, MI or stroke	Despite normalization of plasma [Hcy], B vitamin supplementation did not improve global cognitive performance.	No reported, significant decline in cognition observed in participants randomized to the placebo arm.
WAFACS Trial *Sub-study of HOPE-2 Trial* Kang et al., 2008	n = 2009; 1002 intervention, 1007 placebo	71	Patients with CVD or 3 or more coronary risk factors	Placebo vs. 1 mg B12, 2.5 mg folic acid, 50 mg B6	6	TICS	N/A	B vitamin supplementation failed to delay cognitive decline among patients with CVD or CVD risk factors.	No reported, significant decline in cognition observed in participants randomized to the placebo arm.
Study of the Effectiveness of Additional Reductions in Cholesterol and Homocysteine (SEARCH) Collaborative Group et al., 2010	n = 12064; 6033 interventions, 6031 placebo	64	Patients with history of MI	Placebo + 20 mg or 80 mg simvastatin vs. 1 mg B12, 2 mg folic acid + 20mg or 80 mg simvastatin	7.1	TICS-M, verbal fluency test	Plasma [Hcy], major coronary events, stroke, noncoronary revascularizations, death attributable to vascular or non-vascular causes	Despite normalization of plasma [Hcy], B vitamin supplementation did not improve global cognitive performance.	Baseline cognitive scores not provided.

CH3-THF, methyltetrahydrofolate; CHF, congestive heart failure; CVD, cardiovascular disease; Hcy, homocysteine; MI, myocardial infarction; MMSE, mini-mental state examination; TIA, transient ischemic attack; TICS, telephone interview for cognitive status; TICS-M, modified telephone interview for cognitive status.

normal cognition generally decline only by ~0.1 points on MMSE each year (Hainsworth et al., 2016; Smith and Refsum, 2016). Thus, duration of the intervention must be sufficient to observe cognitive decline, especially if MMSE is to be used as an assessment tool. Three trials represented in **Table 1** and seven of the nine trials examined by Wald et al. (2010) in their meta-analysis were of short duration (<12 months) and therefore too short to identify an effect on cognition. Assessment tools must also be sensitive enough to detect subtle changes over the course of the trial. Collectively, age range of the trial cohort, duration of the intervention, and assessment tools will dictate whether the trial design is sufficient to detect an effect. Finally, the appropriateness of the intervention and whether the chosen cohort is likely to respond to that intervention must be considered. Supplied daily doses of B vitamins should be sufficient to lower plasma homocysteine concentrations by at least 20% (Hainsworth et al., 2016). For example, 1 trial addressed in **Table 1** prescribed doses of folic acid (0.2 mg) and vitamin B12 (1 μg) that were too low to influence plasma homocysteine (McMahon et al., 2006; Hainsworth et al., 2016). Furthermore, the baseline B vitamin status of each potential participant must be considered at the time of enrollment. This relates back to a cardinal principle of nutrition in which the relationship between vitamin status and a given outcome follows a sigmoidal curve. For example, if a participant exhibited low levels of vitamin B6, additional B6 intake would likely be beneficial, with the opposite being true if the participant's B6 intake were already high. Additionally, when at the plateau phase (i.e., adequate B6 intake), additional B6 intake will likely have no effect. Despite having critical implications for clinical trials, this principle is often overlooked. Consideration of the participant's B vitamin status at the time of enrollment would therefore aid in determining whether they are likely to respond to intervention. As such, trial enrollment should only be open to those with insufficient B vitamin status or elevated plasma homocysteine concentration at baseline. Together, these considerations suggest the conclusion that homocysteine-lowering by B vitamin supplementation has no effect on cognition is premature.

Beneficial Effects of B Vitamin Supplementation

As previously mentioned, results from three trials (FACIT, WAFACS, and VITACOG) do support a beneficial effect of B vitamin supplementation on cognition. The FACIT trial showed significant effects of B vitamins on cognition in participants with high plasma homocysteine, while the WAFACS trial showed similarly significant effects in those with inadequate B vitamin status (Durga et al., 2007; Kang et al., 2008). Furthermore, the VITACOG trial revealed strong effects of B vitamins on both rates of brain atrophy and cognition in individuals with mild cognitive impairment (MCI; Douaud et al., 2013). Further data analysis revealed the sevenfold reduction in regional brain atrophy to be significant only in those with plasma homocysteine concentrations above the median (>11.3 μmol/L) (Douaud et al., 2013). Results of the VITACOG trial thereby imply a threshold effect of plasma homocysteine on measures of brain atrophy and cognition. A threshold effect of plasma homocysteine is further supported by results of the OPTIMA study in which only plasma homocysteine concentrations >11 μmol/L were associated with an increased rate of atrophy of the medial temporal lobe (Clarke et al., 1998). The threshold concept is further supported by a study showing a plasma homocysteine concentration-dependent increase in the rate of cognitive decline in AD patients (Oulhaj et al., 2010). Jointly, these studies suggest the threshold for effect of plasma homocysteine lies between 10 and 11 μM, which may explain why studies conducted in countries that employ mandatory folic acid fortification do not find associations between plasma homocysteine and cognition. Retrospective analysis of the VITACOG data revealed that the protective effect of B vitamin supplementation on both brain atrophy and cognition only occurred in those participants with adequate omega-3 fatty acid status (Jerneren et al., 2015). Additionally, the beneficial effect of B vitamin supplementation on brain atrophy was observed only in participants not routinely taking aspirin (Smith et al., 2010). Omega-3 fatty acid and aspirin statuses may therefore contribute to the failure of B vitamin trials.

In all, given the challenges faced by previous trials, further B vitamin supplementation trials are needed. New trials will be most successful if they prescribe a full combination supplement (B6, B12, and folic acid) at high dose (i.e., dosage sufficient to reduce plasma homocysteine by 20%) to at-risk age participants with elevated plasma homocysteine or inadequate B vitamin status at baseline, adequate omega-3 fatty acid status at baseline, and who do not routinely take aspirin.

CONCLUSION

With the number of people aged over 60 expected to increase worldwide by 1.25 billion by 2050, accounting for 22% of the world's population, it is crucial to understand the causes of dementia and develop treatments (Prince et al., 2015). Current clinical and preclinical data provide strong evidence that HHcy is a key risk factor for VCID. With B vitamin supplementation being an inexpensive and safe therapeutic possibility, it would seem that treatment of HHcy-induced VCID would allow for some progress in lowering the number of dementia patients. Unfortunately, the mechanisms through which HHcy induces cognitive impairment remain unclear, with several different mechanisms proposed. In addition, clinical trials aimed at lowering homocysteine levels via B vitamin supplementation have also been lacking in their study design and ability to properly test the hypothesis that lowering homocysteine can slow and/or prevent cognitive decline. Future studies involving preclinical animal models and properly designed clinical trials will be necessary in order to effectively treat HHcy-induced VCID and lower the incidence of dementia.

AUTHOR CONTRIBUTIONS

BP and EW each wrote 50% of the manuscript. DW edited for content, checked for accuracy, and provided guidance in the preparation of the content.

FUNDING

This work was supported by National Institutes of Health grants RO1NS079637 and RO1NS097722 to DW, and fellowship F31NS092202 to EW. The content is solely the responsibility of the authors and does not necessarily represent the official views of the National Institutes of Health.

REFERENCES

Abraham, J. M., and Cho, L. (2010). The homocysteine hypothesis: still relevant to the prevention and treatment of cardiovascular disease? *Cleve. Clin. J. Med.* 77, 911–918. doi: 10.3949/ccjm.77a.10036

Andreeva, V. A., Kesse-Guyot, E., Barberger-Gateau, P., Fezeu, L., Hercberg, S., and Galan, P. (2011). Cognitive function after supplementation with B vitamins and long-chain omega-3 fatty acids: ancillary findings from the SU.FOL.OM3 randomized trial. *Am. J. Clin. Nutr.* 94, 278–286. doi: 10.3945/ajcn.110.006320

Baumbach, G. L., Sigmund, C. D., Bottiglieri, T., and Lentz, S. R. (2002). Structure of cerebral arterioles in cystathionine beta-synthase-deficient mice. *Circ. Res.* 91, 931–937. doi: 10.1161/01.RES.0000041408.64867.1D

Beydoun, M. A., Beydoun, H. A., Gamaldo, A. A., Teel, A., Zonderman, A. B., and Wang, Y. (2014). Epidemiologic studies of modifiable factors associated with cognition and dementia: systematic review and meta-analysis. *BMC Public Health* 14:643. doi: 10.1186/1471-2458-14-643

Bonaa, K. H., Njolstad, I., Ueland, P. M., Schirmer, H., Tverdal, A., Steigen, T., et al. (2006). Homocysteine lowering and cardiovascular events after acute myocardial infarction. *N. Engl. J. Med.* 354, 1578–1588. doi: 10.1056/NEJMoa055227

Bostom, A. G., Rosenberg, I. H., Silbershatz, H., Jacques, P. F., Selhub, J., D'Agostino, R. B., et al. (1999). Nonfasting plasma total homocysteine levels and stroke incidence in elderly persons: the Framingham Study. *Ann. Intern. Med.* 131, 352–355. doi: 10.7326/0003-4819-131-5-199909070-00006

Bowler, J. V., Munoz, D. G., Merskey, H., and Hachinski, V. (1998). Fallacies in the pathological confirmation of the diagnosis of Alzheimer's disease. *J. Neurol. Neurosurg. Psychiatry* 64, 18–24. doi: 10.1136/jnnp.64.1.18

Candelario-Jalil, E., Thompson, J., Taheri, S., Grossetete, M., Adair, J. C., Edmonds, E., et al. (2011). Matrix metalloproteinases are associated with increased blood-brain barrier opening in vascular cognitive impairment. *Stroke* 42, 1345–1350. doi: 10.1161/STROKEAHA.110.600825

Canobbio, I., Abubaker, A. A., Visconte, C., Torti, M., and Pula, G. (2015). Role of amyloid peptides in vascular dysfunction and platelet dysregulation in Alzheimer's disease. *Front. Cell. Neurosci.* 9:65. doi: 10.3389/fncel.2015.00065

Chen, Z., Karaplis, A. C., Ackerman, S. L., Pogribny, I. P., Melnyk, S., Lussier-Cacan, S., et al. (2001). Mice deficient in methylenetetrahydrofolate reductase exhibit hyperhomocysteinemia and decreased methylation capacity, with neuropathology and aortic lipid deposition. *Hum. Mol. Genet.* 10, 433–443. doi: 10.1093/hmg/10.5.433

Clarke, R., Bennett, D., Parish, S., Lewington, S., Skeaff, M., Eussen, S. J., et al. (2014). Effects of homocysteine lowering with B vitamins on cognitive aging: meta-analysis of 11 trials with cognitive data on 22,000 individuals. *Am. J. Clin. Nutr.* 100, 657–666. doi: 10.3945/ajcn.113.076349

Clarke, R., Harrison, G., Richards, S., and Vital Trial Collaborative Group (2003). Effect of vitamins and aspirin on markers of platelet activation, oxidative stress and homocysteine in people at high risk of dementia. *J. Intern. Med.* 254, 67–75.

Clarke, R., Smith, A. D., Jobst, K. A., Refsum, H., Sutton, L., and Ueland, P. M. (1998). Folate, vitamin B12, and serum total homocysteine levels in confirmed Alzheimer disease. *Arch. Neurol.* 55, 1449–1455. doi: 10.1001/archneur.55.11.1449

Clayton, P. T., Smith, I., Harding, B., Hyland, K., Leonard, J. V., and Leeming, R. J. (1986). Subacute combined degeneration of the cord, dementia and parkinsonism due to an inborn error of folate metabolism. *J. Neurol. Neurosurg. Psychiatry* 49, 920–927. doi: 10.1136/jnnp.49.8.920

Crider, K. S., Bailey, L. B., and Berry, R. J. (2011). Folic acid food fortification-its history, effect, concerns, and future directions. *Nutrients* 3, 370–384. doi: 10.3390/nu3030370

Cuenod, M., Do, K. Q., and Streit, P. (1990). Homocysteic acid as an endogenous excitatory amino acid. *Trends Pharmacol. Sci.* 11, 477–478. doi: 10.1016/0165-6147(90)90137-W

de Jager, C. A., Oulhaj, A., Jacoby, R., Refsum, H., and Smith, A. D. (2012). Cognitive and clinical outcomes of homocysteine-lowering B-vitamin treatment in mild cognitive impairment: a randomized controlled trial. *Int. J. Geriatr. Psychiatry* 27, 592–600. doi: 10.1002/gps.2758

Douaud, G., Refsum, H., de Jager, C. A., Jacoby, R., Nichols, T. E., Smith, S. M., et al. (2013). Preventing Alzheimer's disease-related gray matter atrophy by B-vitamin treatment. *Proc. Natl. Acad. Sci. U.S.A.* 110, 9523–9528. doi: 10.1073/pnas.1301816110

Durga, J., van Boxtel, M. P., Schouten, E. G., Kok, F. J., Jolles, J., Katan, M. B., et al. (2007). Effect of 3-year folic acid supplementation on cognitive function in older adults in the FACIT trial: a randomised, double blind, controlled trial. *Lancet* 369, 208–216. doi: 10.1016/S0140-6736(07)60109-3

Eikelboom, J. W., Lonn, E., Genest, J. Jr., Hankey, G., and Yusuf, S. (1999). Homocyst(e)ine and cardiovascular disease: a critical review of the epidemiologic evidence. *Ann. Intern. Med.* 131, 363–375. doi: 10.7326/0003-4819-131-5-199909070-00008

Eussen, S. J., de Groot, L. C., Joosten, L. W., Bloo, R. J., Clarke, R., Ueland, P. M., et al. (2006). Effect of oral vitamin B-12 with or without folic acid on cognitive function in older people with mild vitamin B-12 deficiency: a randomized, placebo-controlled trial. *Am. J. Clin. Nutr.* 84, 361–370. doi: 10.1093/ajcn/84.1.361

Firbank, M. J., Narayan, S. K., Saxby, B. K., Ford, G. A., and O'Brien, J. T. (2010). Homocysteine is associated with hippocampal and white matter atrophy in older subjects with mild hypertension. *Int. Psychogeriatr.* 22, 804–811. doi: 10.1017/S1041610210000499

Ford, A. H., and Almeida, O. P. (2012). Effect of homocysteine lowering treatment on cognitive function: a systematic review and meta-analysis of randomized controlled trials. *J. Alzheimers Dis.* 29, 133–149. doi: 10.3233/JAD-2012-111739

Galis, Z. S., Muszynski, M., Sukhova, G. K., Simon-Morrissey, E., Unemori, E. N., Lark, M. W., et al. (1994). Cytokine-stimulated human vascular smooth muscle cells synthesize a complement of enzymes required for extracellular matrix digestion. *Circ. Res.* 75, 181–189. doi: 10.1161/01.RES.75.1.181

Gibson, J. B., Carson, N. A., and Neill, D. W. (1964). Pathological findings in homocystinuria. *J. Clin. Pathol.* 17, 427–437. doi: 10.1136/jcp.17.4.427

Graham, I. M., Daly, L. E., Refsum, H. M., Robinson, K., Brattstrom, L. E., Ueland, P. M., et al. (1997). Plasma homocysteine as a risk factor for vascular disease. The European Concerted Action Project. *JAMA* 277, 1775–1781. doi: 10.1001/jama.1997.03540460039030

Hainsworth, A. H., Yeo, N. E., Weekman, E. M., and Wilcock, D. M. (2016). Homocysteine, hyperhomocysteinemia and vascular contributions to cognitive impairment and dementia (VCID). *Biochim. Biophys. Acta* 1862, 1008–1017. doi: 10.1016/j.bbadis.2015.11.015

Ho, P. I., Ashline, D., Dhitavat, S., Ortiz, D., Collins, S. C., Shea, T. B., et al. (2003). Folate deprivation induces neurodegeneration: roles of oxidative stress and increased homocysteine. *Neurobiol. Dis.* 14, 32–42. doi: 10.1016/S0969-9961(03)00070-6

Hyland, K., Smith, I., Bottiglieri, T., Perry, J., Wendel, U., Clayton, P. T., et al. (1988). Demyelination and decreased S-adenosylmethionine in 5,10-methylenetetrahydrofolate reductase deficiency. *Neurology* 38, 459–462. doi: 10.1212/WNL.38.3.459

Jakubowski, H. (1999). Protein homocysteinylation: possible mechanism underlying pathological consequences of elevated homocysteine levels. *FASEB J.* 13, 2277–2283. doi: 10.1096/fasebj.13.15.2277

Jakubowski, H., Zhang, L., Bardeguez, A., and Aviv, A. (2000). Homocysteine thiolactone and protein homocysteinylation in human endothelial cells: implications for atherosclerosis. *Circ. Res.* 87, 45–51. doi: 10.1161/01.RES.87.1.45

Janota, C., Lemere, C. A., and Brito, M. A. (2016). Dissecting the contribution of vascular alterations and aging to Alzheimer's disease. *Mol. Neurobiol.* 53, 3793–3811. doi: 10.1007/s12035-015-9319-7

Jellinger, K. A., and Attems, J. (2010). Is there pure vascular dementia in old age? *J. Neurol. Sci.* 299, 150–154. doi: 10.1016/j.jns.2010.08.038

Jerneren, F., Elshorbagy, A. K., Oulhaj, A., Smith, S. M., Refsum, H., and Smith, A. D. (2015). Brain atrophy in cognitively impaired elderly: the importance of long-chain omega-3 fatty acids and B vitamin status in a randomized controlled trial. *Am. J. Clin. Nutr.* 102, 215–221. doi: 10.3945/ajcn.114.103283

Jiang, X., Yang, F., Tan, H., Liao, D., Bryan, R. M. Jr., Randhawa, J. K., et al. (2005). Hyperhomocysteinemia impairs endothelial function and eNOS activity via PKC activation. *Arterioscler. Thromb. Vasc. Biol.* 25, 2515–2521. doi: 10.1161/01.ATV.0000189559.87328.e4

Joosten, E., van den Berg, A., Riezler, R., Naurath, H. J., Lindenbaum, J., Stabler, S. P., et al. (1993). Metabolic evidence that deficiencies of vitamin B-12 (cobalamin), folate, and vitamin B-6 occur commonly in elderly people. *Am. J. Clin. Nutr.* 58, 468–476. doi: 10.1093/ajcn/58.4.468

Kamath, A. F., Chauhan, A. K., Kisucka, J., Dole, V. S., Loscalzo, J., Handy, D. E., et al. (2006). Elevated levels of homocysteine compromise blood-brain barrier integrity in mice. *Blood* 107, 591–593. doi: 10.1182/blood-2005-06-2506

Kang, J. H., Cook, N., Manson, J., Buring, J. E., Albert, C. M., and Grodstein, F. (2008). A trial of B vitamins and cognitive function among women at high risk of cardiovascular disease. *Am. J. Clin. Nutr.* 88, 1602–1610. doi: 10.3945/ajcn.2008.26404

Kim, J. M., Lee, H., and Chang, N. (2002). Hyperhomocysteinemia due to short-term folate deprivation is related to electron microscopic changes in the rat brain. *J. Nutr.* 132, 3418–3421. doi: 10.1093/jn/132.11.3418

Klein, T., and Bischoff, R. (2011). Physiology and pathophysiology of matrix metalloproteases. *Amino Acids* 41, 271–290. doi: 10.1007/s00726-010-0689-x

Langa, K. M., Foster, N. L., and Larson, E. B. (2004). Mixed dementia: emerging concepts and therapeutic implications. *JAMA* 292, 2901–2908. doi: 10.1001/jama.292.23.2901

Lewerin, C., Matousek, M., Steen, G., Johansson, B., Steen, B., and Nilsson-Ehle, H. (2005). Significant correlations of plasma homocysteine and serum methylmalonic acid with movement and cognitive performance in elderly subjects but no improvement from short-term vitamin therapy: a placebo-controlled randomized study. *Am. J. Clin. Nutr.* 81, 1155–1162. doi: 10.1093/ajcn/81.5.1155

Locasale, J. W. (2013). Serine, glycine and one-carbon units: cancer metabolism in full circle. *Nat. Rev. Cancer* 13, 572–583. doi: 10.1038/nrc3557

Lonn, E., Yusuf, S., Arnold, M. J., Sheridan, P., Pogue, J., Micks, M., et al. (2006). Homocysteine lowering with folic acid and B vitamins in vascular disease. *N. Engl. J. Med.* 354, 1567–1577. doi: 10.1056/NEJMoa060900

Maron, B. A., and Loscalzo, J. (2009). The treatment of hyperhomocysteinemia. *Annu. Rev. Med.* 60, 39–54. doi: 10.1146/annurev.med.60.041807.123308

Mattson, M. P., and Shea, T. B. (2003). Folate and homocysteine metabolism in neural plasticity and neurodegenerative disorders. *Trends Neurosci.* 26, 137–146. doi: 10.1016/S0166-2236(03)00032-8

McCully, K. S. (1969). Vascular pathology of homocysteinemia: implications for the pathogenesis of arteriosclerosis. *Am. J. Pathol.* 56, 111–128.

McCully, K. S. (2007). Homocysteine, vitamins, and vascular disease prevention. *Am. J. Clin. Nutr.* 86, 1563S–1568S. doi: 10.1093/ajcn/86.5.1563S

McMahon, J. A., Green, T. J., Skeaff, C. M., Knight, R. G., Mann, J. I., and Williams, S. M. (2006). A controlled trial of homocysteine lowering and cognitive performance. *N. Engl. J. Med.* 354, 2764–2772. doi: 10.1056/NEJMoa054025

Michaluk, P., Kolodziej, L., Mioduszewska, B., Wilczynski, G. M., Dzwonek, J., Jaworski, J., et al. (2007). Beta-dystroglycan as a target for MMP-9, in response to enhanced neuronal activity. *J. Biol. Chem.* 282, 16036–16041. doi: 10.1074/jbc.M700641200

Miller, J. W., Green, R., Mungas, D. M., Reed, B. R., and Jagust, W. J. (2002). Homocysteine, vitamin B6, and vascular disease in AD patients. *Neurology* 58, 1471–1475. doi: 10.1212/WNL.58.10.1471

Moll, S., and Varga, E. A. (2015). Homocysteine and MTHFR mutations. *Circulation* 132, e6–e9. doi: 10.1161/CIRCULATIONAHA.114.013311

Neves, M. F., Endemann, D., Amiri, F., Virdis, A., Pu, Q., Rozen, R., et al. (2004). Small artery mechanics in hyperhomocysteinemic mice: effects of angiotensin II. *J. Hypertens.* 22, 959–966. doi: 10.1097/00004872-200405000-00018

Olney, J. W., Price, M. T., Salles, K. S., Labruyere, J., Ryerson, R., Mahan, K., et al. (1987). L-homocysteic acid: an endogenous excitotoxic ligand of the NMDA receptor. *Brain Res. Bull.* 19, 597–602. doi: 10.1016/0361-9230(87)90077-3

Oulhaj, A., Refsum, H., Beaumont, H., Williams, J., King, E., Jacoby, R., et al. (2010). Homocysteine as a predictor of cognitive decline in Alzheimer's disease. *Int. J. Geriatr. Psychiatry* 25, 82–90. doi: 10.1002/gps.2303

Peng, H. Y., Man, C. F., Xu, J., and Fan, Y. (2015). Elevated homocysteine levels and risk of cardiovascular and all-cause mortality: a meta-analysis of prospective studies. *J. Zhejiang Univ. Sci. B* 16, 78–86. doi: 10.1631/jzus.B1400183

Perla-Kajan, J., Twardowski, T., and Jakubowski, H. (2007). Mechanisms of homocysteine toxicity in humans. *Amino Acids* 32, 561–572. doi: 10.1007/s00726-006-0432-9

Pirchl, M., Ullrich, C., and Humpel, C. (2010). Differential effects of short- and long-term hyperhomocysteinaemia on cholinergic neurons, spatial memory and microbleedings in vivo in rats. *Eur. J. Neurosci.* 32, 1516–1527. doi: 10.1111/j.1460-9568.2010.07434.x

Poloni, S., Sperb-Ludwig, F., Borsatto, T., Weber Hoss, G., Doriqui, M. J. R., Embirucu, E. K., et al. (2018). CBS mutations are good predictors for B6-responsiveness: a study based on the analysis of 35 Brazilian Classical Homocystinuria patients. *Mol. Genet. Genomic Med.* 6, 160–170. doi: 10.1002/mgg3.342

Prince, M., Wimo, A., Guerchet, M., Ali, G., Wu, Y., and Prina, M. (2015). *The Global Impact of Dementia: An Analysis of Prevalence, Incidence, Cost and Trends*. London: Alzheimer's Disease International,

Rasic-Markovic, A., Stanojlovic, O., Hrncic, D., Krstic, D., Colovic, M., Susic, V., et al. (2009). The activity of erythrocyte and brain Na^+/K^+ and Mg^{2+}-ATPases in rats subjected to acute homocysteine and homocysteine thiolactone administration. *Mol. Cell. Biochem.* 327, 39–45. doi: 10.1007/s11010-009-0040-6

Rimm, E. B., Willett, W. C., Hu, F. B., Sampson, L., Colditz, G. A., Manson, J. E., et al. (1998). Folate and vitamin B6 from diet and supplements in relation to risk of coronary heart disease among women. *JAMA* 279, 359–364. doi: 10.1001/jama.279.5.359

Robert, K., Pages, C., Ledru, A., Delabar, J., Caboche, J., and Janel, N. (2005). Regulation of extracellular signal-regulated kinase by homocysteine in hippocampus. *Neuroscience* 133, 925–935. doi: 10.1016/j.neuroscience.2005.03.034

Sacharow, S. J., Picker, J. D., and Levy, H. L. (1993). "Homocystinuria caused by cystathionine beta-synthase deficiency," in *GeneReviews((R))*, eds M. P. Adam, H. H. Ardinger, R. A. Pagon, S. E. Wallace, L. J. H. Bean, K. Stephens, et al. (Seattle, WA: University of Washington).

Schneider, J. A., and Bennett, D. A. (2010). Where vascular meets neurodegenerative disease. *Stroke* 41(Suppl. 10), S144–S146. doi: 10.1161/STROKEAHA.110.598326

Selhub, J. (1999). Homocysteine metabolism. *Annu. Rev. Nutr.* 19, 217–246. doi: 10.1146/annurev.nutr.19.1.217

Selhub, J. (2006). The many facets of hyperhomocysteinemia: studies from the Framingham cohorts. *J. Nutr.* 136(Suppl. 6), 1726S–1730S. doi: 10.1093/jn/136.6.1726S

Shastry, S., and Tyagi, S. C. (2004). Homocysteine induces metalloproteinase and shedding of beta-1 integrin in microvessel endothelial cells. *J. Cell. Biochem.* 93, 207–213. doi: 10.1002/jcb.20137

Simard, M., and Nedergaard, M. (2004). The neurobiology of glia in the context of water and ion homeostasis. *Neuroscience* 129, 877–896. doi: 10.1016/j.neuroscience.2004.09.053

Smith, A. D., and Refsum, H. (2016). Homocysteine, B vitamins, and cognitive impairment. *Annu. Rev. Nutr.* 36, 211–239. doi: 10.1146/annurev-nutr-071715-050947

Smith, A. D., Smith, S. M., de Jager, C. A., Whitbread, P., Johnston, C., Agacinski, G., et al. (2010). Homocysteine-lowering by B vitamins slows the rate of accelerated brain atrophy in mild cognitive impairment: a randomized controlled trial. *PLoS One* 5:e12244. doi: 10.1371/journal.pone.0012244

Stott, D. J., MacIntosh, G., Lowe, G. D., Rumley, A., McMahon, A. D., Langhorne, P., et al. (2005). Randomized controlled trial of homocysteine-lowering vitamin treatment in elderly patients with vascular disease. *Am. J. Clin. Nutr.* 82, 1320–1326. doi: 10.1093/ajcn/82.6.1320

Study of the Effectiveness of Additional Reductions in Cholesterol and Homocysteine (SEARCH) Collaborative Group, Armitage, J. M., Bowman, L., Clarke, R. J., Wallendszus, K., Bulbulia, R., et al. (2010). Effects of homocysteine-lowering with folic acid plus vitamin B12 vs placebo on mortality and major morbidity in myocardial infarction survivors: a randomized trial. *JAMA* 303, 2486–2494. doi: 10.1001/jama.2010.840

Sudduth, T. L., Powell, D. K., Smith, C. D., Greenstein, A., and Wilcock, D. M. (2013). Induction of hyperhomocysteinemia models vascular dementia by induction of cerebral microhemorrhages and neuroinflammation. *J. Cereb. Blood Flow Metab.* 33, 708–715. doi: 10.1038/jcbfm.2013.1

Sudduth, T. L., Weekman, E. M., Price, B. R., Gooch, J. L., Woolums, A., Norris, C. M., et al. (2017). Time-course of glial changes in the hyperhomocysteinemia model of vascular cognitive impairment and dementia (VCID). *Neuroscience* 341, 42–51. doi: 10.1016/j.neuroscience.2016.11.024

Sunden, S. L., Renduchintala, M. S., Park, E. I., Miklasz, S. D., and Garrow, T. A. (1997). Betaine-homocysteine methyltransferase expression in porcine and human tissues and chromosomal localization of the human gene. *Arch. Biochem. Biophys.* 345, 171–174. doi: 10.1006/abbi.1997.0246

Surtees, R., Leonard, J., and Austin, S. (1991). Association of demyelination with deficiency of cerebrospinal-fluid S-adenosylmethionine in inborn errors of methyl-transfer pathway. *Lancet* 338, 1550–1554. doi: 10.1016/0140-6736(91)92373-A

Toole, J. F., Malinow, M. R., Chambless, L. E., Spence, J. D., Pettigrew, L. C., Howard, V. J., et al. (2004). Lowering homocysteine in patients with ischemic stroke to prevent recurrent stroke, myocardial infarction, and death: the Vitamin Intervention for Stroke Prevention (VISP) randomized controlled trial. *JAMA* 291, 565–575. doi: 10.1001/jama.291.5.565

Troen, A. M., Shea-Budgell, M., Shukitt-Hale, B., Smith, D. E., Selhub, J., and Rosenberg, I. H. (2008). B-vitamin deficiency causes hyperhomocysteinemia and vascular cognitive impairment in mice. *Proc. Natl. Acad. Sci. U.S.A.* 105, 12474–12479. doi: 10.1073/pnas.0805350105

Vecil, G. G., Larsen, P. H., Corley, S. M., Herx, L. M., Besson, A., Goodyer, C. G., et al. (2000). Interleukin-1 is a key regulator of matrix metalloproteinase-9 expression in human neurons in culture and following mouse brain trauma in vivo. *J. Neurosci. Res.* 61, 212–224. doi: 10.1002/1097-4547(20000715)61:2<212::AID-JNR12>3.0.CO;2-9

Vemuri, P., and Knopman, D. S. (2016). The role of cerebrovascular disease when there is concomitant Alzheimer disease. *Biochim. Biophys. Acta* 1862, 952–956. doi: 10.1016/j.bbadis.2015.09.013

Vermeer, S. E., van Dijk, E. J., Koudstaal, P. J., Oudkerk, M., Hofman, A., Clarke, R., et al. (2002). Homocysteine, silent brain infarcts, and white matter lesions: the Rotterdam Scan Study. *Ann. Neurol.* 51, 285–289. doi: 10.1002/ana.10111

Vitatops Trial Study Group (2010). B vitamins in patients with recent transient ischaemic attack or stroke in the VITAmins TO Prevent Stroke (VITATOPS) trial: a randomised, double-blind, parallel, placebo-controlled trial. *Lancet Neurol.* 9, 855–865. doi: 10.1016/S1474-4422(10)70187-3

Wald, D. S., Kasturiratne, A., and Simmonds, M. (2010). Effect of folic acid, with or without other B vitamins, on cognitive decline: meta-analysis of randomized trials. *Am. J. Med.* 123, 522–527.e2. doi: 10.1016/j.amjmed.2010.01.017

Watanabe, M., Osada, J., Aratani, Y., Kluckman, K., Reddick, R., Malinow, M. R., et al. (1995). Mice deficient in cystathionine beta-synthase: animal models for mild and severe homocyst(e)inemia. *Proc. Natl. Acad. Sci. U.S.A.* 92, 1585–1589. doi: 10.1073/pnas.92.5.1585

Weiss, N., Heydrick, S. J., Postea, O., Keller, C., Keaney, J. F. Jr., and Loscalzo, J. (2003). Influence of hyperhomocysteinemia on the cellular redox state–impact on homocysteine-induced endothelial dysfunction. *Clin. Chem. Lab. Med.* 41, 1455–1461. doi: 10.1515/CCLM.2003.223

Welch, G. N., and Loscalzo, J. (1998). Homocysteine and atherothrombosis. *N. Engl. J. Med.* 338, 1042–1050. doi: 10.1056/NEJM199804093381507

Yeh, Y. C., Huang, M. F., Hwang, S. J., Tsai, J. C., Liu, T. L., Hsiao, S. M., et al. (2016). Association of homocysteine level and vascular burden and cognitive function in middle-aged and older adults with chronic kidney disease. *Int. J. Geriatr. Psychiatry* 31, 723–730. doi: 10.1002/gps.4383

Zekry, D., Hauw, J. J., and Gold, G. (2002). Mixed dementia: epidemiology, diagnosis, and treatment. *J. Am. Geriatr. Soc.* 50, 1431–1438. doi: 10.1046/j.1532-5415.2002.50367.x

Zou, C. G., and Banerjee, R. (2005). Homocysteine and redox signaling. *Antioxid. Redox Signal.* 7, 547–559. doi: 10.1089/ars.2005.7.547

14

Novel Calibrated Short TR Recovery (CaSTRR) Method for Brain-Blood Partition Coefficient Correction Enhances Gray-White Matter Contrast in Blood Flow Measurements in Mice

*Scott W. Thalman[1,2], David K. Powell[1,3] and Ai-Ling Lin[1,3,4,5]**

[1] F. Joseph Halcomb III, MD Department of Biomedical Engineering, University of Kentucky, Lexington, KY, United States, [2] Sanders-Brown Center on Aging, University of Kentucky, Lexington, KY, United States, [3] Magnetic Resonance Imaging and Spectroscopy Center, University of Kentucky, Lexington, KY, United States, [4] Department of Pharmacology and Nutritional Sciences, University of Kentucky, Lexington, KY, United States, [5] Department of Neuroscience, University of Kentucky, Lexington, KY, United States

***Correspondence:**
Ai-Ling Lin
ailing.lin@uky.edu

The goal of the study was to develop a novel, rapid Calibrated Short TR Recovery (CaSTRR) method to measure the brain-blood partition coefficient (BBPC) in mice. The BBPC is necessary for quantifying cerebral blood flow (CBF) using tracer-based techniques like arterial spin labeling (ASL), but previous techniques required prohibitively long acquisition times so a constant BBPC equal to 0.9 mL/g is typically used regardless of studied species, condition, or disease. An accelerated method of BBPC correction could improve regional specificity in CBF maps particularly in white matter. Male C57Bl/6N mice (n = 8) were scanned at 7T using CaSTRR to measure BBPC determine regional variability. This technique employs phase-spoiled gradient echo acquisitions with varying repetition times (TRs) to estimate proton density in the brain and a blood sample. Proton density weighted images are then calibrated to a series of phantoms with known concentrations of deuterium to determine BBPC. Pseudo-continuous ASL was also acquired to quantify CBF with and without empirical BBPC correction. Using the CaSTRR technique we demonstrate that, in mice, white matter has a significantly lower BBPC ($BBPC_{white} = 0.93 \pm 0.05$ mL/g) than cortical gray matter ($BBPC_{gray} = 0.99 \pm 0.04$ mL/g, $p = 0.03$), and that when voxel-wise BBPC correction is performed on CBF maps the observed difference in perfusion between gray and white matter is improved by as much as 14%. Our results suggest that BBPC correction is feasible and could be particularly important in future studies of perfusion in white matter pathologies.

Keywords: arterial spin labeling, brain-blood partition coefficient, cerebral blood flow, gray-white matter contrast, magnetic resonance imaging

INTRODUCTION

Arterial spin labeling (ASL) is a non-invasive, quantitative magnetic resonance imaging (MRI) technique used to measure cerebral blood flow (CBF) in a wide variety of human conditions. A growing number of studies are using ASL to measure perfusion in a variety of preclinical murine models including, aging (Parikh et al., 2016; Hoffman et al., 2017), Alzheimer's disease (Abrahamson et al., 2013; Lin et al., 2013, 2015), ischemic injury (Pham et al., 2010; Struys et al., 2016; Liu et al., 2017), traumatic brain injury (Foley et al., 2013), and vascular dementia (Hattori et al., 2016). This technique is based on using magnetically labeled protons on water molecules in the blood as a tracer substance to measure perfusion. As in other tracer-based techniques, in order to accurately quantify perfusion it is necessary to determine the partition coefficient of the tracer, which is in this case the relative solubility of water in the brain tissue vs. the blood. The brain-blood partition coefficient (BBPC) is tissue-specific and varies with age, species, pathology, and particularly with brain region (Herscovitch and Raichle, 1985; Kudomi et al., 2005; Leithner et al., 2010; Hirata et al., 2011). Thus the BBPC must be measured directly, and while MRI is well suited to measure water content in the brain, the current techniques to do so have prohibitively long acquisition times (Roberts et al., 1996; Leithner et al., 2010). Because of this, it is standard practice in ASL quantification to assume a BBPC value of 0.9 mL/g based on desiccation experiments performed on *ex vivo* human brain tissue (Herscovitch and Raichle, 1985; Alsop et al., 2015). This global average value is used for all regions of the brain, all ages and pathologies, and is even adopted when performing ASL in mice (Muir et al., 2008; Lei et al., 2011; Chugh et al., 2012; Gao et al., 2014).

Previous studies have determined a wide range of BBPC values in the human brain, particularly between relatively lipophilic white matter (0.82 mL/g) and hydrophilic gray matter (0.99 mL/g) (Bothe et al., 1984; Herscovitch and Raichle, 1985; Iida et al., 1989). Yet even among gray matter regions the BBPC can vary as much as 20% (Iida et al., 1989). Measurements in non-human primates have demonstrated lower BBPC values than humans with an even greater regional variability (Kudomi et al., 2005). An MRI study of BBPC in mice reported an average BBPC of 0.89 mL/g with little regional variability among gray matter regions of interest, but no white matter BBPC values were reported (Leithner et al., 2010). Because ASL has inherently low signal-to-noise ratio and the resolution requirements of scanning mouse brains are particularly high, it is necessary that the quantification methods introduce as little error as possible. Failure to correct for intra-subject regional variability as well as inter-subject variability in BBPC may result in a loss of sensitivity to perfusion deficits when using ASL. This is especially true when studying white matter regions which have both lower perfusion and lower BBPC.

In this study, we used a calibrated short TR recovery (CaSTRR) MRI sequence to measure proton density. This protocol is similar to one used previously by Leithner et al. (2010) to measure BBPC in mice, but has been modified to greatly reduce the acquisition time. Proton density was determined for the brain tissue as well as a fresh sample of each mouse's blood placed adjacent to the animal's head in order to calculate BBPC. Then cerebral perfusion was measured using a pseudo-continuous ASL (pCASL) technique to compare CBF maps that were uncorrected to maps that were corrected for regional BBPC. Particular attention was given to the white matter region of interest in the corpus callosum.

MATERIALS AND METHODS

All animal experiments were performed in accordance with NIH guidelines and approved by the University of Kentucky Institutional Animal Care and Use Committee (Approval number #2014-1264). Male C57Bl/6N mice aged 12 months ($n = 8$) were acquired from the National Institute of Aging colony. MRI experiments were performed using a 7T MR scanner (Clinscan, Brüker BioSpin, Germany) at the MRI and Spectroscopy Center at the University of Kentucky. Mice were anesthetized using a 4% mixture of isoflurane with air for induction and then maintained using 1.2% isoflurane such that the respiration rate was kept within 50–80 breaths/min. Rectal temperature was also monitored continually and maintained at $37 \pm 1°C$ using a water-heated bed.

While under anesthesia a fresh blood sample was taken from the facial vein and sealed in a glass capillary tube with ethylenediaminetetraactetate (EDTA) as an anticoagulant. This sample was then placed adjacent to the head of the mouse in order to measure the proton density of the blood (**Figure 1A**).

Both CaSTRR and pCASL images were acquired consecutively in a single imaging session. Because the CaSTRR acquisitions and the pCASL acquisitions require different receiver coils, a custom 3-D printed nose was developed to accommodate both a birdcage style volume coil and a phased-array surface coil so that the coils could be changed without disturbing the orientation of the mouse. This nose cone also facilitated the placement of phantoms adjacent to the head of the mouse.

Mice were scanned with a series of five phantoms placed alongside their head in the scanner (**Figure 1A**). The phantoms contained a mixture of deuterium oxide with distilled water such that the water contents of the phantoms were 60, 70, 80, 90, and 100% distilled water (Leithner et al., 2010). The phantoms were also doped with 0.07 mM gadobutrol (Gadavist, Bayer Healthcare Pharmaceuticals, Whippany NJ, United States) such that the longitudinal relaxation rate (T_1) was similar to the T_1 of brain tissue (~1.6 s at 7T) (Rohrer et al., 2005).

The CaSTRR proton density measurements were acquired using a 39 mm birdcage transmit/receive coil to ensure the most uniform coil sensitivity profile possible. To measure the proton density a series of image stacks was acquired using a phase-spoiled, fast low-angle shot gradient echo (FLASH-GRE) sequence with varying repetition times (TR = 125, 187, 250, 500, 1000, 2000 ms) (**Figure 1B**). The shortest possible echo time (TE = 3.2 ms) was used to minimize T_2* decay. In order to improve signal to noise, multiple averages were taken for the images with TR = 125 ms (4 averages), 187 ms (4 averages) and 250 ms (2 averages). Image matrix parameters were as follows:

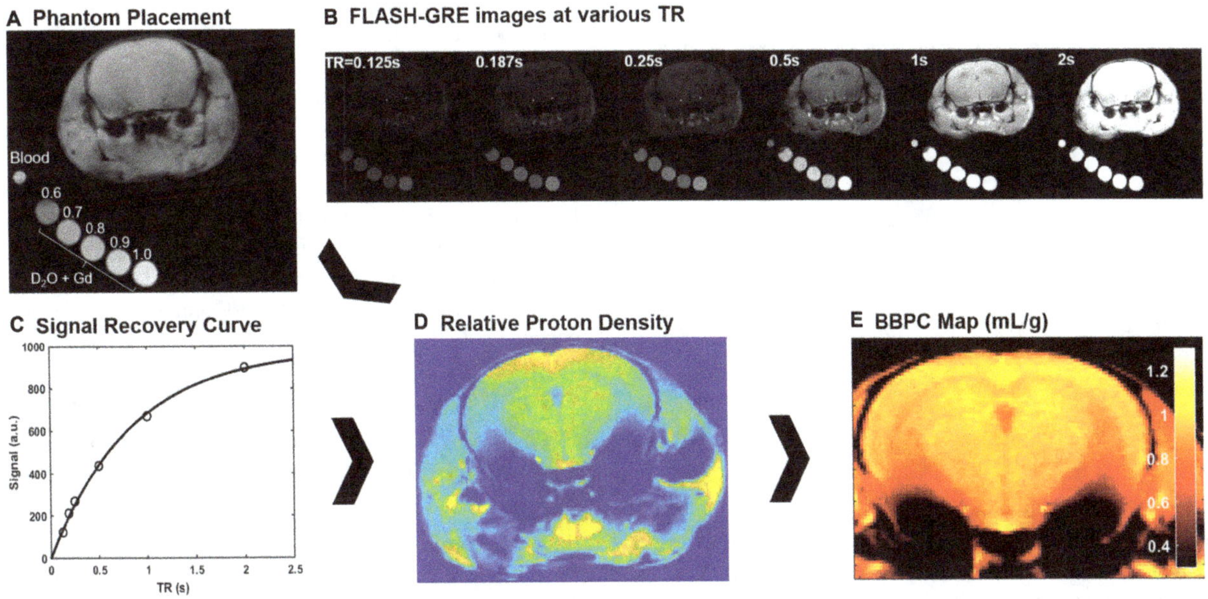

FIGURE 1 | Explanation of the calibrated short repetition time recovery (CaSTRR) imaging protocol to measure BBPC. **(A)** One CaSTRR acquisition showing the placement of blood and gadolinium doped phantoms in relation to the head of the mouse. **(B)** A representative series of FLASH-GRE images used for the CaSTRR method. **(C)** A representative signal recovery curve from a single voxel of brain tissue located in the cortex region of interest (circles) along with the exponential regression used to estimate the relative proton density of the voxel (line). **(D)** A representative map of relative proton density derived from the voxel-wise signal recovery curves. **(E)** The final BBPC map calculated as the ratio of proton density in the brain to the average proton density of the blood phantom and corrected for the density of brain tissue.

field of view = 2.8 cm × 2.8 cm, matrix = 256 × 256, in-plane resolution = 0.11 mm × 0.11 mm, slice thickness = 1 mm, number of slices = 10, flip angle = 90°, acquisition time = 17 min (Leithner et al., 2010).

Brain-blood partition coefficient maps were calculated in a voxel-wise manner by first fitting the signal recovery curve (**Figure 1C**) to the mono-exponential equation $S = M_0*[1 - e^\wedge(TR/T_1)]$ to yield a map of M_0 (**Figure 1D**). Next the M_0 map was normalized to the respective phantom series by fitting a linear regression to the average M_0 value in each phantom. Finally, the proton density in each voxel of the brain was compared to the average proton density of the blood ROI using the equation $BBPC = M_{0,brain}/(M_{0,blood} * 1.04\ g/mL)$ (**Figure 1E**; Roberts et al., 1996; Leithner et al., 2010).

For pCASL acquisitions, paired control and label images were acquired using a four-channel phased-array surface receive coil for increased signal to noise, and a whole body volume transmit coil to improve the tagging efficiency of the blood (Lin et al., 2013). Image pairs were acquired in an interleaved fashion with a train of Hanning window-shaped radiofrequency pulses of duration/spacing = 200/200 μs, flip angle = 25° and slice-selective gradient = 9 mT/m, and a labeling duration = 2100 ms. The images were acquired by 2D multi-slice spin-echo single shot echo planar imaging with FOV = 1.8 cm × 1.3 cm, matrix = 128 × 96, in-plane resolution = 0.14 mm × 0.14 mm, slice thickness = 1 mm, 6 slices, TE/TR = 20/4000 ms, label duration = 1600 ms, post-label delay = 0 s, and averages = 120. A separate, unlabeled acquisition with TR = 10 s and averages = 6 was used to normalize for the receiver coil profile. Total acquisition time for pCASL was 9 min.

When analyzing the CBF maps, the two centermost slices containing the hippocampus were selected for analysis. The brain regions of the CaSTRR and pCASL images were isolated independently using an automated skull-stripping algorithm and then co-registered using an intensity based registration algorithm. The quantitative CBF maps were calculated from the pCASL images according to the equation (Alsop et al., 2015):

$$CBF(mL/g/\min) = \frac{60 * BBPC * e^{(PLD/T_{1,blood})}}{2 * \alpha * \left(1 - e^{(LD/T_{1,blood})}\right)} * \frac{Ctl - Lbl}{M_0}$$

where PLD is post-label delay, LD is label duration, $T_{1,blood}$ is the longitudinal relaxation of blood (2.2 s at 7T), and α is label efficiency (0.85) (Alsop et al., 2015). For standard CBF maps the BBPC was assumed to be a constant 0.9 mL/g. Then a corrected CBF map was calculated by using the CaSTRR derived BBPC maps in place of the assumed constant.

Regions of interest encompassing the superior neocortex, corpus callosum, and hippocampus were drawn manually on each analyzed slice. BBPC, uncorrected CBF, and corrected CBF values were averaged for each region of interest. Gray-white contrast was determined for each slice as the absolute difference of average CBF values in gray and white matter regions of interest. All analysis was performed with in-house written scripts in Matlab (Mathworks, Natick, MA, United States).

TABLE 1 | Mean partition coefficient and perfusion values by region.

Regional Values	Neocortex	Hippocampus	Corpus Callosum
BBPC (mL/g)	0.99 ± 0.04	0.95 ± 0.04	0.93 ± 0.05
CBF, uncorrected (mL/g/min)	2.81 ± 0.4	2.90 ± 0.6	1.44 ± 0.3
CBF, corrected (mL/g/min)	3.09 ± 0.5	3.07 ± 0.7	1.51 ± 0.4
Gray-White Perfusion Contrast	**Neocortex vs. Corpus**		**Hippocampus vs. Corpus**
$\Delta CBF_{Uncorrected}$ (mL/g/min)	1.39 ± 0.4		1.46 ± 0.4
$\Delta CBF_{Corrected}$ (mL/g/min)	1.59 ± 0.5		1.54 ± 0.4
Contrast improvement (%, 95% CI)	14.2%, 9.6–18.8%		5.8%, 1.4–10.1%

Statistical analysis was performed using SPSS (IBM, Armonk, NY, United States). All data are expressed as mean ± standard deviation. Group comparisons were assessed using one- and two-way analysis of variance with Tukey's *post hoc* test. Values of $p < 0.05$ were considered statistically significant.

RESULTS

Corpus Callosum Demonstrates Reduced BBPC Compared to Neocortex

The average BBPC values in the neocortex, corpus callosum, and the hippocampus were determined for each mouse and the average of all mice is reported in **Table 1**. The highest BBPC value was observed in the neocortex (μ_{Ctx} = 0.99 ± 0.04 mL/g) which was significantly higher than the corpus callosum (μ_{CC} = 0.93 ± 0.05 mL/g, p = 0.035), and also higher than the hippocampus, though not significantly (μ_{HC} = 0.95 ± 0.4 mL/g, p = 0.17) (**Figures 2, 3**).

Corpus Callosum Also Demonstrates Lower Perfusion Than Surrounding Gray Matter

Elevated perfusion in gray matter regions was observed relative to the corpus callosum in both uncorrected CBF maps and maps with voxel-wise BBPC correction (**Figure 4**). In the uncorrected maps the hippocampus demonstrated the greatest perfusion (2.90 ± 0.6 mL/g/min) followed by the neocortex (2.81 ± 0.4 mL/g/min) with significantly less perfusion in the corpus callosum (1.44 ± 0.3 mL/g/min, $p < 0.001$). However, when the maps were corrected for BBPC the perfusion in the neocortex was highest (3.09 ± 0.5 mL/g/min) followed by the hippocampus (3.07 ± 0.7 mL/g/min) with significantly less perfusion again in the corpus callosum (1.51 ± 0.4 mL/g/min, $p < 0.001$). None of the regions demonstrated significant changes in average CBF values due to BBPC correction (corrected vs. uncorrected CBF, $p_{Ctx} = 0.31$, $p_{CC} = 0.66$, $p_{HC} = 0.61$).

The Difference in Perfusion Between Gray and White Matter Is Greater in Corrected CBF Maps Than Uncorrected Maps

When perfusion in gray matter regions is compared to the white matter of the corpus callosum for each mouse, the average difference in perfusion for the neocortex is 1.39 ± 0.4 mL/g/min in the uncorrected maps, but it is 1.59 ± 0.5 mL/g/min in the BBPC corrected maps, this constitutes a 14.2% increase in contrast between these regions (95% CI = 9.6–18.8%). For the hippocampus the difference in perfusion is 1.46 ± 0.4 mL/g/min in the uncorrected maps and 1.54 ± 0.4 mL/g/min in the corrected maps, or a 5.8% improvement (95% CI = 1.4–10.1%) (**Figure 5** and **Table 1**).

DISCUSSION

Using CaSTRR imaging we were able to produce high quality BBPC maps suitable for voxel-wise correction of perfusion measurements much faster than previous demonstrated. We determined that the average BBPC in the neocortex was 0.99 ± 0.04 mL/g and in the hippocampus the BBPC was 0.95 ± 0.4 mL/g. We also determined the BBPC in the white matter structure of the corpus callosum to be 0.93 ± 0.05 mL/g which has not previously been reported in mice. We also found significantly lower CBF in the corpus callosum than the neocortex and the hippocampus. Finally, when CBF maps were corrected for regional variability in BBPC the gray-white matter contrast was improved by as much as 14%.

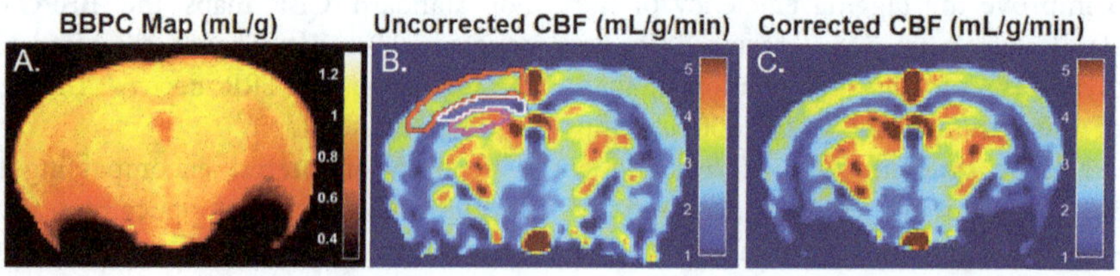

FIGURE 2 | A representative map of blood-brain partition coefficient **(A)** demonstrates elevated BBPC in the neocortex relative to the corpus callosum and hippocampus (μ_{Ctx} = 0.99 ± 0.04 mL/g, μ_{CC} = 0.93 ± 0.05 mL/g, μ_{Hc} = 0.95 ± 0.04 mL/g). Maps of the uncorrected **(B)** and BBPC-corrected **(C)** cerebral blood flow (CBF) demonstrate the improved contrast between gray matter in the neocortex (top) and hippocampus (bottom) and the white matter in the corpus callosum (middle). While only one side is shown, regions of interest were drawn bilaterally and applied equally to all three maps.

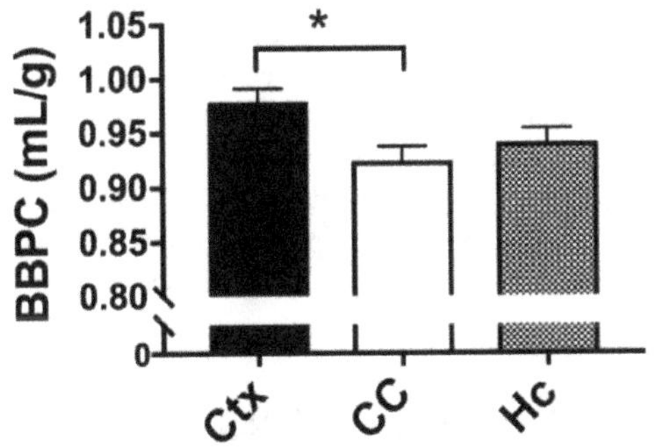

FIGURE 3 | Quantitative analysis of BBPC demonstrates significantly higher BBPC in the neocortex relative to the corpus callosum (μ_{Ctx} = 0.99 ± 0.04 mL/g, μ_{CC} = 0.93 ± 0.05 mL/g, p = 0.035), while the hippocampus had a BBPC of μ_{Hc} = 0.95 ± 0.04 mL/g (* indicates p < 0.05).

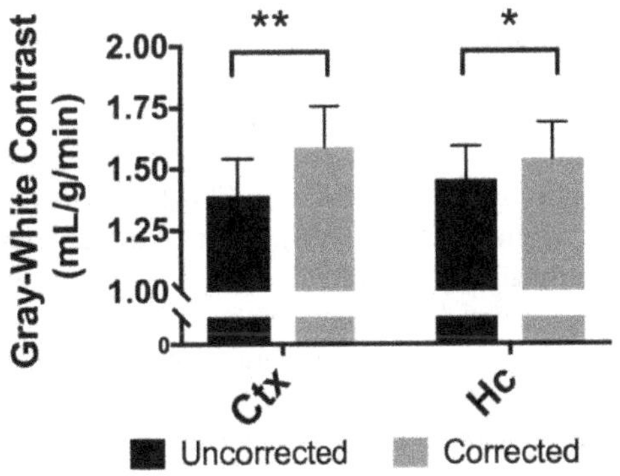

FIGURE 5 | BBPC correction increased the degree of contrast between gray matter regions and the corpus callosum as measured by the absolute difference in CBF between the two regions. Contrast between the neocortex and corpus callosum was improved by 14.2% (95% CI = 9.6–18.8%, $\Delta CBF_{uncorrected}$ = 1.39 ± 0.4 mL/g/min, $\Delta CBF_{corrected}$ = 1.59 ± 0.5 mL/g/min) and between the hippocampus and corpus callosum by 5.8% (95% CI = 1.4–10.1%, $\Delta CBF_{uncorrected}$ = 1.46 ± 0.4 mL/g/min, $\Delta CBF_{corrected}$ = 1.54 ± 0.4 mL/g/min) (* indicates p < 0.05, ** indicates p < 0.01).

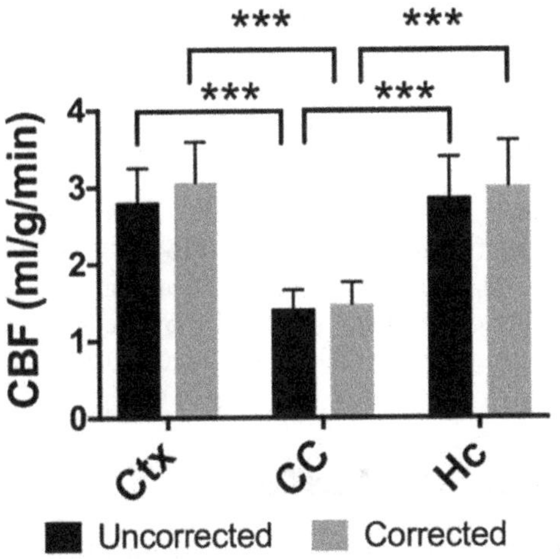

FIGURE 4 | The gray matter regions of the neocortex ($\mu_{uncorrected}$ = 2.81 ± 0.4 mL/g/min, $\mu_{corrected}$ = 3.09 ± 0.5 mL/g/min) and hippocampus ($\mu_{uncorrected}$ = 2.90 ± 0.6 mL/g/min, $\mu_{corrected}$ = 3.07 ± 0.7 mL/g/min) demonstrate significantly higher CBF than the white matter corpus callosum ($\mu_{uncorrected}$ = 1.44 ± 0.3 mL/g/min, $\mu_{corrected}$ = 1.51 ± 0.4 mL/g/min) in both the uncorrected and BBPC-corrected CBF maps (*** indicates p < 0.001).

The significant reduction in the acquisition time of BBPC maps to only 17 min increases the feasibility of including such a scan during an ASL protocol. We were also able to perform a voxel-wise correction due in part to the custom nose cone designed to immobilize the mouse's head while receiver coils are changed. The result of this correction is improved sensitivity to regional perfusion differences in CBF. This study acquired high resolution BBPC maps as was done in previous studies, but those maps had to be down-sampled by 22% to match the resolution of the pCASL acquisition when calculating CBF. This means that further gains could be made in either acquisition time or signal to noise ratio by acquiring CaSTRR images at the same resolution as the ASL image. Furthermore, since the original BBPC mapping technique was adapted to use in mice from a previously established technique in humans, CaSTRR imaging should be rapidly translatable back to the clinical setting (Roberts et al., 1996). In fact, a recently published study on healthy human volunteers demonstrated that an alternative method of correcting CBF maps for BBPC variability also resulted in increased contrast between gray and white matter (Ahlgren et al., 2018). This is consistent with our study and highlights the potential benefit of BBPC correction.

The improved regional specificity of CBF maps that are corrected for BBPC variability will be particularly relevant in the study of white matter pathologies (Mutsaerts et al., 2014). There is growing interest in vascular dysfunctions that accompany commonly observed white matter pathologies like multiple sclerosis (Bester et al., 2015; Sowa et al., 2015), white matter hyperintensities (van Dalen et al., 2016), and schizophrenia (Wright et al., 2014). The inherently low signal to noise of ASL is exacerbated in white matter where there is far less perfusion than gray matter. This means differences in perfusion will be even more subtle and could be confounded by changes in BBPC. While adding a second measurement to the CBF calculation with its inherent noise may introduce more variability in the CBF maps, the ability to account for significant differences in BBPC may increase sensitivity when comparing groups or regions with small perfusion differences.

It should be noted that the CaSTRR technique differs from the one described by Leithner et al. (2010) in a few key aspects. The primary difference is the choice to use logarithmically spaced TRs and omit TRs longer than 2 s. This change reduced the acquisition time by 87% from ~130 to 17 min. In previously published BBPC results, phantoms consisted of pure H_2O/D_2O solutions with very long T_1 recovery times which necessitated long TRs (Roberts et al., 1996; Leithner et al., 2010). By adding gadolinium to the water phantoms we were able to reduce the T_1 of the phantoms to approximately match the tissue thereby obviating the long TR scans that accounted for the vast majority of scan time. It should also be noted that Leithner et al. used 8–16 week old 129S6/SvEv mice. We would expect younger mice to have a higher BBPC than the 12 month-old mice used in our experiment, however, we observed higher BBPC values in our C57Bl/6N mice than were reported by Leithner et al. (2010). Future studies will need to consider the possibility that BBPC could vary with genetic strain.

There are several limitations to this study. While previous studies have used a uniform phantom to try and correct for the field inhomogeneity, variations were typically less than 5% and it is unlikely that the B1 field will be the same in a uniform phantom as it is while scanning a mouse (Roberts et al., 1996; Leithner et al., 2010). For this reason we chose not to perform any *post hoc* field correction and instead assumed a uniform field and receiver profile. More advanced field correction techniques may be useful. Also this study did not include a comparison to a post-mortem desiccation experiment. The standard BBPC mapping technique has been shown to underestimate the BBPC when compared to desiccation because a small fraction of water in the brain tissue does not contribute to the MRI signal (Leithner et al., 2010). Thus the overestimation of BBPC by CaSTRR may compensate for this effect, though not because it is more sensitive to this hidden water. Furthermore, regional analysis is not possible with desiccation, so desiccation could not confirm the regional differences observed by CaSTRR imaging. Finally the gradient echo readout used to acquire CaSTRR images is sensitive to susceptibility artifacts at air-tissue interfaces. This can be seen as a signal loss adjacent to the ear canals, and in this study we were forced to examine only those superior regions of the brain that were not affected by this artifact. For studies involving deep brain structures it may be necessary to separately acquire a B1 field map to correct for susceptibility variation.

In conclusion, the CaSTRR method produced maps of BBPC in mice with quality comparable to the current standard method while requiring far less acquisition time. This enables voxel-wise, empirical correction of CBF maps for regional and inter-subject variability in BBPC. These corrected CBF maps demonstrate improved contrast between gray and white matter regions. With growing interest in using ASL to measure white matter perfusion, this technique may have considerable value in studying pre-clinical models of white matter pathologies as well as potential for rapid translation to use in human studies.

AUTHOR CONTRIBUTIONS

ST was responsible for experimental and scanning protocol design, analysis software development, image acquisition, data and statistical analyses, and manuscript preparations. DP contributed to sequence development, scanning protocol design, technical support, and manuscript editing. A-LL was the primary investigator and contributed to project design, interpretation of results, and manuscript preparation.

FUNDING

This research was supported by the National Institute of Health (NIH) (Grant Nos. K01AG040164, R01AG054459, and T32AG057461). The 7T ClinScan small animal MRI scanner of the University of Kentucky was funded by the S10 NIH Shared Instrumentation Program (Grant No. 1S10RR029541-01).

ACKNOWLEDGMENTS

We thank Jared D. Hoffman for assisting with the MRI experiments and Dr. Ishita Parikh for statistical analysis.

REFERENCES

Abrahamson, E. E., Foley, L. M., Dekosky, S. T., Hitchens, T. K., Ho, C., Kochanek, P. M., et al. (2013). Cerebral blood flow changes after brain injury in human amyloid-beta knock-in mice. *J. Cereb. Blood Flow Metab.* 33, 826–833. doi: 10.1038/jcbfm.2013.24

Ahlgren, A., Wirestam, R., Knutsson, L., and Petersen, E. T. (2018). Improved calculation of the equilibrium magnetization of arterial blood in arterial spin labeling. *Magn. Reson. Med.* 80, 2223–2231. doi: 10.1002/mrm.27193

Alsop, D. C., Detre, J. A., Golay, X., Gunther, M., Hendrikse, J., Hernandez-Garcia, L., et al. (2015). Recommended implementation of arterial spin-labeled perfusion MRI for clinical applications: a consensus of the ISMRM perfusion study group and the European consortium for ASL in dementia. *Magn. Reson. Med.* 73, 102–116. doi: 10.1002/mrm.25197

Bester, M., Forkert, N. D., Stellmann, J. P., Sturner, K., Aly, L., Drabik, A., et al. (2015). Increased perfusion in normal appearing white matter in high inflammatory multiple sclerosis patients. *PLoS One* 10:e0119356. doi: 10.1371/journal.pone.0119356

Bothe, H. W., Bodsch, W., and Hossmann, K. A. (1984). Relationship between specific gravity, water content, and serum protein extravasation in various types of vasogenic brain edema. *Acta Neuropathol.* 64, 37–42. doi: 10.1007/bf00695604

Chugh, B. P., Bishop, J., Zhou, Y. Q., Wu, J., Henkelman, R. M., and Sled, J. G. (2012). Robust method for 3D arterial spin labeling in mice. *Magn. Reson. Med.* 68, 98–106. doi: 10.1002/mrm.23209

Foley, L. M., Iqbal O'meara, A. M., Wisniewski, S. R., Hitchens, T. K., Melick, J. A., Ho, C., et al. (2013). MRI assessment of cerebral blood flow after experimental traumatic brain injury combined with hemorrhagic shock in mice. *J. Cereb. Blood Flow Metab.* 33, 129–136. doi: 10.1038/jcbfm.2012.145

Gao, Y., Goodnough, C. L., Erokwu, B. O., Farr, G. W., Darrah, R., Lu, L., et al. (2014). Arterial spin labeling-fast imaging with steady-state free precession (ASL-FISP): a rapid and quantitative perfusion technique for high-field MRI. *NMR Biomed.* 27, 996–1004. doi: 10.1002/nbm.3143

Hattori, Y., Enmi, J., Iguchi, S., Saito, S., Yamamoto, Y., Tsuji, M., et al. (2016). Gradual carotid artery stenosis in mice closely replicates hypoperfusive vascular dementia in humans. *J. Am. Heart Assoc.* 5:e002757. doi: 10.1161/JAHA.115.002757

Herscovitch, P., and Raichle, M. E. (1985). What is the correct value for the brain-blood partition coefficient for water? *J. Cereb. Blood Flow Metab.* 5, 65–69. doi: 10.1038/jcbfm.1985.9

Hirata, K., Hattori, N., Katoh, C., Shiga, T., Kuroda, S., Kubo, N., et al. (2011). Regional partition coefficient of water in patients with cerebrovascular disease and its effect on rCBF assessment. *Nucl. Med. Commun.* 32, 63–70. doi: 10.1097/MNM.0b013e3283412106

Hoffman, J. D., Parikh, I., Green, S. J., Chlipala, G., Mohney, R. P., Keaton, M., et al. (2017). Age drives distortion of brain metabolic, vascular and cognitive functions, and the gut microbiome. *Front. Aging Neurosci.* 9:298. doi: 10.3389/fnagi.2017.00298

Iida, H., Kanno, I., Miura, S., Murakami, M., Takahashi, K., and Uemura, K. (1989). A determination of the regional brain/blood partition coefficient of water using dynamic positron emission tomography. *J. Cereb. Blood Flow Metab.* 9, 874–885. doi: 10.1038/jcbfm.1989.121

Kudomi, N., Hayashi, T., Teramoto, N., Watabe, H., Kawachi, N., Ohta, Y., et al. (2005). Rapid quantitative measurement of CMRO(2) and CBF by dual administration of (15)O-labeled oxygen and water during a single PET scan-a validation study and error analysis in anesthetized monkeys. *J. Cereb. Blood Flow Metab.* 25, 1209–1224. doi: 10.1038/sj.jcbfm.9600118

Lei, H., Pilloud, Y., Magill, A. W., and Gruetter, R. (2011). Continuous arterial spin labeling of mouse cerebral blood flow using an actively-detuned two-coil system at 9.4T. *Conf. Proc. IEEE Eng. Med. Biol. Soc.* 2011, 6993–6996. doi: 10.1109/IEMBS.2011.6091768

Leithner, C., Muller, S., Fuchtemeier, M., Lindauer, U., Dirnagl, U., and Royl, G. (2010). Determination of the brain-blood partition coefficient for water in mice using MRI. *J. Cereb. Blood Flow Metab.* 30, 1821–1824. doi: 10.1038/jcbfm.2010.160

Lin, A. L., Jahrling, J. B., Zhang, W., Derosa, N., Bakshi, V., Romero, P., et al. (2015). Rapamycin rescues vascular, metabolic and learning deficits in apolipoprotein E4 transgenic mice with pre-symptomatic Alzheimer's disease. *J. Cereb. Blood Flow Metab.* 37, 217–226.

Lin, A. L., Zheng, W., Halloran, J. J., Burbank, R. R., Hussong, S. A., Hart, M. J., et al. (2013). Chronic rapamycin restores brain vascular integrity and function through NO synthase activation and improves memory in symptomatic mice modeling Alzheimer's disease. *J. Cereb. Blood Flow Metab.* 33, 1412–1421. doi: 10.1038/jcbfm.2013.82

Liu, S., Dai, Q., Hua, R., Liu, T., Han, S., Li, S., et al. (2017). Determination of brain-regional blood perfusion and endogenous cpkcgamma impact on ischemic vulnerability of mice with global ischemia. *Neurochem. Res.* 42, 2814–2825. doi: 10.1007/s11064-017-2294-9

Muir, E. R., Shen, Q., and Duong, T. Q. (2008). Cerebral blood flow MRI in mice using the cardiac-spin-labeling technique. *Magn. Reson. Med.* 60, 744–748. doi: 10.1002/mrm.21721

Mutsaerts, H. J., Richard, E., Heijtel, D. F., Van Osch, M. J., Majoie, C. B., and Nederveen, A. J. (2014). Gray matter contamination in arterial spin labeling white matter perfusion measurements in patients with dementia. *Neuroimage Clin.* 4, 139–144. doi: 10.1016/j.nicl.2013.11.003

Parikh, I., Guo, J., Chuang, K. H., Zhong, Y., Rempe, R. G., Hoffman, J. D., et al. (2016). Caloric restriction preserves memory and reduces anxiety of aging mice with early enhancement of neurovascular functions. *Aging* 8, 2814–2826. doi: 10.18632/aging.101094

Pham, M., Helluy, X., Braeuninger, S., Jakob, P., Stoll, G., Kleinschnitz, C., et al. (2010). Outcome of experimental stroke in C57Bl/6 and Sv/129 mice assessed by multimodal ultra-high field MRI. *Exp. Transl. Stroke Med.* 2:6. doi: 10.1186/2040-7378-2-6

Roberts, D. A., Rizi, R., Lenkinski, R. E., and Leigh, J. S. Jr. (1996). Magnetic resonance imaging of the brain: blood partition coefficient for water: application to spin-tagging measurement of perfusion. *J. Magn. Reson. Imaging* 6, 363–366. doi: 10.1002/jmri.1880060217

Rohrer, M., Bauer, H., Mintorovitch, J., Requardt, M., and Weinmann, H. J. (2005). Comparison of magnetic properties of MRI contrast media solutions at different magnetic field strengths. *Invest. Radiol.* 40, 715–724. doi: 10.1097/01.rli.0000184756.66360.d3

Sowa, P., Bjornerud, A., Nygaard, G. O., Damangir, S., Spulber, G., Celius, E. G., et al. (2015). Reduced perfusion in white matter lesions in multiple sclerosis. *Eur. J. Radiol.* 84, 2605–2612. doi: 10.1016/j.ejrad.2015.09.007

Struys, T., Govaerts, K., Oosterlinck, W., Casteels, C., Bronckaers, A., Koole, M., et al. (2016). In vivo evidence for long-term vascular remodeling resulting from chronic cerebral hypoperfusion in mice. *J. Cereb. Blood Flow Metab.* 37, 726–739. doi: 10.1177/0271678X16638349

van Dalen, J. W., Mutsaerts, H. J., Nederveen, A. J., Vrenken, H., Steenwijk, M. D., Caan, M. W., et al. (2016). White matter hyperintensity volume and cerebral perfusion in older individuals with hypertension using arterial spin-labeling. *AJNR Am. J. Neuroradiol.* 37, 1824–1830. doi: 10.3174/ajnr.A4828

Wright, S., Kochunov, P., Chiappelli, J., Mcmahon, R., Muellerklein, F., Wijtenburg, S. A., et al. (2014). Accelerated white matter aging in schizophrenia: role of white matter blood perfusion. *Neurobiol. Aging* 35, 2411–2418. doi: 10.1016/j.neurobiolaging.2014.02.016

15

Pericyte Structural Remodeling in Cerebrovascular Health and Homeostasis

*Andrée-Anne Berthiaume [1], David A. Hartmann [1], Mark W. Majesky [2,3], Narayan R. Bhat [1] and Andy Y. Shih [1,2,4]**

[1]Department of Neuroscience, Medical University of South Carolina, Charleston, SC, United States, [2]Center for Developmental Biology and Regenerative Medicine, Seattle Children's Research Institute, Seattle, WA, United States, [3]Departments of Pediatrics and Pathology, University of Washington, Seattle, WA, United States, [4]Center for Biomedical Imaging, Medical University of South Carolina, Charleston, SC, United States

***Correspondence:**
Andy Y. Shih
andy.shih@seattlechildrens.org

The biology of brain microvascular pericytes is an active area of research and discovery, as their interaction with the endothelium is critical for multiple aspects of cerebrovascular function. There is growing evidence that pericyte loss or dysfunction is involved in the pathogenesis of Alzheimer's disease, vascular dementia, ischemic stroke and brain injury. However, strategies to mitigate or compensate for this loss remain limited. In this review, we highlight a novel finding that pericytes in the adult brain are structurally dynamic *in vivo*, and actively compensate for loss of endothelial coverage by extending their far-reaching processes to maintain contact with regions of exposed endothelium. Structural remodeling of pericytes may present an opportunity to foster pericyte-endothelial communication in the adult brain and should be explored as a potential means to counteract pericyte loss in dementia and cerebrovascular disease. We discuss the pathophysiological consequences of pericyte loss on capillary function, and the biochemical pathways that may control pericyte remodeling. We also offer guidance for observing pericytes *in vivo*, such that pericyte structural remodeling can be more broadly studied in mouse models of cerebrovascular disease.

Keywords: pericyte, two-photon imaging, capillary blood flow, blood-brain barrier, Alzheimer's disease, mural cell, stroke, neurovascular coupling

INTRODUCTION

Brain pericytes nurture the development and maintenance of a healthy cerebrovascular system. In concert with endothelial cells, they support numerous vascular functions including blood-brain barrier (BBB) integrity, cerebral blood flow regulation, vessel stability, angiogenesis and immune cell trafficking (Sweeney et al., 2016). Pericytes have also been suggested as a source of adult multipotent stem cells (Dore-Duffy, 2008; Nakagomi et al., 2015), although whether this attribute persists *in vivo* was recently questioned (Guimarães-Camboa et al., 2017). The coordination of molecular signaling between pericytes and endothelial cells is crucial for a properly organized microvascular network, a subject which has been extensively studied in the context of brain development (Armulik et al., 2005, 2011). However, less is known about pericyte-endothelial communication in the adult brain and the implications of disrupted signaling in age-related cerebrovascular diseases such as dementia and stroke.

The purpose of this review is to describe "pericyte structural remodeling," a novel facet of pericyte biology we have recently observed in the adult mouse brain using long-term high-resolution optical imaging (Berthiaume et al., 2018). Pericyte structural remodeling is the adaptive extension of pericyte processes along microvessel walls on the time-scale of days. It is an under-explored mechanism by which pericytes react on-demand to preserve endothelial contact in the adult brain. As a prelude to further discussion of this topic, we briefly describe the importance of pericyte-endothelial signaling during vascular development and maturation, followed by an account of the current knowledge on pericyte changes during aging. Specifically, we emphasize the vulnerability of pericytes in age-related cerebrovascular and neurodegenerative diseases, particularly Alzheimer's disease. Next, we focus on the structural remodeling of pericytes that we have visualized using *in vivo* two-photon imaging of the adult mouse cortex. This includes an updated view of the identity and topography of pericytes and smooth muscle cells (SMCs) in the adult brain vasculature, which is an evolving topic in the cerebrovascular field. Finally, we discuss potential mechanisms underlying the control of pericyte structural remodeling, which may be targeted for experimental exploration or potential therapeutic benefit in the adult or aging brain. We would like to emphasize that the phenomenon discussed in this article refers specifically to the dynamic remodeling of pericyte shape and size rather than the oft-discussed phenotypic (cell fate) or functional plasticity of these cells (Lange et al., 2013; Holm et al., 2018).

PERICYTE-ENDOTHELIAL DYNAMICS FROM DEVELOPMENT TO MATURATION

How is a capillary bed established in the developing brain? The complexity of this task cannot be understated, as it involves the coordinated layering of different vascular cell types and structures to establish critical properties, such as BBB integrity and the microvascular tone needed to regulate blood flow in a limited cranial space. It further involves a delicate balance between angiogenesis and microvascular pruning to shape the angioarchitecture in a way that ensures nutrient supply to all brain cells. At the heart of this immense task is the dynamic interplay between pericytes and endothelial cells, which lays the foundation for the microvascular network.

Multiple pericyte-endothelial signaling pathways are involved in the transition of dynamic, growing vasculature in the developing brain to stable, mature networks of the adult brain. These pathways have been described in detail by excellent reviews (Armulik et al., 2005), and are only selectively discussed here as a preamble to the topic of pericyte structural remodeling. During angiogenesis, endothelial cells proliferate and migrate to form a nascent capillary tube. At the end of each new vascular stalk is an endothelial tip cell that guides vessel growth, stimulated by the release of vascular endothelial growth factor (VEGF; Gerhardt et al., 2003). New endothelial tubes are permeable and unstable until covered by pericytes. A key step in coordinating this coverage is an increase in PDGF-B/PDGFR-β signaling, which promotes the co-migration of pericytes (or pericyte precursors) to populate nascent capillaries and offsets the expression of VEGF (Hellström et al., 1999). The growth factor PDGF-B is secreted by endothelial cells, dimerizes to form PDGF-BB, and binds to the vascular extracellular matrix. PDGF-BB is sensed by pericytes, which express PDGFR-β, initiating pericyte proliferation and migration. Recruited pericytes promote the growth arrest and survival of endothelial cells, partially through TGFβ signaling (Goumans et al., 2002; Walshe et al., 2009), and by doing so, ensure vessel stability and homeostasis. While difficult to observe in developing mammals, the highly dynamic co-migration of pericytes and endothelial cells was recently captured by elegant live imaging studies using *ex utero* developing zebrafish (Ando et al., 2016). Pericytes appeared to "crawl" along endothelial tubes with peristaltic activity involving extension and contraction of long processes extending from the cell soma.

The importance of pericyte-endothelial signaling to cerebrovascular health is underscored in seminal studies involving congenital deletion of platelet-derived growth factor receptor-β (PDGFR-β) or its ligand PDGF-B. Deletion of either receptor or ligand is embryonic lethal, and the microvasculature develops aberrantly because of an inability to recruit pericytes to the endothelium (Lindahl et al., 1997). The resulting dearth of pericyte coverage is associated with endothelial hyperplasia, increased lumen diameters, and greater vascular permeability than wild-type mice (Hellström et al., 2001). Subsequent studies have used mice with varying levels of PDGF-B/PDGFR-β deficiency to show that the degree of pericyte coverage is strongly correlated with capillary BBB integrity in both developing and adult brains (Armulik et al., 2010; Daneman et al., 2010). Pericytes influence endothelial permeability by suppressing the formation of endothelial caveolae as well as the expression of leukocyte adhesion molecules (Armulik et al., 2010; Daneman et al., 2010; Ben-Zvi et al., 2014). They further influence astrocytes by modifying the polarization of their end-feet along the abluminal side of the capillary wall (Armulik et al., 2010).

Another pathway relevant to our topic is Eph-ephrin signaling, which plays a key role in tissue patterning processes during developmental morphogenesis (Kania and Klein, 2016). Eph receptor tyrosine kinases and their membrane bound ligands, called ephrins, are involved in short-range cell-cell communication. These are well-characterized as a source of cell repulsion and adhesion signaling in axon guidance, which continue to be relevant for the maintenance of cell-to-cell boundaries in adulthood (Yamaguchi and Pasquale, 2004; Evans et al., 2007). Interestingly, there also appears to be a role for these bidirectional signaling partners in blood vessel assembly (Wang et al., 1998; Salvucci et al., 2009). Though better understood as a determinant of endothelial cell arteriovenous identity, mural cell-specific consequences of impaired Eph-ephrin signaling was demonstrated by genetic deletion of a floxed *Efnb2* allele (encoding the Eph receptor ligand Ephrin B2) in mural cells of the dermal vasculature (Foo et al., 2006). This deletion did not affect mural cell numbers but resulted in pericytes and SMCs that were loosely attached to the endothelium, rounded in morphology, and improperly spread along the vasculature. Thus, EphB/ephrin-B2 signaling is required for the proper integration and organization of pericytes along the microvasculature following their recruitment. However, whether this type of signaling is as influential in the context of adult central nervous system microvasculature has yet to be determined.

As the vasculature matures in the healthy brain, the presence of pericytes continues to promote endothelial cell quiescence and vessel stabilization. The sustained activation of endothelial cell Tie2 receptors by mural cell-expressed ligand angiopoietin 1 (Ang1) contributes to the maintenance of a stable, non-leaky endothelium throughout adulthood (Augustin et al., 2009). Furthermore, the vascular basement membrane, which pericytes help to generate (Stratman et al., 2009), completely surrounds the pericytes and adds to the barrier properties of the vascular wall (Gautam et al., 2016). Direct pericyte-endothelial contact is made through the basement membrane at peg-and-socket junctions, which are inter-digitations of the pericyte and endothelial membranes bound by adhesion molecules, notably N-cadherin. The adhesion of pericytes and upregulation and translocation of endothelial N-cadherin involves a variety of signaling pathways, including TGF-β, Notch and sphingosine-1-phosphate signaling (Armulik et al., 2011). Consistent with a stabilized microvascular system in the adult brain, long-term imaging of adult mouse cerebral cortex has shown only rare formations and eliminations of capillary branches (Lam et al., 2010). This stability is further extended to pericytes, as studies from our lab, and others, have shown that pericyte cell bodies are immobile over months of imaging (Cudmore et al., 2017; Berthiaume et al., 2018). Thus, pericytes migrate to vessels during development, but are fixed in place in healthy adult brain capillaries.

PERICYTE PATHOLOGY IN AGING AND AGE-RELATED BRAIN DISEASES

Recently, there has been a strong push to understand how dysfunction of small brain vessels contributes to cognitive decline within the context of cerebrovascular and neurodegenerative disease (Snyder et al., 2015; Corriveau et al., 2016). Studies suggest that the BBB deteriorates progressively in the aging brain due to structural, cellular and molecular deficits in the neurovascular unit. These abnormalities include endothelial atrophy, thickening and irregularity of basement membranes, microvessel thinning (string vessels), increased capillary tortuosity, as well as capillary rarefaction and degeneration (Brown and Thore, 2011; Hunter et al., 2012; Bhat, 2015). With regard to pericyte pathology, a decrease in pericyte numbers has been reported with aging in both human and preclinical models, as well as ultrastructural changes, suggestive of pericyte degeneration (Erdő et al., 2017). Consistent with these observations, a recent transcriptomic and histological study of neurovasculature in the aged mouse brain (18–24 months) showed significant pericyte loss, reduced basement membrane integrity and increased endothelial transcytosis (Soto et al., 2015). Moreover, pericyte-deficient genetic mouse lines with less severe phenotypes often survive to adulthood, and have been useful in implicating pericyte loss as an accelerator of age-dependent BBB breakdown and cerebral hypoperfusion, which precede neurodegeneration and cognitive impairment (Bell et al., 2010; Kisler et al., 2017).

Pericyte status in the aging human brain has also been examined in relation to BBB function using dynamic contrast-enhanced MRI, revealing that an early degeneration of pericytes (as determined by pericyte markers in the cerebral spinal fluid) correlates with increased BBB permeability within the hippocampus (Montagne et al., 2015). Further, *post-mortem* analyses in a number of recent studies have confirmed loss of pericyte number and coverage in the cortex, hippocampus and white matter of AD subjects, compared with age-matched controls (Sengillo et al., 2013; Halliday et al., 2016; Miners et al., 2018; Schultz et al., 2018). Pericytes are highly susceptible to the toxic effects of Aβ, likely because of their ability to internalize the protein for attempted clearance across the BBB (Verbeek et al., 1997; Wilhelmus et al., 2007). This toxicity affects their overall survival as well as their structure. For example, in a mouse model of cerebral amyloid angiopathy affecting microvessels, not only were pericytes progressively lost with age, but the surviving pericytes were found to have unusually short processes, suggesting impairment in structural remodeling (Park et al., 2014). Since pericytes are also involved in removal of Aβ from the brain (Wilhelmus et al., 2007; Sagare et al., 2013; Candela et al., 2015), pericyte loss can initiate a "snowballing" effect to further increase Aβ burden, ultimately worsening microvascular injury in AD. This was exemplified through the accelerated Aβ accumulation, tau pathology, and worsened cognitive decline observed when cross-breeding a mouse model of AD pathology with a model of progressive pericyte deficiency (Sagare et al., 2013).

Aging is also a risk factor for small-vessel disease (SVD), which accounts for approximately 50% of all dementias including AD (Iadecola, 2013; Snyder et al., 2015). SVD is characterized by white matter hyperintensities (leukoaraiosis), lacunar infarcts, and microbleeds (Wardlaw et al., 2013). A recent study using a pericyte-deficient mouse model revealed pericyte loss as a mechanism of white matter degeneration (Montagne et al., 2018). In line with this idea, the walls of microvessels in human white matter become thinner with age, in part due to increased pericyte loss (Stewart et al., 1987). Genetic factors such as mutations in the NOTCH3, a cell surface receptor expressed by mural cells, cause a genetic form of SVD termed cerebral autosomal dominant arteriopathy with subcortical infarcts leukoencephalopathy (CADASIL). A recent study identified pericyte pathology as a primary source of vascular dysfunction in a mouse model of CADASIL (Ghosh et al., 2015).

Finally, it is worth mentioning that the description of pericyte pathology in the literature encompasses, besides cell death, a range of cellular abnormalities including detachment from the endothelium, migration, shape change, and in the case of brain injury, trauma and stroke, their phenotypic transformation. As noted by Kalaria, "it is likely that the brain vasculature is continually modified by growth and repair mechanisms in attempts to maintain perfusion during ageing and disease" (Kalaria, 1996). However, it is yet unknown if, and to what extent, pericytes can adapt in the face of vascular degeneration during aging and age-related diseases.

IDENTIFYING PERICYTES IN THE ADULT MOUSE BRAIN

A key step in understanding the physiological roles of pericytes is the ability to visualize the cells in real time *in vivo*. Two-photon imaging now allows researchers to both observe and manipulate fluorescently-tagged pericytes in cerebrovascular networks of the intact mouse brain (**Figure 1**). However, despite the precision with which pericytes can be visualized, there remains ambiguity on what to call a "pericyte" (Attwell et al., 2016). It is therefore important to first clarify the different microvascular zones in cerebral cortex, and mural cell types that reside within these zones. We consider seven different microvascular zones that connect pial arterioles to pial venules in cerebral cortex, including: (1) pial arterioles, (2) penetrating arterioles, (3) pre-capillary arterioles, (4) capillaries, (5) post-capillary venules, (6) ascending venules, and (7) pial venules (**Figure 2A**). Along this arteriovenous route, there are genes that mural cells in all zones express at high levels, such as *Pdgfrb* (PDGFRβ) and *Cspg4* (NG2). However, recent single-cell transcriptomic data has also revealed zonation in gene expression (Vanlandewijck et al., 2018). At the junction between pre-capillary arterioles and capillaries, there is a sharp transition in expression profile that punctuates mural cells into two broad groups. Upstream to this transition, pial arteriole to pre-capillary arteriole zones highly express proteins related to contractile machinery, such as *Acta2* (α-smooth muscle actin; α-SMA), *Tagln* (smooth muscle protein 22-α), and *Cnn1* (calponin 1). In contrast, downstream mural cells from capillary to venule zones are characterized by high expression of membrane transporters, such as *abcc9* (ATP binding cassette subfamily C member 9), consistent with roles in BBB transport. This may explain why pericytes at the capillary zone preferentially uptake the FluoroNissl dye Neurotrace 500/525 when applied to the brain surface (Damisah et al., 2017).

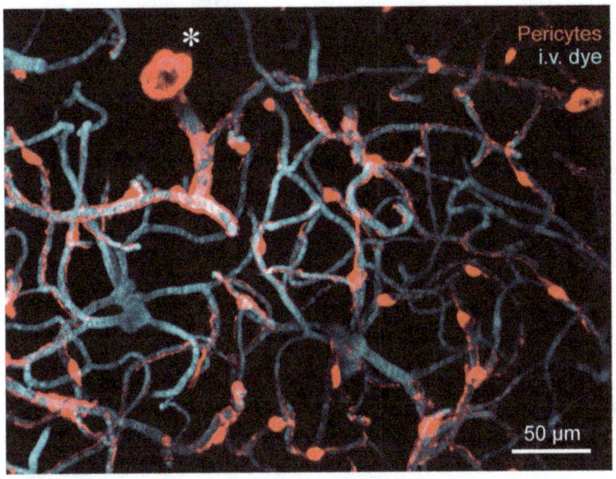

FIGURE 1 | *In vivo* two-photon microscopy of adult mouse cerebrovasculature. High-resolution image of the capillary network surrounding a penetrating arteriole (*) in the mouse cortex. Mural cells are labeled red through expression of tdTomato driven under the control of the Myosin heavy chain 11 (Myh11) promoter. The vasculature is labeled with intravenously administered 2-MDa FITC-dextran, and pseudo-colored blue. Many inducible and constitutively active Cre drivers are suitable for imaging brain mural cells. For more information, see Hartmann et al. (2015a,b).

We next focus on the subsurface network of pre-capillary, capillary and post-capillary zones, where vessels are typically ≤12 μm. Mural cells of varying morphology line these zones (**Figures 2B**, **3A**; Hartmann et al., 2015a; Grant et al., 2017). Most groups use a vessel branch order system to navigate the tortuous subsurface network, where branch order refers to the number of vessel bifurcations between the capillary of interest and a penetrating arteriole, which is denoted 0th branch order. Through detailed analyses of cortical vascular topology in mouse, we recently showed that the capillary zone can be reliably identified and distinguished from α-SMA expressing pre-capillary zone by examining capillaries that are more than four branch points from a penetrating arteriole (Grant et al., 2017).

We refer to pericytes of the capillary zone as "capillary pericytes." These pericytes have conspicuous ovoid cell bodies that intermittently protrude from the vascular wall (**Figures 2B**, **3B**). They extend thin, meandering processes that run along the vessel lumen for hundreds of micrometers (thin-strand pericyte). On the arteriolar pole of the capillary zone, capillary pericyte processes can adopt a mesh-like appearance that covers more of the abluminal surface area (mesh pericyte; Hartmann et al., 2015a; Grant et al., 2017). Critically, all capillary pericytes in the brain appear to express little to no α-SMA, and this has been verified by transcriptional analyses (Vanlandewijck et al., 2018).

Mural cells of the pre-capillary arterioles, a transitional zone between arteriole and capillary, are distinct from capillary pericytes. They are shorter in length, offer greater coverage of the endothelial surface, and like SMCs of pial and penetrating arterioles, are rich in α-SMA (**Figure 2B**). We have referred to these cells as "ensheathing pericytes," i.e., a sub-type of pericyte, because they possess the hallmark protruding cell body of pericytes, and because α-SMA expression has historically been a marker for a subset of pericytes (Grant et al., 2017). Other groups have called these cells simply "pericytes" without distinguishing from capillary pericytes (Hall et al., 2014; Cai et al., 2018), transitional pericytes (Sweeney et al., 2016), pre-capillary SMCs (Hill et al., 2015), or aaSMCs (Vanlandewijck et al., 2018). The shifting nomenclature of these cells has been the root of recent controversy on pericyte roles in blood flow control (discussed further below), and a consensus on naming needs to be established.

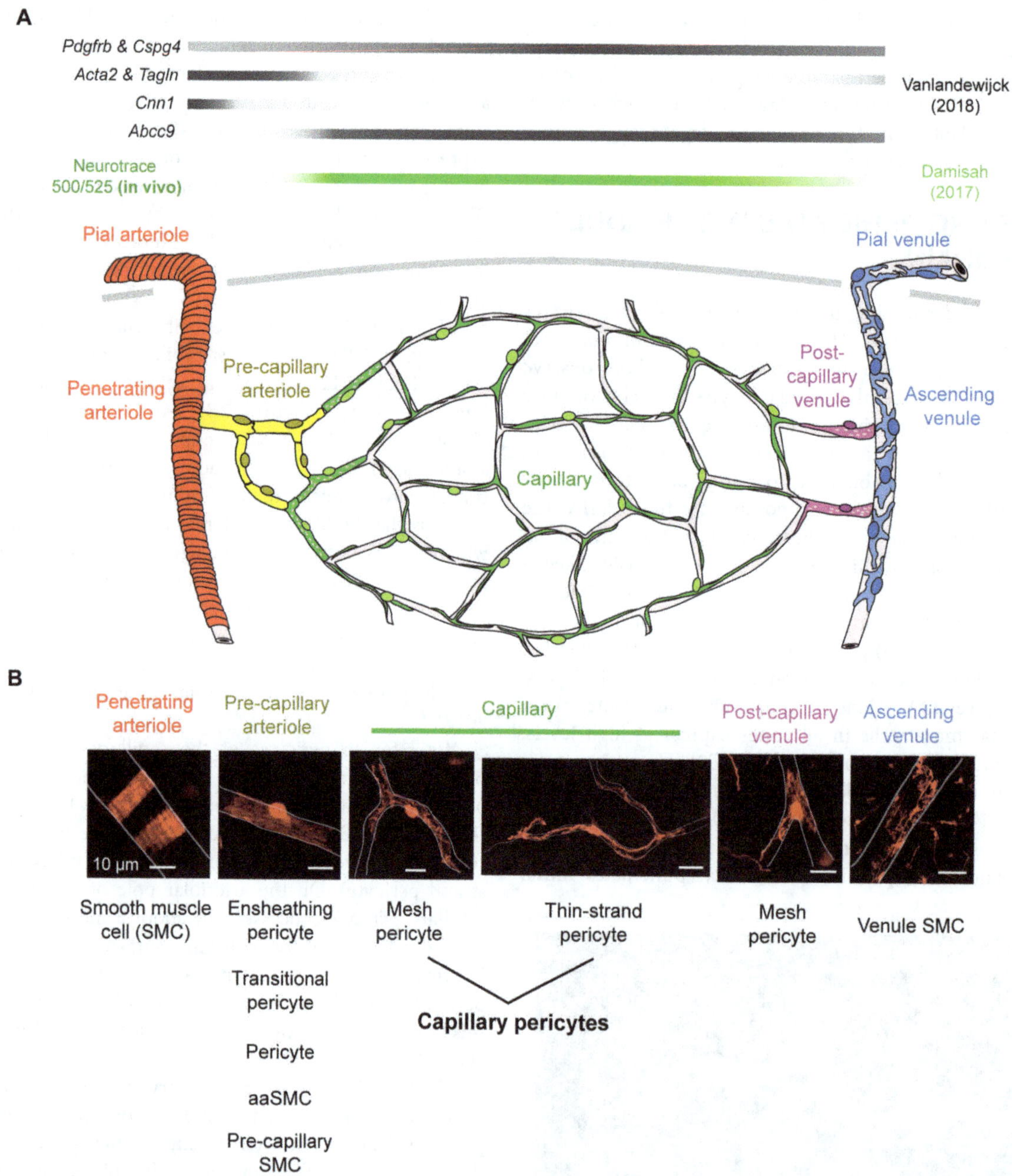

FIGURE 2 | Mural cell heterogeneity in the adult mouse cerebrovascular network. **(A)** (Top) Mural cell gene expression in different zones of the microvasculature in cerebral cortex. Adapted from Vanlandewijck et al. (2018). Neurotrace 500/525 is specifically taken up by capillary pericytes, providing a cell-specific fluorescent label for *in vivo* imaging (Damisah et al., 2017). (Bottom) Schematic depicting mural cells in seven microvascular zones from pial arterioles to pial venule of cerebral cortex. **(B)** (Top) Representative images showing morphology of mural cells in five zones below the cortical surface. All scale bars are 10 μm, except the penetrating venule image, which is 50 μm. Adapted from Hartmann et al. (2015a) and Grant et al. (2017). (Bottom) The evolving nomenclature for each cell type. Note that naming of mural cells in the pre-capillary arteriole zone is not universally agreed upon and has become a source of controversy.

The term "post-capillary venules" has been used in past literature, but whether this should represent a distinct microvascular zone with pericytes performing unique functions remains unclear. Pericytes of post-capillary venules have mesh-like processes, express little to no α-SMA, and are shorter than capillary pericytes (Hartmann et al., 2015a). There is evidence that venular pericytes of the cremaster muscle play a role in immune cell migration (Proebstl et al., 2012), but a similar role for venular pericytes in the brain remains to be examined.

Capillary pericytes are arranged along the capillary bed in a chain-like network, with the majority of the vasculature being contacted by their long cellular processes rather than

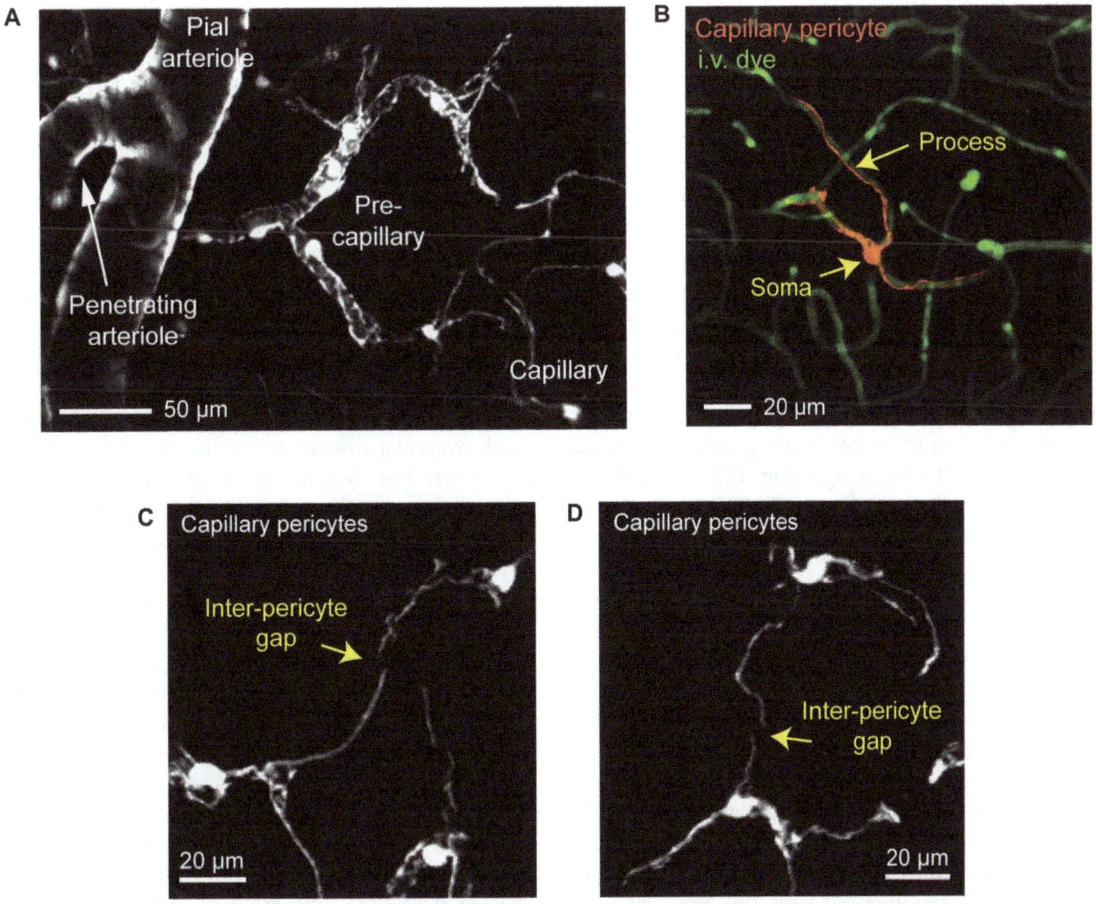

FIGURE 3 | Visualizing capillary pericytes with *in vivo* two-photon imaging. **(A)** An *in vivo* image showing shift in mural cell appearance as a pial arteriole branches into an underlying penetrating arteriole, which then ramifies into the pre-capillary arteriole and capillary bed. The image was captured in the cortex of a Myh11-tdTomato mouse and is a maximal projection over 150 μm of cortical thickness. **(B)** *In vivo* image of an isolated capillary pericyte following intravenous injection of 2 MDa FITC-dextran to co-label the microvasculature. Image was captured from a NG2-tdTomato mouse. **(C,D)** Examples of the non-overlapping territories of adjacent capillary pericytes from a Myh11-tdTomato mouse. The location of gaps between two pericyte territories are denoted with arrows.

cell bodies (Berthiaume et al., 2018). In fact, over 90% of the vasculature in the mouse cerebral cortex is contacted by pericyte processes, suggesting that pericyte-endothelial signaling may occur primarily through these processes (Underly et al., 2017). Interestingly, each pericyte occupies a defined territory that does not overlap with the territories of neighboring pericytes (Hill et al., 2015; Berthiaume et al., 2018). Pericyte territories are so precisely arranged that it is usually difficult to determine where one pericyte ends and the next begins, but for the occasional gap between processes of neighboring cells (**Figures 3C,D**).

PERICYTE REMODELING IN THE ADULT BRAIN

In a recent long-term *in vivo* imaging study, we showed that capillary pericytes under basal conditions negotiate their individual territories with neighboring pericytes through slight extensions and retractions of their terminal processes (Berthiaume et al., 2018). When inter-pericyte gaps were visible, the push-pull interplay between adjacent pericytes could be observed, suggesting that pericyte domains might be maintained throughout adulthood by repulsive pericyte-pericyte interactions (**Figure 4A**). The extent to which neighboring pericytes make direct contact with each other remains unclear. However, recent studies in the retina have suggested gap junction communication between neighboring pericytes involved in conductive vasomotor constrictions (Ivanova et al., 2017).

While the basal changes in pericyte structure we observed were small, it nonetheless raised the question of whether mature brain pericytes are structurally plastic, and if this plasticity could be further induced. To examine this idea, we ablated single capillary pericytes using precise two-photon laser irradiation. This enabled the specific and immediate deletion of individual cells anywhere within the cortical capillary network. In the days to weeks following ablation, the processes of neighboring pericytes extended into the territories uncovered by the ablated pericyte with ~10-fold greater speed and magnitude than dynamics observed under basal conditions (**Figures 4B,C**). Process extension occurred while the pericyte somata remained firmly affixed, indicating no overt cell migration or proliferation. New cytoplasmic material was added to the growing pericyte process, enabling contact with hundreds of micrometers of extra capillary length. Importantly, this work demonstrated that pericytes can remodel their shape and grow in size in the adult brain and are inherently programed to maintain coverage of the endothelium. Yet, the mechanism appears imperfect, as the need to increase cytoplasmic volume suggests a limit to growth, and many days were required to regain endothelial coverage. Whether this reparative process can be pharmacologically enhanced to promote continued pericyte-endothelial contact in the adult brain will be important to explore.

A logical molecular target to modulate pericyte structural remodeling is PDGF-B/PDGFR-β signaling. PDGF-B delivery is neuroprotective in stroke models and PDGFR-β expression in pericytes increases progressively following cerebral ischemia in the adult brain (Arimura et al., 2012), likely reflecting a reparative response. Also relating to PDGF-B/PDGFR-β signaling, Lebrin et al. (2010) showed that the drug thalidomide reduced bleeding in patients with hereditary hemorrhagic telangiectasia (HHT), a disease involving vascular malformations and bleeds in multiple organs. Using a mouse model of HHT, the benefit of thalidomide was shown to be partly due to the enhancement of endothelial PDGF-B expression leading to increase of pericyte recruitment/coverage. Similarly, thalidomide was reported to promote PDGF-B/PDGFR-β signaling, increase pericyte coverage, and reduce bleeding in a mouse model of brain arteriovenous malformation (bAVM; Zhu et al., 2018), a cerebrovascular disease with marked pericyte loss in humans (Winkler et al., 2018). Whether enhanced pericyte structural remodeling is a salutary effect of thalidomide needs further investigation. However, it seems likely in light of recent work reporting increased pericyte process growth following treatment with PDGF-BB in a mouse model of epilepsy (Arango-Lievano et al., 2018).

A second molecular interaction that may be at play in adult pericyte structural remodeling is Eph-ephrin signaling. It is currently unknown whether this bidirectional signaling pathway acts basally as a repulsion and/or cell-spreading signal for defining pericyte territories in the adult brain. If so, pericyte loss in the adult brain could disrupt pericyte-to-pericyte Eph-ephrin repulsive signaling, essentially disinhibiting the growth of pericyte processes. This, in conjunction with the expression of other directional growth cues (i.e., PDGF-B), could help explain our observation following single pericyte ablation, where neighboring processes robustly spread into vacated territories until contact with another pericyte is made.

CONSEQUENCES OF PERICYTE LOSS IN THE ADULT BRAIN

The ability to selectively remove pericytes from an existing vascular network and then track recovery over time provided insight into the physiological consequence of pericyte loss in the adult brain. We examined three modes of pericyte function that are well-established from studies of developing organisms, including regulation of: (1) capillary network structure, (2) BBB integrity, and (3) capillary lumen diameter.

First, we found that single pericyte loss in mature vascular networks had no overt effect on capillary structure. That is, no formation or elimination of new capillary branches was observed in regions without pericyte coverage. This was an unexpected finding, as pericyte loss could conceivably lead to capillary pruning due to loss of endothelial support, or aberrant angiogenesis by alleviating the suppression of endothelial proliferation. Thus, capillaries in the adult brain can be structurally stable with transient loss of pericyte coverage *in vivo*. It will be important to determine if and how aging or cerebrovascular disease makes the vasculature more vulnerable to pericyte loss. Second, we were unable to detect acute BBB leakage from uncovered capillary segments following single pericyte ablation. This was also surprising, as pericyte loss in the developing brain is strongly associated with increased endothelial transcytosis. Even with the use of small molecular weight dyes (1 kDa), which have been previously shown to permeate through a trans-cellular route (Armulik et al., 2010), we found no evidence of plasma extravasation at capillary regions lacking pericyte coverage. In line with this lack of BBB leakage, a recent study using an inducible diphtheria toxin strategy to acutely kill mural cells, including pericytes, in adult mice reported intact blood-retinal and blood-brain barriers, despite vascular leakage in peripheral tissues (Park et al., 2017). Furthermore, mouse models of mild pericyte deficiency retaining approximately 70% of normal pericyte coverage in the adult cerebral neocortex do not present BBB leakage, while a drop to 45% coverage results in a modest BBB leak (Armulik et al., 2010). Collectively, these findings suggest that BBB integrity in the adult brain can be resilient to some degree of pericyte loss.

One consistent alteration we did observe after single pericyte ablation, however, was the sustained dilation of the capillary lumen in regions lacking pericyte contact (**Figures 4B–D**). This dilation persisted until pericyte processes grew back into the exposed territory, at which point capillary diameter returned to basal levels. This finding was mirrored in a study examining the dynamic loss and gain of mural cell coverage induced by seizure activity (Arango-Lievano et al., 2018). This implies that pericytes at the capillary level exert a steady-state vascular tone that may behave like a tension clamp on the endothelial tube either mechanically or through constant molecular signaling with the endothelium.

The idea that pericytes regulate blood flow has persisted through the literature since their discovery by Rouget in the late 1800s (Rouget, 1873), but has remained a controversial topic to this day (Attwell et al., 2016). The majority of *in vivo* imaging studies to date have focused on whether pericytes are involved in the second-to-second diameter changes need for blood flow control during neurovascular coupling. This issue is challenging to address because constriction or relaxation of upstream arterioles will influence blood flow into downstream capillaries, making it very difficult to attribute changes in capillary blood

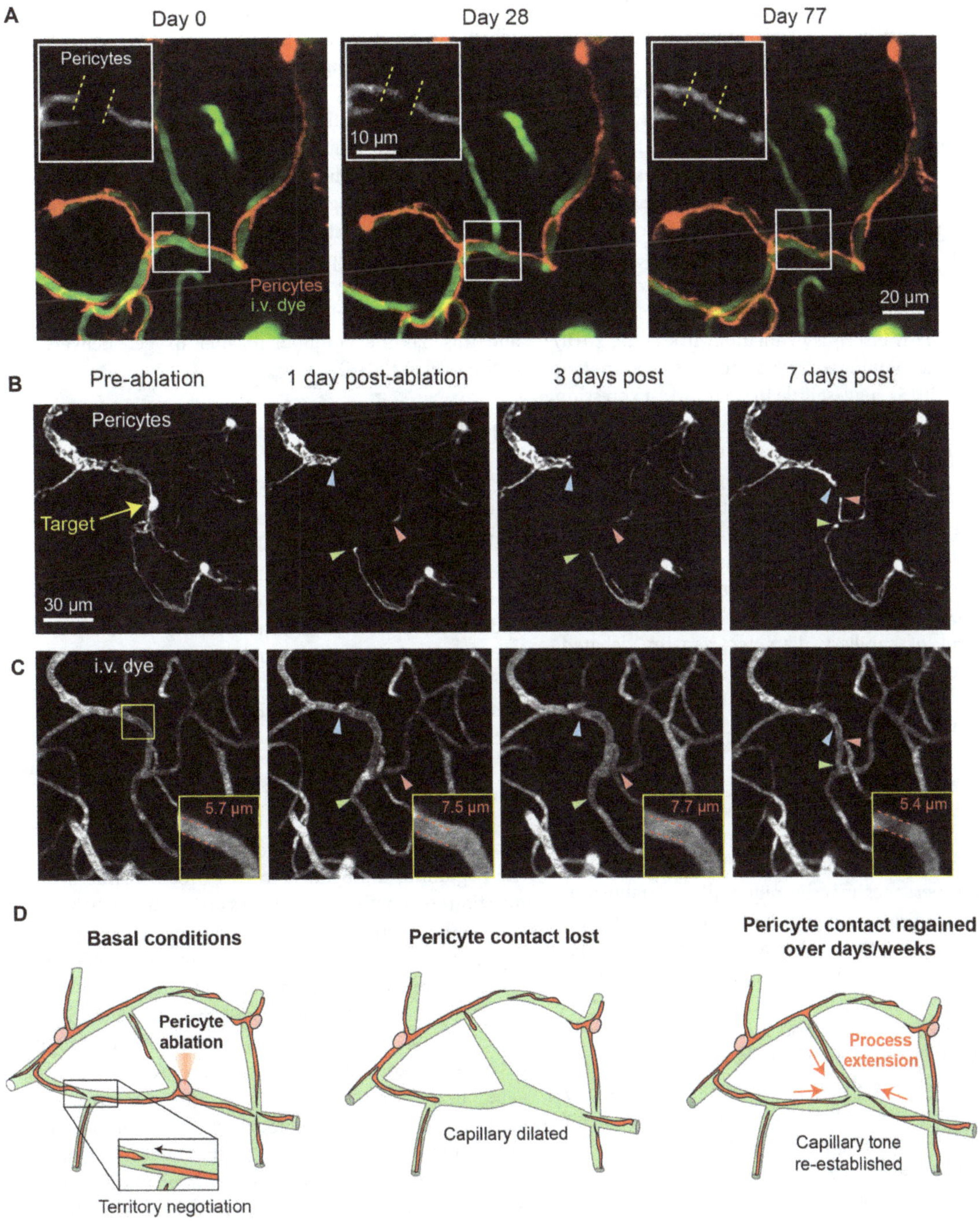

FIGURE 4 | Pericyte structural remodeling captured with chronic *in vivo* 2-photon imaging. **(A)** An example of the structural dynamics of adjacent pericytes under basal conditions. Inset shows the extension of a pericyte process beyond its territory at Day 0, and the corresponding retraction of a neighboring pericyte process. Images are from a Myh11-tdTomato mouse. Adapted from Berthiaume et al. (2018). **(B)** Two-photon laser ablation of a single pericyte results in the robust extension of immediately adjacent pericyte processes into the vacated territory over 7 days. The image shows the extension of two thin-strand pericytes (green and red arrowheads) and one mesh pericyte (blue arrowhead). Images are from a Myh11-tdTomato mouse. **(C)** Images of the vasculature, labeled by 2 MDa FITC-dextran, at the site of pericyte ablation (same region as panel **B**). Inset shows an increased capillary diameter in the vessel segment lacking pericyte coverage, which returns to baseline diameter once pericyte contact is regained suggesting vascular tone. **(D)** Schematic of pericyte structural remodeling under basal conditions and following acute pericyte ablation.

flow to autonomous action by capillary pericytes *in vivo*. Many have circumvented this issue by studying pericyte contractility *ex vivo* in a variety of CNS tissues, such as cortical/cerebellar slices and isolated retina. These studies agree that pericytes of capillary and pre-capillary zones can respond to electrical (Peppiatt et al., 2006; Mishra et al., 2016; Ivanova et al., 2017), pharmacological (Peppiatt et al., 2006; Fernández-Klett et al., 2010; Hall et al., 2014) and neural stimuli (Hall et al., 2014; Biesecker et al., 2016; Mapelli et al., 2017). However, some caution needs to be taken for interpretation as *ex vivo* systems exhibit capillary diameter changes on much longer timescales (2 min), with relevance to neurovascular coupling less certain. Further, mixing pericytes functions across different tissues (brain vs. retina) is problematic because pericytes functions and vascular architecture differ. In fact, a recent study using modified tissue fixation procedures suggests that retinal capillary pericytes express high α-SMA (Alarcon-Martinez et al., 2018). However, measurements of *acta2* transcripts (Vanlandewijck et al., 2018) and use of *acta2* Cre-recombinase drivers combined with potent reporters (Hill et al., 2015) suggest little to no α-SMA expression in brain capillary pericytes.

In vivo imaging studies agree that mural cells of pre-capillary arterioles support rapid diameter changes required for neurovascular coupling, though nomenclature for these cells differ between labs (Hall et al., 2014; Hill et al., 2015). In fact, dilatory and constrictive responses may initiate at pre-capillary arterioles and then conduct upstream to penetrating arterioles (Cai et al., 2018). However, the role of capillary pericytes in dynamic control of capillary diameter remains debated. Some groups have reported no capillary diameter changes with optogenetic stimulation (Hill et al., 2015), neural activity (Fernández-Klett et al., 2010; Hill et al., 2015; Wei et al., 2016) or ischemia (Hill et al., 2015), while other groups have observed diameter changes with neural activity (Hall et al., 2014; Kisler et al., 2017).

One way to reconcile these data is that capillary pericytes are contractile, but much less so than their counterparts on upstream arterioles. Capillary pericytes may be required for establishing basal, long-term equilibrium and optimum flow through the capillary bed, whereas upstream mural cells are responsible for initiating rapid moment-to-moment changes in blood flow. A constant, steady-state tone imparted by capillary pericytes is a less studied aspect of cerebral blood flow control. However, it is critical for brain function as all blood entering the brain must percolate through the dense, pericyte-covered capillary bed, irrespective of local neuronal activity. Given that red blood cells are larger than the average diameter of the capillary lumen and must deform to pass through (Secomb, 1991), even small alterations in basal capillary diameter will have a significant effect on capillary transit time and oxygen availability (Jespersen and Østergaard, 2012). An estimated 40% of total cerebrovascular resistance exists at the level of penetrating arterioles, capillaries, and venules Iadecola (2017), and modeling studies suggest that the capillaries confer a sizable proportion of this resistance (Gould et al., 2017).

Little is known about how age or disease-dependent pericyte loss affects basal capillary diameter, blood flow and oxygen delivery. One recent study examined young *pdgfrb*$^{+/-}$ mice, which exhibit a moderate loss of pericyte coverage (from 77% coverage in wild-type to ~55% in knockouts), and showed impaired basal tissue oxygen supply using a novel oxygen-sensitive imaging probe (Kisler et al., 2017), but no change in basal capillary diameter. However, in adult *pdgfrb*$^{ret/ret}$ mice, which exhibit more severe loss of pericyte coverage (from ~90% coverage in wild-type to ~25% in knockouts), capillary diameters became significantly larger, consistent with the idea of altered basal tone with sufficient pericyte loss (Armulik et al., 2010). Further, a study of human bAVMs showed increased blood flow within the AVM nidus (shorter mean transit time), as measured by pre-operative angiograms, when pericyte coverage dropped below 40%, suggestive of capillary dilation. Like capillary constriction and impedance of flow (Yemisci et al., 2009; Hall et al., 2014), capillary dilation can disrupt normal blood flow rate and blood cell distribution within the microvascular network, and this has the potential to alter oxygen delivery to tissues (Schmid et al., 2015).

OUTLOOK

The structural remodeling of pericytes in the adult mouse brain may be essential for maintenance of cerebrovascular health and needs to be broadly explored in models of cerebrovascular disease. This task is facilitated by long-term *in vivo* imaging methods that allow quantification of pericyte growth, coverage, and capillary flow over time. Among the critical next steps are the need to examine the physiological consequence of pericyte ablation at the *adult* stage using either precise optical methods (Hill et al., 2017; Berthiaume et al., 2018), or novel pericyte-specific Cre drivers to delete or modify capillary pericytes (Zlokovic et al., 2015; Park et al., 2017). While many studies have used mice with congenital deficiency in pericyte-endothelial signaling, very little is known about the impact of pericyte loss in models where pericytes develop normally at the beginning. Embedded in this broader issue are intriguing questions of whether all pericytes are functionally homogeneous, or whether pericytes in some microvascular zones lack the capacity to remodel and are more vulnerable to vascular disease. More work is also needed to determine the threshold for pericyte loss that surpasses the compensatory ability of pericyte process growth, which presumably contributes to the development of neurovascular pathologies in the adult and aging brain. The effects of age and cerebrovascular disease on pericyte structural remodeling will be important areas of future inquiry as well. Lastly, the molecular signaling that governs pericyte remodeling in adulthood requires further study, with PDGF-B/PDGFR-β and Eph-ephrin signaling as logical targets for pharmacological or genetic manipulation in the adult brain.

AUTHOR CONTRIBUTIONS

A-AB wrote the review with feedback from MM, NB and AS.

FUNDING

AS is supported by grants from the National Institutes of Health (NIH)/NINDS (R01NS085402, R21NS096997, P20GM109040), the National Science Foundation (1539034), American Heart Association (14GRNT20480366), and the Alzheimer's Association (2016-NIRG-397149). DH is supported by the NIH/NINDS (F30NS096868). NB is supported by the NIH/NIA (R21AG052321). MM is supported by the NIH/NHLBI grants (R01HL123650, R01HL121877, R01HL133723), the Loie Power Robinson Stem Cell and Regenerative Medicine Fund, and the Seattle Children's Research Institute.

REFERENCES

Alarcon-Martinez, L., Yilmaz-Ozcan, S., Yemisci, M., Schallek, J., Kılıç, K., Can, A., et al. (2018). Capillary pericytes express α-smooth muscle actin, which requires prevention of filamentous-actin depolymerization for detection. *Elife* 7:e34861. doi: 10.7554/eLife.34861

Ando, K., Fukuhara, S., Izumi, N., Nakajima, H., Fukui, H., Kelsh, R. N., et al. (2016). Clarification of mural cell coverage of vascular endothelial cells by live imaging of zebrafish. *Development* 143, 1328–1339. doi: 10.1242/dev.132654

Arango-Lievano, M., Boussadia, B., De Terdonck, L. D. T., Gault, C., Fontanaud, P., Lafont, C., et al. (2018). Topographic reorganization of cerebrovascular mural cells under seizure conditions. *Cell Rep.* 23, 1045–1059. doi: 10.1016/j.celrep.2018.03.110

Arimura, K., Ago, T., Kamouchi, M., Nakamura, K., Ishitsuka, K., Kuroda, J., et al. (2012). PDGF receptor β signaling in pericytes following ischemic brain injury. *Curr. Neurovasc. Res.* 9, 1–9. doi: 10.2174/156720212799297100

Armulik, A., Abramsson, A., and Betsholtz, C. (2005). Endothelial/pericyte interactions. *Circ. Res.* 97, 512–523. doi: 10.1161/01.res.0000182903.16652.d7

Armulik, A., Genové, G., and Betsholtz, C. (2011). Pericytes: developmental, physiological, and pathological perspectives, problems and promises. *Dev. Cell* 21, 193–215. doi: 10.1016/j.devcel.2011.07.001

Armulik, A., Genové, G., Mäe, M., Nisancioglu, M. H., Wallgard, E., Niaudet, C., et al. (2010). Pericytes regulate the blood-brain barrier. *Nature* 468, 557–561. doi: 10.1038/nature09522

Attwell, D., Mishra, A., Hall, C. N., O'Farrell, F. M., and Dalkara, T. (2016). What is a pericyte? *J. Cereb. Blood Flow Metab.* 36, 451–455. doi: 10.1177/0271678X15610340

Augustin, H. G., Koh, G. Y., Thurston, G., and Alitalo, K. (2009). Control of vascular morphogenesis and homeostasis through the angiopoietin-Tie system. *Nat. Rev. Mol. Cell Biol.* 10, 165–177. doi: 10.1038/nrm2639

Bell, R. D., Winkler, E. A., Sagare, A. P., Singh, I., LaRue, B., Deane, R., et al. (2010). Pericytes control key neurovascular functions and neuronal phenotype in the adult brain and during brain aging. *Neuron* 68, 409–427. doi: 10.1016/j.neuron.2010.09.043

Ben-Zvi, A., Lacoste, B., Kur, E., Andreone, B. J., Mayshar, Y., Yan, H., et al. (2014). Mfsd2a is critical for the formation and function of the blood-brain barrier. *Nature* 509, 507–511. doi: 10.1038/nature13324

Berthiaume, A. A., Grant, R. I., McDowell, K. P., Underly, R. G., Hartmann, D. A., Levy, M., et al. (2018). Dynamic remodeling of pericytes *in vivo* maintains capillary coverage in the adult mouse brain. *Cell Rep.* 22, 8–16. doi: 10.1016/j.celrep.2017.12.016

Bhat, N. R. (2015). Vasculoprotection as a convergent, multi-targeted mechanism of Anti-AD therapeutics and interventions. *J. Alzheimers Dis.* 46, 581–591. doi: 10.3233/JAD-150098

Biesecker, K. R., Srienc, A. I., Shimoda, A. M., Agarwal, A., Bergles, D. E., Kofuji, P., et al. (2016). Glial cell calcium signaling mediates capillary regulation of blood flow in the retina. *J. Neurosci.* 36, 9435–9445. doi: 10.1523/JNEUROSCI.1782-16.2016

Brown, W. R., and Thore, C. R. (2011). Review: cerebral microvascular pathology in ageing and neurodegeneration. *Neuropathol. Appl. Neurobiol.* 37, 56–74. doi: 10.1111/j.1365-2990.2010.01139.x

Cai, C., Fordsmann, J. C., Jensen, S. H., Gesslein, B., Lønstrup, M., Hald, B. O., et al. (2018). Stimulation-induced increases in cerebral blood flow and local capillary vasoconstriction depend on conducted vascular responses. *Proc. Natl. Acad. Sci. U S A* 115, E5796–E5804. doi: 10.1073/pnas.1707702115

Candela, P., Saint-Pol, J., Kuntz, M., Boucau, M. C., Lamartiniere, Y., Gosselet, F., et al. (2015). *In vitro* discrimination of the role of LRP1 at the BBB cellular level: focus on brain capillary endothelial cells and brain pericytes. *Brain Res.* 1594, 15–26. doi: 10.1016/j.brainres.2014.10.047

Corriveau, R. A., Bosetti, F., Emr, M., Gladman, J. T., Koenig, J. I., Moy, C. S., et al. (2016). The science of vascular contributions to cognitive impairment and dementia (VCID): a framework for advancing research priorities in the cerebrovascular biology of cognitive decline. *Cell. Mol. Neurobiol.* 36, 281–288. doi: 10.1007/s10571-016-0334-7

Cudmore, R. H., Dougherty, S. E., and Linden, D. J. (2017). Cerebral vascular structure in the motor cortex of adult mice is stable and is not altered by voluntary exercise. *J. Cereb. Blood Flow Metab.* 37, 3725–3743. doi: 10.1177/0271678x16682508

Damisah, E. C., Hill, R. A., Tong, L., Murray, K. N., and Grutzendler, J. (2017). A fluoro-Nissl dye identifies pericytes as distinct vascular mural cells during *in vivo* brain imaging. *Nat. Neurosci.* 20, 1023–1032. doi: 10.1038/nn.4564

Daneman, R., Zhou, L., Kebede, A. A., and Barres, B. A. (2010). Pericytes are required for blood-brain barrier integrity during embryogenesis. *Nature* 468, 562–566. doi: 10.1038/nature09513

Dore-Duffy, P. (2008). Pericytes: pluripotent cells of the blood brain barrier. *Curr. Pharm. Des.* 14, 1581–1593. doi: 10.2174/138161208784705469

Erdő, F., Denes, L., and De Lange, E. (2017). Age-associated physiological and pathological changes at the blood-brain barrier: a review. *J. Cereb. Blood Flow Metab.* 37, 4–24. doi: 10.1177/0271678x16679420

Evans, I. R., Renne, T., Gertler, F. B., and Nobes, C. D. (2007). Ena/VASP proteins mediate repulsion from ephrin ligands. *J. Cell Sci.* 120, 289–298. doi: 10.1242/jcs.03333

Fernández-Klett, F., Offenhauser, N., Dirnagl, U., Priller, J., and Lindauer, U. (2010). Pericytes in capillaries are contractile *in vivo*, but arterioles mediate functional hyperemia in the mouse brain. *Proc. Natl. Acad. Sci. U S A* 107, 22290–22295. doi: 10.1073/pnas.1011321108

Foo, S. S., Turner, C. J., Adams, S., Compagni, A., Aubyn, D., Kogata, N., et al. (2006). Ephrin-B2 controls cell motility and adhesion during blood-vessel-wall assembly. *Cell* 124, 161–173. doi: 10.1016/j.cell.2005.10.034

Gautam, J., Zhang, X., and Yao, Y. (2016). The role of pericytic laminin in blood brain barrier integrity maintenance. *Sci. Rep.* 6:36450. doi: 10.1038/srep36450

Gerhardt, H., Golding, M., Fruttiger, M., Ruhrberg, C., Lundkvist, A., Abramsson, A., et al. (2003). VEGF guides angiogenic sprouting utilizing endothelial tip cell filopodia. *J. Cell Biol.* 161, 1163–1177. doi: 10.1083/jcb.200302047

Ghosh, M., Balbi, M., Hella, F., Dichgans, M., Lindauer, U., and Plesnila, N. (2015). Pericytes are involved in the pathogenesis of cerebral autosomal dominant arteriopathy with subcortical infarcts and leukoencephalopathy. *Ann. Neurol.* 78, 887–900. doi: 10.1002/ana.24512

Gould, I. G., Tsai, P. S., Kleinfeld, D., and Linninger, A. (2017). The capillary bed offers the largest hemodynamic resistance to the cortical blood supply. *J. Cereb. Blood Flow Metab.* 37, 52–68. doi: 10.1177/0271678x16671146

Goumans, M. J., Valdimarsdottir, G., Itoh, S., Rosendahl, A., Sideras, P., and Ten Dijke, P. (2002). Balancing the activation state of the endothelium via two distinct TGF-α type I receptors. *EMBO J.* 21, 1743–1753. doi: 10.1093/emboj/21.7.1743

Grant, R. I., Hartmann, D. A., Underly, R. G., Berthiaume, A.-A., Bhat, N. R., and Shih, A. Y. (2017). Organizational hierarchy and structural diversity of microvascular pericytes in adult mouse cortex. *J. Cereb. Blood Flow Metab.* doi: 10.1177/0271678X17732229 [Epub ahead of print].

Guimarães-Camboa, N., Cattaneo, P., Sun, Y., Moore-Morris, T., Gu, Y., Dalton, N. D., et al. (2017). Pericytes of multiple organs do not behave as mesenchymal stem cells *in vivo*. *Cell Stem Cell* 20, 345–359. doi: 10.1016/j.stem.2016.12.006

Hall, C. N., Reynell, C., Gesslein, B., Hamilton, N. B., Mishra, A., Sutherland, B. A., et al. (2014). Capillary pericytes regulate cerebral blood flow in health and disease. *Nature* 508, 55–60. doi: 10.1038/nature13165

Halliday, M. R., Rege, S. V., Ma, Q., Zhao, Z., Miller, C. A., Winkler, E. A., et al. (2016). Accelerated pericyte degeneration and blood-brain barrier breakdown in apolipoprotein E4 carriers with Alzheimer's disease. *J. Cereb. Blood Flow Metab.* 36, 216–227. doi: 10.1038/jcbfm.2015.44

Hartmann, D. A., Underly, R. G., Grant, R. I., Watson, A. N., Lindner, V., and Shih, A. Y. (2015a). Pericyte structure and distribution in the cerebral cortex revealed by high-resolution imaging of transgenic mice. *Neurophotonics* 2:041402. doi: 10.1117/1.nph.2.4.041402

Hartmann, D. A., Underly, R. G., Watson, A. N., and Shih, A. Y. (2015b). A murine toolbox for imaging the neurovascular unit. *Microcirculation* 22, 168–182. doi: 10.1111/micc.12176

Hellström, M., Gerhardt, H., Kalén, M., Li, X., Eriksson, U., Wolburg, H., et al. (2001). Lack of pericytes leads to endothelial hyperplasia and abnormal vascular morphogenesis. *J. Cell Biol.* 153, 543–553. doi: 10.1083/jcb.153.3.543

Hellström, M., Kalén, M., Lindahl, P., Abramsson, A., and Betsholtz, C. (1999). Role of PDGF-B and PDGFR-α in recruitment of vascular smooth muscle cells and pericytes during embryonic blood vessel formation in the mouse. *Development* 126, 3047–3055.

Hill, R. A., Damisah, E. C., Chen, F., Kwan, A. C., and Grutzendler, J. (2017). Targeted two-photon chemical apoptotic ablation of defined cell types *in vivo*. *Nat. Commun.* 8:15837. doi: 10.1038/ncomms15837

Hill, R. A., Tong, L., Yuan, P., Murikinati, S., Gupta, S., and Grutzendler, J. (2015). Regional blood flow in the normal and ischemic brain is controlled by arteriolar smooth muscle cell contractility and not by capillary pericytes. *Neuron* 87, 95–110. doi: 10.1016/j.neuron.2015.06.001

Holm, A., Heumann, T., and Augustin, H. G. (2018). Microvascular mural cell organotypic heterogeneity and functional plasticity. *Trends Cell Biol.* 28, 302–316. doi: 10.1016/j.tcb.2017.12.002

Hunter, J. M., Kwan, J., Malek-Ahmadi, M., Maarouf, C. L., Kokjohn, T. A., Belden, C., et al. (2012). Morphological and pathological evolution of the brain microcirculation in aging and Alzheimer's disease. *PLoS One* 7:e36893. doi: 10.1371/journal.pone.0036893

Iadecola, C. (2013). The pathobiology of vascular dementia. *Neuron* 80, 844–866. doi: 10.1016/j.neuron.2013.10.008

Iadecola, C. (2017). The neurovascular unit coming of age: a journey through neurovascular coupling in health and disease. *Neuron* 96, 17–42. doi: 10.1016/j.neuron.2017.07.030

Ivanova, E., Kovacs-Oller, T., and Sagdullaev, B. T. (2017). Vascular pericyte impairment and connexin43 gap junction deficit contribute to vasomotor decline in diabetic retinopathy. *J. Neurosci.* 37, 7580–7594. doi: 10.1523/JNEUROSCI.0187-17.2017

Jespersen, S. N., and Østergaard, L. (2012). The roles of cerebral blood flow, capillary transit time heterogeneity, and oxygen tension in brain oxygenation and metabolism. *J. Cereb. Blood Flow Metab.* 32, 264–277. doi: 10.1038/jcbfm.2011.153

Kalaria, R. N. (1996). Cerebral vessels in ageing and Alzheimer's disease. *Pharmacol. Ther.* 72, 193–214. doi: 10.1016/s0163-7258(96)00116-7

Kania, A., and Klein, R. (2016). Mechanisms of ephrin-Eph signalling in development, physiology and disease. *Nat. Rev. Mol. Cell Biol.* 17, 240–256. doi: 10.1038/nrm.2015.16

Kisler, K., Nelson, A. R., Rege, S. V., Ramanathan, A., Wang, Y., Ahuja, A., et al. (2017). Pericyte degeneration leads to neurovascular uncoupling and limits oxygen supply to brain. *Nat. Neurosci.* 20, 406–416. doi: 10.1038/nn.4489

Lam, C. K., Yoo, T., Hiner, B., Liu, Z., and Grutzendler, J. (2010). Embolus extravasation is an alternative mechanism for cerebral microvascular recanalization. *Nature* 465, 478–482. doi: 10.1038/nature09001

Lange, S., Trost, A., Tempfer, H., Bauer, H. C., Bauer, H., Rohde, E., et al. (2013). Brain pericyte plasticity as a potential drug target in CNS repair. *Drug Discov. Today* 18, 456–463. doi: 10.1016/j.drudis.2012.12.007

Lebrin, F., Srun, S., Raymond, K., Martin, S., van den Brink, S., Freitas, C., et al. (2010). Thalidomide stimulates vessel maturation and reduces epistaxis in individuals with hereditary hemorrhagic telangiectasia. *Nat. Med.* 16, 420–428. doi: 10.1038/nm.2131

Lindahl, P., Johansson, B. R., Levé, P., and Betsholtz, C. (1997). Pericyte loss and microaneurysm formation in PDGF-B-deficient mice. *Science* 277, 242–245. doi: 10.1126/science.277.5323.242

Mapelli, L., Gagliano, G., Soda, T., Laforenza, U., Moccia, F., and D'Angelo, E. U. (2017). Granular layer neurons control cerebellar neurovascular coupling through an NMDA receptor/NO-dependent system. *J. Neurosci.* 37, 1340–1351. doi: 10.1523/JNEUROSCI.2025-16.2016

Miners, J. S., Schulz, I., and Love, S. (2018). Differing associations between Aβ accumulation, hypoperfusion, blood-brain barrier dysfunction and loss of PDGFRB pericyte marker in the precuneus and parietal white matter in Alzheimer's disease. *J. Cereb. Blood Flow Metab.* 38, 103–115. doi: 10.1177/0271678X17690761

Mishra, A., Reynolds, J. P., Chen, Y., Gourine, A. V., Rusakov, D. A., and Attwell, D. (2016). Astrocytes mediate neurovascular signaling to capillary pericytes but not to arterioles. *Nat. Neurosci.* 19, 1619–1627. doi: 10.1038/nn.4428

Montagne, A., Barnes, S. R., Sweeney, M. D., Halliday, M. R., Sagare, A. P., Zhao, Z., et al. (2015). Blood-brain barrier breakdown in the aging human hippocampus. *Neuron* 85, 296–302. doi: 10.1016/j.neuron.2014.12.032

Montagne, A., Nikolakopoulou, A. M., Zhao, Z., Sagare, A. P., Si, G., Lazic, D., et al. (2018). Pericyte degeneration causes white matter dysfunction in the mouse central nervous system. *Nat. Med.* 24, 326–337. doi: 10.1038/nm.4482

Nakagomi, T., Kubo, S., Nakano-Doi, A., Sakuma, R., Lu, S., Narita, A., et al. (2015). Brain vascular pericytes following ischemia have multipotential stem cell activity to differentiate into neural and vascular lineage cells. *Stem Cells* 33, 1962–1974. doi: 10.1002/stem.1977

Park, L., Koizumi, K., El Jamal, S., Zhou, P., Previti, M. L., Van Nostrand, W. E., et al. (2014). Age-dependent neurovascular dysfunction and damage in a mouse model of cerebral amyloid angiopathy. *Stroke* 45, 1815–1821. doi: 10.1161/STROKEAHA.114.005179

Park, D. Y., Lee, J., Kim, J., Kim, K., Hong, S., Han, S., et al. (2017). Plastic roles of pericytes in the blood-retinal barrier. *Nat. Commun.* 8:15296. doi: 10.1038/ncomms15296

Peppiatt, C. M., Howarth, C., Mobbs, P., and Attwell, D. (2006). Bidirectional control of CNS capillary diameter by pericytes. *Nature* 443, 642–643. doi: 10.1038/nature05193

Proebstl, D., Voisin, M. B., Woodfin, A., Whiteford, J., D'Acquisto, F., Jones, G. E., et al. (2012). Pericytes support neutrophil subendothelial cell crawling and breaching of venular walls *in vivo*. *J. Exp. Med.* 209, 1219–1234. doi: 10.1084/jem.20111622

Rouget, C. (1873). Memoire sur le developpement la structure et les proprietes physiologiques des capillaires sanguins et lymphatiques. *Arch. Physiol. Norm. Path.* 5, 603–663.

Sagare, A. P., Bell, R. D., Zhao, Z., Ma, Q., Winkler, E. A., Ramanathan, A., et al. (2013). Pericyte loss influences Alzheimer-like neurodegeneration in mice. *Nat. Commun.* 4:2932. doi: 10.1038/ncomms3932

Salvucci, O., Maric, D., Economopoulou, M., Sakakibara, S., Merlin, S., Follenzi, A., et al. (2009). EphrinB reverse signaling contributes to endothelial and mural cell assembly into vascular structures. *Blood* 114, 1707–1716. doi: 10.1182/blood-2008-12-192294

Schmid, F., Reichold, J., Weber, B., and Jenny, P. (2015). The impact of capillary dilation on the distribution of red blood cells in artificial networks. *Am. J. Physiol. Heart Circ. Physiol.* 308, H733–H742. doi: 10.1152/ajpheart.00335.2014

Schultz, N., Brännström, K., Byman, E., Moussaud, S., Nielsen, H. M., Bank, N. B., et al. (2018). Amyloid α 1-40 is associated with alterations in NG2+ pericyte population *ex vivo* and *in vitro*. *Aging Cell* 17:e12728. doi: 10.1111/acel.12728

Secomb, T. W. (1991). Red blood cell mechanics and capillary blood rheology. *Cell Biophys.* 18, 231–251. doi: 10.1007/bf02989816

Sengillo, J. D., Winkler, E. A., Walker, C. T., Sullivan, J. S., Johnson, M., and Zlokovic, B. V. (2013). Deficiency in mural vascular cells coincides with blood-brain barrier disruption in Alzheimer's disease. *Brain Pathol.* 23, 303–310. doi: 10.1111/bpa.12004

Snyder, H. M., Corriveau, R. A., Craft, S., Faber, J. E., Greenberg, S. M., Knopman, D., et al. (2015). Vascular contributions to cognitive impairment and dementia including Alzheimer's disease. *Alzheimers Dement.* 11, 710–717. doi: 10.1016/j.jalz.2014.10.008

Soto, I., Graham, L. C., Richter, H. J., Simeone, S. N., Radell, J. E., Grabowska, W., et al. (2015). APOE stabilization by exercise prevents aging neurovascular dysfunction and complement induction. *PLoS Biol.* 13:e1002279. doi: 10.1371/journal.pbio.1002279

Stewart, P. A., Magliocco, M., Hayakawa, K., Farrell, C. L., Del Maestro, R. F., Girvin, J., et al. (1987). A quantitative analysis of blood-brain barrier ultrastructure in the aging human. *Microvasc. Res.* 33, 270–282. doi: 10.1016/0026-2862(87)90022-7

Stratman, A. N., Malotte, K. M., Mahan, R. D., Davis, M. J., and Davis, G. E. (2009). Pericyte recruitment during vasculogenic tube assembly stimulates endothelial basement membrane matrix formation. *Blood* 114, 5091–5101. doi: 10.1182/blood-2009-05-222364

Sweeney, M. D., Ayyadurai, S., and Zlokovic, B. V. (2016). Pericytes of the neurovascular unit: key functions and signaling pathways. *Nat. Neurosci.* 19, 771–783. doi: 10.1038/nn.4288

Underly, R. G., Levy, M., Hartmann, D. A., Grant, R. I., Watson, A. N., and Shih, A. Y. (2017). Pericytes as inducers of rapid, matrix metalloproteinase-9 dependent capillary damage during ischemia. *J. Neurosci.* 37, 129–140. doi: 10.1523/JNEUROSCI.2891-16.2016

Vanlandewijck, M., He, L., Mäe, M. A., Andrae, J., Ando, K., Del Gaudio, F., et al. (2018). A molecular atlas of cell types and zonation in the brain vasculature. *Nature* 554, 475–480. doi: 10.1038/nature25739

Verbeek, M. M., de Waal, R. M., Schipper, J. J., and Van Nostrand, W. E. (1997). Rapid degeneration of cultured human brain pericytes by amyloid α protein. *J. Neurochem.* 68, 1135–1141. doi: 10.1046/j.1471-4159.1997.68031135.x

Walshe, T. E., Saint-Geniezm, M., Maharaj, A. S., Sekiyama, E., Maldonado, A. E., and D'Amore, P. A. (2009). TGF-α is required for vascular barrier function, endothelial survival and homeostasis of the adult microvasculature. *PLoS One* 4:e5149. doi: 10.1371/journal.pone.0005149

Wang, H. U., Chen, Z. F., and Anderson, D. J. (1998). Molecular distinction and angiogenic interaction between embryonic arteries and veins revealed by ephrin-B2 and its receptor Eph-B4. *Cell* 93, 741–753. doi: 10.1016/s0092-8674(00)81436-1

Wardlaw, J. M., Smith, E. E., Biessels, G. J., Cordonnier, C., Fazekas, F., Frayne, R., et al. (2013). Neuroimaging standards for research into small vessel disease and its contribution to ageing and neurodegeneration. *Lancet Neurol.* 12, 822–838. doi: 10.1016/S1474-4422(13)70124-8

Wei, H. S., Kang, H., Rasheed, I. Y., Zhou, S., Lou, N., Gershteyn, A., et al. (2016). Erythrocytes are oxygen-sensing regulators of the cerebral microcirculation. *Neuron* 91, 851–862. doi: 10.1016/j.neuron.2016.07.016

Wilhelmus, M. M., Otte-Höller, I., van Triel, J. J., Veerhuis, R., Maat-Schieman, M. L., Bu, G., et al. (2007). Lipoprotein receptor-related protein-1 mediates amyloid-α-mediated cell death of cerebrovascular cells. *Am. J. Pathol.* 171, 1989–1999. doi: 10.2353/ajpath.2007.070050

Winkler, E. A., Birk, H., Burkhardt, J. K., Chen, X., Yue, J. K., Guo, D., et al. (2018). Reductions in brain pericytes are associated with arteriovenous malformation vascular instability. *J. Neurosurg.* doi: 10.3171/2017.6.JNS17860 [Epub ahead of print].

Yamaguchi, Y., and Pasquale, E. B. (2004). Eph receptors in the adult brain. *Curr. Opin. Neurobiol.* 14, 288–296. doi: 10.1016/j.conb.2004.04.003

Yemisci, M., Gursoy-Ozdemir, Y., Vural, A., Can, A., Topalkara, K., and Dalkara, T. (2009). Pericyte contraction induced by oxidative-nitrative stress impairs capillary reflow despite successful opening of an occluded cerebral artery. *Nat. Med.* 15, 1031–1037. doi: 10.1038/nm.2022

Zhu, W., Chen, W., Zou, D., Wang, L., Bao, C., Zhan, L., et al. (2018). Thalidomide reduces hemorrhage of brain arteriovenous malformations in a mouse model. *Stroke* 49, 1232–1240. doi: 10.1161/STROKEAHA.117.020356

Zlokovic, B., Zhao, Z., Nikolakopoulou, A. M., Kong, P., Sagare, A. P., and Makshanoff, J. (2015). "Pericyte ablation in a pericyte-specific inducible Cre mouse," in *Society for Neuroscience*, ed. P. 436.03/Y40. Available online at: http://www.abstractsonline.com/Plan/ViewAbstract.aspx?sKey=9d652d83-67f8-4780-9581-5cc072a7d1be&cKey=e0765062-c7c1-4abf-b446-17d281f83845&mKey=d0ff4555-8574-4fbb-b9d4-04eec8ba0c84

16

Trajectories of Brain Lactate and Re-Visited Oxygen-Glucose Index Calculations do not Support Elevated Non-Oxidative Metabolism of Glucose Across Childhood

Helene Benveniste[1], Gerald Dienel[2,3]*, Zvi Jacob[4], Hedok Lee[1], Rany Makaryus[4], Albert Gjedde[5], Fahmeed Hyder[6] and Douglas L. Rothman[6]**

[1] Department of Anesthesiology, Yale School of Medicine, Yale University, New Haven, CT, United States, [2] Department of Neurology, University of Arkansas for Medical Sciences, Little Rock, AR, United States, [3] Department of Cell Biology and Physiology, University of New Mexico, Albuquerque, NM, United States, [4] Department of Anesthesiology, Stony Brook University, Stony Brook, NY, United States, [5] Department of Translational Neurobiology, University of Southern Denmark, Odense, Denmark, [6] Department of Biomedical Engineering & Radiology and Biomedical Imaging, Yale School of Medicine, Yale University, New Haven, CT, United States

Correspondence:
Helene Benveniste
helene.benveniste@yale.edu
Gerald Dienel
gadienel@uams.edu
Douglas L. Rothman
douglas.rothman@yale.edu

Brain growth across childhood is a dynamic process associated with specific energy requirements. A disproportionately higher rate of glucose utilization ($CMR_{glucose}$) compared with oxygen consumption (CMR_{O2}) was documented in children's brain and suggestive of non-oxidative metabolism of glucose. Several candidate metabolic pathways may explain the $CMR_{glucose}$-CMR_{O2} mismatch, and lactate production is considered a major contender. The ~33% excess $CMR_{glucose}$ equals 0.18 μmol glucose/g/min and predicts lactate release of 0.36 μmol/g/min. To validate such scenario, we measured the brain lactate concentration ([Lac]) in 65 children to determine if indeed lactate accumulates and is high enough to (1) account for the glucose consumed in excess of oxygen and (2) support a high rate of lactate efflux from the young brain. Across childhood, brain [Lac] was lower than predicted, and below the range for adult brain. In addition, we re-calculated the $CMR_{glucose}$-CMR_{O2} mismatch itself by using updated lumped constant values. The calculated cerebral metabolic rate of lactate indicated a net influx of 0.04 μmol/g/min, or in terms of $CMR_{glucose}$, of 0.02 μmol glucose/g/min. Accumulation of [Lac] and calculated efflux of lactate from brain are not consistent with the increase in non-oxidative metabolism of glucose. In addition, the value for the lumped constant for [^{18}F]fluorodeoxyglucose has a high impact on calculated $CMR_{glucose}$ and use of updated values alters or eliminates the $CMR_{glucose}$-CMR_{O2} mismatch in developing brain. We conclude that the presently-accepted notion of non-oxidative metabolism of glucose during childhood must be revisited and deserves further investigations.

Keywords: non-oxidative metabolism, aerobic glycolysis, brain, child, development, lactate, bioenergetics

INTRODUCTION

Understanding the metabolic needs of the developing brain is essential for maintaining brain health across childhood and during adolescence. Information on the bioenergetic state of normal children's brain during development remains limited due to ethical concerns and overall complexity of conducting quantitative cerebral metabolic studies using positron emission tomography (PET) or magnetic resonance spectroscopy (MRS). Filling this gap in knowledge may shed light on several clinical predicaments and disease states including understanding the high incidence of benign febrile seizures in children 18 month of age (Pavlidou et al., 2013), the increased risk of long-term cognitive sequelae from multiple anesthesia and surgeries exposures before age 4 years (Glatz et al., 2017), and the higher rate of brain overgrowth observed in children with autism spectrum disorder (Hazlett et al., 2005; Sacco et al., 2015).

In humans, brain growth is rapid after birth and the young brain reaches adult-sized volume around age six (Giedd et al., 1999; Lenroot and Giedd, 2006; Semple et al., 2013). Neuronal maturational processes and myelination rates are dynamic and varying across the cortex (Bauernfeind and Babbitt, 2014). Synaptic density peaks at 2–3 years of age followed by pruning and decreased number (Huttenlocher, 1990; Semple et al., 2013). Myelination rate remains high until age 10 years (Miller et al., 2012). The growth pattern of brain development is paralleled by age-varying energy requirements.

The brain relies predominantly on glucose for energy, and PET is used to measure rates of glucose consumption ($CMR_{glucose}$) with the glucose analog [^{18}F]fluorodeoxyglucose (FDG) and oxygen consumption (CMR_{O2}) with $^{15}O\text{-}O_2$ (Raichle et al., 1976; Mintun et al., 1984; Reivich et al., 1985; Ohta et al., 1992; Gjedde and Marrett, 2001), allowing for calculation of the oxygen-glucose index (OGI = $CMR_{O2}/CMR_{glucose}$). The theoretical maximum for OGI is 6.0 ($6O_2$ + 1 glucose $\rightarrow$ $6CO_2 + 6H_2O$) when no other substrates are utilized, and the OGI therefore falls below 6 when glucose is consumed but not oxidized. The disproportionate utilization of glucose compared with oxygen *in the presence of normal oxygen delivery* is a phenomenon often called "aerobic glycolysis" in the literature (Hertz et al., 1998; Vaishnavi et al., 2010; Goyal et al., 2014; Dienel and Cruz, 2016; Hyder et al., 2016). However, to avoid confusion, since glycolysis can be upregulated under either aerobic or hypoxic/anaerobic conditions, we refer here to non-oxidative metabolism of glucose as glycolytic production of lactate that is not oxidized and/or of utilization of glucose by any other pathways that do not consume oxygen via the mitochondrial electron transport chain (e.g., glycogen synthesis, pentose phosphate shunt activity, biosynthetic reactions, etc.).

Chugani et al. reported that cortical $CMR_{glucose}$ in newborns was ~20–35% lower than in adults, and increased rapidly over the first 1–3 years (Chugani et al., 1987). In 3–8 year old children, $CMR_{glucose}$ was twice adult values, followed by a gradual decrease from 4 to 15 years to attain lower adult levels (Chugani et al., 1987). These values have become widely accepted and form the basis of proposals regarding metabolic adaptations in the developing human brain. Goyal et al. (2014) recently extended these findings by performing a meta-analysis based on the data from Chugani et al. and other studies to map trajectories of $CMR_{glucose}$ and CMR_{O2}, across the human lifespan and reported a 33% peak of excess $CMR_{glucose}$ over CMR_{O2} at 3–5 years of age (Goyal et al., 2014) and an OGI of ~4.1, inferring enhanced non-oxidative metabolism of glucose during early childhood (Goyal et al., 2014). By analogy to cancer cell growth—where an elevated non-oxidative metabolism of glucose is thought to support accelerated uptake and incorporation of nutrients into the growing cancer biomass (Vander Heiden et al., 2009)—it has been proposed that an elevated non-oxidative metabolism of glucose in the developing brain would support growth, axonal elongation synaptogenesis, and remodeling (Bauernfeind et al., 2014; Goyal et al., 2014).

However, conversion of all of the glucose consumed in excess of oxygen into brain biomass would cause an impossibly large increase in brain size, doubling within a month. It is necessary, therefore, to search for potential explanations for the large magnitudes of non-oxidative metabolism of glucose reported by Goyal et al. (2014), which is several-fold higher than in the adult brain (Hyder et al., 2016). Although a lower than normal OGI in children's brain is suggestive of increased glycolytic flux or non-oxidative metabolism of glucose, the downstream fate of the glucose carbon has not been established. In other words, the "OGI" by itself provides no information about the fate of excess glucose utilization which can involve many pathways as shown in **Figure 1**.

A possibility is that a higher-than-normal lactate production may explain the elevated non-oxidative metabolism of glucose reported in the developing brain (Goyal et al., 2014). To assess this concept, we measured steady state lactate concentrations ([Lac]) from brains of 87 children who underwent routine MRI examination under anesthesia (Jacob et al., 2012) using proton magnetic resonance spectroscopy (^{1}H MRS), and found that lactate accumulation and efflux could not explain the excess non-oxidative utilization of glucose. We, therefore, also evaluated several other possibilities including the storage of the excess glucose uptake into glycogen, and its complete oxidation or shunting away from lactate via the pentose phosphate pathway. At present there is no strong evidence for these possibilities although they will need to be directly measured before definite conclusions can be made. We then examined the alternate possibilities of age dependence on the conversion of the FDG PET measurement into a calculated rate of $CMR_{glucose}$ and the impact of plasma ketones, lactate, and other non-glucose substrates on the OGI calculation. We found that the "lumped constant," which is the constant used for the conversion of FDG phosphorylation to $CMR_{glucose}$, of Chugani et al. (1987) was considerably lower than modern accepted values and tested the impact of updated values on OGI.

Based on our direct measurements of brain [Lac] and calculations as well as mass balance considerations, we conclude that the claims of net lactate efflux and/or conversion of glucose into brain mass explaining the enhanced non-oxidative metabolism of glucose in children compared to adults are incorrect. There are several other potential metabolic sources of the reported glucose uptake/oxidation mismatch, including

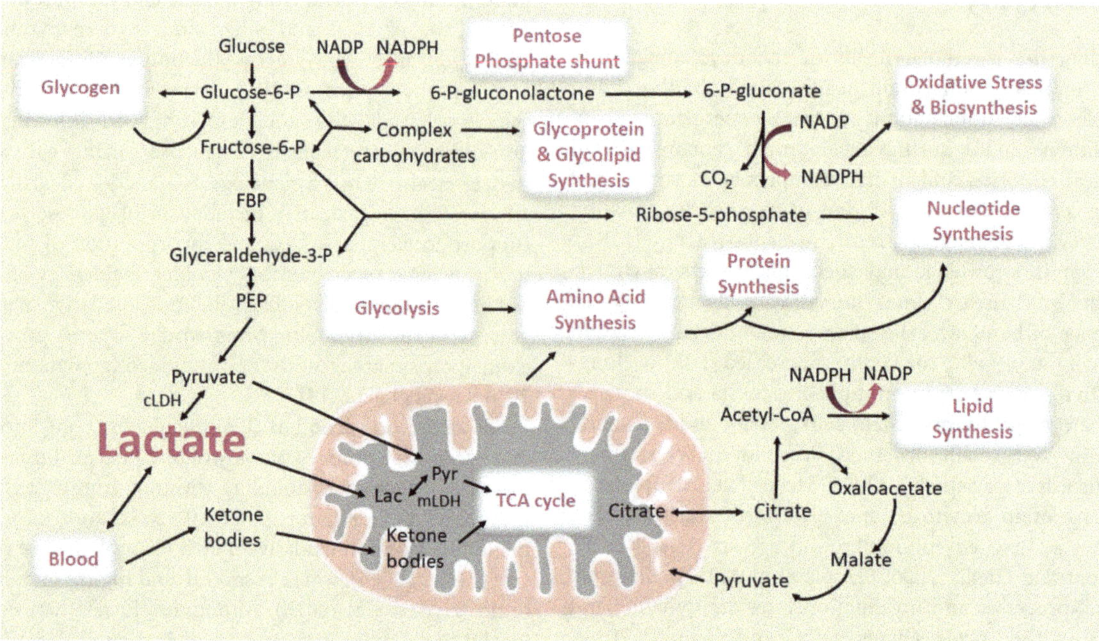

FIGURE 1 | Metabolic pathways of importance for the developing brain. Glycolysis, oxidative phosphorylation via the citric acid (TCA) cycle and the pentose phosphate pathway generating NADPH, and the use of ketone bodies as supplemental fuel are shown. The connections between glycolysis, complex carbohydrate, amino acid, protein, lipid, and nucleotide synthesis are also illustrated. The pathway fluxes that change during brain development to cause glucose utilization in excess of oxygen (enhanced non-oxidative metabolism of glucose) are not known. Glucose can be converted to lactate directly via the glycolytic pathway or after shunting through glycogen or the pentose shunt pathway, then either oxidized in the mitochondria or released from brain. Our diagram shows two pathways for mitochondrial lactate oxidation, direct lactate transport into the mitochondria and oxidation as has been reported in studies of muscle and brain (Brooks, 1986, 2000, 2018; Schurr, 2006; Passarella et al., 2014; Rogatzki et al., 2015) and conversion of lactate to pyruvate in the cytosol by cytosolic lactate dehydrogenase (cLDH) and subsequent transport into inner matrix of the mitochondria through pyruvate transporters. Although in muscle it has been reported that the large majority of lactate is directly oxidized in the mitochondria by mitochondrial LDH (mLDH), the effective blocking of glucose oxidation in brain cell cultures, synaptosomes, and brain slices by inhibition of the malate aspartate shuttle (MAS) (which transports the redox equivalent from NADH produced by cLDH into the mitochondria) (Fitzpatrick et al., 1983; Kauppinen et al., 1987; Cheeseman and Clark, 1988; Mckenna et al., 1993) and the inability of L-lactate to rescue glutamate toxicity in MAS-knockout neurons whereas it does in wild type (Llorente-Folch et al., 2016) suggests that brain mitochondria mainly use cytosolic pyruvate as an oxidative source. Also, LDH is considered to be a cytoplasmic marker in subcellular fractionation studies of brain (Johnson and Whittaker, 1963; Tamir et al., 1972), and <1% of the LDH in a brain homogenate is recovered in purified mitochondria (Lai and Clark, 1976; Lai et al., 1977). However, from the standpoint of this study the two pathways of lactate oxidation would lead to the same OGI as shown in **Figure 2**. Glucose can also be used for synthesis of glycogen, amino acids, proteins, complex carbohydrates, lipids, glycolipids, and glycoproteins, and nucleotides. The flux of the pentose shunt in developing brain is higher than in adult brain even though maximal capacity is similar at all ages (Baquer et al., 1977). The illustration is based metabolic pathways active in proliferative cells to explain the Warburg effect that involves aerobic glycolysis and lactate efflux (Vander Heiden et al., 2009). Warburg theories for cancer cells state that the increased glucose uptake is shunted through the pentose phosphate pathway for the additional NADPH needed for biosynthetic reactions. Theoretically, 5/6 of the glucose entering the oxidative branch of the pentose phosphate pathway should end up as lactate and be exported from the brain. However, if recycling of Fru-6-P back into the pentose shunt is complete, this pathway can contribute a higher fraction to the consumption of glucose in excess of oxygen (see text). It is an open question how much NADPH is needed to meet the biosynthetic needs for synaptogenesis. CoA, Coenzyme A; P, phosphate; FBP, fructose-1,6-P_2; PEP, phosphoenolpyruvate. Modified from Figure 3 of Vander Heiden et al. (2009) with permission of the authors. Reprinted with permission from AAAS.

alternate pathways of glucose metabolism or even other substrates. For example, ketone metabolism is known to be higher in children, but this would reduce the measured rate of non-oxidative metabolism of glucose by increasing the OGI. However, there are limited measurements available on these alternate pathways. We show through simulations that a more likely explanation, at present, is the use of different lump constants in PET $CMR_{glucose}$ data in children and adults. When modern LC values are used with the originally reported Chugani et al. results (Chugani et al., 1987), the difference in non-oxidative metabolism of glucose between adults and children disappears. However, until the necessary studies are performed, our present understanding of glucose metabolism in the developing brain, despite being widely accepted, is at best incomplete and potentially largely incorrect and deserves further investigation. The non-oxidative metabolism of glucose "story" is more complex than conversion of glucose into brain mass or lactate.

MATERIALS AND METHODS

De-identified ^{1}H MRS spectra and anatomical T1-weighted scans from 87 children (age: 2–7 years, 38 females and 49 males) undergoing diagnostic MRI under anesthesia were included in the analysis. ^{1}H MRS metabolite data from 60 of the 87 children included were previously reported in a study not focused on lactate but documenting cerebral metabolomic profiles during different anesthesia regimens; and study procedures are described in detail in Jacob et al. (2012). Briefly, after IRB approval [Committees on Research Involving Human Subjects (CORIHS), Stony Brook University] and parental consent, children (2–7 years) were anesthetized with sevoflurane (N = 37) or propofol (N = 50) and underwent routine MRI imaging for clinical evaluation. Common clinical indications for the diagnostic MRI scans included seizures, headache, and potential developmental delay (Jacob et al., 2012). Exclusion criteria were acute brain trauma, stroke or hemorrhage or any confirmed diagnosis of elevated intracranial pressure (Jacob et al., 2012). Scanning was performed on a 3.0T Philips Achieva whole body scanner, and high resolution T1-weighted and single voxel ^{1}H MRS were performed in each session. A T1-weighted turbo field echo sequence was acquired in the sagittal plane at voxel dimensions of $0.94 \times 0.94 \times 1.00$ mm.

Data Analysis

For gray matter and white matter analysis, the T1-weighted scans were segmented using SPM8 (Ashburner and Friston, 2000). The ^{1}H MRS single-voxel point-resolved sequence (PRESS) was acquired in the cortex (e.g., parietal or temporal lobes) with following parameters voxel size of $1.5 \times 1.5 \times 1.5$ cm^3, TR/TE/2000 ms/32 ms, receiver bandwidth = 1200/2000 Hz, number of points = 1024/2048, and averages = 256. In the current analysis, the following metabolite concentrations were quantified and extracted from the spectra by linear combination of model (LCModel) analysis using the water concentration as an internal reference (Provencher, 2001): N-acetylaspartate (NAA) + N-acetylaspartylglutamate (NAAG) = tNAA; phosphorylcholine + glycerophosphorylcholine = total choline (tCh); creatine + phosphocreatine = total creatine (tCr); glutamate + glutamine = tGlx, and lactate (Lac). Partial volume effect in the water concentration was also considered in the concentration calculation (Lee et al., 2013).

Calculation of the Cerebral Metabolic Rate of Lactate

To assess the degree of $CMR_{glucose}$-CMR_{O2} uncoupling consistent with the measured lactate levels and to compare with previous reported $CMR_{glucose}$ and CMR_{O2} in early childhood, we calculated the cerebral metabolic rate of lactate, CMR_{lac}, as the difference between the unidirectional transport of lactate into the brain (V_{in}) and the lactate efflux (V_{out}) from the brain, Equation 1 (Boumezbeur et al., 2010), i.e., it is net lactate carbon flux across the blood-brain barrier. CMR_{lac} is defined as the cerebral metabolic rate of either net lactate production or consumption of plasma lactate by the brain. The two parameters V_{in} and V_{out} can be calculated based on Equation 2, 3, and CMR_{Lac}, $[Lac]_p$, and $Lac]_B$ can be calculated with Equation 4 when different values for lactate concentrations or V_{MAX} are used:

$$CMR_{Lac} = V_{in} - V_{out} \tag{1a}$$

$$CMR_{Lac} = -2\,(CMR_{glucose} - CMR_{O2}/6) \tag{1b}$$

$$V_{in} = V_{MAX}\frac{[Lac]_p}{K_T + [Lac]_p + [Lac]_B} \tag{2}$$

$$V_{out} = V_{MAX}\frac{[Lac]_B}{K_T + [Lac]_p + [Lac]_B} \tag{3}$$

$$CMR_{Lac} = V_{MAX}([Lac]_p - [Lac]_B)/(K_T + [Lac]_p + [Lac]_B) \tag{4}$$

Where $[Lac]_p$ and $[Lac]_B$ are the concentrations of lactate in arterial plasma and brain, respectively. Since we did not measure $[Lac]_p$ in the children we set it to be 0, 1, or 2 mM for the calculations, which is a reasonable range for the estimate since the clinical guides report normal plasma [Lac] in children in the range of 0.5–2 mM (Agrawal et al., 2004) and none of the children in our study was acutely sick or suffering from chronic infections (Jacob et al., 2012). Lactate transport kinetic parameters V_{MAX} and K_T determined previously in adult brain of 0.4 μmol/g/min and 5.1 mM, respectively were used for the calculations (Boumezbeur et al., 2010). We also examined the impact of a 3, 5, and 10-fold higher V_{MAX}, based on studies of neonatal rats demonstrating that transport kinetics are elevated in young rat brain when compared to adult brain (Cremer et al., 1979).

Calculation of the Effect of Different Substrates on the Measured OGI

Figure 2 shows the stoichiometries used in order to calculate the effect of different substrates on the measured OGI. We also give the equations (**Figure 2**; **Table 4**) for the oxygen-carbohydrate index (OCI) and oxygen carbohydrate ketone index (OCKI) which take into account the oxidation of lactate and lactate plus ketones, respectively, as opposed to only glucose in the OGI. As illustrated in **Figure 2**, oxygen consumed by complete oxidation of different substrates varies with the number of carbon atoms (and oxidation of β-hydroxybutyrate to acetoacetate before entering the TCA cycle), and it is necessary to take the stoichiometry into account when calculating molar oxygen/substrate ratios. When all substrates are included in the same calculation, the molar equivalent carbon each substrate is expressed relative to the oxygen consumed by glucose. For example, lactate and pyruvate would consume $3O_2$, and are equivalent to 0.5 glucose. Use of these calculations emphasizes the stoichiometry of net utilization of substrate(s) compared with oxygen, and has been used in OCI calculations during exercise to exhaustion (Quistorff et al., 2008; van Hall et al., 2009). Thus, if glucose is taken up into brain and converted to pyruvate that is transported into and oxidized in mitochondria or converted to lactate in cytoplasm, followed by its uptake and oxidation in mitochondria, the same number of moles of oxygen will be consumed per glucose. On the other hand, if lactate is released from brain or if non-oxidative metabolism predominates, the oxygen/substrate index falls below the theoretical maximum. In addition, if brain glycogen is consumed, as during hypoglycemia (Oz et al., 2009) or brain activation (Swanson et al., 1992; Cruz and Dienel, 2002), the additional carbon fuel must also be taken into account. In the present study, the children were anesthetized and glycogenolysis is not anticipated to be increased, since glycogen turnover in resting brain is very slow (Watanabe and Passonneau, 1973). However, glycogen may have contributed to brain metabolism during the $CMR_{glucose}$ and CMR_{O2} assays,

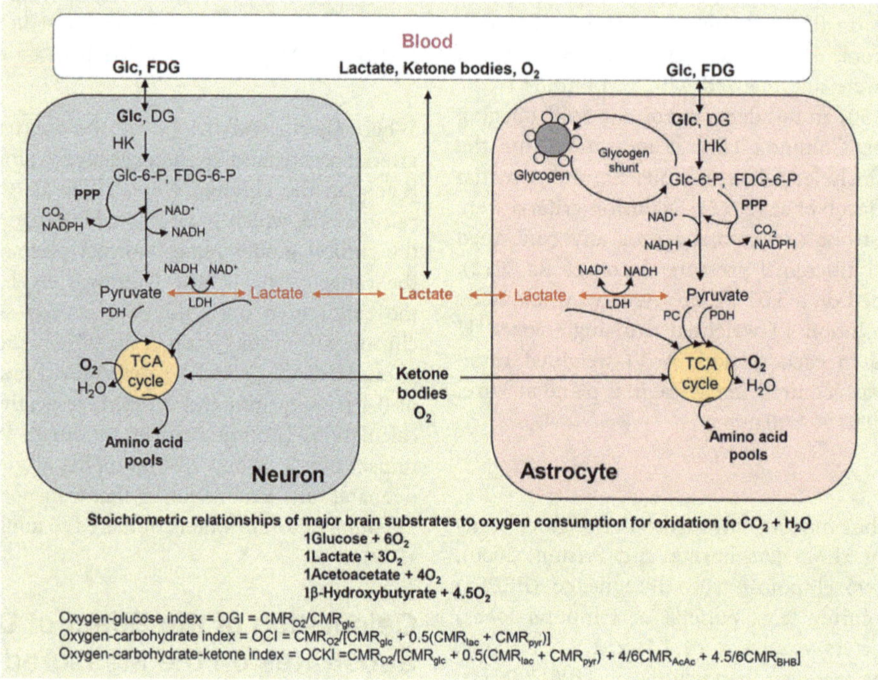

FIGURE 2 | Oxygen-substrate stoichiometry in brain. Substrates are delivered to brain by blood where they are metabolized by brain cells that consume oxygen. Glucose (Glc) and the glucose analog fluorodeoxyglucose (FDG) are phosphorylated by hexokinase (HK) to their respective hexose-6-phosphate (P). FDG-6-P is trapped in the cell where phosphorylated, whereas Glc-6-P is further metabolized via the glycolytic pathway to a 3-carbon product that can be oxidized in mitochondria as either as pyruvate (Pyr) via pyruvate dehydrogenase (PDH) in all cells and pyruvate carboxylase (PC) in astrocytes, or as lactate (Lac) that may be taken up into mitochondria and converted to Pyr by mitochondrial lactate dehydrogenase (LDH) (see text and legend to **Figure 1**). Glc-6-P can also enter the pentose phosphate shunt pathway (PPP) to generate NADPH for management of oxidative stress or for use in biosynthetic reactions. The PPP also generates ribulose-5-P that is a precursor for nucleic acid synthesis and intermediates are rearranged to produce fructose-6-P and glyceraldehyde-3-P that can re-enter the glycolytic pathway and fructose-6-P may recycled into the PPP. In astrocytes, Glc-6-P is also stored as glycogen. Lactate can be released from brain when non-oxidative metabolism is upregulated more than the oxidative pathways. Lactate and ketone bodies can also be taken up from blood and oxidized, particularly in suckling mammals during development, as well as during exercise and starvation, respectively, when their blood levels rise. Different substrates consume different amounts of oxygen when completely oxidized, and the relationship between total oxygen consumption and total utilization of various substrates is illustrated. The oxygen-glucose index (OGI) is based on the stoichiometry of glucose oxidation, and assumes no other substrates are metabolized. The same OGI will be obtained whether Lac or Pyr is oxidized, as long as there is no uptake of these substrates from blood. Metabolism of other substrates is taken into account by the oxygen-carbohydrate (OCI) and oxygen-carbohydrate-ketone body (OCKI) indicies. Note that Lac and Pyr are converted to glucosyl units. Ketone bodies, acetoacetate (AcAc) and β-hydroxybutyrate (BHB), are metabolized in mitochondria.

especially if the subjects were stimulated or stressed, and it would cause errors in calculated OGI.

Statistical Analysis

We analyzed associations between brain volumes and age using Analysis of Covariance (ANCOVA) with adjustment for gender. To examine the relation between LCModel-derived metabolite concentrations and age, an Analysis of Covariance (ANCOVA) with adjustment for anesthesia regimen (Sevoflurane or Propofol) and gender was employed. Analysis was conducted using XLSTAT (Version 2011.4.03).

RESULTS

MRS Spectral Quality

In order to assess spectral quality the ^{1}H MRS spectra were checked for poor signal-to-noise ratio (SNR), spectral line width via full width at half maximum (FWHM) and baseline fluctuations estimated from LCModel analysis (Provencher, 2001), and 13 spectra were excluded. The average FWHM and SNR of the spectral NAA peaks were 0.028 ± 0.006 ppm and 22.3 ± 4.2, respectively indicating excellent spectral resolution and sensitivity. **Figure 3** shows representative ^{1}H MRS spectra from the cortex of a 3-year-old child (top) and a 7 year old child (bottom); and the LCModel-determined lactate peak is also depicted (blue, scaled $\times$ 4 for enhancing the peak). The Cramer–Rao lower bounds (CRLBs) which are the standard error estimates expressed in percent of the estimated concentrations (%SD) calculated by LCModel analysis (Provencher, 2001) for [tCr], [tNAA], [tCh] were 2–5%SD; and CRLB's for [tGlx] were 8–14%SD. The CRLB's for [Lac] were considerably higher and [Lac] $<$0.1 mM were discarded leaving 65 subjects with [Lac] for analysis, and the average CRLB for these was 80 ± 35%SD. The high CRLB for [Lac] was due to its low concentration in the brain being on the order of the noise level in some subjects.

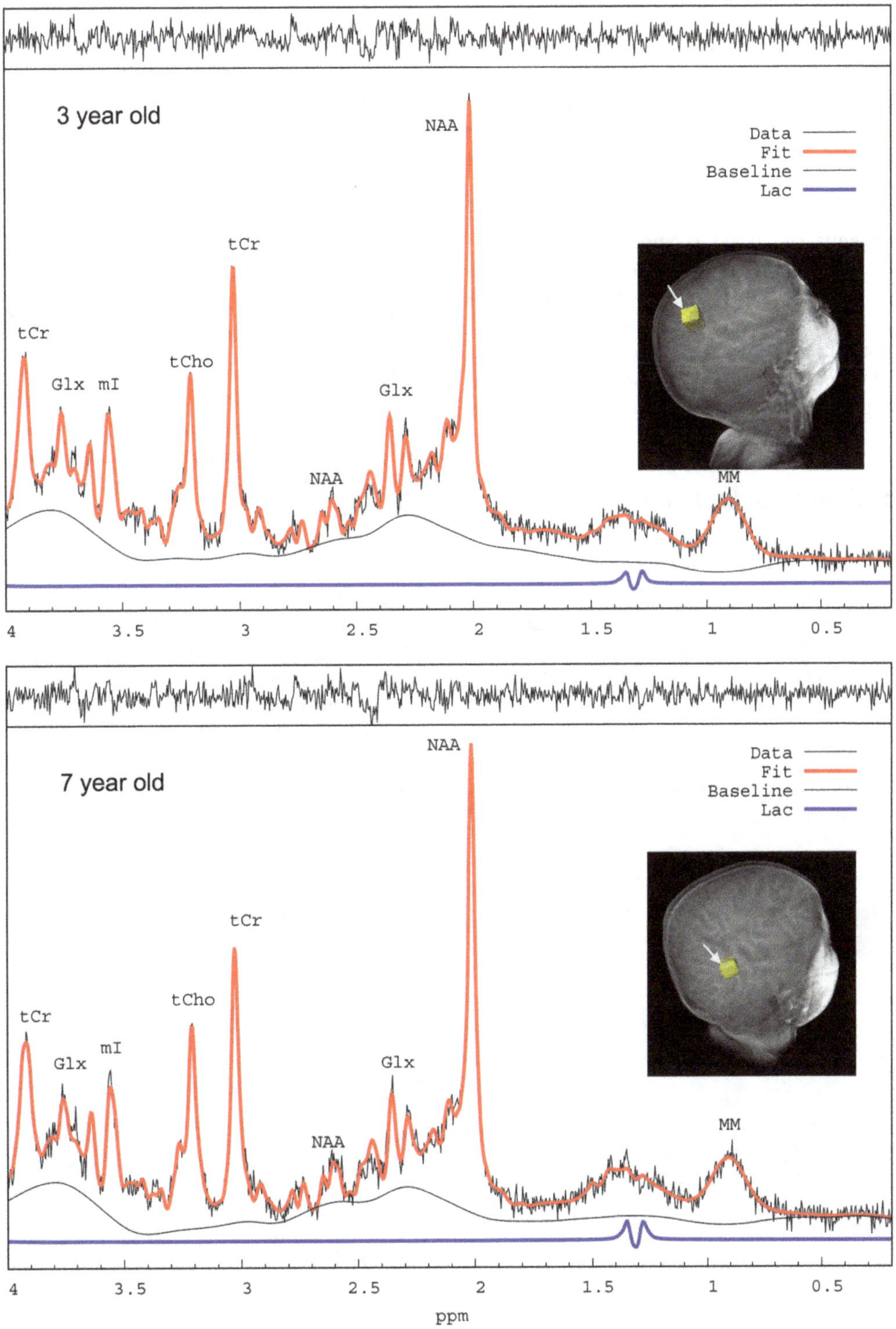

FIGURE 3 | ^{1}H MRS spectra from a 3-year-old and a 7-year-old child. Representative proton magnetic resonance spectroscopic (^{1}H MRS) spectra from parietal cortex of children anesthetized with sevoflurane and analyzed by LCModel. The spectra are of excellent quality with sufficient water suppression and spectral resolution to resolve at least 6–10 metabolites. The raw unsmoothed spectra are shown (black) in addition to the LCModel-fitted output (red solid lines). NAA, N-acetylaspartate; Glx, glutamate + glutamine; tCr, total creatine; ml, myo-inositol; tCho, total choline; MM, macromolecules. The LCModel- defined lactate peaks on the two spectra are shown in blue (scaled x4 for enhancing visualization of the peaks).

Brain Morphometry and Metabolites Across Early Childhood (2–7 Years)

Global brain morphometric analysis revealed that total gray matter (GM) and white matter (WM) in the children significantly correlated with age in the expected, positive direction (GM $R^2 = 0.14$ WM $R^2 = 0.36$, $p < 0.001$, **Figure 4**). For GM, 15% of the variability was explained by the two variables, with age being significant ($p = 0.003$) but not gender ($p = 0.082$). For WM, 39% of the variability was explained by the two variables, with age being more influential ($p < 0.0001$) compared to gender ($p < 0.001$). The concentration of tNAA ([tNAA], a neuronal marker) was in the range of 5–6 mM and also positively correlated with the children's age in agreement with a previous report (Kadota et al., 2001), but not with gender (**Table 1**). However, in contrast to [tNAA], none of the other metabolites including [tCr], [tCho], [Lac], or [tGlx] appeared to follow a linear age-dependency pattern (**Table 1**).

Trajectory of Brain Lactate in Early Childhood

We characterized the trajectory of the brain concentration of lactate, [Lac] across the children's ages, because previous reports documented enhanced levels of non-oxidative metabolism of glucose in early childhood and the peak excess $CMR_{glucose}$ over CMR_{O2} occurred at 3–5 years of age (Goyal et al., 2014). **Figure 5** shows the mean cortical [Lac] for each year of children aged 2–7 years, anesthetized with either sevoflurane or propofol and demonstrates that in all children, regardless of age and anesthetic, [Lac] is <1 mM. Further, we did not observe a $[Lac]_B$ peak at ~ at 3–5 years, however, $[Lac]_B$ in children anesthetized with sevoflurane was noted to be highest at ~5 years of age and reached a level of 0.28 ± 0.20 mM. Thus, mean cortical [Lac] in children is lower than the reported [Lac] values in brain of unanesthetized adults (0.5–1.0 mM) (Prichard et al., 1991; Bednarik et al., 2015; Rowland et al., 2016). Second, to explore the age-dependent relation with the AG trajectory (Goyal et al., 2014), we performed a Lowess, non-parametric regression of [Lac] from children anesthetized with sevoflurane which is shown in **Figure 6A**.

Calculation of CMR_{Lac} and Quantitative Evaluation of its Contribution to Elevated Non-oxidative Metabolism of Glucose

Using the standard reversible Michaelis-Menten model for brain lactate transport (Simpson et al., 2007; Boumezbeur et al., 2010) we calculated the magnitude and direction of brain lactate transport. **Table 2** presents the calculated CMR_{Lac} for brain [Lac] for 4 year old children anesthetized with sevoflurane [average brain [Lac] was 0.28 ± 0.20 mM (range: 0.12–0.54 mM)]. Using previously measured plasma lactate concentrations in children of ~1 mM (Agrawal et al., 2004) and the kinetic constants for lactate transport measured previously in adults the calculated value of CMR_{Lac} was for net entry into the brain at a relatively low rate (0.04 μmol/g/min). The lactate that entered the brain would be oxidized, raising CMR_{O2} and causing errors in calculated OGI that does not account for lactate oxidation, as does the oxygen-carbohydrate index (OCI, **Figure 2**, **Table 4**). A net efflux of lactate only occurred if plasma lactate were assumed to be 0 mM and also would be at a very low rate (−0.02 μmol/g/min, **Table 2**) and much lower than the lactate efflux rate needed to account for

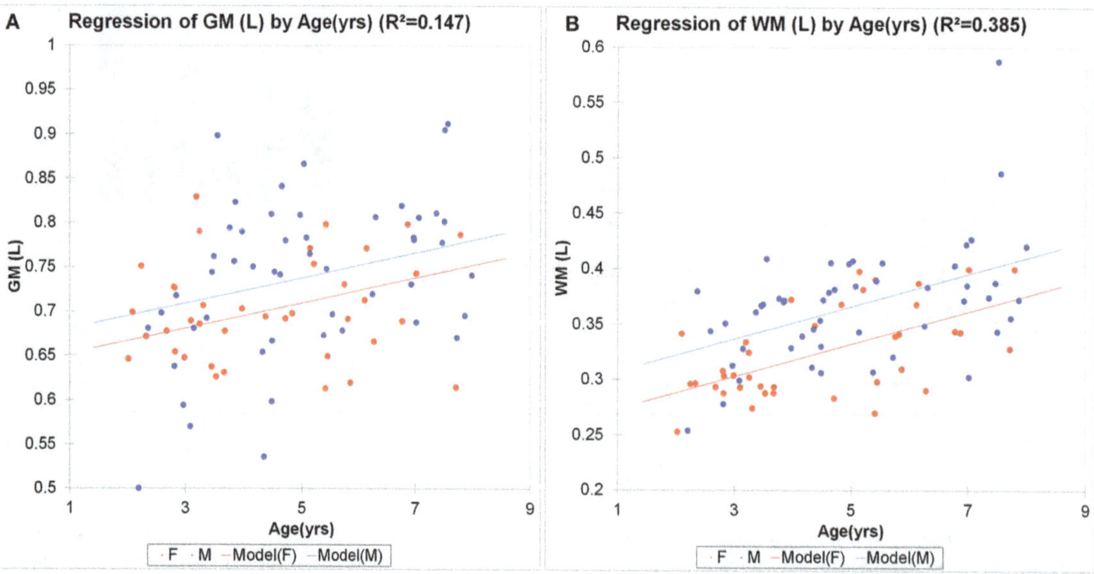

FIGURE 4 | Morphometric brain analysis across childhood. Total brain gray **(A)** and white **(B)** matter volumes in male (M, blue circles) and female (F, red circles) children as a function of age. Linear regression analysis shows significant brain growth in gray matter (GM $R^2 = 0.147$, $p < 0.001$; WM $R^2 = 0.385$, $p < 0.0001$). For GM, 15% of the variability was explained by the two variables, with age being significant ($p = 0.003$) but not gender ($p = 0.082$). For WM, 39% of the variability was explained by the two variables, with age being more influential ($p < 0.0001$) compared to gender ($p < 0.001$).

TABLE 1 | Analysis of energy metabolites by age with gender and anesthesia regimen as covariates.

		[Lac]	[tCho]	[tNAA]	[tCr]	[tGlx]
R^2		0.021	0.030	0.180	0.061	0.034
F		0.437	0.862	6.066	1.801	0.970
P-value		0.727	0.464	**0.001**	0.153	0.411
Age	F	0.513	0.474	7.459	0.007	2.133
	P-value	0.477	0.493	**0.008**	0.935	0.148
Gender	F	0.354	2.311	1.538	0.040	0.657
	P-value	0.554	0.132	0.218	0.841	0.420
Anesthesia	F	0.122	0.062	10.281	5.355	0.120
	P-value	0.728	0.803	**0.002**	**0.023**	0.730

ANCOVA (Analysis of COVAriance) was used to analyze interactions between brain metabolites and age and anesthesia regimen. Given the R^2 for [tNAA], 18% of the variability of the dependent variable—[tNAA]—is explained by the three explanatory variables. Among the explanatory variables, the anesthesia regimen and age are the most influential. Bold values are statistically significant.

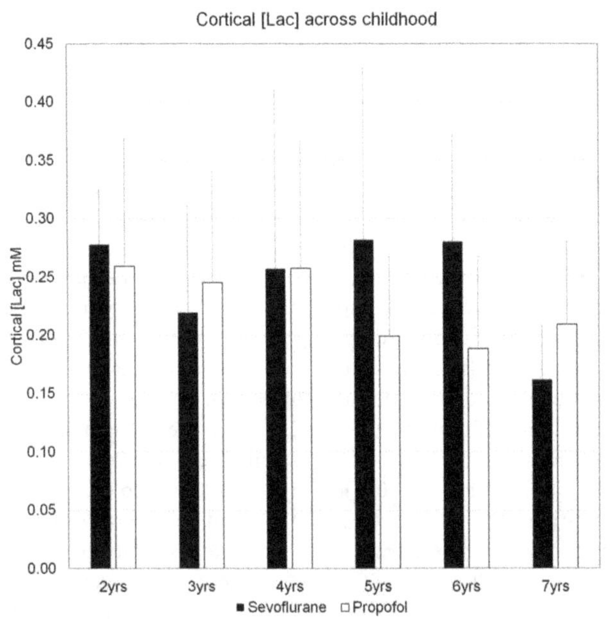

FIGURE 5 | The concentrations of cerebral cortical lactate in children aged 2–7 years. Concentrations of lactate, [Lac], for each year of children aged 2–7 years, anesthetized with either sevoflurane or propofol are means + SD. For sevoflurane the ranges of [Lac] are given below: Age 2 years: 0.24–0.35 mM; Age 3 years: 0.13–0.37 mM; Age 4 years: 0.12–0.54 mM; Age 5 years: 0.15–0.51 mM; Age 6 years: 0.16–0.39 mM; Age 7 years: 0.11–0.20 mM. The number of subjects in each age group for the two anesthetics are as follows: Sevoflurane group: Age 2 (*N* = 5); Age 3 (*N* = 5); Age 4 (*N* = 6); Age 5 (*N* = 5); Age 6 (*N* = 6); Age 7 (*N* = 3). Propofol group: Age 2 (*N* = 5); Age 3 (*N* = 10); Age 4 (*N* = 6); Age 5 (*N* = 7); Age 6 (*N* = 4); Age 7 (*N* = 3). Please note that "Age 2," children ≥2 yrs, <3 yrs; "Age 3 yrs," children ≥3 yrs, <4 yrs; "Age 4 yrs," children ≥4 yrs, <5 yrs; "Age 5 yrs," children ≥5 yrs, <6 yrs; "Age 6 yrs," children ≥6 yrs, <7 yrs; "Age 7 yrs," children ≥7 yrs, <8 yrs.

the mismatch between glucose uptake and oxygen consumption derived by Goyal et al. of −0.36 µmol/g/min.

To assess the impact of the kinetic constants used from adult brain on the calculations we also examined the impact of increasing the Vmax for lactate transport by a factor of 3, 5, and 10. At typical plasma lactate levels of 1 mM the calculated CMR_{lac} increased but the directionality (into the brain) remained the same. Based on studies in animal models (Cremer et al., 1979) the maximum anticipated increase in lactate transport in children was 3-fold and assuming 0 plasma lactate the efflux of lactate would only be −0.07 µmol/gm/min which again is well-below the predicted −0.36 µmol/g/min. Note that, based on Equation 4 lactate efflux can only occur when $[Lac]_B$ exceeds $[Lac]_P$.

In order to assess the concentration of brain lactate which would be required to account for the reported mismatch we calculated brain lactate concentration $[Lac]_B$ for a CMR_{lac} of −0.36 µmol/g/min (**Table 2**). Using the V_{MAX} measured in adults and varying the plasma lactate concentration from 0 to 2 mM yielded a predicted brain [Lac] ranging from 46 to 84 mM. Even with a 5-fold increase in V_{MAX} assumed the brain [Lac] would have to be between 2.6 and 4.0 mM which is 8–12 times higher than the measured value.

Re-calculating $CMR_{glucose}$ and OGI Across Childhood Using Updated Values for the Lumped Constant

Because brain lactate levels and calculated lactate efflux rates based on our data were too low to explain the low OGI reported in children (Goyal et al., 2014), we considered and evaluated an alternative explanation for low OGI. The FDG-PET literature has reported and discussed updated values for the lumped constant (LC), the factor that accounts for kinetic differences in rates of transport and phosphorylation between FDG and glucose and is used to convert [18F]FDG phosphorylation rate to $CMR_{glucose}$. Based on our review of the Supplemental Table 1 of Goyal et al. (2014) the $CMR_{glucose}$ data were taken from **Table 1** of Chugani et al. (1987) in which a LC of 0.42 was used for subjects of all ages as originally published for adult brain by Phelps and coworkers (Phelps et al., 1979; Huang et al., 1980). Since that time higher values for adult brain have been found with recent values close to 0.8–0.85 (Graham et al., 2002; Hyder et al., 2016).

Due to the uncertainty regarding the true value of the LC, we re-calculated the $CMR_{glucose}$ using LC = 0.65, a value subsequently determined in the Phelps laboratory for adult brain (Wu et al., 2003) that also determined LC = 0.42, the value used by Chugani et al. (1987), as well as LC = 0.80, a value determined by Hyder et al. (2016) that is within the range of the higher values noted above. We performed the calculations based on the peak $CMR_{glucose}$ = 0.58 µmol/g/min and OGI = 4.1 in the loessR plot in Figure 2A of Goyal et al. (2014). When LC = 0.80 was used, $CMR_{glucose}$ fell and approached $CMR_{glucose}$ for normal adults (**Table 3**). Importantly, the OGI increased from 4.1 to 6.4 and 7.9 when higher values for the LC were used, and the magnitude of non-oxidative metabolism of glucose representing ∼33% $CMR_{glucose}$ in excess of CMR_{O2} was reversed. When LC was increased by 55% from 0.42 to 0.65, CMR_{O2} and $CMR_{glucose}$ were nearly stoichiometrically matched because the calculated $CMR_{glucose}$ was reduced by a corresponding percentage (**Table 3**). There was no excess glucose consumed and the predicted lactate uptake agrees with calculated

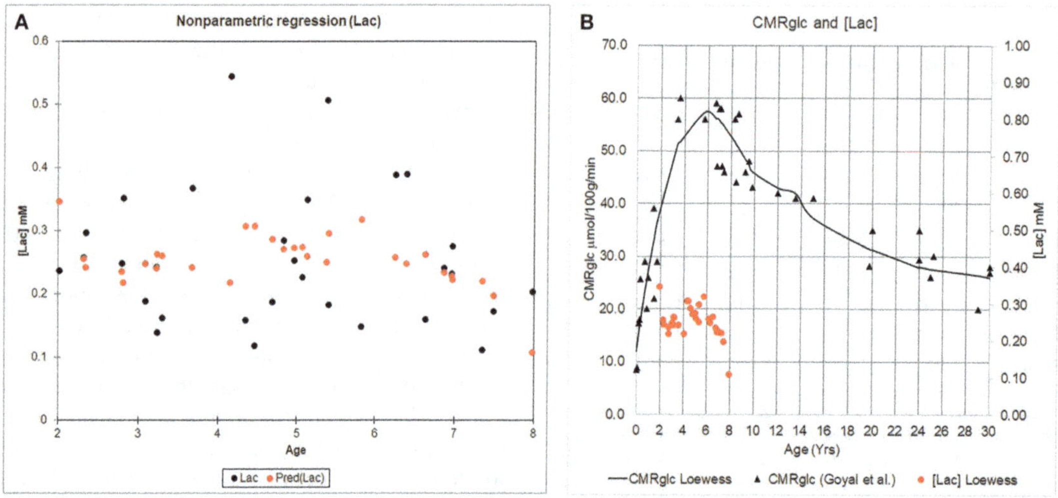

FIGURE 6 | The concentration of cerebral cortical [Lac] and $CMR_{glucose}$ across childhood. **(A)** Cerebral cortical [Lac] from children anesthetized with sevoflurane is plotted as a function of age (black circles). A Lowess regression (locally weighted regression and smoothing scatter plot) was fitted to the data using XLSTAT (Version 18.07); and is represented by the red circles. **(B)** Whole brain $CMR_{glucose}$ data as reported by Goyal et al. (2014) (black triangles) is shown in relation to the Lowess fit of the [Lac] data (red circles).

CMR_{Lac} of +0.04 µmol/g/min based on measured brain [Lac] (**Figures 5, 6; Table 2**).

Goyal et al. (2014) strongly emphasized the temporal profile of enhanced non-oxidative metabolism of glucose (higher $CMR_{glucose}$ compared with CMR_{O2}) in children 1–10 years of age, with a peak at about 5 years of age (as illustrated in **Figure 6B**). However, due to the uncertainty in the true value for the LC and its high impact on OGI and therefore on the magnitude of non-oxidative metabolism of glucose revealed by calculations as illustrated in **Table 3**, we recalculated the $CMR_{glucose}$ trajectories with updated values for the LC along with CMR_{O2}. **Figure 6A** shows the age-dependent changes for the Goyal data for $CMR_{glucose}$ (blue) and CMR_{O2} (red, expressed in glucose equivalents as calculated by Goyal et al., $CMR_{O2}/6$, a calculation that assumes all oxygen consumed is due to glucose oxidation), and for re-calculated values with LC = 0.65 (green), and LC = 0.80 (brown). When higher LC values were used the discrepancy between $CMR_{glucose}$ and CMR_{O2} was age-dependent, with CMR_{O2} exceeding $CMR_{glucose}$ in 1–2 year old children, and nearly-stoichiometric rates at ages 5–10 years (**Figure 6A**).

DISCUSSION

In this study we measured brain [Lac] in 65 children across 2–7 years and documented that $[Lac]_B$ on average was <0.3 mM throughout and below previous MRS measurements in the adult brain (0.5–0.7 mM). In addition, $[Lac]_B$ did not peak at 3–5 years inconsistent with the peak excess $CMR_{glucose}$ over CMR_{O2} and low OGI documented at 3–5 years of age (Goyal et al., 2014), which they ascribed to the needs of increased synaptogenesis. However, there are other potential reasons for the fall in OGI, including lactate release from brain. This possibility was ruled out because the brain [Lac] we measured was many fold below what is needed to explain the quantitative drop in the OGI and was consistent with small net brain uptake as opposed to efflux of lactate. We discuss these findings below in light of what is known about fuel consumption in the developing brain and evaluate potential metabolic and methodological explanations for the discrepancy between the reported low OGI and the brain [Lac] measured. Previous studies have discussed the quantitative contribution of lactate uptake into resting adult brain (Boumezbeur et al., 2010), the oxygen/substrate stoichiometry in brain of non-stimulated, sedentary human subjects (Hyder et al., 2016), decreases in the ratio during brain activation (Dienel and Cruz, 2016), and the contributions of glucose and lactate during exhaustive exercise (Quistorff et al., 2008; van Hall et al., 2009). The present study examines the basis for decreases in this ratio in brains of children during development.

Enhanced Aerobic Non-oxidative Metabolism of Glucose in the Developing Brain and Relation to Brain Lactate

To assess whether lactate efflux could account for the low OGI reported in early childhood we calculated CMR_{Lac} based upon the measured concentration of brain lactate and literature values for plasma lactate concentration and transport kinetics. As shown in **Table 2** these calculations indicate that based on the measured brain [Lac] an inflow of plasma lactate is predicted. In order to obtain lactate efflux sufficient to account for the reported elevated non-oxidative metabolism of glucose (and low OGI) brain [Lac] ranging from 46 to 84 mM (with the range based upon the concentration of plasma lactate and adult brain kinetic constants) were calculated which is two orders of magnitude above the measured values.

TABLE 2 | Calculated values for CMR_{Lac}, $[Lac]_P$, and $[Lac]_B$.

Calculated value	Fixed values				
	CMR_{Lac} (μmol/g/min)	$[Lac]_P$ (mM)	$[Lac]_B$ (mM)	V_{MAX} (μmol/g/min)	K_T (mM)
$CMR_{Lac} = -0.02$	–	0	0.28	0.4	5.1
$CMR_{Lac} = +0.05$	–	1	0.28	0.4	5.1
$CMR_{Lac} = +0.09$	–	2	0.28	0.4	5.1
$CMR_{Lac} = -0.06$	–	0	0.28	1.2	5.1
$CMR_{Lac} = +0.14$	–	1	0.28	1.2	5.1
$CMR_{Lac} = +0.23$	–	1	0.28	2.0	5.1
$CMR_{Lac} = +0.45$	–	1	0.28	4.0	5.1
$[Lac]_B = 46$	−0.36	0	–	0.4	5.1
$[Lac]_B = 65$	−0.36	1	–	0.4	5.1
$[Lac]_B = 84$	−0.36	2	–	0.4	5.1
$[Lac]_B = 2.6$	−0.36	1	–	2	5.1
$[Lac]_B = 4.0$	−0.36	2	–	2	5.1

*Values were calculated with Equation 4: $CMR_{Lac} = V_{MAX}$ ($[Lac]_P$ - $[Lac]_B$)/(K_T + $[Lac]_P$ + $[Lac]_B$). The present study measured brain lactate concentration ($[Lac]_B$) = 0.28 mM in 5-year-old sevoflurane anesthetized children (**Figure 5**), but their plasma lactate concentrations ($[Lac]_P$), the kinetic constants for lactate transport across the blood-brain barrier (V_{MAX} and K_T), and the rate of lactate utilization (CMR_{Lac}) are not known. Two questions were, therefore, posed: (1) What is calculated CMR_{Lac} based on measured brain [Lac] and different values for plasma lactate concentration and V_{MAX}? (2) What is brain lactate level when CMR_{Lac} is fixed and plasma lactate level and V_{MAX} are varied? Positive or negative values for CMR_{Lac} denote net influx or efflux of lactate into or from brain, respectively. Measured values for V_{MAX} (0.4 μmol/g/min) and K_T (5.1 mM) in normal adult human brain are from Boumezbeur et al. (2010) Because V_{MAX} is higher in developing rodent brain (but not known in human children), values were increased 3, 5, or 10-fold for the calculations. Note: (i) net lactate uptake occurs when plasma lactate level exceeds that in brain, and lactate efflux occurs when brain lactate level exceeds that in plasma, and (ii) calculated values for brain lactate levels based on adult kinetic constants are not realistic.*

An alternate possibility to explain our data in relation to previously-reported data (Goyal et al., 2014) is that children have several-fold higher lactate transport activity through the monocarboxylate transporter (MCT) system than adults. Preclinical data in rodents show that the expression of MCTs is higher in neonates than in adults (Gerhart et al., 1997). Cremer et al. measured MCT transport in neonatal and adult rats and the transport kinetics were found to be ~3-fold higher in the neonates (Cremer et al., 1979). Assuming that V_{MAX} is 5-fold higher we calculated a minimum brain [Lac] needed to account for elevated non-oxidative metabolism of glucose of 2.6 mM which, is 9-fold greater than the measured values. Using the measured value of brain [Lac] the impact of a higher V_{MAX} would be to increase lactate influx (**Table 2**). We note that a 3-fold higher value is most likely, well-above the elevation, if any, in the children studied since it was obtained from rat pups that were not yet weaned, during which time there is a much higher percentage of ketones and other monocarboxylic acid substrates consumed by the brain (Chowdhury et al., 2007).

Overall our ^{1}H MRS data - which were not supportive of lactate efflux from children's brain - are in agreement with previous data reporting a cerebral arterio-venous (AV) difference for lactate of ~0 in seven anesthetized children (Persson et al., 1972). In another study which documented AV-differences of glucose and oxygen in children, OGI was close to the expected theoretical value of 6:1 (Settergren et al., 1976) (see ketones as alternate fuels and **Table 4**, below).

Alternate Metabolic Pathways to Explain High Non-oxidative Metabolism of Glucose in Early Childhood, a Complex Phenomenon

The concept of enhanced "aerobic glycolysis" (Goyal et al., 2014) (i.e., enhanced non-oxidative metabolism of glucose) is derived from consumption of more glucose than oxygen in the presence of abundant oxygen. The inference is that glycolytic flux is increased but the downstream fate of the glucose carbon is not established. Flux of glucose into many pathways could contribute to the CMR_{O2}-$CMR_{glucose}$ mismatch (**Figure 1**). We assess below possible contributions from these pathways.

Pentose Phosphate Pathway

One alternate possibility to explain the elevated non-oxidative metabolism of glucose is the pentose phosphate pathway. The use of glucose for biosynthesis involves both energy production, production of NADPH via the pentose phosphate pathway, and use of different pathways to incorporate glucose carbon into macromolecules that might be used for synaptic remodeling (**Figure 1**). Studies of the pentose phosphate pathway in adults (Baquer et al., 1988) suggest that it works primarily in the direction of NADPH production in which 1 carbon is lost per glucose that goes through the pathway with the remainder of the carbons reentering glycolysis and being converted to pyruvate and lactate. Therefore, even if all the glucose phosphorylated into glucose-6-phosphate (Glc-6-P) enters the pentose shunt it would only reduce the rate of glycolysis by 1/6 unless there is a very large ribose synthesis flux.

However, pentose phosphate pathway activity is higher during brain development (Baquer et al., 1977, 1988), and a greater fraction of glucose carbons may not enter glycolysis immediately [either being removed as riboses or lost through extensive cycling at the level of fructose-6-phosphate (Fru-6-P) which can be in relatively fast exchange with Glc-6-P via phosphoglucose isomerase (Rodriguez-Rodriguez et al., 2013); **Figure 1**] resulting in a larger underestimate of the CMR_{O2}-$CMR_{glucose}$ mismatch based on lactate production and levels. In fact, if recycling is complete, the shunt could explain most or all of the fall in OGI. The stoichiometry of the pentose shunt is 3 Glc-6-P → 3 CO_2 + 2 Fru-6-P + 1 glyceraldehyde-3-phosphate (GAP). If *all of the Fru-6-P* is recycled by conversion to Glc-6-P that re-enters the shunt pathway, then one "new" Glc-6-P from glucose (or glycogen) is required per cycle, with the net result that for each glucose that enters as Glc-6-P, 3 CO_2 + 1 GAP are produced. If the GAP is oxidized, the OGI would be 3 because half of the equivalents of the incoming glucose are converted to CO_2 without oxygen consumption. If the GAP is converted to lactate and released from brain, OGI = 0. High activity of the pentose shunt in young children coupled with complete Fru-6-P recycling could explain both the low OGI and

TABLE 3 | Estimates of changes in OGI and lactate efflux rates from brain of children when updated values for the lumped constant are used to calculate $CMR_{glucose}$.

Lumped constant	$CMR_{glucose}$ (μmol/g/min)	OGI	$CMR_{O2}/6$ (μmol/g/min)	CMR_{O2}-$CMR_{glucose}$ stoichiometric mismatch	
				$CMR_{glucose}$-($CMR_{O2}/6$) (μmol/g/min)	Equivalent CMR_{Lac} (μmol/g/min)
0.42	0.58	4.1	0.4	0.18	−0.36
0.65	0.37	6.4	0.4	−0.03	+0.06
0.80	0.30	7.9	0.4	−0.10	+0.20

*Analysis of the stoichiometric mismatch between oxygen and glucose was evaluated using equation 1b: $CMR_{Lac} = -2[CMR_{glucose} - (CMR_{O2}/6)]$ for different values for the lumped constant that alter calculated $CMR_{glucose}$. CMR_{Lac} is assigned a negative value to denote release of glucose equivalents from brain when $CMR_{glucose}$ exceeds CMR_{O2}; positive values are obtained when CMR_{O2} exceeds $CMR_{glucose}$ and indicate oxidation of other substrates (carbohydrate or ketone bodies) that were not taken into account in the OGI calculation. Maximal values of CMR_{O2} and $CMR_{glucose}$ in the loessR plots for ~3–5 year old children in **Figure 2A** of Goyal et al. (2014) i.e., 2.4 and 0.58 μmol/g/min, respectively, were used to calculate OGI = CMR_{O2}/ $CMR_{glucose}$. $CMR_{glucose}$ for updated values of the lumped constant was calculated by multiplying $CMR_{glucose}$ = 0.58 by 0.42/0.65 or 0.42/0.80 and used to calculate updated OGIs. Stoichiometric balance between $CMR_{glucose}$ and CMR_{O2} was determined by subtracting the glucose equivalents of maximal CMR_{O2} (i.e., $CMR_{O2}/6 = 2.4/6 = 0.4$) from $CMR_{glucose}$. For comparison to values in brain of normal resting awake adults, OGI determined in 8 independent studies by arteriovenous differences, was 5.95 ± 0.27 (mean ± SD) (Quistorff et al., 2008). This value for OGI was determined by a method independent of the value of the lumped constant. Whole-brain $CMR_{glucose}$ in normal resting awake adult human brain was 0.26 ± 0.07 μmol/g/min when calculated using the lumped constant = 0.80, whole brain CMR_{O2} was 1.36 ± 0.37 μmol/g/min, and whole-brain OGI was 5.17 + 0.95 (Hyder et al., 2016).*

inability to account for the additional glucose carbon consumed in excess of oxygen because it is released as CO_2. A caveat is that CO_2 production without oxygen consumption via the pentose shunt would *increase* the respiratory quotient (RQ—see legend to **Table 4** for definitions and discussion below) above 1.0, the value determined in young children that is indicative of carbohydrate utilization (**Table 4**). However, oxidation of ketone bodies has an RQ of 0.7, and the combination of high pentose shunt activity plus oxidation of blood-borne ketone bodies in brain of young children may explain the net RQ = 1. Future studies in children using ^{13}C MRS technology to directly measure the pentose phosphate pathway and ketone body utilization could potentially distinguish these possibilities (Rothman et al., 2011).

Use of Glucose Carbons as Biosynthesis Precursors

In addition to ribose formation from the pentose phosphate pathway there are many other pathways by which carbons derived from glucose can be used for net biosynthesis, such as for lipids and amino acids. In order to assess this possibility, we calculated the approximate rate of increase in biomass implied by the non-oxidative metabolism of glucose mismatch using the following expression based on the "aerobic glycolysis" data of Goyal et al. (2014) (see **Table 3**)

Rate of biomass increase = the rate of "aerobic glycolysis" (μmol glucose/min/g brain)*brain weight

For the reported excess of glucose consumption over oxidation at 5 years old of 0.18 μmol/g/min and an average brain weight of 1300 g this calculation yields ~1800 g per month of additional carbon incorporation. This amount is well-over the total brain weight (which is ~70% water) and clearly not possible.

An alternate possibility, discussed by Goyal et al. (2014), is that there is a high level of synaptic turnover so that the carbon incorporated from glucose into nucleotides, lipids and proteins in the building of new synapses is largely matched by synapse breakdown and catabolism of the structural components. However, if this were the case then the released carbon building blocks would be oxidized at the same rate as new carbons are incorporated resulting in a normal OGI value.

Ketones and Lactate as Alternate Fuels in Early Childhood

A limitation of the OGI is that it only takes into account the relationship between oxygen and glucose. The oxidation of non-glucose substrates is assumed to be negligible in adult brain, which may not be the case in children. Accurate values for the oxygen-fuel index would require measurement of net uptake into brain of all alternate substrates (e.g., β-hydroxybutyrate, acetoacetate, lactate) in plasma plus utilization of brain glycogen. It is well-known that in the developing brain lactate and ketones serves as fuel and substrates during the suckling period and beyond and ketones are essential for brain lipid synthesis (Settergren et al., 1976). For example, children 2–6 years of age have been reported to have significantly higher overnight fasting values of β-hydroxybutyrate and acetoacetate than older children and adults (Persson et al., 1972). Also, in a study where children were anesthetized (with N_2O) the cerebral uptake of ketones (acetoacetate and β-hydroxybutyrate) accounted for ~13% of the measured oxygen uptake, assuming complete oxidation of the ketones (Settergren et al., 1976). In addition to ketones our calculations suggest that plasma lactate could be a net oxidative energy source in the developing brain, albeit at a low level. The effect of net lactate oxidation would be to increase the measured OGI due to the increase in oxygen consumption for the same amount of glucose uptake. As shown in **Figure 2** and **Table 4** alternate carbohydrate indicies can be defined that takes glucose, lactate, and ketone body net uptake into account (excluding brain glycogen consumption that cannot be measured in young children and is very difficult to measure in adults).

Table 4 summarizes results from metabolic studies in awake and N_2O-anesthetized children and reveals the impact of inclusion of inclusion of lactate and ketone body fluxes on calculated oxygen/substrate ratios. If lactate efflux is not taken into account in study 1, OGI is too low compared with OCI (oxygen-carbohydrate index; see legend to **Table 4** for definitions and equations for calculation). When lactate and ketone bodies are included in the calculation of OCKI (oxygen-carbohydrate-ketone index), the general trend is for OCI to exceed OGI due

TABLE 4 | Blood flow, metabolic rates, and calculated oxygen/substrate utilization ratios and brain lactate concentration in brain of young children.

Reference	1[a]	2[b]		3[d]	4[e]	5[f]	6[g]	7[h]	8[i]				
Age range (years)	0.5–3.3	3–11	Adults	0.58–14	0.08–0.58	10–15	1–15	21–24 55–65	0–1	1–2	3–8	9–15	19–30
Mean age (years)	0.92	6.1	24.5			12							
Number of subjects	10	9	12	7	17	7	42–65	10	7	4	12	6	7
Duration of fasting (h)	3				9		10	15	4	4	4	4	4
Physiological status during assay	Awake, 15% N_2O	Awake, 15% N_2O	Awake, 15% N_2O	70%N2O	awake	75→ 50% N_2O	75→ 50% N_2O	awake	All groups awake				
Anesthesia duration (min)							20–40						
CBF (ml/g/min)	0.903	1.064	0.601				0.68	0.64					
Arterial conc. (μmol/ml)													
Glucose				4.18	5.21		5.27	4.57					
Lactate	1.80			1.52	1.25		1.13	0.61					
Pyruvate	0.094			0.08			0.104	0.065					
Acetoacetate				0.60	0.12		0.273	0.159					
β-hydroxybutyrate				1.75	0.28		0.890	0.347					
(A-V) (μmol/ml)													
O_2	2.87			1.49	2.23	2.08	2.17						
Glucose	0.726			0.29	0.48	0.33	0.36						
Lactate	−0.507			−0.03	−0.27	0.012	−0.07						
Pyruvate	−0.0085			−0.01		0.014	−0.01						
Acetoacetate				0.08	0.03		0.018						
β-hydroxybutyrate				0.09	0.04		0.049						
CMR (μmol/g/min)													
O_2	2.59	2.31[c]	1.86				1.35	1.72					
Glucose	0.656						0.248	0.248	0.204	0.274	0.481	0.392	0.243
Lactate	−0.458						−0.048	−0.028					
Pyruvate	−0.008						−0.008	−0.004					
Acetoacetate							0.012	0.004					
β-Hydroxybutyrate							0.034	0.006					
Respiratory quotient	1.00	0.97	0.94										
OGI	3.95			5.14	4.65	6.3	6.03	6.94	11.3[j] 6.62[k]	8.4[j] 4.93[k]	4.8[j] 2.81[k]	5.9[j] 3.44[k]	7.7[j] 6.91[k]
OCI	6.13			5.52	6.46	6.3	6.78	7.41					
OCKI				3.81	4.56	4.04	5.88	7.19					
Calculated O_2 uptake	2.81			2.35	2.37	2.09	2.21	1.44					
%O_2 from ketone oxidation				30.9	12.7	5.3	13.2	3.0					
Lac+Pyr release (% Glc)	−35.5			−6.9	−28.1	0	−11.3	−6.5					
Calc.$[Lac]_B$: V_{MAX} = 0.4	−64.8						2.14	1.08					
V_{MAX} = 2.0	4.4						1.31	0.70					
V_{MAX} = 4.0	2.9						1.22	0.65					

Values are means; those not included were not determined/reported by the tabulated studies.

CBF, cerebral blood flow; (A-V), arteriovenous difference that is positive when there is net uptake into brain and negative when there is net efflux; Glc, glucose; Lac, lactate; Pyr, pyruvate; AcAc, acetoacetate; BHB, β-hydroxybutyrate; KB, ketone bodies (AcAc + BHB); CMR, cerebral metabolic rate; OGI, oxygen-glucose index; OCI, oxygen-carbohydrate index; OCKI, oxygen-carbohydrate-ketone index.

Metabolic rates and oxygen/substrate ratios:

$CMR_{substrate} = CBF(A\text{-}V)_{substrate}$.

$OGI = CMR_{O2}/CMR_{glucose} = (A\text{-}V)_{O2}/(A\text{-}V)_{glucose}$ *and assumes no other substrates are oxidized.*

$OCI = CMR_{O2}/[CMR_{glucose} + 0.5(CMR_{lac} + CMR_{pyr})] = (A\text{-}V)_{O2}/[(A\text{-}V)_{glucose} + 0.5((A\text{-}V)_{lac} + (A\text{-}V)_{pyr})]$, *where pyruvate and lactate are expressed in glucose equivalents 1 glucose = 2 pyruvate or 2 lactate. OCI takes into account lactate + pyruvate uptake or efflux from brain and assumes no other substrates are consumed, which is generally valid for normal, non-fasted adults during rest or graded exercise to exhaustion.*

$OCKI = CMR_{O2}/[CMR_{glucose} + 0.5(CMR_{lac} + CMR_{pyr}) + 4/6CMR_{AcAc} + 4.5/6CMR_{BHB}] = (A\text{-}V)_{O2}/[(A\text{-}V)_{glucose} + 0.5((A\text{-}V)_{lac} + (A\text{-}V)_{pyr}) + 4/6(A\text{-}V)_{AcAc} + 4.5/6(A\text{-}V)_{BHB}]$, *where utilization of other substrates are expressed in glucose equivalents for oxygen utilization. Oxidative metabolism of one glucose, one AcAc, or one BHB molecule consumes 6, 4, or 4.5 molecules of O_2 (Hawkins et al., 1971). The OCKI calculation accounts for the major substrates consumed or released from brain relative to oxygen.*

(Continued)

TABLE 4 | Continued

Ketone body (KB) oxidation as percent of calculated O_2 utilization: *Calculated O_2 uptake = $6^*[(A\text{-}V)_{glc}+0.5((A\text{-}V)lac + (A\text{-}V)_{pyr})] + 4(A\text{-}V)_{AcAc} + 4.5(A\text{-}V)_{BHB}$, assuming complete oxidation of ketone bodies. Calculated %KB oxidation = $100^*(4(A\text{-}V)_{AcAc}+4.5(A\text{-}V)_{BHB})$/calculated $(A\text{-}V)_{O2}$. For adults, CMR values replaced (A-V) in the equations.*
Lactate-pyruvate release/glucose uptake: *Lactate + pyruvate release/uptake from brain (negative value if release) is expressed in glucose equivalents as % of glucose uptake = $100^*0.5[(A\text{-}V)_{lac} + (A\text{-}V)_{pyr}]/(A\text{-}V)_{glc}$.*
Respiratory quotient (RQ): *RQ = volume of CO_2 produced/volume of O_2 consumed = $(A\text{-}V)_{CO2}/(A\text{-}V)_{O2}$. An RQ of 1.0, 0.8 or 0.7 indicates that carbohydrates, proteins, or lipids/ketones, respectively, are metabolized, with intermediate values indicating mixed fuel utilization.*
Calculated brain lactate concentrations: *$[Lac]_B$ was calculated (Calc.) with Equation 4: $CMR_{Lac} = V_{MAX}$ $([Lac]_p - [Lac]_B)/(K_T + [Lac]_p + [Lac]_B)$ using measured $[Lac]_p$ and CMR_{lac} and different values for V_{MAX}. Positive or negative values for CMR_{Lac} denote net influx into or net efflux of lactate from brain, respectively. Measured values for V_{MAX} (0.4 μmol/g/min) and K_T (5.1 mM) for plasma-brain lactate transport in normal adult human brain are from (Boumezbeur et al., 2010). For calculations V_{MAX} values 5 or 10 times higher were also used because based on rodent studies the developing brain may have a higher V_{MAX} for blood-brain barrier lactate transport (Cremer et al., 1979).*
[a] *Most children cried and required some restraint during the procedure, especially at time of needle punctures. PCO_2 did not change significantly during the procedures.*
[b] *The authors stated that great pains were taken to minimize anxiety in the children, including having the dim lighting, minimal stimulation, and providing a movie on the ceiling that was considered to be unlikely to influence the global CBF or $CMRO_2$. Low anxiety is supported by recording of mean pulse rates and mean arterial blood pressures were in the range of normal, resting 6-year-old children. Also, one child that had 4 repeated determinations with no significant changes due to familiarity with the procedure. The authors' subjective opinion was that the children were less anxious than the adults.*
[c] *Global CMR_{O2} had no significant correlation, positive or negative, with age between age 3 to 10 years.*
[d] *Children were pre-medicated with morphine and atropine, anesthesia induced with thiopentane, intubated, ventilated with 70% N_2O/30%O_2. Data for mild hypercapnia were also reported but not tabulated.*
[e] *Data for infants <0.15 years old were also reported but not tabulated. If the infants completely oxidized the ketone bodies they would account for 13% of total oxygen consumption, with glucose corrected for lactate efflux accounting for 87%.*
[f] *Children were pre-medicated with morphine, anesthesia induced with thiopentane, general anesthesia with pancuronium (prior to intubation) and 75% N_2O/25%O_2 that was abruptly reduced to 50% N_2O during the CBF assay. More detailed data for infants <1 year old were also reported but not tabulated. In these infants, blood ketone body concentrations were much higher than in 12-year-old children, and (A-V) differences for AcAc and BHB were greater in the infants in whom net ketone body uptake accounted for 13% of measured oxygen uptake, assuming complete oxidation. However, less oxygen was consumed compared to calculated oxidation of glucose corrected for lactate + pyruvate release and ketone bodies, and this discordance could not be explained. Infants released lactate + pyruvate from brain to blood, equivalent to 6% of glucose uptake. Equally-detailed assays were not reported for the children.*
[g] *Children were pre-medicated with morphine and atropine, anesthesia induced with thiopentane, general anesthesia with pancuronium and 75% N_2O/25%O_2 that was abruptly reduced to 50% N_2O during the CBF assay. (A-V) Differences were measured in 42 children (age range 1–15 years old), whereas CBF and O_2 were measured in more children, including those at younger ages. Uptake of the ketone bodies was positively correlated with arterial concentration. CBF and the metabolic rates for oxygen, glucose, lactate, pyruvate, acetoacetate, and β-hydroxybutyrate were not correlated with age. However, the relationship between measured oxygen consumption and the amount needed for complete oxidation of glucose, acetoacetate, and β-hydroxybutyrate minus release of lactate + pyruvate was poor, as reported in Settergren et al. (1976); the basis for this finding is unknown. The authors reported considerable variability in CBF, so OGI, OCI, OCKI, and %lactate released were calculated from (A-V) differences. To calculate $[Lac]_B$ for different V_{MAX} values it was necessary to use CMR_{Lac}.*
[h] *Subjects were calm and relaxed after catheter insertion. Data were obtained for two groups of adults (21–24 and 55–65 years old; n = 5/group) that were not significantly different, and results were pooled.*
[i] *$CMR_{glucose}$ is for cerebral hemispheres in children who had transient neurological events that did not significantly affect neurodevelopment and were considered to be reasonably representative of normal children. Some children had medication on the day of the study. Children that became drowsy during the assay were tapped on the shoulder but other stimuli were minimized. Regional values for $CMR_{glucose}$ were also reported but are not tabulated.*
[j] *Global CMR_{O2} = 2.31 from Kennedy and Sokoloff (1957) was used to calculate OGI in awake children because no correlation with age (3–11 years old) was reported, whereas OGI in awake adults was based on CMR_{O2} = 1.86 determined in adults.*
[k] *Global CMR_{O2} = 1.35 from Settergren et al. was used to calculate OGI because no correlation with age was reported in anesthetized children (1–15 years old), whereas CMR_{O2} = 1.68 for awake adults was used to calculate OGI for adults. Settergren et al. also reported no age-related correlation of $CMR_{glucose}$, CMR_{Lac}, CMR_{pyr}, CMR_{AcAc}, or CMR_{BHB} across age between 1–15 years old in anesthetized children, contrasting the results of Chugani et al. (1987) in awake subjects. Note that global $CMRO_2$ in 1–15-year-old anesthetized children the study by Settergren et al. (1980) is lower than that of awake adults the Lying-Tunell et al. (1980) and Kennedy and Sokoloff (1957) studies, whereas awake children age 3–11 years old had higher global $CMRO_2$ than awake adults.*
1. Mehta et al. (1977); 2. Kennedy and Sokoloff (1957); 3. Settergren et al. (1973); 4. Kraus et al. (1974); 5. Settergren et al. (1976); 6. Settergren et al. (1980); 7. Lying-Tunell et al. (1980); 8. Chugani et al. (1987).

to correction of glucose uptake for lactate efflux in all studies where measured, then OCKI is falls below OCI due to inclusion of ketone body uptake (**Table 4**). In most cases, the calculated oxygen uptake is similar to the measured oxygen uptake value, and oxidation of ketone bodies accounted for 3–13% of total oxygen consumption except for study 3 where calculated oxygen uptake was 59% higher than the measured value and ketones accounted for 30% of oxygen uptake. Lactate *efflux* accounted for 0–11% of glucose uptake in the 0.6–15-year-old N_2O-anesthetized children and 28–36% in children <3.3 years old when awake, suggesting stress-induced glycolysis/glycogenolysis and enhanced release. Of interest, OCI in study 1 is 6.1 and the respiratory quotient (RQ $=(A\text{-}V)_{CO2}/(A\text{-}V)_{O2}$) is 1.00 indicating strictly carbohydrate oxidation, whereas the RQ in older children was slightly <1, suggesting some ketone body use. (See discussion above regarding the potential balancing of pentose shunt and ketone body oxidation to influence the RQ).

Glycogen and the Glycogen Shunt

Little is known about the role of glycogen in energy metabolism during brain development (Rust, 1994). However, glycogen turnover with lactate release from brain in conjunction with synaptic activity would consume glucose without oxygen. Previous studies have considered the role of the glycogen shunt (i.e., the cycling of glucose-6-phosphate from the glycolytic pathway into glycogen and its return upon glycogenolysis) to explain, in part, the $CMR_{glucose}$-CMR_{O2} mismatch observed during brain activation studies (Shulman et al., 2001). However, in this case the enhanced glucose uptake relative to oxidation would result in increased lactate production which would have been seen in the present study.

Alternatively, net glycogen synthesis could be occurring in which case there would be an equivalent increase in glucose uptake resulting in a lower OGI without an increase in lactate production. In the early preparative aspects of the PET studies of awake children, glycogen could have been depleted prior to the $CMR_{glucose}$ measurement due to stress, sensory stimulation, or alerting, then re-synthesized during the assay interval. Evidence exists from animal models supporting enhanced glycogen breakdown under conditions of stress and increased arousal (Dienel and Cruz, 2016). In the present study, however, the children were anesthetized and glycogenolysis is not likely to contribute to lactate production above the low basal level.

Metabolic Studies in Children Underscore the Difficulty and Complexity of Accurate, Fully-Quantitative Determinations of Non-oxidative Metabolism of Glucose With Developmental Age

Due to the invasive nature of methods for measuring brain glucose and oxygen consumption as well as concerns regarding radiation the number of brain metabolic studies in children is highly limited. The reports by Kennedy and Sokoloff (1957) and Mehta et al. (1977) (**Table 4**) were the only ones (to our knowledge) to measure CMR_{O2} in awake children. Kennedy and Sokoloff stated that there was no correlation of CMR_{O2} with age between 3 and 11 years, and dividing the Chugani values for $CMR_{glucose}$ into the mean CMR_{O2} gives results (**Table 4**) similar to the OGI profile shown for LC = 0.65 in **Figure 7B**. In sharp contrast, use of the lower value for CMR_{O2} from N_2O-anesthesized children resulted in much lower OGI values due to low CMR_{O2} in the anesthetized children (**Table 4**). In both cases, the OGIs do not reflect the true oxygen/substrate ratio because the contributions of lactate efflux and ketone body influx are not included. Notably, CBF in awake children (studies 1 and 2, **Table 4**), exceeded that in awake adults, whereas CBF in N_2O-anesthetized children was lower than in awake adults and was 58% that of awake children in the same age range (studies 2, 6, and 7, **Table 4**).

Inspection of **Figure 2A** and Supplemental Table 1 of Goyal et al. indicates that most of the data for the 3–10-year-old children came from two studies: Kennedy and Sokoloff (1957) and Chugani et al. (1987). Kennedy and Sokoloff reported *whole-brain* CMR_{O2}, whereas Chugani et al. reported *regional* $CMR_{glucose}$ (also see **Table 4**) so the regional or global metabolic rates are not congruent, as required for an accurate OGI. Use of higher cerebral cortical values for $CMR_{glucose}$ compared with lower whole-brain CMR_{O2} will artifactually inflate the magnitude of the CMR_{O2}-$CMR_{glucose}$ mismatch. Regional variations in $CMR_{glucose}$ and CMR_{O2} and stability of regional OGI in normal resting adult brain (Hyder et al., 2016) support the conclusion that errors will be incurred by combined use of global and regional data to calculate OGI.

A caveat to the majority of studies looking at metabolic changes during development is that often sedation or anesthesia must be used to study young children. Of importance, N_2O stimulates brain norepinephrine release in a time- and concentration-dependent manner, with 60% N_2O increasing norepinephrine levels by about 3-fold at 50 min (Yoshida et al., 2001, 2010), and may influence brain glucose and glycogen metabolism and brain metabolite levels (Dienel and Cruz, 2016).

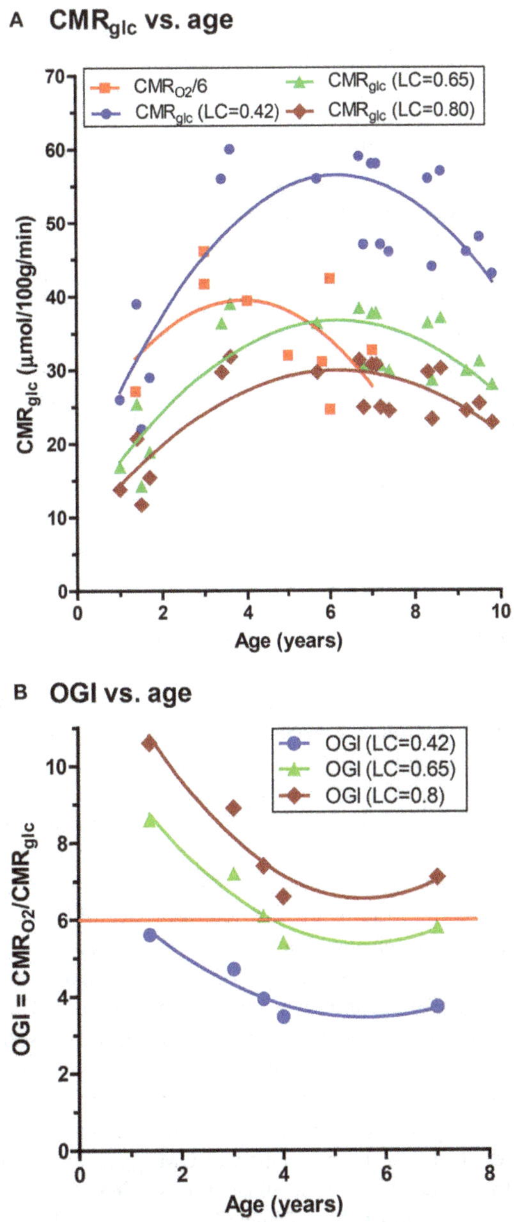

FIGURE 7 | Calculated $CMR_{glucose}$ and OGI as function of age in children. Values for children from age 1-10 years were taken from Supplementary Table 1 of Goyal et al. **(A)** Based on the ages of the subjects in the Goyal et al. (2014) and Chugani et al. (1987) all $CMR_{glucose}$ data for this age group were assumed to be from the study of Chugani et al. who used a value of the lumped constant (LC) of 0.42 to calculate $CMR_{glucose}$ in their [^{18}F]FDG-PET studies (blue symbols and lines). For comparison, values at each age were recalculated using updated values for the LC, i.e., LC = 0.65 (Wu et al., 2003) (green) and LC = 0.80 (Wienhard, 2002; Hyder et al., 2016) (brown). To directly compare the different $CMR_{glucose}$ data sets to the CMR_{O2} values reported by Goyal et al. each CMR_{O2} was converted to glucose equivalents (red squares) by dividing by 6 (which assumes all oxygen consumed is due to glucose oxidation–see text), with the caveat that correction for lactate fluxes and ketone body utilization that were not measured in these studies will alter these values (see **Table 4**). **(B)** OGI values tabulated by Goyal et al. were similarly corrected using LC = 0.65 or 0.8. The horizontal red line represents the theoretical maximum of 6.0 (see text). The solid curved lines are quadratic nonlinear regression lines calculated with GraphPad Prism 5.

Lumped Constant and Accurate $CMR_{glucose}$ Values

Calculation of OGI requires *accurate* and *absolute* values for both rates to obtain a valid molar ratio of oxygen to glucose utilization. However, as previously mentioned, the OGI does not have any information about the fate of the glucose carbon consumed in excess of oxygen. During development, there is growth and remodeling of brain structures such as synapses, and Goyal et al. emphasized this process as an explanation for excess glucose consumption (Goyal et al., 2014). However, the studies used in the meta-analysis did not measure fluxes of metabolic pathways, and the fate of glucose is unknown and remains speculative. The results of the present study demonstrate that lactate levels are far, far lower than expected in developing brain, ruling out glycolysis with lactate accumulation as a major contributor to a fall in OGI in children. Re-calculation of $CMR_{glucose}$ and OGI with updated values for the LC strongly suggests that calculated $CMR_{glucose}$ is not as accurate as required, causing errors in OGI. The OGI variability in **Figure 7B** is probably due, in part, to the reported CMR_{O2} values that have fewer data points than $CMR_{glucose}$ within this age range. These data would be most accurate if CMR_{O2} and $CMR_{glucose}$ were sequentially determined in the same brain regions of the same awake subjects, which is extremely difficult, if not impossible, to carry out in young children. In addition, determination of the net utilization of lactate, ketone bodies, and other potential substrates in blood and inclusion in the oxygen/substrate indicies is necessary to obtain accurate measures of brain metabolism during development.

Another caveat is that the LC may change with age and also depends on the model (Kuwabara et al., 1990). One component of the LC is the ratio of the distribution space of FDG to that for glucose. Conceivably, the distribution spaces may change during maturation as astrocytes, neurons, and oligodendrocytes increase transporters and metabolic enzymes, but the LC may be relatively stable because it is a ratio. The LC has been shown to be similar in fetal and neonatal sheep (Abrams et al., 1984) and studies in developing brain have assumed that the LC is constant during development (Kennedy et al., 1978, 1982; Kato et al., 1980; Nehlig et al., 1988). Re-calculation of $CMR_{glucose}$ with updated values for the LC does not invalidate the age-dependent changes in $CMR_{glucose}$ reported by Chugani et al. (1987). In fact our measured brain [Lac] values, while consistently low at all ages, do reach a maximum at ~5 years which is the maximum $CMR_{glucose}$ reported by Chugani et al. (1987).

However, and most importantly, any departure from the true value of the LC for FDG and from the true absolute rate of $CMR_{glucose}$ will invalidate the calculated OGI across all ages, not just in young children. The analyses presented in **Figure 7** and **Tables 3**, **4** raise serious concerns about the accuracy of the OGI profiles in developing brain and aging brain reported by Goyal et al. because they did not take the use of different LC values and utilization of supplemental substrates into account in their meta-analysis (Goyal et al., 2014). Note that if ketone body oxidation were measured and included in the OGI calculations for the youngest children in **Figure 7B**, the values for OGI > 6 would be reduced to close to or below 6 (see **Table 4**). Furthermore, Goyal et al. divided CMR_{O2} by 6 to get glucose equivalents, which assumes no other substrates are oxidized. If ketones are consumed this calculation introduces an error into the comparison of $CMR_{glucose}$ and CMR_{O2} in their **Figure 2A** because ketone bodies have different O_2 - substrate stoichiometries than glucose (legend, **Table 4**). While recognizing this issue, the same calculation was used in **Figure 7** in the present study so the data sets in their and our studies could be compared. Even if the LC = 0.42 and calculated $CMR_{glucose}$ are appropriate and valid in the study by Chugani et al., regional CMR_{O2} was not measured in the same brain regions in the same subjects at the same time, seriously weakening conclusions related to the magnitude of aerobic glycolysis in children. Moreover, as we show in this study, the commensurate lactate levels do not match their predictions based on non-oxidative metabolism of glucose, and thus it is premature to conclude that 33% of the glucose consumed by 3-8-year old children is not metabolized via the tricarboxylic acid cycle to consume proportionate amounts of oxygen.

The brain glucose in children in the present study measured by the LC model analysis was in the range of about 1.7–2.2 mM (results not shown), ~2 times higher than anticipated in adults at a similar plasma glucose level based on ^{13}C MRS measurements and ^{1}H MRS measurements at higher fields using pulse sequences optimized for glucose detection (Gruetter et al., 1992, 1998; de Graaf et al., 2001; Shestov et al., 2011). From four studies in normal adults (Gruetter et al., 1992, 1998; de Graaf et al., 2001; Shestov et al., 2011), the brain/plasma ratio for glucose is about 0.2, and if this ratio is the same in children and we use the mean value for brain glucose for children aged 0.5–15 years old (under N_2O) of 4.89 mM (**Table 4**), the expected brain glucose level would be 0.98 mM. Plasma glucose levels in adults in which the LC of 0.42 (Phelps et al., 1979; Huang et al., 1980) and 0.65 (Wu et al., 2003) were within the range 5.1–5.5 mM, with an anticipated brain concentration range of 1.0–1.1 mM. Due to limitations in the pulse sequence for measuring brain glucose in our study, the glucose values can be deceptive in that there can be poor accuracy but good precision (low Cramer Rao bounds, which in our study was in the range of 10–30% for glucose), and it is likely that the brain glucose concentrations in children are not accurate and are overestimated. Nevertheless, addressing this question in future studies is of importance for obtaining accurate $CMR_{glucose}$ assays in children. Both brain and plasma glucose levels will impact the value of LC, with higher brain levels of glucose leading to somewhat lower LC values and correspondingly-higher calculated $CMR_{glucose}$, as shown for [^{14}C]deoxyglucose in adult animal studies (Schuier et al., 1990; Suda et al., 1990; Dienel et al., 1991). The relationships between the LC for FDG and brain and plasma glucose levels need to be determined in humans across age.

To summarize, the use of supplemental fuel and metabolic assays in different brain regions in different cohorts in which nutritional status was not matched will cause errors in calculated OGI. Higher metabolism of glucose via the pentose shunt in young children with Fru-6-P recycling and release of glucose carbon as CO_2 is an important potential contributor to consumption of glucose in excess of oxygen. These issues must be evaluated quantitatively before the validity of the DG method is challenged. In this regard, regional CMR_{glc} reported by Chugani et al. (1987) for normal adult brain (0.2–0.27 μmol/g/min) with LC=0.42 determined in adult brain in a separate cohort is similar to the whole brain CMR_{glc} (0.26 μmol/g/min) reported by Hyder et al. (2016) using FDT-PET and LC=0.8 determined in the same subjects, and adult whole brain CMR_{glc} reported by Madsen et al. (1995) (0.23 μmol/g/min), calculated from measurements of cerebral blood flow and arteriovenous differences. As discussed above, the updated values for the LC can arise for various technical reasons, and their use in the present study illustrates the effects of uncertainties in the true value of the LC in young children on the temporal profile of OGI. Changing the value of the LC increases OGI, which would be too high when supplemental fuels are used but not taken into account.

Limitations of the Study

The ability to measure resting lactate by ^1H MRS has been criticized based on its low levels and contamination from brain macromolecules and lipids from the skull (arising due to incomplete volume localization). However, based on examination of spectra (**Figure 3**) the outer volume lipid contamination was minimal. Furthermore, excellent Bo homogeneity was achieved so that the lactate methyl group doublet at 1.33 ppm was well-resolved from the broad macromolecule peak at 1.3 ppm underlying lactate which would minimize the possibility of lactate spectral intensity being assigned to the macromolecule peak in the fitting process. Furthermore, if all the resonance intensity at 1.3 ppm were due to lactate, its concentration would be at most ~1 mM (**Figure 3**), which is still well-below what would be needed to explain the reported OGI.

The measured values of lactate as a function of age could potentially be influenced by changes in water and metabolite relaxation as a result of changes in water content and the cellular microstructural environment. Due to the challenges of studying young children there are only a limited number of studies looking at T2 relaxation. However, an extensive study at 1.5 T by Leppert and coworkers found that the T2 of water in gray and white matter rapidly decreased after birth reaching a constant value between 10 months and 5 years (Leppert et al., 2009) which encompasses the age range of children in our study (and at values of T2 similar to those measured in adults). Although there are no studies of lactate T2 changes with age it is unlikely that it would be more sensitive than H_2O which undergoes extensive exchange with macromolecules and other compounds. Furthermore, the T2 of lactate in adults at 3T is ~200 msec (Cady et al., 1996) so that even if it is higher in children there would be little impact on the relative quantitation of lactate for a TE of 32 msec. Although the macromolecule T2 is on the order of the TE (Behar et al., 1994) there is no evidence of a change in the linewidth or relative intensity of the 1.3 ppm macromolecule peak with age so that the effectiveness of the LC model in separating lactate from macromolecules would not be age dependent.

A possible confound of the present study is that the children were studied under sevoflurane or propofol anesthesia (Jacob et al., 2012). However a recent ^1H MRS study has shown that lactate is, in fact, elevated in mice anesthetized with volatile halogenated anesthetics (Boretius et al., 2013), suggesting that the awake $[Lac]_B$ values may be lower. Thus, the measured $[Lac]_B$ in the current study, and therefore the CMR_{Lac} determined from it, should be considered as maximal estimates. Furthermore, our results are similar to a 3T study recently published using ^1H MRS to measure brain [Lac] in a smaller group of neonates and children (Tomiyasu et al., 2016). Another possible confound could be attributed to the variable anatomical voxel location for the ^1HMRS spectra which was not consistent across subjects. We therefore acknowledge that there might have been minor variance in the data due to region dependent differences in metabolite levels.

Dienel and colleagues (Ball et al., 2010) have shown that during activation up to 25% of lactate can diffuse out of regions where it is produced by mechanisms independent of blood flow and, therefore, lead to an underestimate of regional brain lactate efflux from lactate levels alone. However, given the non-activated (anesthetized) conditions such as the present study it is unlikely that these mechanisms would lead to a significant underestimate since the entire cerebral cortex of anesthetized children is at a similar level of activity and presumably lactate production. Future studies using MRS imaging could further address the issue of lactate concentration heterogeneity.

Metabolic studies in children are particularly difficult to interpret because the duration of fasting influences plasma ketone body levels (the longer the fast, the higher the plasma ketone levels), brain ketone body utilization is linearly related to plasma level, and younger children take up ketones better than older children or adults at the same plasma level. Notably, Kennedy and Sokoloff reported no age-dependence of CMR_{O2} in their awake 3–11-year-old cohort, and Settergren et al. (1980) also reported no age correlation with CBF, CMR_{O2}, $CMR_{glucose}$, $CMR_{lactate}$, and $CMR_{ketones}$, in 1–15-year-old N_2O-anesthetized children (study 6, **Table 4**) contrasting the age-dependence of $CMR_{glucose}$ in the awake children in the Chugani study (study 8). To summarize, the contributions of N_2O, alerting, stress, fear, and other factors on these metabolic differences remain to be evaluated, underscoring the need for caution in interpreting results of a meta-analysis in which oxygen and total substrate utilization were not measured in the same subjects and brain regions at the same time. Many factors complicate interpretation of metabolic rates and OGI in children.

CONCLUSIONS

Using ^1H MRS we found that [Lac] in cerebral cortex of young children was very low, and that the maximal calculated efflux of lactate cannot explain the mismatch between $CMR_{glucose}$ and CMR_{O2} previously reported, in agreement with results of the previous metabolic studies in 3-15-year-old children summarized in **Table 4**. Depending on plasma lactate levels it is possible that there was a net small influx of lactate. The results of this study rule out an increase in glycolytic rate and accumulation and release of lactate as a primary cause of elevated non-oxidative metabolism of glucose reported in young children. Possible explanations for utilization of the "missing" glucose in excess of oxygen are carbon loss as CO_2 via the pentose phosphate pathway, use of carbon for nucleotide synthesis, protein synthesis, lipid synthesis, and glycogen turnover with lactate efflux. However, the most significant sources of disagreement are likely the (i) validity of assumptions made in PET studies regarding the true value of the LC, which we believe requires that the present understanding of how OGI and $CMR_{glucose}$ change with age be reexamined, (ii) use of fuel in addition to glucose, and (iii) assays of $CMR_{glucose}$ and CMR_{O2} in different brain regions of different subjects. To summarize, enhanced non-oxidative metabolism of glucose during brain maturation is a complex phenomenon to which many metabolic pathways, fuel sources, and technical issues have a strong influence. Brain developmental progress certainly plays a role in metabolic changes with age, but their quantitative contributions remain to be established. In spite of these interpretive limitations, ^{1}H MRS provides a potentially valuable new biomarker for assessing non-oxidative metabolism of glucose in infants and children and studying its relationship to brain development in health and disease.

ETHICS STATEMENT

The study uses de-identified data from a previous published human IRB approved study (Jacob et al., 2012). The original study by Jacob et al. (2012) was carried out in accordance with the recommendations of Federal Regulations Department of Health and Human Services (DHHS)/Office for Human Research Protections (OHRP), USA. The protocol was approved by the IRB committee at Stony Brook University (CORIHS). All parents of the children gave written informed consent in accordance with the Declaration of Helsinki.

AUTHOR CONTRIBUTIONS

HB and DR conceived the study. HB, DR, and GD performed the analyses; GD conceived the revisiting of the lumped constant for FDG conversion and calculation of OGI. HB, ZJ, and RM designed the original ^{1}HMRs experiments. HL performed the LCModel analysis on ^{1}H MRS spectra and the volumetric analysis. HB, DR, and GD wrote the paper. AG and FH posed scientific questions, read and revised the manuscript. All authors edited and reviewed the paper.

FUNDING

DR - 1- R01NS087568A, R01NS100106; HB - R21HD080573; FH - R01MH067528, P30NS052519.

REFERENCES

Abrams, R. M., Ito, M., Frisinger, J. E., Patlak, C. S., Pettigrew, K. D., and Kennedy, C. (1984). Local cerebral glucose utilization in fetal and neonatal sheep. *Am. J. Physiol.* 246, R608–R618. doi: 10.1152/ajpregu.1984.246.4.R608

Agrawal, S., Sachdev, A., Gupta, D., and Chugh, K. (2004). Role of lactate in critically ill children. *Indian J. Crit. Care Med.* 8, 173–181.

Ashburner, J., and Friston, K. J. (2000). Voxel-based morphometry–the methods. *Neuroimage* 11, 805–821. doi: 10.1006/nimg.2000.0582

Ball, K. K., Cruz, N. F., Mrak, R. E., and Dienel, G. A. (2010). Trafficking of glucose, lactate, and amyloid-beta from the inferior colliculus through perivascular routes. *J. Cereb. Blood Flow Metab.* 30, 162–176. doi: 10.1038/jcbfm.2009.206

Baquer, N. Z., Hothersall, J. S., and Mclean, P. (1988). Function and regulation of the pentose phosphate pathway in brain. *Curr. Top. Cell. Regul.* 29, 265–289. doi: 10.1016/B978-0-12-152829-4.50008-2

Baquer, N. Z., Hothersall, J. S., Mclean, P., and Greenbaum, A. L. (1977). Aspects of carbohydrate metabolism in developing brain. *Dev. Med. Child Neurol.* 19, 81–104. doi: 10.1111/j.1469-8749.1977.tb08027.x

Bauernfeind, A. L., and Babbitt, C. C. (2014). The appropriation of glucose through primate neurodevelopment. *J. Hum. Evol.* 77, 132–140. doi: 10.1016/j.jhevol.2014.05.016

Bauernfeind, A. L., Barks, S. K., Duka, T., Grossman, L. I., Hof, P. R., and Sherwood, C. C. (2014). Aerobic glycolysis in the primate brain: reconsidering the implications for growth and maintenance. *Brain Struct. Funct.* 219, 1149–1167. doi: 10.1007/s00429-013-0662-z

Bednarik, P., Tkac, I., Giove, F., Dinuzzo, M., Deelchand, D. K., Emir, U. E., et al. (2015). Neurochemical and BOLD responses during neuronal activation measured in the human visual cortex at 7 Tesla. *J. Cereb. Blood Flow Metab.* 35, 601–610. doi: 10.1038/jcbfm.2014.233

Behar, K. L., Rothman, D. L., Spencer, D. D., and Petroff, O. A. (1994). Analysis of macromolecule resonances in 1H NMR spectra of human brain. *Magn. Reson. Med.* 32, 294–302. doi: 10.1002/mrm.19103 20304

Boretius, S., Tammer, R., Michaelis, T., Brockmoller, J., and Frahm, J. (2013). Halogenated volatile anesthetics alter brain metabolism as revealed by proton magnetic resonance spectroscopy of mice *in vivo*. *Neuroimage* 69, 244–255. doi: 10.1016/j.neuroimage.2012.12.020

Boumezbeur, F., Petersen, K. F., Cline, G. W., Mason, G. F., Behar, K. L., Shulman, G. I., et al. (2010). The contribution of blood lactate to brain energy metabolism in humans measured by dynamic 13C nuclear magnetic resonance spectroscopy. *J. Neurosci.* 30, 13983–13991. doi: 10.1523/JNEUROSCI.2040-10.2010

Brooks, G. A. (1986). The lactate shuttle during exercise and recovery. *Med. Sci. Sports Exerc.* 18, 360–368. doi: 10.1249/00005768-198606000-00019

Brooks, G. A. (2000). Intra- and extra-cellular lactate shuttles. *Med. Sci. Sports Exerc.* 32, 790–799. doi: 10.1097/00005768-200004000-00011

Brooks, G. A. (2018). The science and translation of lactate shuttle theory. *Cell Metab.* 27, 757–785. doi: 10.1016/j.cmet.2018.03.008

Cady, E. B., Penrice, J., Amess, P. N., Lorek, A., Wylezinska, M., Aldridge, R. F., et al. (1996). Lactate, N-acetylaspartate, choline and creatine concentrations, and spin-spin relaxation in thalamic and occipito-parietal regions of developing human brain. *Magn. Reson. Med.* 36, 878–886. doi: 10.1002/mrm.1910360610

Cheeseman, A. J., and Clark, J. B. (1988). Influence of the malate-aspartate shuttle on oxidative metabolism in synaptosomes. *J. Neurochem.* 50, 1559–1565. doi: 10.1111/j.1471-4159.1988.tb03044.x

Chowdhury, G. M., Patel, A. B., Mason, G. F., Rothman, D. L., and Behar, K. L. (2007). Glutamatergic and GABAergic neurotransmitter cycling and energy metabolism in rat cerebral cortex during postnatal development. *J. Cereb. Blood Flow Metab.* 27, 1895–1907. doi: 10.1038/sj.jcbfm.9600490

Chugani, H. T., Phelps, M. E., and Mazziotta, J. C. (1987). Positron emission tomography study of human brain functional development. *Ann. Neurol.* 22, 487–497. doi: 10.1002/ana.410220408

Cremer, J. E., Cunningham, V. J., Pardridge, W. M., Braun, L. D., and Oldendorf, W. H. (1979). Kinetics of blood-brain barrier transport of pyruvate, lactate and glucose in suckling, weanling and adult rats. *J. Neurochem.* 33, 439–445. doi: 10.1111/j.1471-4159.1979.tb05173.x

Cruz, N. F., and Dienel, G. A. (2002). High glycogen levels in brains of rats with minimal environmental stimuli: implications for metabolic contributions of working astrocytes. *J. Cereb. Blood Flow Metab.* 22, 1476–1489. doi: 10.1097/01.WCB.0000034362.37277.C0

de Graaf, R. A., Pan, J. W., Telang, F., Lee, J. H., Brown, P., Novotny, E. J., et al. (2001). Differentiation of glucose transport in human brain gray and white matter. *J. Cereb. Blood Flow Metab.* 21, 483–492. doi: 10.1097/00004647-200105000-00002

Dienel, G. A., and Cruz, N. F. (2016). Aerobic glycolysis during brain activation: adrenergic regulation and influence of norepinephrine on astrocytic metabolism. *J. Neurochem.* 138, 14–52. doi: 10.1111/jnc.13630

Dienel, G. A., Cruz, N. F., Mori, K., Holden, J. E., and Sokoloff, L. (1991). Direct measurement of the lambda of the lumped constant of the deoxyglucose method in rat brain: determination of lambda and lumped constant from tissue glucose concentration or equilibrium brain/plasma distribution ratio for methylglucose. *J. Cereb. Blood Flow Metab.* 11, 25–34. doi: 10.1038/jcbfm.1991.3

Fitzpatrick, S. M., Cooper, A. J., and Duffy, T. E. (1983). Use of beta-methylene-D,L-aspartate to assess the role of aspartate aminotransferase in cerebral oxidative metabolism. *J. Neurochem.* 41, 1370–1383. doi: 10.1111/j.1471-4159.1983.tb00835.x

Gerhart, D. Z., Enerson, B. E., Zhdankina, O. Y., Leino, R. L., and Drewes, L. R. (1997). Expression of monocarboxylate transporter MCT1 by brain endothelium and glia in adult and suckling rats. *Am. J. Physiol.* 273, E207–E213. doi: 10.1152/ajpendo.1997.273.1.E207

Giedd, J. N., Blumenthal, J., Jeffries, N. O., Castellanos, F. X., Liu, H., Zijdenbos, A., et al. (1999). Brain development during childhood and adolescence: a longitudinal MRI study. *Nat. Neurosci.* 2, 861–863. doi: 10.1038/13158

Gjedde, A., and Marrett, S. (2001). Glycolysis in neurons, not astrocytes, delays oxidative metabolism of human visual cortex during sustained checkerboard stimulation *in vivo*. *J. Cereb. Blood Flow Metab.* 21, 1384–1392. doi: 10.1097/00004647-200112000-00002

Glatz, P., Sandin, R. H., Pedersen, N. L., Bonamy, A. K., Eriksson, L. I., and Granath, F. (2017). Association of anesthesia and surgery during childhood with long-term academic performance. *JAMA Pediatr.* 171:e163470. doi: 10.1001/jamapediatrics.2016.3470

Goyal, M. S., Hawrylycz, M., Miller, J. A., Snyder, A. Z., and Raichle, M. E. (2014). Aerobic glycolysis in the human brain is associated with development and neotenous gene expression. *Cell Metab.* 19, 49–57. doi: 10.1016/j.cmet.2013.11.020

Graham, M. M., Muzi, M., Spence, A. M., O'sullivan, F., Lewellen, T. K., Link, J. M., et al. (2002). The FDG lumped constant in normal human brain. *J. Nucl. Med.* 43, 1157–1166.

Gruetter, R., Novotny, E. J., Boulware, S. D., Rothman, D. L., Mason, G. F., Shulman, G. I., et al. (1992). Direct measurement of brain glucose concentrations in humans by 13C NMR spectroscopy. *Proc. Natl. Acad. Sci. U.S.A.* 89, 1109–1112. doi: 10.1073/pnas.89.3.1109

Gruetter, R., Ugurbil, K., and Seaquist, E. R. (1998). Steady-state cerebral glucose concentrations and transport in the human brain. *J. Neurochem.* 70, 397–408. doi: 10.1046/j.1471-4159.1998.70010397.x

Hawkins, R. A., Williamson, D. H., and Krebs, H. A. (1971). Ketone-body utilization by adult and suckling rat brain *in vivo*. *Biochem. J.* 122, 13–18. doi: 10.1042/bj1220013

Hazlett, H. C., Poe, M., Gerig, G., Smith, R. G., Provenzale, J., Ross, A., et al. (2005). Magnetic resonance imaging and head circumference study of brain size in autism: birth through age 2 years. *Arch. Gen. Psychiatry* 62, 1366–1376. doi: 10.1001/archpsyc.62.12.1366

Hertz, L., Swanson, R. A., Newman, G. C., Marrif, H., Juurlink, B. H., and Peng, L. (1998). Can experimental conditions explain the discrepancy over glutamate stimulation of aerobic glycolysis?. *Dev. Neurosci.* 20, 339–347.

Huang, S. C., Phelps, M. E., Hoffman, E. J., Sideris, K., Selin, C. J., and Kuhl, D. E. (1980). Noninvasive determination of local cerebral metabolic rate of glucose in man. *Am. J. Physiol.* 238, E69–E82. doi: 10.1152/ajpendo.1980.238.1.E69

Huttenlocher, P. R. (1990). Morphometric study of human cerebral cortex development. *Neuropsychologia* 28, 517–527. doi: 10.1016/0028-3932(90)90031-I

Hyder, F., Herman, P., Bailey, C. J., Moller, A., Globinsky, R., Fulbright, R. K., et al. (2016). Uniform distributions of glucose oxidation and oxygen extraction in gray matter of normal human brain: no evidence of regional differences of aerobic glycolysis. *J. Cereb. Blood Flow Metab.* 36, 903–916. doi: 10.1177/0271678X15625349

Jacob, Z., Li, H., Makaryus, R., Zhang, S., Reinsel, R., Lee, H., et al. (2012). Metabolomic profiling of children's brains undergoing general anesthesia with sevoflurane and propofol. *Anesthesiology* 117, 1062–1071. doi: 10.1097/ALN.0b013e31826be417

Johnson, M. K., and Whittaker, V. P. (1963). Lactate dehydrogenase as a cytoplasmic marker in brain. *Biochem. J.* 88, 404–409. doi: 10.1042/bj0880404

Kadota, T., Horinouchi, T., and Kuroda, C. (2001). Development and aging of the cerebrum: assessment with proton MR spectroscopy. *Am. J. Neuroradiol.* 22, 128–135.

Kato, M., Malamut, B. L., Caveness, W. F., Hosokawa, S., Wakisaka, S., and O'neill, R. R. (1980). Local cerebral glucose utilization in newborn and pubescent monkeys during focal motor seizures. *Ann. Neurol.* 7, 204–212. doi: 10.1002/ana.410070303

Kauppinen, R. A., Sihra, T. S., and Nicholls, D. G. (1987). Aminooxyacetic acid inhibits the malate-aspartate shuttle in isolated nerve terminals and prevents the mitochondria from utilizing glycolytic substrates. *Biochim. Biophys. Acta* 930, 173–178. doi: 10.1016/0167-4889(87)90029-2

Kennedy, C., Sakurada, O., Shinohara, M., Jehle, J., and Sokoloff, L. (1978). Local cerebral glucose utilization in the normal conscious macaque monkey. *Ann. Neurol.* 4, 293–301. doi: 10.1002/ana.410040402

Kennedy, C., Sakurada, O., Shinohara, M., and Miyaoka, M. (1982). Local cerebral glucose utilization in the newborn macaque monkey. *Ann. Neurol.* 12, 333–340. doi: 10.1002/ana.410120404

Kennedy, C., and Sokoloff, L. (1957). An adaptation of the nitrous oxide method to the study of the cerebral circulation in children; normal values for cerebral blood flow and cerebral metabolic rate in childhood. *J. Clin. Invest.* 36, 1130–1137. doi: 10.1172/JCI103509

Kraus, H., Schlenker, S., and Schwedesky, D. (1974). Developmental changes of cerebral ketone body utilization in human infants. *Hoppe Seylers Z. Physiol. Chem.* 355, 164–170. doi: 10.1515/bchm2.1974.355.1.164

Kuwabara, H., Evans, A. C., and Gjedde, A. (1990). Michaelis-Menten constraints improved cerebral glucose metabolism and regional lumped constant measurements with [18F]fluorodeoxyglucose. *J. Cereb. Blood Flow Metab.* 10, 180–189. doi: 10.1038/jcbfm.1990.33

Lai, J. C., and Clark, J. B. (1976). Preparation and properties of mitochondria derived from synaptosomes. *Biochem. J.* 154, 423–432. doi: 10.1042/bj1540423

Lai, J. C., Walsh, J. M., Dennis, S. C., and Clark, J. B. (1977). Synaptic and non-synaptic mitochondria from rat brain: isolation and characterization. *J. Neurochem.* 28, 625–631. doi: 10.1111/j.1471-4159.1977.tb10434.x

Lee, H., Caparelli, E., Li, H., Mandal, A., Smith, S. D., Zhang, S., et al. (2013). Computerized MRS voxel registration and partial volume effects in single voxel 1H-MRS. *Magn. Reson. Imaging* 31, 1197–1205. doi: 10.1016/j.mri.2013.04.001

Lenroot, R. K., and Giedd, J. N. (2006). Brain development in children and adolescents: insights from anatomical magnetic resonance imaging. *Neurosci. Biobehav. Rev.* 30, 718–729. doi: 10.1016/j.neubiorev.2006.06.001

Leppert, I. R., Almli, C. R., Mckinstry, R. C., Mulkern, R. V., Pierpaoli, C., Rivkin, M. J., et al. (2009). T(2) relaxometry of normal pediatric brain development. *J. Magn. Reson. Imaging* 29, 258–267. doi: 10.1002/jmri.21646

Llorente-Folch, I., Rueda, C. B., Perez-Liebana, I., Satrustegui, J., and Pardo, B. (2016). L-Lactate-mediated neuroprotection against glutamate-induced excitotoxicity requires ARALAR/AGC1. *J. Neurosci.* 36, 4443–4456. doi: 10.1523/JNEUROSCI.3691-15.2016

Lying-Tunell, U., Lindblad, B. S., Malmlund, H. O., and Persson, B. (1980). Cerebral blood flow and metabolic rate of oxygen, glucose, lactate, pyruvate, ketone bodies and amino acids. *Acta Neurol. Scand.* 62, 265–275. doi: 10.1111/j.1600-0404.1980.tb03035.x

Madsen, P. L., Hasselbalch, S. G., Hagemann, L. P., Olsen, K. S., Bulow, J., Holm, S., et al. (1995). Persistent resetting of the cerebral oxygen/glucose uptake ratio by brain activation: evidence obtained with the Kety-Schmidt technique. *J. Cereb. Blood Flow Metab.* 15, 485–491. doi: 10.1038/jcbfm.1995.60

Mckenna, M. C., Tildon, J. T., Stevenson, J. H., Boatright, R., and Huang, S. (1993). Regulation of energy metabolism in synaptic terminals and cultured rat brain astrocytes: differences revealed using aminooxyacetate. *Dev. Neurosci.* 15, 320–329. doi: 10.1159/000111351

Mehta, S., Kalsi, H. K., Nain, C. K., and Menkes, J. H. (1977). Energy metabolism of brain in human protein-calorie malnutrition. *Pediatr. Res.* 11, 290–293. doi: 10.1203/00006450-197704000-00006

Miller, D. J., Duka, T., Stimpson, C. D., Schapiro, S. J., Baze, W. B., Mcarthur, M. J., et al. (2012). Prolonged myelination in human neocortical evolution. *Proc. Natl. Acad. Sci. U.S.A.* 109, 16480–16485. doi: 10.1073/pnas.1117943109

Mintun, M. A., Raichle, M. E., Martin, W. R., and Herscovitch, P. (1984). Brain oxygen utilization measured with O-15 radiotracers and positron emission tomography. *J. Nucl. Med.* 25, 177–187.

Nehlig, A., De Vasconcelos, A. P., and Boyet, S. (1988). Quantitative autoradiographic measurement of local cerebral glucose utilization in freely moving rats during postnatal development. *J. Neurosci.* 8, 2321–2333. doi: 10.1523/JNEUROSCI.08-07-02321.1988

Ohta, S., Meyer, E., Thompson, C. J., and Gjedde, A. (1992). Oxygen consumption of the living human brain measured after a single inhalation of positron emitting oxygen. *J. Cereb. Blood Flow Metab.* 12, 179–192. doi: 10.1038/jcbfm.1992.28

Oz, G., Kumar, A., Rao, J. P., Kodl, C. T., Chow, L., Eberly, L. E., et al. (2009). Human brain glycogen metabolism during and after hypoglycemia. *Diabetes* 58, 1978–1985. doi: 10.2337/db09-0226

Passarella, S., Paventi, G., and Pizzuto, R. (2014). The mitochondrial L-lactate dehydrogenase affair. *Front. Neurosci.* 8:407. doi: 10.3389/fnins.2014.00407

Pavlidou, E., Hagel, C., and Panteliadis, C. (2013). Febrile seizures: recent developments and unanswered questions. *Childs. Nerv. Syst.* 29, 2011–2017. doi: 10.1007/s00381-013-2224-3

Persson, B., Settergren, G., and Dahlquist, G. (1972). Cerebral arterio-venous difference of acetoacetate and D- β -hydroxybutyrate in children. *Acta Paediatr. Scand.* 61, 273–278. doi: 10.1111/j.1651-2227.1972.tb16098.x

Phelps, M. E., Huang, S. C., Hoffman, E. J., Selin, C., Sokoloff, L., and Kuhl, D. E. (1979). Tomographic measurement of local cerebral glucose metabolic rate in humans with (F-18)2-fluoro-2-deoxy-D-glucose: validation of method. *Ann. Neurol.* 6, 371–388. doi: 10.1002/ana.410060502

Prichard, J., Rothman, D., Novotny, E., Petroff, O., Kuwabara, T., Avison, M., et al. (1991). Lactate rise detected by 1H NMR in human visual cortex during physiologic stimulation. *Proc. Natl. Acad. Sci. U.S.A.* 88, 5829–5831. doi: 10.1073/pnas.88.13.5829

Provencher, S. W. (2001). Automatic quantitation of localized *in vivo* 1H spectra with LCModel. *NMR Biomed.* 14, 260–264. doi: 10.1002/nbm.698

Quistorff, B., Secher, N. H., and Van Lieshout, J. J. (2008). Lactate fuels the human brain during exercise. *FASEB J.* 22, 3443–3449. doi: 10.1096/fj.08-106104

Raichle, M. E., Grubb, R. L. Jr., Gado, M. H., Eichling, J. O., and Ter-Pogossian, M. M. (1976). Correlation between regional cerebral blood flow and oxidative metabolism. *In vivo* studies in man. *Arch. Neurol.* 33, 523–526. doi: 10.1001/archneur.1976.00500080001001

Reivich, M., Alavi, A., Wolf, A., Fowler, J., Russell, J., Arnett, C., et al. (1985). Glucose metabolic rate kinetic model parameter determination in humans: the lumped constants and rate constants for [18F]fluorodeoxyglucose and [11C]deoxyglucose. *J. Cereb. Blood Flow Metab.* 5, 179–192. doi: 10.1038/jcbfm.1985.24

Rodriguez-Rodriguez, P., Fernandez, E., and Bolanos, J. P. (2013). Underestimation of the pentose-phosphate pathway in intact primary neurons as revealed by metabolic flux analysis. *J. Cereb. Blood Flow Metab.* 33, 1843–1845. doi: 10.1038/jcbfm.2013.168

Rogatzki, M. J., Ferguson, B. S., Goodwin, M. L., and Gladden, L. B. (2015). Lactate is always the end product of glycolysis. *Front. Neurosci.* 9:22. doi: 10.3389/fnins.2015.00022

Rothman, D. L., De Feyter, H. M., De Graaf, R. A., Mason, G. F., and Behar, K. L. (2011). 13C MRS studies of neuroenergetics and neurotransmitter cycling in humans. *NMR Biomed.* 24, 943–957. doi: 10.1002/nbm.1772

Rowland, L. M., Pradhan, S., Korenic, S., Wijtenburg, S. A., Hong, L. E., Edden, R. A., et al. (2016). Elevated brain lactate in schizophrenia: a 7 T magnetic resonance spectroscopy study. *Transl. Psychiatry* 6:e967. doi: 10.1038/tp.2016.239

Rust, R. S. (1994). Energy metabolism of developing brain. *Curr. Opin. Neurol.* 7, 160–165. doi: 10.1097/00019052-199404000-00013

Sacco, R., Gabriele, S., and Persico, A. M. (2015). Head circumference and brain size in autism spectrum disorder: a systematic review and meta-analysis. *Psychiatry Res.* 234, 239–251. doi: 10.1016/j.pscychresns.2015.08.016

Schuier, F., Orzi, F., Suda, S., Lucignani, G., Kennedy, C., and Sokoloff, L. (1990). Influence of plasma glucose concentration on lumped constant of the deoxyglucose method: effects of hyperglycemia in the rat. *J. Cereb. Blood Flow Metab.* 10, 765–773. doi: 10.1038/jcbfm.1990.134

Schurr, A. (2006). Lactate: the ultimate cerebral oxidative energy substrate?. *J. Cereb. Blood Flow Metab.* 26, 142–152. doi: 10.1038/sj.jcbfm.9600174

Semple, B. D., Blomgren, K., Gimlin, K., Ferriero, D. M., and Noble-Haeusslein, L. J. (2013). Brain development in rodents and humans: identifying benchmarks of maturation and vulnerability to injury across species. *Prog. Neurobiol.* 106–107, 1–16. doi: 10.1016/j.pneurobio.2013.04.001

Settergren, G., Lindblad, B. S., and Persson, B. (1976). Cerebral blood flow and exchange of oxygen, glucose, ketone bodies, lactate, pyruvate and amino acids in infants. *Acta Paediatr. Scand.* 65, 343–353. doi: 10.1111/j.1651-2227.1976.tb04896.x

Settergren, G., Lindblad, B. S., and Persson, B. (1980). Cerebral blood flow and exchange of oxygen, glucose ketone bodies, lactate, pyruvate and amino acids in anesthetized children. *Acta Paediatr. Scand.* 69, 457–465. doi: 10.1111/j.1651-2227.1980.tb07114.x

Settergren, G., Persson, B., and Dahlquist, G. (1973). The effect of moderate hypocapnia on the cerebral arterio-venous difference of acetoacetate, D- -hydroxybutyrate and oxygen in children. *Acta Paediatr. Scand.* 62, 141–145. doi: 10.1111/j.1651-2227.1973.tb08081.x

Shestov, A. A., Emir, U. E., Kumar, A., Henry, P. G., Seaquist, E. R., and Oz, G. (2011). Simultaneous measurement of glucose transport and utilization in the human brain. *Am. J. Physiol. Endocrinol. Metab.* 301, E1040–E1049. doi: 10.1152/ajpendo.00110.2011

Shulman, R. G., Hyder, F., and Rothman, D. L. (2001). Lactate efflux and the neuroenergetic basis of brain function. *NMR Biomed.* 14, 389–396. doi: 10.1002/nbm.741

Simpson, I. A., Carruthers, A., and Vannucci, S. J. (2007). Supply and demand in cerebral energy metabolism: the role of nutrient transporters. *J. Cereb. Blood Flow Metab.* 27, 1766–1791. doi: 10.1038/sj.jcbfm.9600521

Suda, S., Shinohara, M., Miyaoka, M., Lucignani, G., Kennedy, C., and Sokoloff, L. (1990). The lumped constant of the deoxyglucose method in hypoglycemia: effects of moderate hypoglycemia on local cerebral glucose utilization in the rat. *J. Cereb. Blood Flow Metab.* 10, 499–509. doi: 10.1038/jcbfm.1990.92

Swanson, R. A., Morton, M. M., Sagar, S. M., and Sharp, F. R. (1992). Sensory stimulation induces local cerebral glycogenolysis: demonstration by autoradiography. *Neuroscience* 51, 451–461. doi: 10.1016/0306-4522(92)90329-Z

Tamir, H., Kaufman, H., and Rapport, M. M. (1972). Subcellular distribution of pyruvate kinase (EC 2.7.1.40) in cerebral cortex. *J. Neurochem.* 19, 1759–1768. doi: 10.1111/j.1471-4159.1972.tb06220.x

Tomiyasu, M., Aida, N., Shibasaki, J., Tachibana, Y., Endo, M., Nozawa, K., et al. (2016). Normal lactate concentration range in the neonatal brain. *Magn. Reson. Imaging* 34, 1269–1273. doi: 10.1016/j.mri.2016.07.006

Vaishnavi, S. N., Vlassenko, A. G., Rundle, M. M., Snyder, A. Z., Mintun, M. A., and Raichle, M. E. (2010). Regional aerobic glycolysis in the human brain. *Proc. Natl. Acad. Sci. U.S.A.* 107, 17757–17762. doi: 10.1073/pnas.1010459107

van Hall, G., Stromstad, M., Rasmussen, P., Jans, O., Zaar, M., Gam, C., et al. (2009). Blood lactate is an important energy source for the human brain. *J. Cereb. Blood Flow Metab.* 29, 1121–1129. doi: 10.1038/jcbfm.2009.35

Vander Heiden, M. G., Cantley, L. C., and Thompson, C. B. (2009). Understanding the Warburg effect: the metabolic requirements of cell proliferation. *Science* 324, 1029–1033. doi: 10.1126/science.1160809

Watanabe, H., and Passonneau, J. V. (1973). Factors affecting the turnover of cerebral glycogen and limit dextrin *in vivo*. *J. Neurochem.* 20, 1543–1554. doi: 10.1111/j.1471-4159.1973.tb00272.x

Wienhard, K. (2002). Measurement of glucose consumption using [(18)F]fluorodeoxyglucose. *Methods* 27, 218–225. doi: 10.1016/S1046-2023(02)00077-4

Wu, H. M., Bergsneider, M., Glenn, T. C., Yeh, E., Hovda, D. A., Phelps, M. E., et al. (2003). Measurement of the global lumped constant for 2-deoxy-2-[18F]fluoro-D-glucose in normal human brain using [15O]water and 2-deoxy-2-[18F]fluoro-D-glucose positron emission tomography imaging. A method with validation based on multiple methodologies. *Mol. Imaging Biol.* 5, 32–41. doi: 10.1016/S1536-1632(02)00122-1

Yoshida, H., Kushikata, T., Kubota, T., Hirota, K., Ishihara, H., and Matsuki, A. (2001). Xenon inhalation increases norepinephrine release from the anterior and posterior hypothalamus in rats. *Can. J. Anaesth.* 48, 651–655. doi: 10.1007/BF03016198

Yoshida, H., Kushikata, T., Tose, R., Kudo, M., Kudo, T., and Hirota, K. (2010). Nitrous oxide and xenon increase noradrenaline release in the cerebral cortex *in vivo* and *in vitro*. *Neurosci. Lett.* 469, 199–203. doi: 10.1016/j.neulet.2009.11.074

17

Manganese-Enhanced Magnetic Resonance Imaging: Overview and Central Nervous System Applications With a Focus on Neurodegeneration

Ryan A. Cloyd[1,2,3], *Shon A. Koren*[1,3,4] *and Jose F. Abisambra*[1,3,4,5]*

[1]Department of Physiology, University of Kentucky, Lexington, KY, United States, [2]College of Medicine, University of Kentucky, Lexington, KY, United States, [3]Sanders-Brown Center on Aging, University of Kentucky, Lexington, KY, United States, [4]Department of Neuroscience & Center for Translational Research in Neurodegenerative Disease, University of Florida, Gainesville, FL, United States, [5]Spinal Cord and Brain Injury Research Center, University of Kentucky, Lexington, KY, United States

***Correspondence:**
Jose F. Abisambra
joe.abisambra@uky.edu;
j.abisambra@ufl.edu

Manganese-enhanced magnetic resonance imaging (MEMRI) rose to prominence in the 1990s as a sensitive approach to high contrast imaging. Following the discovery of manganese conductance through calcium-permeable channels, MEMRI applications expanded to include functional imaging in the central nervous system (CNS) and other body systems. MEMRI has since been employed in the investigation of physiology in many animal models and in humans. Here, we review historical perspectives that follow the evolution of applied MRI research into MEMRI with particular focus on its potential toxicity. Furthermore, we discuss the more current *in vivo* investigative uses of MEMRI in CNS investigations and the brief but decorated clinical usage of chelated manganese compound mangafodipir in humans.

Keywords: manganese, MEMRI, MRI, mangafodipir, CNS imaging

INTRODUCTION

The use of manganese and similar paramagnetic contrast agents began shortly after the development of magnetic resonance imaging (MRI). Manganese (II) chloride is the most commonly utilized manganese species for manganese-enhanced MRI (MEMRI). Though MEMRI has been widely employed in imaging studies of various investigative directions, the primary focus of this review will be the role of functional MEMRI in the nervous system beginning with a brief historical introduction.

History

Some of the earliest work into MRI was performed by Paul Lauterbur in 1973 (Lauterbur, 1973). This work contributed to the basis of nuclear magnetic resonance (NMR) and MRI studies as they exist today and resulted in Lauterbur receiving the 2003 Nobel Prize in Physiology and Medicine with Peter Mansfield. Lauterbur et al. (1980) showed that manganese enhanced magnetic images by shortening proton relaxation time, and soon manganese contrast grew into a common imaging staple in living systems. Early uses of manganese contrast were aimed at delineating normal and abnormal tissue. For example, early studies used manganese MRI to study ischemic myocardium in dogs (Brady et al., 1982; Goldman et al., 1982), cerebral edema in cats (Shirakuni et al., 1985) and human tumor xenografts in mice (Ogan et al., 1987). The discovery of paramagnetic enhancement in MRI also lead to research into other paramagnetic contrast agents including gadolinium (Couet et al., 1984; Runge et al., 1984; Fornasiero et al., 1987).

Lin and Koretsky (1997) first demonstrated manganese contrast can be used as a noninvasive, direct measurement of neuronal function. Lin and Koretsky (1997) administered manganese chloride via a peripheral intravenous injection and reported imaging enhancement in stimulated brain regions not affected by changes in blood flow, strongly supporting MEMRI as a direct functional imaging measure. The major advantage of Lin and Koretsky's (1997) novel application of manganese enhancement was the ability to measure neuronal function *in vivo*. However, this initial application of MEMRI was limited by the need to co-administer mannitol to disrupt the blood-brain barrier. Subsequent studies have refined MEMRI to visualize neuronal activity. A recent study demonstrated that with a sufficiently strong magnetic field (17.1T), MEMRI can be used to visualize action potentials in individual Aplysia buccal neurons (Svehla et al., 2018). Following the discovery that radioactive manganese transports along neural tracts in a microtubule-dependent fashion (Sloot and Gramsbergen, 1994), Koretsky's group used manganese as a non-radioactive neuronal connection tracer (Pautler et al., 1998). Manganese-enhanced tract tracing has since been used in conjunction with techniques such as diffusion tensor imaging (DTI) to study brain region connectivity and validate tractography studies (Lin et al., 2001; Knosche et al., 2015).

Today, MEMRI is used in three major types of MRI protocols: anatomic studies, functional studies and tractography studies. In the case of anatomic studies, manganese functions much like gadolinium or other paramagnetic contrast agents, and such studies will not be a major focus of this review. In contrast, unique properties of manganese compared to other paramagnetic agents (which will be discussed in more detail in section "Pharmacodynamics" of this review) allow MEMRI to provide information about the function and connectivity of brain regions. Specific instances of these studies will be discussed in regard to specific fields of study in section "MEMRI in CNS imaging" of this review. The ability to perform anatomical, functional and connectivity studies with a single technique has allowed MEMRI to be used to describe dynamic systems *in vivo*. A series of studies from the Van der Linden group used several different types of manganese enhanced MRI protocols to describe the song generation and control in songbirds (Van der Linden et al., 2002; Tindemans et al., 2003, 2006; Van Meir et al., 2004). This demonstrates how all three major types of MEMRI applications can be used to study a single topic. Van der Linden et al. (2004) group developed a technique to allow long term study of a single anatomical region (repeated dynamic MEMRI) through the use of a permanent cannula.

These types of studies can be performed via other types of MRI experiments such as blood-oxygen level dependent (BOLD) contrast or DTI/diffusion kurtosis imaging (DKI). While these types of studies are more widely used, they are less direct measurements of activity/connectivity in the brain than MEMRI. MEMRI should not be seen as a replacement for other types of MRI studies but rather as another tool to provide a more complete understanding of *in vivo* brain function. One study that compared functional measurements obtained via BOLD imaging and MEMRI found that the techniques produce consistent results, demonstrating the potential for them to be used in conjunction (Duong et al., 2000).

MRI Background

A basic understanding of the principles underlying manganese and other paramagnetic contrast agents aids in understanding their enhancement of magnetic images. MRI depends on the spin, charge and magnetism of specific atomic nuclei, particularly ^{1}H but also ^{31}P, ^{23}Na, ^{19}F and ^{13}C (Jackson et al., 2005). Application of an external magnetic field reorients these species' axes of spin approximately with the axis of the field. Each species has a unique frequency of rotation around the magnetic field, termed precession (**Figure 1**). Since precession is linearly proportional to the strength of the magnetic field, stronger applied magnetic fields produce greater precession, resulting in higher signal-to-noise ratios (SNR). For this reason, the strength of the magnetic field defines the resolution of MR imaging.

Under the main magnetic field force (B_0) and a secondary set of field gradients, each nucleus rotates so it reorients itself with the field, adopting either an aligned or anti-aligned state (Jackson et al., 2005). Most nuclei reside in the lower energy aligned state with a smaller proportion populating the high energy anti-aligned state. The difference in these populations is the basis of NMR. These aligned and anti-aligned systems absorb electromagnetic energy from a third magnetic force

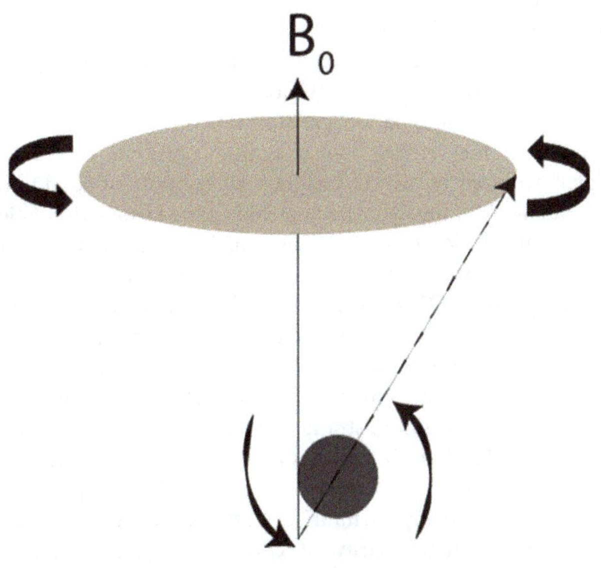

FIGURE 1 | Visual demonstration of precession. Redrawn from **Figure 2** of Jackson et al. (2005). The nucleus's axis of rotation (dotted line) does not exactly align with the magnetic field B_0 (solid line). As the nucleus rotates around the B_0, it also spins on its own axis. The frequency with which the nucleus rotates around B_0, termed the precession, is inherent to each species and scales linearly with the strength of the magnetic field.

(the radiofrequency (RF) pulse), which briefly equalizes the two nuclear alignment states. As the applied perturbation resolves, the energy emitted is detected by a receiver coil and interpreted to generate the MRI. The gradient fields and RF pulse can be altered to suit the needs of the current experiment. A single scan protocol includes repeated RF pulses in rapid succession.

A major variable measured in MR experiments is relaxation time, defined as the time required to reestablish equilibrium between alignment states. Relaxation time is divided into the spin-lattice (T_1) relaxation time and the spin-spin (T_2) relaxation time. T_1 represents the time required for the axis of the nucleus to realign with the main field in the z-direction. A sample with a longer T_1 time requires a slower rate of RF pulses to allow for recovery between pulses. T_2 is based on changes in the rates of rotation that occur following termination of the RF pulse. When nuclei are aligned in the same plane, they initially rotate in phase with each other. After the pulse is removed, the nuclei begin rotating at different rates and the amount of time required for the nuclei to lose phase is the T_2 relaxation time (Jackson et al., 2005). A single scan protocol measures either T1 or T2. In either case, the signal intensity of the final image is determined by the relaxation time. Both relaxation times are determined by a number of intrinsic and environmental factors, and of particular note, the T_1 is influenced by the presence of paramagnetic species as discovered by Paul Lauterbur's group in 1980. Paramagnetic agents cause the nuclei to realign more rapidly resulting in shortening of the T_1 time, which increases the signal intensity on MR images (Mendonça-Dias et al., 1983).

MEMRI vs. BOLD

Currently, the most common method used for function MR imaging is BOLD. BOLD uses paramagnetic deoxygenated hemoglobin as a natural contrast agent to measure changes in cerebral blood oxygenation (Ogawa et al., 1990). Oxygenated hemoglobin is non-paramagnetic; therefore, under normoxic conditions, the arterial flow does not contribute to the MR signal acquired by BOLD imaging. Under normal conditions, essentially all of the deoxyhemoglobin in the venous circulation is generated by local tissue metabolism. As a result, BOLD signal provides a measure of total metabolism of brain regions.

While both BOLD and MEMRI allow functional MRI, each technique has strengths and weaknesses that must be considered when designing experiments. One major advantage of BOLD over other types of contrast-enhanced MRI protocols is that it does not require administration of exogenous contrast agents (Ogawa et al., 1990). It provides a rapid assessment of regional and global brain metabolism without exposing the patient or animal to potentially harmful contrast agents. Given concerns over the potential toxicity of chronic manganese exposure (discussed more in section "Toxicity"), BOLD may be preferable for long-term studies requiring repeated exposure to manganese.

The BOLD signal is an aggregate of the metabolism of all the cells in the region and therefore the relative contributions of neurons cannot be distinguished from that of glia or other cells. Furthermore, BOLD implementation is complicated during conditions of generalized hypoxia in the area of interest because of the presence of paramagnetic deoxyhemoglobin in the arterial blood supply (Michaely et al., 2012; Taylor et al., 2015; Wang et al., 2017). Similarly, disruptions in regional hemodynamics caused by tumors or arteriovenous malformations can produce artifacts on BOLD (Zaca et al., 2014). In contrast, manganese enhancement is much more specific for neuronal activity and the signal is less susceptible to contributions from non-neuron cells (discussed in section "Mechanism of Entry and Dispersion of Manganese"). Whereas BOLD indirectly measures brain activity through changes in metabolism, MEMRI directly measures activity through changes in calcium dynamics.

PHARMACODYNAMICS

As with any contrast agent, manganese is influenced and limited by how the body alters it (pharmacokinetics) and how it alters the body (pharmacodynamics). The pharmacokinetic properties of manganese were recently reviewed elsewhere (Chen et al., 2018). To understand the toxic limitations of manganese, potential administration routes into the body, and downstream applications, it is critical to first understand the biological mechanism of action and transport of manganese.

Mechanism of Entry and Dispersion of Manganese

Out of all paramagnetic contrast agents used as MRI contrasts, manganese has unique application capabilities based on its ability to form a divalent cation with an ionic radius similar to that of calcium. The ability of manganese ions to impede calcium transportation has been recognized since the 1960s (Hubbard et al., 1968), although the precise mechanism (now known to be due to competition for transport) would not be recognized until later. Understanding of the biological mechanisms of manganese developed in conjunction with advances in its uses for imaging purposes, beginning in the early 1980s when its accumulation (Hunter et al., 1980), permeability (Ribalet and Beigelman, 1980) and calcium channel competition (in cardiac tissue; Payet et al., 1980), in nerve terminals (Kita et al., 1981) was discovered. The passage of manganese ions through calcium channels was further supported by the prevention of Mn^{2+}-induced changes in nerve terminal activity caused by administration of the calcium channel blockers verapamil (Narita et al., 1990) and later diltiazem, which was found to suppress MEMRI changes following forepaw stimulation in rats (Lu et al., 2007). These studies by Narita et al. (1990) and Lu et al. (2007) as well as others (Carlson et al., 1994) support the hypothesis that the primary entry point for manganese into neurons is through L-type calcium channels; though other studies from as early as 1987 (Mayer and Westbrook, 1987) show evidence manganese may also transverse through other channel types such as NMDA and AMPA receptors.

For example, Itoh et al. (2008) studied the effects of NMDA modulation on MEMRI signal and found drug-induced activation of NMDA receptors increased signal intensity while non-competitive antagonism of the receptors reduced signal intensity, suggesting NMDA receptors play a role in facilitating manganese transport. They found no changes associated with AMPA modulation. A later study by Hankir et al. (2012) further supported the hypothesis that manganese can pass through NMDA receptors, with contrasting evidence suggesting that AMPA receptors mediate manganese enhancement in certain brain structures. However, the two studies used substantially different dosages of AMPA receptor antagonist NBQX (Hankir et al., 2012 used a dose of approximately 40 mg/kg compared to the 10 mg/kg dose used by Itoh et al., 2008), possibly accounting for differences between the two studies. Given this difference, it seems plausible that AMPA receptors do contribute to the transport of manganese through the blood brain barrier, but the role is smaller than that of the NMDARs. Recent work has supported the role of NMDARs in controlling blood brain barrier permeability (Vazana et al., 2016), however the reliance on NMDA of manganese penetrance into the brain was not studied. Though the exact mechanism of calcium channel entry of manganese into the brain is not understood, it is this capacity that facilitates the usage of manganese as a more direct functional imaging method in MEMRI.

Recently, the Turnbull group showed that manganese uptake is also mediated by the divalent metal transporter, DMT1 (Bartelle et al., 2013). By inducing DMT1 expression, Bartelle et al. (2013) achieved MEMRI signal in cell populations (human embryonic kidney, glioma and melanoma) that would not normally be susceptible to manganese enhancement. After this finding, Turnbull's group induced expression of the bacterial manganese-binding protein MntR in mammalian cells to increase signal enhancement (Bartelle et al., 2015). Expression of MntR, which can be targeted to the Golgi apparatus, endoplasmic reticulum, or cytosol, increases intracellular manganese concentration by preventing efflux of manganese from cells. This paradigm allows for any tissue type to potentially be specifically enhanced via MEMRI. For example, transplanted cells expressing DMT1 can be effectively tracked via MEMRI (Lewis et al., 2015). Future development of the DMT1 MRI reporter system will likely lead to more widespread use. While the role of DMT1 presents potential new avenues for MEMRI, it also adds additional variables to the system that must be studied further to clearly understand the extent to which MEMRI measures calcium dynamics from L-type calcium channels separate from other types of ion channels and transporters.

Nearly 30 years following the discovery that manganese impedes calcium dynamics, evidence of intracellular manganese trafficking in vesicles by a microtubule-dependent mechanism was reported in a series of studies (Sloot and Gramsbergen, 1994; Pautler et al., 1998; Takeda et al., 1998). Functionally, this mechanism allows the usage of MEMRI for neuronal tract tracing, a crucial investigative method when considering the methods of manganese administration (discussed later in this section). By nature of being packaged into vesicles similar to neurotransmitters, manganese transports trans-synaptically following fusion of its carrier vesicle with the axon terminal membrane (Serrano et al., 2008). Synaptic manganese is then taken up by the post-synaptic neuron as discussed previously through any of a number of potential calcium-permeable channels or receptors and is then repackaged for further transport propagation. For these mechanistic similarities of manganese and calcium, manganese provides valuable tools for imaging applications but may be limited by substantial toxicity.

Toxicity

Along with other organ system toxicity, excessive manganese exposure is particularly neurotoxic. These neurotoxic effects include dystonia, impaired speech and poor cognition, and they have been shown to be a particular threat to the developing central nervous system (CNS) throughout childhood (Zoni and Lucchini, 2013; Bjørklund et al., 2017; Lao et al., 2017). Adults are less susceptible to manganese toxicity than children[1], although neurotoxic (Olanow, 2004; Bowler et al., 2016; Schuh, 2016) and carcinogenic/teratogenic (Gerber et al., 2002) effects have been documented following moderate chronic exposure in adults. Manganism, the classic picture of chronic manganese toxicity in humans, is characterized by motor deficits that closely resemble Parkinson's disease (PD) in the early stages (Andruska and Racette, 2015). Animal studies have supported the adverse effect findings of chronic manganese exposure. Further neurotoxic potential of manganese is extensively reviewed elsewhere (Chen et al., 2015).

Systemic Administration of Manganese

For imaging studies, manganese solutions are most commonly administered via injections. Koretsky's early experiments used 25% D-mannitol to break the blood-brain barrier and increase penetration of manganese into the brain (Lin and Koretsky, 1997). Later studies by Koretsky and others determined that MEMRI can be performed in animals with an intact blood-brain barrier, although generally more time and a larger dose of manganese is required to achieve similar enhancement, as demonstrated in **Figure 2** (Watanabe et al., 2002; Aoki et al., 2004; Lee et al., 2005; Yu et al., 2005; Kuo et al., 2006). These initial experiments advanced the usage of manganese as a systemically-injected contrast agent for widespread use in imaging.

In the context of MEMRI, the toxicity threshold of manganese remains contested. Since MEMRI studies typically involve a single exposure of moderate to high doses of manganese, these differ from previously described reports on chronic or repeated exposures (Takács et al., 2012; Okada et al., 2016). A study by Eschenko et al. (2010a) looked for signs of toxicity following a single low (0.1 mmol/kg, 16 mg/kg) or high (0.5 mmol/kg, 80 mg/kg) dosage subcutaneous injection of manganese chloride. While the group found no histopathologic differences at either dose, moderate synaptic and motor behavior deficits were observed in rats at the higher dose. Another study by the same group found the synaptic and motor deficits persisted through 1 week following exposure (Eschenko et al., 2010b). These and other studies

[1] Agency for Toxic Substances and Disease Registry, *Manganese*, https://www.atsdr.cdc.gov/toxprofiles/tp151-c2.pdf

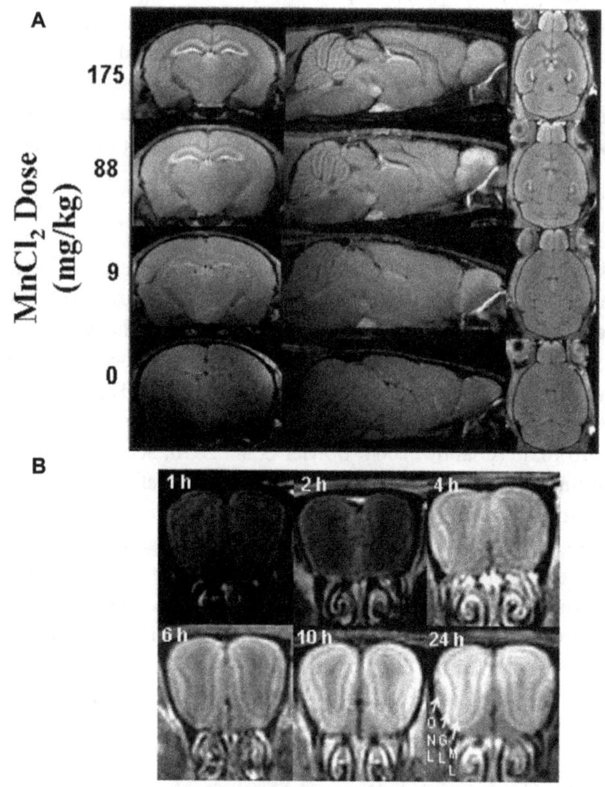

FIGURE 2 | Signal intensity depends on dose and time. Adapted with permission from Lee et al. (2005). Scans performed in mice with intact blood-brain barrier showing the dependence of signal enhancement on **(A)** dose and **(B)** time. **(A)** Manganese produces global enhancement that scales with dose. Enhancement is most significant in the hippocampus, interpeduncular nucleus, pituitary, and olfactory bulb. **(B)** Enhancement of signal increases over time as demonstrated in the olfactory bulb (ONL, olfactory nerve layer; GL, glomerular layer; ML, mitral cell layer).

(Liu et al., 2004; Alaverdashvili et al., 2017) use ranges at or lower than doses typically used for MEMRI, raising concern over potential toxicity and confounding effects of MEMRI.

Other studies found little to no neurotoxicity in mice after single intraperitoneal (IP) doses of manganese chloride at 66 mg/kg (Fontaine et al., 2017), or short-term repeated IP injection in rats reaching final doses of 60 mg/kg (Galosi et al., 2017). To date, many studies have investigated alternative administration paradigms (see next section), alternative manganese-containing compounds (discussed in section "Mangafodipir") and co-administration of additional compounds (Alahmari et al., 2015; Johnson et al., 2018) to mitigate any potential toxic effects of manganese in MEMRI and still retain useful imaging enhancement.

Fractionated and continuous infusion doses of manganese have been investigated as systemic administration routes that limit toxic effects and exposure for imaging studies. Many studies have noted sufficient manganese enhancement of imaging from fractionated doses, often with no to mild and reversible side effects identified (Bock et al., 2008b; Grünecker et al., 2010; Galosi et al., 2017). One study by Bock et al. (2008a) found fractionated doses of manganese in a non-human primate model has increased longevity of manganese in the brain, notably in the visual cortex and basal ganglia, compared to the rat brain following a similar administration. The authors suggest this species difference may be similar across all mammals, suggesting fractionated dosages may be a viable method in humans using similar manganese-based agents. Similarly, continuous IP infusion of manganese was also found to reduce toxicity relative to a single dose while retaining imaging enhancement (Eschenko et al., 2010a).

Sepúlveda et al. (2012) reported pumps implanted subcutaneously achieve comparable results to fractionated dosing, which allows less invasive implementation of continuous manganese delivery. A more recent study by Vousden et al. (2018) has shown that continuous infusion of manganese via subcutaneous pumps achieves image enhancement without affecting spatial learning or memory. However, this study reported severe and dose-dependent skin ulcerations at the site of implantation in most of the manganese treated mice, whereas control IP injected and saline treated mice did not develop such adverse effects. The authors suggest ulceration may develop due to manganese-induced itching, but this does not sufficiently explain why ulceration has not occurred in more studies investigating subcutaneous manganese pumps. Poole et al. (2017) compared the two methods and found that continuous infusion produced less toxic effects than fractionated injections. However, as this study was published prior to the Vousden et al. (2018) study, it does not consider skin ulcerations. To date, no study has systematically compared fractionated or continuous injection administration of manganese which considers all currently known adverse effects.

The contention on the toxicity threshold and systemic injection method of manganese highlights the importance in considering previous studies along with the chosen animal model, administration route and dose in determining experimental parameters of manganese for MRI studies. A review from Koretsky's group demonstrates the variability in dosing and routes of administration used in the first years of modern MEMRI research as summarized in **Figure 3** (Silva et al., 2004). If possible, piloting toxicity studies on a per-study basis may provide the only truly sufficient data on toxicity until further investigations reveal consistent thresholds.

Localized Administration and Applications

As a viable alternative to systemic routes of manganese administration, a variety of non-systemic administration methods are also successfully used to limit any potential toxic effects. Perhaps the most common non-injection route for manganese exposure is through oral administration. Early studies of oral administration showed sufficient bioavailability of manganese for imaging studies in livers of rats following manganese chloride feeding (Cory et al., 1987). Digested manganese is circulated through and filtered out by the hepatic portal system (i.e., the first past effect), severely reducing systemic distribution of manganese and limiting potential toxicity (Hauser et al., 1994). More recently, oral administration

A **Toxicity data (LD_{50}) for $MnCl_2$**

Species	Route	Dose	Remarks
Rat	Oral	250 mg/kg	
	Intraperitoneal	147 mg/kg	Behavioral: somnolence (general depressed activity) Behavioral: convulsions or effect on seizure threshold
	Intravenous	92.6 mg/kg	Behavioral: somnolence (general depressed activity) Behavioral: convulsions or effect on seizure threshold
	Intramuscular	700 mg/kg	
Mouse	Oral	1031 mg/kg	Behavioral: tremor Behavioral: convulsions or effect on seizure threshold Lungs, thorax or respiration: other changes
	Intraperitoneal	121 mg/kg	
	Intravenous	38 mg/kg	Behavioral: somnolence (general depressed activity) Behavioral: ataxia Lungs, thorax or respiration: respiratory stimulation
	Intramuscular	255 mg/kg	
Dog	Intravenous	202 mg/kg	
Guinea pig	Oral	916 mg/kg	Behavioral: tremor Behavioral: convulsions or effect on seizure threshold Lungs, thorax or respiration: other changes

Source: MSDS for $MnCl_2$ (product number 244589, Sigma-Adrich, St Louis, MO, USA).

B **Systemic doses of $MnCl_2$ used in current MEMRI experiments**

Species	Route	Dose	Reference
Rat	Intravenous	54 mg/kg	Lin and Koretsky 1997
	Intravenous	60 mg/kg	Duong *et al.* 2000
	Intra-arterial	53 mg/kg	Aoki *et al.* 2002
	Intravenous	175 mg/kg	Aoki *et al.* 2004
Mouse	Nasal	65 mg/kg	Pautler *et al.* 1998
	Intravenous	175 mg/kg	Lee *et al.* 2004
	Intravenous	6.6 mg/kg	Hu *et al.* 2001
	Intraperitoneal	20 mg/kg	Watanabe *et al.* 2002

FIGURE 3 | Toxicity data and common doses used in early manganese-enhanced magnetic resonance imaging (MEMRI) experiments. Adapted with permission from Silva et al. (2004). **(A)** Summary of toxic manganese doses and associated effects as reported on the MSDS. **(B)** Manganese doses used in several early MEMRI studies in rats and mice. With some exceptions, the dose of manganese used in imaging studies is much lower than the accepted toxic level.

of manganese chloride has been used as an effective and well-tolerated agent for hepatic and hepatobiliary imaging (Leander et al., 2010; Albiin et al., 2012; Marugami et al., 2013). Although manganese removal from the blood is highly efficient, its sensitivity as a contrast agent still facilitates imaging studies in non-privileged body compartments following oral administration (Jacobs et al., 2012). To date, no studies recorded successful MEMRI of CNS structures after oral manganese administration, although manganese reportedly accumulates to levels sufficient to enhance T1 weighted images in patients with cholestatic disease (Ikeda et al., 2000). Given the importance of manganese penetration into the CNS for proper imaging described by Lee et al. (2005), it is still unknown whether oral administration of manganese produces sufficient, safe exposure for clinical MEMRI studies.

One potential method for CNS MEMRI is intranasal administration, which was first reported to deliver manganese to the brains of pike (Tjälve et al., 1995) and rats (Tjälve et al., 1996) sufficient for enhanced imaging. More commonly used today for olfactory imaging studies (Cross et al., 2006; Lehallier et al., 2012b), nasal instillation of manganese reportedly also sufficiently enhances visual cortex imaging in rats (Fa et al., 2010). Though nasal instillation of manganese bypasses the need for systemic administration and may reduce the risk of toxicity, an unintended byproduct is significant nonspecific enhancement (Pautler et al., 1998; Cross et al., 2004). However, later reports suggest this nonspecific enhancement may be reduced with experimental tradeoffs (Chuang and Koretsky, 2009). Additionally, olfactory impairment may occur at doses higher than typically required for imaging (Lehallier et al., 2012a) and moderate inflammation was reported following nasal instillation of manganese solutions (Foster et al., 2018), highlighting potential limitations for its use in CNS MEMRI.

As in the olfactory system, the visual system lends itself to relatively non-invasive methods of manganese administration. Intravitreal injections enhance the retina and visual pathways without the need for systemic administration of manganese. Although intravitreal injection of manganese may result in loss of retinal ganglion cell density at relatively low doses (Thuen et al., 2008), smaller doses provide good enhancement without major signs of damage to retina or other ocular structures (Lindsey et al., 2013).

Topical application of manganese has been investigated as an alternative to intravitreal injection. Topically applied manganese resulted in strong enhancement of ocular structures and the superior colliculus without diffusing into the vitreous space (Sun et al., 2011). The authors posit that the manganese may absorb into the iris and enter the capillary circulation to reach the retina. This hypothesis is supported by the fact that the enhancement was attenuated when retinal ischemia was induced by increasing the intraocular pressure. No adverse changes were observed in the mice 1 week after topical administration of manganese. Similarly, in Sun et al. (2012) the authors administered topical manganese biweekly or monthly in groups of mice. While they found significant retinal ganglion loss and corneal thickening in the biweekly treatment paradigm, no adverse effects were observed when manganese was applied monthly. This was further supported by a later study (Liang et al., 2015) and suggests long-term MEMRI is possible with topical administration of manganese.

Other methods of administration of manganese by bypassing the blood brain barrier into the CNS have been investigated, stemming from early experiments of injections directly into cerebrospinal fluid (CSF). The earliest application of direct CSF injections involved stereotaxic injection of manganese chloride into the lateral ventricles of rats (Wan et al., 1991). Later, a similar experiment by Liu et al. (2004) achieved measurable enhancement of brain parenchyma 24–96 h following injection of manganese chloride into the cisterna magna (**Figure 4**). Liu et al. (2004) injected mice with the analogous paramagnetic contrast agent GdDTPA and found no parenchymal enhancement suggesting that the described effect was dependent on cellular uptake of manganese (described in section "Mechanism of Entry and Dispersion of Manganese"). Remarkably, transcranial injection of manganese chloride showed detectable manganese signal in the brain parenchyma within 2 h of administration (Roth et al.,

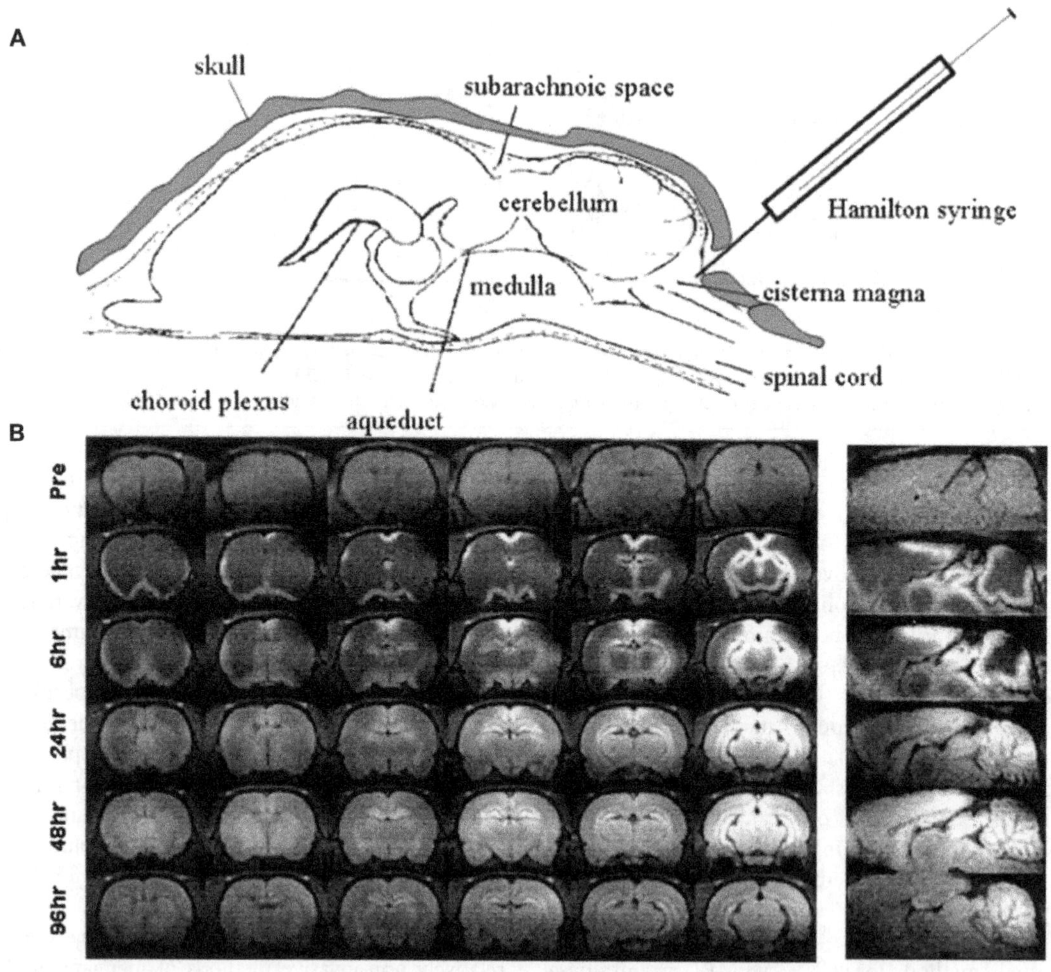

FIGURE 4 | Intrathecal injection of manganese chloride. Adapted with permission from Liu et al. (2004). **(A)** Injection scheme for intrathecal manganese injection. **(B)** Serial images show the spread of enhancement from the ventricles throughout the cortex, subcortex, and cerebellum.

2014). More recently, the Koretsky group expanded upon this technique by showing that manganese penetrates into underlying brain structures when applied transcranially by passing through brain suture lines (Atanasijevic et al., 2017). While transcranial application of manganese for MEMRI requires further optimization before widespread use, its potential in relatively noninvasive MEMRI studies are becoming extremely valuable.

Effect of Blood Brain Barrier Permeability

Poor blood-brain barrier permeability has been a major obstacle in MEMRI studies of the CNS. Several MEMRI protocols call for chemical (Lin and Koretsky, 1997; Lu et al., 2010) or mechanical (Howles et al., 2012) disruption of the blood-brain barrier to improve penetration of manganese into the CNS. The integrity of the blood-brain barrier has a significant effect on the penetrance of manganese into the CNS, and because of this several studies have used manganese to evaluate changes in blood-brain barrier permeability (Fitsanakis et al., 2006; Grillon et al., 2008; Nischwitz et al., 2008). It may be advisable to evaluate animals for blood-brain barrier damage to eliminate potential confounding variables that could arise from differential penetrance of manganese into the CNS as this could result in apparent differences in MEMRI signal. Furthermore, animals with possible blood-brain barrier dysfunction should be monitored more closely for signs of manganese-related injury as they are more likely to reach toxic accumulation of manganese in the brain.

MEMRI IN CNS IMAGING

One major application of MEMRI is functional imaging of the CNS. The technique has been applied to a variety of CNS pathologies including traumatic brain injury, epilepsy, neurodegeneration and pain. Additionally, MEMRI has been used heavily in studies of the olfactory and visual systems. These areas of study are by no means mutually exclusive, and recurrent patterns will emerge between areas of MEMRI implementation that may suggest future avenues for investigation.

Traumatic Brain Injury

Traumatic brain injury (TBI) is a serious threat to health, contributing to 30% of all injury related deaths in the United States according to the CDC[2]. Glutamate increases sharply in animal models following acute TBI (Palmer et al., 1993), a finding that's been supported in human studies (Brown et al., 1998; Yamamoto et al., 1999; Ruppel et al., 2001). Excitotoxicity leads to activation of voltage-gated calcium channels, increasing intracellular calcium concentration (Young, 1992). High intracellular calcium concentrations play a significant role in cell injury and death (Trump and Berezesky, 1995). As discussed previously, manganese influx can occur concurrently with calcium influx, which allows MEMRI to monitor changes in calcium dynamics after TBI.

The first study to apply MEMRI to TBI measured changes after diffuse TBI in rats (Cernak et al., 2004). Subsequent studies found varying patterns of signal enhancement following TBI, which is potentially due to disturbances in the blood-brain barrier (Bouilleret et al., 2009; Rodriguez et al., 2016). Talley Watts et al. (2015) found that manganese-enhanced images showed crescent-shaped areas of hyperintensity at the impact site corresponding to areas of reactive gliosis, a finding that was further supported by positive GFAP staining. Comparisons between these studies are difficult due to inherent differences in the particular models of TBI employed, but despite these differences, MEMRI is effective to measure changes in brain function after injury. Of particular note, one study by Tang et al. (2011) used MEMRI to successfully track migration and function of human neural stem cells implanted in rats after TBI. They went on to show that this activity was attenuated by treatment with the calcium channel blocker diltiazem, which supports the findings of Lu et al. (2007) discussed previously.

Epilepsy

Epilepsy is a neurological condition characterized by recurrent seizures. It is estimated to affect 50 million people worldwide[3]. In humans, temporal lobe epilepsy (TLE) is the most common type of focal epilepsy (Asadi-Pooya et al., 2017). Status epilepticus (SE), defined as a seizure lasting more than 30 min, is a medical emergency that can result in significant morbidity and mortality (Cherian and Thomas, 2009). Currently, electroencephalogram (EEG) is the most commonly used modality for monitoring epilepsy, and MRI plays a crucial role during diagnosis (Rüber et al., 2018).

One of the most consistent features of TLE and SE in human and animal models is mossy fiber sprouting in the dentate gyrus of the hippocampus beginning in the first week following epileptogenesis and continuing to develop for months after (Mathern et al., 1995; Smith and Dudek, 2001; Scharfman et al., 2003; Shetty et al., 2003). Nairismägi et al. (2006) showed *in vivo* MEMRI evidence of mossy fiber sprouting following drug-induced SE in rats, which was later confirmed via histopathology. This finding has since been replicated in multiple models of TLE and SE (Immonen et al., 2008; Malheiros et al., 2012) and studies have used MEMRI to detect focal edema, neuronal death and astrocyte proliferation in the hippocampus of rats as a result of sustained seizure activity (Hsu et al., 2007; Malheiros et al., 2014). One study found a negative correlation between hippocampus signal intensity and seizure frequency, suggesting a role for MEMRI in preclinical assessment of epileptogenesis severity in future studies (Dedeurwaerdere et al., 2013).

Sudden unexplained death in epilepsy (SUDEP) is a major concern for people with epilepsy, and it accounts for approximately 15% of epilepsy related deaths (Tomson et al., 2016). As the name suggests, SUDEP is difficult to

[2]Centers for Disease Control and Prevention, TBI: Get the Stats on Traumatic Brain Injury in the United States, https://www.cdc.gov/traumaticbraininjury/get_the_facts.html [Accessed March 12, 2018].

[3]World Health Organization, *Epilepsy Fact Sheet*. http://www.who.int/news-room/fact-sheets/detail/epilepsy [Accessed March 12, 2018].

predict although seizure frequency is positively correlated to risk. Recently, MEMRI was used to show changes in an audiogenic seizure mouse model consistent with human SUDEP (Kommajosyula et al., 2017). This model develops tonic seizures leading to respiratory arrest that is fatal without resuscitation. MEMRI performed during seizure-induced respiratory arrest showed increased signal intensity in regions of the superior colliculus, periaqueductal gray and amygdala, brain regions previously implicated in SUDEP in humans (Mueller et al., 2014; Tang et al., 2014; Wandschneider et al., 2015). Future studies will be needed to better adapt MEMRI to the study of SUDEP, but continued efforts may provide better risk stratification and preventative measures.

Neurodegeneration

Neurodegenerative diseases are a debilitating class of conditions involving progressive brain atrophy and loss of cognitive and/or motor function. This class comprises tauopathies (including Alzheimer's disease (AD) and frontotemporal dementia), PD, Lewy body disease, amyotrophic lateral sclerosis (ALS) and Huntington's disease. Despite years of ongoing research, the prognosis for patients diagnosed with these conditions is generally poor. To date, studies have explored the role of MEMRI in context of tauopathies, PD and ALS. No studies are currently available describing the use of MEMRI to investigate Huntington's disease or Lewy body disease; however, given the relative youth of the field and the rapid expansion over the past two decades, future research may find utility of MEMRI in studying these conditions.

Alzheimer's Disease and Other Tauopathies

AD, the most common cause of dementia, is part of the class of related diseases termed tauopathies (Bertram and Tanzi, 2005). These diseases vary widely in geographic involvement and symptomatic presentation, but all share underlying tau pathology as a basis for neurodegeneration. Tau protein is classically involved with stabilizing microtubules and loss of tau function mediates axonal degeneration in many tauopathy cases (Kneynsberg et al., 2017). Confirmed diagnoses for tauopathies cannot be made until post-mortem examination confirms histopathology. This major obstacle in the diagnosis of tauopathies compounds with the problem that appropriate therapies for one type of tauopathy likely will not be effective for another (Coughlin and Irwin, 2017), establishing the importance of identifying the tauopathy as early as possible.

The first application of MEMRI for research into tauopathies quantified differences in axonal transport (Smith et al., 2007). In this study, it was shown that MEMRI could detect decreased rates of axonal transport in the Swedish mutant APP mouse, a model of AD characterized by secondary tau pathology. Many other studies have since used MEMRI to show impairments or therapy-related improvements in axonal transport in mouse models of AD or tauopathies (Massaad et al., 2010; Smith et al., 2010, 2011; Gallagher et al., 2012; Wang et al., 2012; Majid et al., 2015; Saar et al., 2015). MEMRI has also been used to demonstrate axonal deficits in the olfactory pathways of tau-transgenic JNPL3 (Bertrand et al., 2013) and rTg4510 (Majid et al., 2014) mouse models. Further supporting these findings, Fontaine et al. (2017) showed broad changes in neuronal function in preclinical rTg4510 mice following systemic administration of manganese. With detectable changes in the asymptomatic stage of the disease, these studies highlight the potential application of MEMRI in preclinical identification of tau pathology *in vivo*.

Parkinson's Disease

PD is the second most common neurodegenerative condition (Bertram and Tanzi, 2005) and involves the progressive loss of dopaminergic neurons in the substantia nigra leading to a characteristic pattern of impaired movement (Hughes et al., 1992). Neurological manifestations of PD include cognitive impairment, impulse control disorders and circadian rhythm dysfunction (Mantovani et al., 2018; Marques et al., 2018; Weil et al., 2018; Weintraub et al., 2018).

Initiation and control of movement relies on close communication between the basal ganglia and substantia nigra (Lanciego et al., 2012). Manganese deposits in the basal ganglia (Nelson et al., 1993; Fredstrom et al., 1995; Nagatomo et al., 1999), and this is the basis for motor deficits associated with manganese toxicity as previously discussed and may explain the relative paucity of studies employing MEMRI to investigate PD.

The earliest study to use MEMRI in the context of PD supported previous observations that interhemispheric cortical connectivity observed in humans and rats is mediated through the basal ganglia (Pelled et al., 2007). Direct injection of manganese chloride into the subthalamic nucleus in rat of the 6-hydroxydopmaine model of PD reveals impaired transport of manganese throughout the basal ganglia-substantia nigra circuit indicating impaired axonal transport (Soria et al., 2011). In addition to establishing connectivity between brain regions in PD, two recent studies highlighted the potential for MEMRI in monitoring response to novel therapeutics (Olson et al., 2016; Weng et al., 2016).

Amyotrophic Lateral Sclerosis

ALS is characterized by progressive degeneration of upper (cortical) and lower (spinal) motor neurons leading to generalized weakness (Peters and Brown, 2015). Patients gradually become weaker and succumb to respiratory failure. The current standard therapy for ALS is riluzole, which appears to slow progression of the disease, as well as physical and speech therapy and respiratory support[4]. While the exact etiology of ALS is currently unknown, deficits in axonal transport have been identified (Collard et al., 1995).

To date, only one study could be found which applied MEMRI to ALS (Jouroukhin et al., 2013). In this study, davunetide was shown to slow disease progression in a mouse model of ALS, thereby increasing the speed of axonal transport and protecting against neuronal loss. Davunetide functions

[4]National Institute of Neurological Disorders and Stroke, *Amyotrophic Lateral Sclerosis (ALS) Fact Sheet.* https://www.ninds.nih.gov/Disorders/Patient-Caregiver-Education/Fact-Sheets/Amyotrophic-Lateral-Sclerosis-ALS-Fact-Sheet [Accessed March 13, 2018].

by stabilizing microtubules, thereby preventing colchicine-mediated degradation (Jouroukhin et al., 2013; Magen and Gozes, 2013). Interestingly, davunetide was previously evaluated for therapeutic effects in the tauopathy progressive supranacular palsy, although it ultimately proved to be ineffective for this use. Given the common involvement of axonal deficits and the overlap between therapeutic approaches, one could expect more studies to employ MEMRI in the context of ALS in the future.

Pain

Chronic pain is a complex condition that causes significant loss of quality of life in approximately 7%–8% of adults worldwide[5]. Neuropathic pain, which arises from damage to the somatosensory system, takes many forms including central neuropathic pain, polyneuropathy, post-amputation pain and HIV-associated neuropathy. For many years, opioid analgesics have been the standard therapy for chronic pain. Given the current rates of opioid abuse facing the United States, there is a significant effort to develop alternate approaches to treat chronic pain (Downes et al., 2018; Morad et al., 2018). Furthermore, pain is known to adversely affect the mental health of affected patients (Goesling et al., 2018). One aspect of chronic pain that complicates development of a comprehensive therapeutic approach is that many of the pathways underlying the development and maintenance of pain are not well understood.

The earliest studies to use MEMRI in a pain-related setting examined the use of acupuncture for analgesia (Chiu et al., 2001). After showing changes in brain activity after acupuncture via MEMRI, Chiu et al. (2001) compared activation patterns between electroacupuncture at points associated with analgesic or non-analgesic properties (Chiu et al., 2003). While acupuncture at either site was associated with activity in the somatosensory cortex and hypothalamus, acupuncture at the analgesic site also increased activation in the periaqueductal gray and median raphe nucleus; these regions specifically involved in the processing of pain. This study was the first to demonstrate the use of MEMRI in identifying pain pathways.

Later, Yang et al. (2011) published the first report to use MEMRI to study pain specifically. After injecting manganese chloride into the thalamus, electrical current was applied to the forepaw of a rat to induce pain. Subsequent imaging showed the strong activation in the anterior cingulate and midcingulate cortex, areas that were previously well-established in pain processing. This study also identified the ventral medial caudate-putamen and nucleus accumbens as possible components of pain processing circuitry. Pain-induced activation in each of these areas was attenuated by pretreatment with morphine. Recently, Sperry et al. (2017) performed similar imaging in perfused brains, allowing much longer scan times to improve resolution.

Since Yang et al. (2011) first used MEMRI to map pain circuits, the technique has been used in several studies of pain. MEMRI has proved effective for studying irritant injection (Devonshire et al., 2017; Sperry et al., 2017), nerve injury (Behera et al., 2013; Jeong and Kang, 2018) and thermal (Lei et al., 2014) models of pain. Interestingly, in an investigation into the difference between processing of neuropathic pain and pathological itching using MEMRI, Jeong et al. (2016) found differences in processing for each stimulus in the limbic systems. However, further studies are needed to better describe this process.

Olfactory System

MEMRI studies have long been employed for use in studying the olfactory system, owing largely to the ease with which manganese can be applied via the nasal mucosa. The first study to demonstrate tract tracing via MEMRI were performed in the olfactory bulb after nasal instillation of manganese (Pautler et al., 1998). As previously described, tract tracing requires introduction of manganese solutions to specific regions of the CNS, typically via intracranial or intravitreal injection. The olfactory receptors in the nasal mucosa project directly to the olfactory bulb, allowing tract tracing in this region with a less invasive route of administration. Pautler and Koretsky (2002) later showed region specific activation in the mouse olfactory bulb in response to aerosolized urine odorants. Subsequent work used the rodent olfactory system to refine the process of tract tracing (Lehallier et al., 2011).

Since these early reports many additional reports have used MEMRI to map circuits in rodent olfactory systems. Chen et al. (2007) observed differences in activation patterns between unconditioned arousal (lemon) and fear (fox) odorant stimuli. Work from the Koretsky lab found specific activation patterns in the olfactory bulb corresponding to different odorants achieving resolution of individual glomerular cells (Chuang et al., 2009, 2010). Gutman et al. (2013) combined MEMRI with DTI and found the imaging modalities compatible and complementary for the purpose of tracing neural circuits.

MEMRI studies of the olfactory system have also been used in disease-specific context. Several studies showed deficits in axonal transport in the olfactory bulb of neurodegenerative mice, as previously described in the context of tauopathy (Smith et al., 2007, 2010, 2011; Wang et al., 2012; Bertrand et al., 2013; Majid et al., 2014; Saar et al., 2015) and ALS (Jouroukhin et al., 2013). MEMRI has similarly shown changes in olfactory function in animal models of cerebral palsy (Drobyshevsky et al., 2006, 2012), neuropsychiatric lupus (Kivity et al., 2010) and diabetes (Sharma et al., 2010). Gobbo et al. (2012) used MEMRI to study the effects of glutamate excitotoxicity in the olfactory bulb, modeling a possible mechanism of atrophy associated with diseases such as AD or stroke. These studies demonstrate the utility of MEMRI to detect neuronal changes in the olfactory bulb that may represent disease specific processes or broader changes in neuronal function.

Visual System

As discussed previously (section "Localized Administration and Applications"), the visual system lends itself to relatively noninvasive methods of manganese administration. Historically, MEMRI was first used to study the mapping of the visual

[5]International Association for the Study of Pain. Fact Sheets. https://www.iasp-pain.org/Advocacy/Content.aspx?ItemNumber=3934 [Accessed March 14, 2018].

pathway from retina to superior colliculus (Watanabe et al., 2001; **Figure 5**). With this study supporting the theoretical role of MEMRI in visual system further investigations have delved into the structure, function and tractographical details and diseases in a variety of animal models.

Mapping the Visual System

Following successful mapping of the visual system by Watanabe et al. (2001), studies used manganese to show finely-tuned changes in functional differences of the visual system. For example, Bissig and Berkowitz (2009) showed systemic manganese administration and visual stimulation revealed discrete layer-specific changes in function in the visual cortex of rats.

Subsequent research by Chan et al. (2011b, 2014) and Chan and Wu (2012) expanded these previous studies to assess neuroarchitecture and functional relationships in the rat visual system using a variety of manganese injection techniques. They first investigated visual system development and found faster axonal transport of manganese in the developing rats, attributed to higher permeability of the blood-ocular and blood-brain barriers in the immature rat (Chan et al., 2011a). With an increase in detectable projections from both the retina and visual cortex following enucleation, this study demonstrates the ability of MEMRI to not only map the visual system, but also to detect finer neuroplastic changes. Other studies have since demonstrated the ability of MEMRI to detect sensory system-wide neuroplastic changes (Tang et al., 2017a,b).

Chan et al. (2014) conducted additional experiments to more fully characterize the normally functioning rat visual system. They partially transected the optic nerve near the optic head to show retinotopic attenuation of signal in the superior colliculus. Later studies further expanded the connectivity work previously performed, using varied injection techniques (intravitreal, intracortical, subcortical) to provide more detailed descriptions of the connections between parts of the visual system (Chan and Wu, 2012).

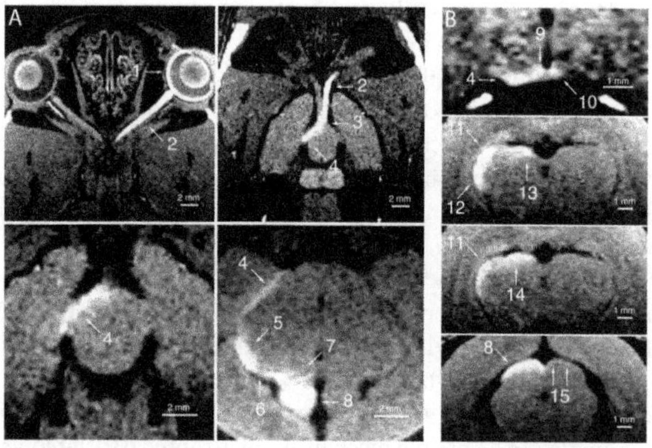

FIGURE 5 | Manganese enhanced tracing of the rat visual system. Adapted with permission from Watanabe et al. (2001). Enhancement of the visual pathway 24 h after intravitreal injection of manganese. Images were collected in the **(A)** horizontal and **(B)** coronal planes. 1 = left retina, 2 = left optic nerve, 3 = optic chiasm, 4 = right optic tract, 5 = right lateral geniculate nucleus, 6 = right brachium of the superior colliculus, 7 = right pretectal region, 8 = right superior colliculus, 9 = right suprachiasmatic nucleus, 10 = left suprachiasmatic nucleus, 11 = right dorsal geniculate nucleus, 12 = right ventral lateral geniculate nucleus, 13 = right olivary pretectal nucleus, 14 = right nucleus of the optic tract, 15 = superficial part of the superficial gray layer of the left superior colliculus.

Retinal Structure and Function

Another area of vision-related research that has benefitted greatly from application of MEMRI is the study of retinal function. The first application of MEMRI to the retina measured differences in ion demand between light- and dark-adapted rats (Berkowitz et al., 2006), an application which has since been replicated (De La Garza et al., 2012). Subsequent studies from Berkowitz and colleagues provided *in vivo* descriptions of ion regulation through the visual cycle (Berkowitz et al., 2009b), activity of channelrhodopsin-2 (Ivanova et al., 2010) and horizontal cell inhibitory signaling (Berkowitz et al., 2015b). These experiments established MEMRI as a sensitive technique capable of producing *in vivo* resolution of retinal layers to establish biochemical understandings.

Additional studies have demonstrated that MEMRI can be used to study degenerative pathology associated with the retina. Berkowitz and colleagues used MEMRI to show changes in retinal ion demand in models of ocular injury (Berkowitz et al., 2007a), retinopathy of prematurity (Berkowitz et al., 2007b) and retinal thinning (Berkowitz et al., 2008). Nair et al. (2011) showed layer resolution and lamina-specific structures in degenerating rat retina, which highlighted the potential for disease monitoring via MEMRI. This potential was further expanded when another group used MEMRI to show the effects of prophylactic retinylamine therapy in a mouse model of retinal degeneration (Schur et al., 2015).

Optic Nerve Injury and Regeneration

In addition to investigating the retina, MEMRI can be applied to study injury and regeneration of the optic nerve. The capacity for MEMRI studies to detect injury-related changes in optic nerve function has been well-established (Ryu et al., 2002; Thuen et al., 2005) and MEMRI can be used in conjunction with DTI to provide more detailed evaluation (Thuen et al., 2009). Work from Sandvig et al. (2011) used MEMRI to monitor optic nerve regeneration in four different animal models longitudinally. Shortly after, they showed evidence that transplanted olfactory ensheathing cells mediate repair and remyelination in damaged optic nerves (Sandvig et al., 2012). Additional studies have further demonstrated the use of MEMRI in assessing optic nerve injury and repair (Haenold et al., 2012; Fischer et al., 2014; Yang et al., 2016).

Diabetic Retinopathy

Diabetes is a chronic, systemic condition characterized by persistent high blood sugar associated with a variety of negative conditions including heart disease, stroke, kidney failure, peripheral neuropathy and impaired vision or blindness[6]. Ocular

[6]Centers for Disease Control and Preventions, *At a Glance 2016: Diabetes*. https://www.cdc.gov/diabetes/library/factsheets.html [Accessed March 15, 2018].

manifestations of diabetes, particularly diabetic retinopathy, are a leading cause of visual impairment and preventable blindness worldwide (Lee et al., 2015). Diabetic retinopathy can be detected reliably via fundoscopic examination; however, due to the asymptomatic early stages and limited ophthalmologic care in developing nations, many cases remain undiagnosed until permanent damage has occurred (Viswanath and McGavin, 2003).

MEMRI has been suggested as a viable method to study the processes associated with the development of diabetic retinopathy and to monitor therapeutic responses. For example, manganese-enhanced imaging shows *in vivo* ion dysregulation (Berkowitz et al., 2009a) and oxidative stress (Berkowitz et al., 2015a) in diabetic mice, providing potential mechanistic insight into the disease. Furthermore, MEMRI detects changes in retinal function 14 days after induction of hyperglycemia, earlier than any previous time point in literature (Muir et al., 2015). In addition to studying disease progression, MEMRI has been used to assess several potential therapeutic approaches for diabetic retinopathy (Berkowitz et al., 2007c, 2012; Giordano et al., 2015).

Glaucoma

Glaucoma is a group of related diseases that result in abnormally high intraocular pressure. Left untreated, the high pressure can damage the optic nerve, leading to permanent impairment or loss of vision[7]. Like diabetic retinopathy, glaucoma is a major cause of vision loss worldwide (Tham et al., 2014). The prevalence of glaucoma increases with age and the number of people affected by glaucoma is projected to double by 2040. Therefore, continued research is necessary to adapt to the increasing health challenges faced by an increasingly aged population.

Though limited in number, the studies employing MEMRI nevertheless demonstrate a role for MEMRI in assessing glaucoma pathology. Studies using MEMRI identified impaired axonal transport in glaucomatous eyes of rats compared to normal prior to the development of changes in retinal thickness (Chan et al., 2007, 2008; Calkins et al., 2008). Data collected via MEMRI suggest the development of glaucoma may be more complicated than previously thought (Fiedorowicz et al., 2018). Therefore, more research in this field will be required to better understand progression of the disease as well as the optimal methods to study it *in vivo*.

Auditory System

The first studies to use MEMRI in the study of the auditory system came from the Turnbull group. They generated the first tonotopic map of the inferior colliculus, showing functional changes associated with varying degrees of hearing loss (Yu et al., 2005). Subsequent studies applied MEMRI to describe development and plasticity of the auditory system (Yu et al., 2007) and to examine the effect of frequency and amplitude on auditory processing in the inferior colliculus (Yu et al., 2008). In these studies, manganese was administered to mice immediately before a sound exposure experiment. Because neuronal activity correlates with manganese uptake, this paradigm allows for brain responses to be encoded away from the noisy environment of the MRI scanner. Manganese in the stimulated brainstem regions persisted long enough to allow the activation pattern to be measured 24 h later.

MEMRI studies of the auditory system can be performed following intratympanic injection of manganese chloride. Analogous to the tracing of the visual pathways performed by Thuen et al. (2005), intratympanic administration of manganese produces sequential enhancement of the auditory system from cochlea to inferior colliculus (Lee et al., 2012). Subsequent work found that auditory pathway tracing is sensitive to changes in the frequency and amplitude of the sound stimulus (Jin et al., 2013) and this mapping technique had been applied to disease models (Jung et al., 2014).

In addition to mapping the auditory system, MEMRI has been used to study auditory disorders including hearing loss and tinnitus. Using MEMRI, Gröschel et al. (2011) identified changes in calcium-dependent activity in the central auditory system associated with noise-induced, age-related (Gröschel et al., 2014) and drug-induced hearing loss (Gröschel et al., 2016), thereby providing novel insights into these conditions and suggesting that multiple mechanisms may produce similar symptoms across different modalities of hearing loss. MEMRI studies have also demonstrated abnormal neuronal function in animal models of tinnitus. Brozoski et al. (2007) measured hyperactivity in brain regions including the cochlear nucleus, inferior colliculus, cerebellar paraflocculus and amygdala. This study was the first to identify abnormal cerebellar function associated with tinnitus. A follow-up study attributed the tinnitus-related hyperactivity to abnormal NMDA activity, demonstrating the NMDA blockade improves symptoms (Brozoski et al., 2013). These studies from Brozoski et al. (2007, 2013) described a previously unidentified interaction between the paraflocculus and cochlear nucleus as a necessary component of noise-induced tinnitus. Subsequent work has expanded these findings to include drug induced models of tinnitus and implicated additional brain regions in the pathology (Holt et al., 2010; Muca et al., 2018). Consistent with previous work, these studies strongly implicate brain stem structures (particularly the inferior colliculus) in the development of tinnitus and found no tinnitus-related changes in function in the auditory cortex.

MANGAFODIPIR

Chelated manganese compounds such as mangafodipir (MnDPDP, Teslascan) provide an alternative to potentially toxic manganese chloride solutions for use in clinical applications of MEMRI. Mangafodipir is prepared by chelating ionic manganese with the organic ligand fodipir (Rocklage et al., 1989) producing a complex metabolized in humans to release manganese ions for enhancement in MR imaging studies (Toft et al., 1997a,b). Mangafodipir was first used to show ischemia associated with myocardial infarctions (Pomeroy et al., 1989; Saeed et al., 1989), but its primary usage has been as a contrast for hepatobiliary imaging (Rofsky and Weinreb, 1992). Its use expanded considerably since FDA approval in 1997.

[7]National Eye Institute, *Facts About Glaucoma*. https://nei.nih.gov/health/glaucoma/glaucoma_facts [Accessed March 16, 2018].

Animal Studies With Mangafodipir

Quickly following its original intended use, mangafodipir substantially enhanced hepatobiliary imaging without significant toxicity. Studies in rats evaluating its toxicity for MEMRI reported toxicity at high doses but with a high therapeutic index (Elizondo et al., 1991). A later study showed that mangafodipir was not associated with injection site or dermal hypersensitivity reactions (Larsen and Grant, 1997), which is in contrast to later studies of manganese injections. The potential negative ionotropic effects of manganese in the heart were balanced by a release of catecholamines triggered by MnDPDP *in vivo* (Jynge et al., 1997). Furthermore, unlike manganese chloride, mangafodipir does not cause higher levels of manganese accumulation in the brain in animals with biliary obstruction compared to control (Grant et al., 1997b). It should be noted, however, that mangafodipir induced skeletal abnormalities in fetal rats, suggesting teratogenicity (Grant et al., 1997a).

For the purposes of imaging, the major differences observed between MEMRI studies with manganese chloride and mangafodipir is the time to maximal enhancement. The slow release of manganese during mangafodipir metabolism compared to solutions of manganese chloride produces a more gradual rise in manganese concentration (Ni et al., 1997) with no loss of enhancement (Southon et al., 2016). A later study of retinal function after systemic mangafodipir administration and MEMRI detected changes in retinal function consistent with previous studies done with manganese chloride (Tofts et al., 2010).

Human Studies With Mangafodipir

The use of mangafodipir in human MRI studies began shortly following successful animal imaging studies and focused on tumor and lesion identification in the hepatobiliary system. The first use of mangafodipir MEMRI in human subjects demonstrated enhancement of the liver parenchyma within 15 min of intravenous injection without major adverse effects (Lim et al., 1991). The most commonly reported effect of mangafodipir injection is facial flushing and warmth and minor adverse events including nausea, headache, elevated blood pressure and accelerated heart rate (Lim et al., 1991; Wang et al., 1997b).

Several stage II clinical trials and other studies have shown mangafodipir-enhanced MRI to be effective for identifying tumors and metastases in the human hepatobiliary system (Bernardino et al., 1991, 1992; Rummeny et al., 1991, 1997; Hamm et al., 1992; Wang et al., 1997a). The sensitivity of mangafodipir enhanced MRI is highest for tumors or hepatocellular origin (Aicher et al., 1993; Rofsky et al., 1993; Vogl et al., 1993).

Following these successful studies, several stage III clinical trials compared mangafodipir enhanced MRI with human-approved contrast agents and found that it improved identification of hepatocellular carcinoma (Kettritz et al., 1996) and detection of focal lesions (Diehl et al., 1999) over gadolinium based contrasts, but no difference was found in the ability to detect liver metastases or other masses (Kettritz et al., 1996; Schima et al., 1997).

Other studies have compared mangafodipir-enhanced MRI with other methods of clinical imaging modalities such as computed tomography (CT). Several have reported greater efficacy of mangafodipir enhanced MRI to contrast enhanced CT imaging for detection of hepatocellular lesions (Bartolozzi et al., 2000; Federle et al., 2000; Oudkerk et al., 2002). Mangafodipir-enhanced MRI has additionally shown similar accuracy for diagnosis and staging of pancreatic cancer compared to contrast enhanced CT, but neither modality demonstrated a clear advantage (Rieber et al., 2000; Romijn et al., 2000).

Non-imaging Uses of Mangafodipir

Despite these promising clinical trials, mangafodipir was removed from the European market in 2012[8] due to poor sales and is similarly listed as discontinued by the FDA[9]. We found limited evidence of non-marketing related reasons behind these regulatory decisions. However, research using mangafodipir has been ongoing. Two metabolites of mangafodipir, MnPLED and ZnPLED, have exhibit antioxidant properties through actions mimicking superoxide dismutase (SOD) in rats (Brurok et al., 1999). When donor rats were pretreated with MnDPDP before liver transplant, the recipient experienced reduced ischemic injury after transplantation (Ben Mosbah et al., 2012). Later studies in humans reported mangafodipir administration reduces cardiac injury associated with chemotherapy (Yri et al., 2009) and post-myocardial infarction reperfusion (Karlsson et al., 2015).

Recently, the efficacy of mangafodipir as an adjunct to chemotherapy has been established. In culture, co-administration of mangafodipir with the anti-cancer drugs oxaliplatin or 5-fluorouracil resulted in increased killing of mouse colon cancer cells and improved survival of human leukocytes *ex vivo* (Alexandre et al., 2006). The mechanisms of this differential targeting are unclear, but the authors speculate that the increased oxidative stress at baseline in the cancer cells compared to normal is a contributing factor. A preliminary trial in human subjects similarly preserved leukocyte counts during treatment with oxaliplatin and 5-fluorouracil (Karlsson et al., 2012a). Calmangafodipir, a derivative complex of mangafodipir in which some of the manganese is replaced by calcium, exhibits a greater degree of myelo-preservation while still enhancing antitumor effects (Karlsson et al., 2012b). Two additional studies show that mangafodipir reduces the occurrence of oxaliplatin-induced peripheral neuropathy in human patients (Coriat et al., 2014; Karlsson et al., 2017) and is an active area of interest. Future studies are needed to better characterize how mangafodipir and related compounds interact with anti-cancer therapies, but current research shows promise.

[8]European Medicines Agency, *Public statement on Mangafodipir*, EMA/486286/2012 (London, UK, 2012)

[9]U.S. Food and Drug Administration, FDA approved drug products: Teslascan. https://www.accessdata.fda.gov/scripts/cder/daf/index.cfm?event=overview.process&ApplNo=020652. [Accessed March 22, 2018].

CONCLUSION

Manganese provides useful enhancement of MR images by nature of its paramagnetic properties. Augmented by having cell permeability like that of calcium, manganese application for MRI provides unique functional imaging capacities. Over the last 40 years, research using applied MEMRI has delved into the structure, function and tractography in a wide variety of investigative areas. In the CNS, the functional component of MEMRI provides unique insight into the cellular mechanisms of brain disorders and neurodegenerative diseases like AD. Concerns over the toxicity and administrative methods of manganese *in vivo* have spurred the use of manganese-chelated compounds such as mangafodipir for MEMRI clinically, though no recorded studies have reported uses in human CNS imaging. Current applications show renewed promise of manganese- and chelated MEMRI usage for research questions.

AUTHOR CONTRIBUTIONS

RC, SK and JA wrote and edited the manuscript.

FUNDING

This work was supported by National Institutes of Health (NIH)/NINDS award 1R01NS091329-01A1, U.S. Department of Defense award AZ140097, NIH/NIMH L32 MD009205-01, NIH/NCATS 5UL1TR000117-04 and NIH/NIGMS 5P30GM110787-Pilot.

ACKNOWLEDGMENTS

We thank Dr. Moriel Vandsburger for drawing our initial attention to the vast advantage of MEMRI in neuroscience research. We also thank Dr. David Powell for his intellectual and technical support in understanding and performing MEMRI.

REFERENCES

Aicher, K. P., Laniado, M., Kopp, A. F., Grönewäller, E., Duda, S. H., and Claussen, C. D. (1993). Mn-DPDP-enhanced MR imaging of malignant liver lesions: efficacy and safety in 20 patients. *J. Magn. Reson. Imaging* 3, 731–737. doi: 10.1002/jmri.1880030507

Alahmari, K. A., Prabhakaran, H., Prabhakaran, K., Chandramoorthy, H. C., and Ramugounder, R. (2015). Antioxidants and NOS inhibitors selectively targets manganese-induced cell volume via Na-K-Cl cotransporter-1 in astrocytes. *Brain Res.* 1610, 69–79. doi: 10.1016/j.brainres.2015.03.035

Alaverdashvili, M., Lapointe, V., Whishaw, I. Q., and Cross, A. R. (2017). Manganese-enhanced magnetic resonance imaging and studies of rat behavior: transient motor deficit in skilled reaching, rears, and activity in rats after a single dose of $MnCl_2$. *Magn. Reson. Insights* 10:1178623X17706878. doi: 10.1177/1178623x17706878

Albiin, N., Kartalis, N., Bergquist, A., Sadigh, B., and Brismar, T. B. (2012). Manganese chloride tetrahydrate (CMC-001) enhanced liver MRI: evaluation of efficacy and safety in healthy volunteers. *MAGMA* 25, 361–368. doi: 10.1007/s10334-012-0307-x

Alexandre, J., Nicco, C., Chéreau, C., Laurent, A., Weill, B., Goldwasser, F., et al. (2006). Improvement of the therapeutic index of anticancer drugs by the superoxide dismutase mimic mangafodipir. *J. Natl. Cancer Inst.* 98, 236–244. doi: 10.1093/jnci/djj049

Andruska, K. M., and Racette, A. B. (2015). Neuromythology of manganism. *Curr. Epidemiol. Rep.* 2, 143–148. doi: 10.1007/s40471-015-0040-x

Aoki, I., Wu, Y. J., Silva, A. C., Lynch, R. M., and Koretsky, A. P. (2004). *In vivo* detection of neuroarchitecture in the rodent brain using manganese-enhanced MRI. *Neuroimage* 22, 1046–1059. doi: 10.1016/j.neuroimage.2004.03.031

Asadi-Pooya, A. A., Stewart, G. R., Abrams, D. J., and Sharan, A. (2017). Prevalence and incidence of drug-resistant mesial temporal lobe epilepsy in the united states. *World Neurosurg.* 99, 662–666. doi: 10.1016/j.wneu.2016.12.074

Atanasijevic, T., Bouraoud, N., McGavern, D. B., and Koretsky, A. P. (2017). Transcranial manganese delivery for neuronal tract tracing using MEMRI. *Neuroimage* 156, 146–154. doi: 10.1016/j.neuroimage.2017.05.025

Bartelle, B. B., Mana, M. D., Suero-Abreu, G. A., Rodriguez, J. J., and Turnbull, D. H. (2015). Engineering an effective Mn-binding MRI reporter protein by subcellular targeting. *Magn. Reson. Med.* 74, 1750–1757. doi: 10.1002/mrm.25566

Bartelle, B. B., Szulc, K. U., Suero-Abreu, G. A., Rodriguez, J. J., and Turnbull, D. H. (2013). Divalent metal transporter, DMT1: a novel MRI reporter protein. *Magn. Reson. Med.* 70, 842–850. doi: 10.1002/mrm.24509

Bartolozzi, C., Donati, F., Cioni, D., Crocetti, L., and Lencioni, R. (2000). MnDPDP-enhanced MRI vs. dual-phase spiral CT in the detection of hepatocellular carcinoma in cirrhosis. *Eur. Radiol.* 10, 1697–1702. doi: 10.1007/s003300000564

Behera, D., Behera, S., Jacobs, K. E., and Biswal, S. (2013). Bilateral peripheral neural activity observed *in vivo* following unilateral nerve injury. *Am. J. Nucl. Med. Mol. Imaging* 3, 282–290.

Ben Mosbah, I., Mouchel, Y., Pajaud, J., Ribault, C., Lucas, C., Laurent, A., et al. (2012). Pretreatment with mangafodipir improves liver graft tolerance to ischemia/reperfusion injury in rat. *PLoS One* 7:e50235. doi: 10.1371/journal.pone.0050235

Berkowitz, B. A., Bissig, D., Patel, P., Bhatia, A., and Roberts, R. (2012). Acute systemic 11-*cis*-retinal intervention improves abnormal outer retinal ion channel closure in diabetic mice. *Mol. Vis.* 18, 372–376.

Berkowitz, B. A., Gradianu, M., Bissig, D., Kern, T. S., and Roberts, R. (2009a). Retinal ion regulation in a mouse model of diabetic retinopathy: natural history and the effect of Cu/Zn superoxide dismutase overexpression. *Invest. Ophthalmol. Vis. Sci.* 50, 2351–2358. doi: 10.1167/iovs.08-2918

Berkowitz, B. A., Roberts, R., Oleske, D. A., Chang, M., Schafer, S., Bissig, D., et al. (2009b). Quantitative mapping of ion channel regulation by visual cycle activity in rodent photoreceptors *in vivo*. *Invest. Ophthalmol. Vis. Sci.* 50, 1880–1885. doi: 10.1167/iovs.08-2958

Berkowitz, B. A., Grady, E. M., Khetarpal, N., Patel, A., and Roberts, R. (2015a). Oxidative stress and light-evoked responses of the posterior segment in a mouse model of diabetic retinopathy. *Invest. Ophthalmol. Vis. Sci.* 56, 606–615. doi: 10.1167/iovs.14-15687

Berkowitz, B. A., Murphy, G. G., Craft, C. M., Surmeier, D. J., and Roberts, R. (2015b). Genetic dissection of horizontal cell inhibitory signaling in mice in complete darkness *in vivo*. *Invest. Ophthalmol. Vis. Sci.* 56, 3132–3139. doi: 10.1167/iovs.15-16581

Berkowitz, B. A., Gradianu, M., Schafer, S., Jin, Y., Porchia, A., Iezzi, R., et al. (2008). Ionic dysregulatory phenotyping of pathologic retinal thinning with manganese-enhanced MRI. *Invest. Ophthalmol. Vis. Sci.* 49, 3178–3184. doi: 10.1167/iovs.08-1720

Berkowitz, B. A., Roberts, R., Luan, H., Bissig, D., Bui, B. V., Gradianu, M., et al. (2007a). Manganese-enhanced MRI studies of alterations of intraretinal ion demand in models of ocular injury. *Invest. Ophthalmol. Vis. Sci.* 48, 3796–3804. doi: 10.1167/iovs.06-1278

Berkowitz, B. A., Roberts, R., Penn, J. S., and Gradianu, M. (2007b). High-resolution manganese-enhanced MRI of experimental retinopathy of prematurity. *Invest. Ophthalmol. Vis. Sci.* 48, 4733–4740. doi: 10.1167/iovs.06-1516

Berkowitz, B. A., Roberts, R., Stemmler, A., Luan, H., and Gradianu, M. (2007c). Impaired apparent ion demand in experimental diabetic retinopathy:

correction by lipoic Acid. *Invest. Ophthalmol. Vis. Sci.* 48, 4753–4758. doi: 10.1167/iovs.07-0433

Berkowitz, B. A., Roberts, R., Goebel, D. J., and Luan, H. (2006). Noninvasive and simultaneous imaging of layer-specific retinal functional adaptation by manganese-enhanced MRI. *Invest. Ophthalmol. Vis. Sci.* 47, 2668–2674. doi: 10.1167/iovs.05-1588

Bernardino, M. E., Young, S. W., Lee, J. K., and Weinreb, J. C. (1992). Hepatic MR imaging with Mn-DPDP: safety, image quality, and sensitivity. *Radiology* 183, 53–58. doi: 10.1148/radiology.183.1.1549694

Bernardino, M. E., Young, S. W., Lee, J. K., and Weinreb, J. (1991). Contrast-enhanced magnetic resonance imaging of the liver with Mn-DPDP for known or suspected focal hepatic disease. *Am. J. Med. Genet. A* 26, S148–S149; discussion S50–S55. doi: 10.1097/00004424-199111001-00050

Bertram, L., and Tanzi, R. E. (2005). The genetic epidemiology of neurodegenerative disease. *J. Clin. Invest.* 115, 1449–1457. doi: 10.1172/jci24761

Bertrand, A., Khan, U., Hoang, D. M., Novikov, D. S., Krishnamurthy, P., Rajamohamed Sait, H. B., et al. (2013). Non-invasive, *in vivo* monitoring of neuronal transport impairment in a mouse model of tauopathy using MEMRI. *Neuroimage* 64, 693–702. doi: 10.1016/j.neuroimage.2012.08.065

Bissig, D., and Berkowitz, B. A. (2009). Manganese-enhanced MRI of layer-specific activity in the visual cortex from awake and free-moving rats. *Neuroimage* 44, 627–635. doi: 10.1016/j.neuroimage.2008.10.013

Bjørklund, G., Chartrand, M. S., and Aaseth, J. (2017). Manganese exposure and neurotoxic effects in children. *Environ. Res.* 155, 380–384. doi: 10.1016/j.envres.2017.03.003

Bock, N. A., Paiva, F. F., Nascimento, G. C., Newman, J. D., and Silva, A. C. (2008a). Cerebrospinal fluid to brain transport of manganese in a non-human primate revealed by MRI. *Brain Res.* 1198, 160–170. doi: 10.1016/j.brainres.2007.12.065

Bock, N. A., Paiva, F. F., and Silva, A. C. (2008b). Fractionated manganese-enhanced MRI. *NMR Biomed.* 21, 473–478. doi: 10.1002/nbm.1211

Bouilleret, V., Cardamone, L., Liu, Y. R., Fang, K., Myers, D. E., and O'Brien, T. J. (2009). Progressive brain changes on serial manganese-enhanced MRI following traumatic brain injury in the rat. *J. Neurotrauma* 26, 1999–2013. doi: 10.1089/neu.2009.0943

Bowler, R. M., Beseler, C. L., Gocheva, V. V., Colledge, M., Kornblith, E. S., Julian, J. R., et al. (2016). Environmental exposure to manganese in air: associations with tremor and motor function. *Sci. Total Environ.* 541, 646–654. doi: 10.1016/j.scitotenv.2015.09.084

Brady, T. J., Goldman, M. R., Pykett, I. L., Buonanno, F. S., Kistler, J. P., Newhouse, J. H., et al. (1982). Proton nuclear magnetic resonance imaging of regionally ischemic canine hearts: effect of paramagnetic proton signal enhancement. *Radiology* 144, 343–347. doi: 10.1148/radiology.144.2.6283594

Brown, J. I., Baker, A. J., Konasiewicz, S. J., and Moulton, R. J. (1998). Clinical significance of CSF glutamate concentrations following severe traumatic brain injury in humans. *J. Neurotrauma* 15, 253–263. doi: 10.1089/neu.1998.15.253

Brozoski, T. J., Ciobanu, L., and Bauer, C. A. (2007). Central neural activity in rats with tinnitus evaluated with manganese-enhanced magnetic resonance imaging (MEMRI). *Hear. Res.* 228, 168–179. doi: 10.1016/j.heares.2007.02.003

Brozoski, T. J., Wisner, K. W., Odintsov, B., and Bauer, C. A. (2013). Local NMDA receptor blockade attenuates chronic tinnitus and associated brain activity in an animal model. *PLoS One* 8:e77674. doi: 10.1371/journal.pone.0077674

Brurok, H., Ardenkjær-Larsen, J. H., Hansson, G., Skarra, S., Berg, K., Karlsson, J. O., et al. (1999). Manganese dipyridoxyl diphosphate: MRI contrast agent with antioxidative and cardioprotective properties? *Biochem. Biophys. Res. Commun.* 254, 768–772. doi: 10.1006/bbrc.1998.0131

Calkins, D. J., Horner, P. J., Roberts, R., Gradianu, M., and Berkowitz, B. A. (2008). Manganese-enhanced MRI of the DBA/2J mouse model of hereditary glaucoma. *Invest. Ophthalmol. Vis. Sci.* 49, 5083–5088. doi: 10.1167/iovs.08-2205

Carlson, R. O., Masco, D., Brooker, G., and Spiegel, S. (1994). Endogenous ganglioside GM1 modulates L-type calcium channel activity in N18 neuroblastoma cells. *J. Neurosci.* 14, 2272–2281. doi: 10.1523/JNEUROSCI.14-04-02272.1994

Cernak, I., Vink, R., Zapple, D. N., Cruz, M. I., Ahmed, F., Chang, T., et al. (2004). The pathobiology of moderate diffuse traumatic brain injury as identified using a new experimental model of injury in rats. *Neurobiol. Dis.* 17, 29–43. doi: 10.1016/j.nbd.2004.05.011

Chan, K. C., Cheng, J. S., Fan, S., Zhou, I. Y., and Wu, E. X. (2011a). *In vivo* manganese-enhanced MRI and diffusion tensor imaging of developing and impaired visual brains. *Conf. Proc. IEEE Eng. Med. Biol. Soc.* 2011, 7005–7008. doi: 10.1109/iembs.2011.6091771

Chan, K. C., Li, J., Kau, P., Zhou, I. Y., Cheung, M. M., Lau, C., et al. (2011b). *In vivo* retinotopic mapping of superior colliculus using manganese-enhanced magnetic resonance imaging. *Neuroimage* 54, 389–395. doi: 10.1016/j.neuroimage.2010.07.015

Chan, K. C., Fan, S. J., Chan, R. W., Cheng, J. S., Zhou, I. Y., and Wu, E. X. (2014). *In vivo* visuotopic brain mapping with manganese-enhanced MRI and resting-state functional connectivity MRI. *Neuroimage* 90, 235–245. doi: 10.1016/j.neuroimage.2013.12.056

Chan, K. C., Fu, Q. L., Hui, E. S., So, K. F., and Wu, E. X. (2008). Evaluation of the retina and optic nerve in a rat model of chronic glaucoma using *in vivo* manganese-enhanced magnetic resonance imaging. *Neuroimage* 40, 1166–1174. doi: 10.1016/j.neuroimage.2008.01.002

Chan, K. C., Fu, Q. L., So, K. F., and Wu, E. X. (2007). Evaluation of the visual system in a rat model of chronic glaucoma using manganese-enhanced magnetic resonance imaging. *Conf. Proc. IEEE Eng. Med. Biol. Soc.* 2007, 67–70. doi: 10.1109/iembs.2007.4352224

Chan, K. C., and Wu, E. X. (2012). *In vivo* manganese-enhanced MRI for visuotopic brain mapping. *Conf. Proc. IEEE Eng. Med. Biol. Soc.* 2012, 2279–2282. doi: 10.1109/embc.2012.6346417

Chen, P., Bornhorst, J., and Aschner, M. (2018). Manganese metabolism in humans. *Front. Biosci.* 23, 1655–1679. doi: 10.2741/4665

Chen, P., Chakraborty, S., Peres, T. V., Bowman, A. B., and Aschner, M. (2015). Manganese-induced neurotoxicity: from C. elegans to humans. *Toxicol. Res.* 4, 191–202. doi: 10.1039/c4tx00127c

Chen, W., Tenney, J., Kulkarni, P., and King, J. A. (2007). Imaging unconditioned fear response with manganese-enhanced MRI (MEMRI). *Neuroimage* 37, 221–229. doi: 10.1016/j.neuroimage.2007.05.001

Cherian, A., and Thomas, S. V. (2009). Status epilepticus. *Ann. Indian Acad. Neurol.* 12, 140–153. doi: 10.4103/0972-2327.56312

Chiu, J.-H., Cheng, H.-C., Tai, C.-H., Hsieh, J.-C., Yeh, T.-C., Cheng, H., et al. (2001). Electroacupuncture-induced neural activation detected by use of manganese-enhanced functional magnetic resonance imaging in rabbits. *Am. J. Vet. Res.* 62, 178–184. doi: 10.2460/ajvr.2001.62.178

Chiu, J.-H., Chung, M.-S., Cheng, H.-C., Yeh, T.-C., Hsieh, J.-C., Chang, C.-Y., et al. (2003). Different central manifestations in response to electroacupuncture at analgesic and nonanalgesic acupoints in rats: a manganese-enhanced functional magnetic resonance imaging study. *Can. J. Vet. Res.* 67, 94–101.

Chuang, K.-H., Belluscio, L., and Koretsky, A. P. (2010). *In vivo* detection of individual glomeruli in the rodent olfactory bulb using manganese enhanced MRI. *Neuroimage* 49, 1350–1356. doi: 10.1016/j.neuroimage.2009.09.060

Chuang, K.-H., Lee, J. H., Silva, A. C., Belluscio, L., and Koretsky, A. P. (2009). Manganese enhanced MRI reveals functional circuitry in response to odorant stimuli. *Neuroimage* 44, 363–372. doi: 10.1016/j.neuroimage.2008.08.046

Chuang, K.-H., and Koretsky, A. P. (2009). Accounting for nonspecific enhancement in neuronal tract tracing using manganese enhanced magnetic resonance imaging. *Magn. Reson. Imaging* 27, 594–600. doi: 10.1016/j.mri.2008.10.006

Collard, J. F., Côté, F., and Julien, J.-P. (1995). Defective axonal transport in a transgenic mouse model of amyotrophic lateral sclerosis. *Nature* 375, 61–64. doi: 10.1038/375061a0

Coriat, R., Alexandre, J., Nicco, C., Quinquis, L., Benoit, E., Chereau, C., et al. (2014). Treatment of oxaliplatin-induced peripheral neuropathy by intravenous mangafodipir. *J. Clin. Invest.* 124, 262–272. doi: 10.1172/JCI68730

Cory, D. A., Schwartzentruber, D. J., and Mock, B. H. (1987). Ingested manganese chloride as a contrast agent for magnetic resonance imaging. *Magn. Reson. Imaging* 5, 65–70. doi: 10.1016/0730-725x(87)90485-1

Couet, W. R., Eriksson, U. G., Tozer, T. N., Tuck, L. D., Wesbey, G. E., Nitecki, D., et al. (1984). Pharmacokinetics and metabolic fate of two nitroxides potentially useful as contrast agents for magnetic resonance imaging. *Pharm. Res.* 1, 203–209. doi: 10.1023/A:1016317212601

Coughlin, D., and Irwin, D. J. (2017). Emerging diagnostic and therapeutic strategies for tauopathies. *Curr. Neurol. Neurosci. Rep.* 17:72. doi: 10.1007/s11910-017-0779-1

Cross, D. J., Flexman, J. A., Anzai, Y., Morrow, T. J., Maravilla, K. R., and Minoshima, S. (2006). *In vivo* imaging of functional disruption, recovery and alteration in rat olfactory circuitry after lesion. *Neuroimage* 32, 1265–1272. doi: 10.1016/j.neuroimage.2006.04.229

Cross, D. J., Minoshima, S., Anzai, Y., Flexman, J. A., Keogh, B. P., Kim, Y., et al. (2004). Statistical mapping of functional olfactory connections of the rat brain *in vivo*. *Neuroimage* 23, 1326–1335. doi: 10.1016/j.neuroimage.2004.07.038

De La Garza, B. H., Li, G., Shih, Y. Y., and Duong, T. Q. (2012). Layer-specific manganese-enhanced MRI of the retina in light and dark adaptation. *Invest. Ophthalmol. Vis. Sci.* 53, 4352–4358. doi: 10.1167/iovs.11-8826

Dedeurwaerdere, S., Fang, K., Chow, M., Shen, Y. T., Noordman, I., van Raay, L., et al. (2013). Manganese-enhanced MRI reflects seizure outcome in a model for mesial temporal lobe epilepsy. *Neuroimage* 68, 30–38. doi: 10.1016/j.neuroimage.2012.11.054

Devonshire, I. M., Burston, J. J., Xu, L., Lillywhite, A., Prior, M. J., Watson, D. J. G., et al. (2017). Manganese-enhanced magnetic resonance imaging depicts brain activity in models of acute and chronic pain: a new window to study experimental spontaneous pain? *Neuroimage* 157, 500–510. doi: 10.1016/j.neuroimage.2017.06.034

Diehl, S. J., Lehmann, K. J., Gaa, J., McGill, S., Hoffmann, V., and Georgi, M. A. X. (1999). MR imaging of pancreatic lesions: comparison of manganese-DPDP and gadolinium chelate. *Invest. Radiol.* 34:589. doi: 10.1097/00004424-199909000-00007

Downes, J. M., Klepser, D. G., Foster, J., and Nelson, M. (2018). Development of a standardized approach for managing opioids in adults with chronic noncancer pain. *Am. J. Health Syst. Pharm.* 75, 321–326. doi: 10.2146/ajhp161012

Drobyshevsky, A., Robinson, A. M., Derrick, M., Wyrwicz, A. M., Ji, X., Englof, I., et al. (2006). Sensory deficits and olfactory system injury detected by novel application of MEMRI in newborn rabbit after antenatal hypoxia-ischemia. *Neuroimage* 32, 1106–1112. doi: 10.1016/j.neuroimage.2006.06.002

Drobyshevsky, A., Yu, L., Yang, Y., Khalid, S., Luo, K., Jiang, R., et al. (2012). Antenatal insults modify newborn olfactory function by nitric oxide produced from neuronal nitric oxide synthase. *Exp. Neurol.* 237, 427–434. doi: 10.1016/j.expneurol.2012.07.006

Duong, T. Q., Silva, A. C., Lee, S.-P., and Kim, S.-G. (2000). Functional MRI of calcium-dependent synaptic activity: cross correlation with CBF and BOLD measurements. *Magnetic Resonance in Medicine* 43, 383–392. doi: 10.1002/(sici)1522-2594(200003)43:3<383::aid-mrm10>3.0.co;2-q

Elizondo, G., Fretz, C. J., Stark, D. D., Rocklage, S. M., Quay, S. C., Worah, D., et al. (1991). Preclinical evaluation of MnDPDP: new paramagnetic hepatobiliary contrast agent for MR imaging. *Radiology* 178, 73–78. doi: 10.1148/radiology.178.1.1898538

Eschenko, O., Canals, S., Simanova, I., Beyerlein, M., Murayama, Y., and Logothetis, N. K. (2010a). Mapping of functional brain activity in freely behaving rats during voluntary running using manganese-enhanced MRI: implication for longitudinal studies. *Neuroimage* 49, 2544–2555. doi: 10.1016/j.neuroimage.2009.10.079

Eschenko, O., Canals, S., Simanova, I., and Logothetis, N. K. (2010b). Behavioral, electrophysiological and histopathological consequences of systemic manganese administration in MEMRI. *Magn. Reson. Imaging* 28, 1165–1174. doi: 10.1016/j.mri.2009.12.022

Fa, Z., Zhang, P., Huang, F., Li, P., Zhang, R., Xu, R., et al. (2010). Activity-induced manganese-dependent functional MRI of the rat visual cortex following intranasal manganese chloride administration. *Neurosci. Lett.* 481, 110–114. doi: 10.1016/j.neulet.2010.06.063

Federle, M., Chezmar, J., Rubin, D. L., Weinreb, J., Freeny, P., Schmiedl, U. P., et al. (2000). Efficacy and safety of mangafodipir trisodium (MnDPDP) injection for hepatic MRI in adults: results of the U.S. Multicenter phase III clinical trials. Efficacy of early imaging. *J. Magn. Reson. Imaging* 12, 689–701. doi: 10.1002/1522-2586(200011)12:5<689::aid-jmri5>3.0.co;2-z

Fiedorowicz, M., Orzel, J., Kossowski, B., Welniak-Kaminska, M., Choragiewicz, T., Swiatkiewicz, M., et al. (2018). Anterograde transport in axons of the retinal ganglion cells and its relationship to the intraocular pressure during aging in mice with hereditary pigmentary glaucoma. *Curr. Eye Res.* 43, 539–546. doi: 10.1080/02713683.2017.1416147

Fischer, S., Engelmann, C., Herrmann, K. H., Reichenbach, J. R., Witte, O. W., Weih, F., et al. (2014). *In vivo* imaging of optic nerve fiber integrity by contrast-enhanced MRI in mice. *J. Vis. Exp.* 22:89. doi: 10.3791/51274

Fitsanakis, V. A., Piccola, G., Aschner, J. L., and Aschner, M. (2006). Characteristics of manganese (Mn) transport in rat brain endothelial (RBE4) cells, an *in vitro* model of the blood-brain barrier. *Neurotoxicology* 27, 60–70. doi: 10.1016/j.neuro.2005.06.004

Fontaine, S. N., Ingram, A., Cloyd, R. A., Meier, S. E., Miller, E., Lyons, D., et al. (2017). Identification of changes in neuronal function as a consequence of aging and tauopathic neurodegeneration using a novel and sensitive magnetic resonance imaging approach. *Neurobiol. Aging* 56, 78–86. doi: 10.1016/j.neurobiolaging.2017.04.007

Fornasiero, D., Bellen, J. C., Baker, R. J., and Chatterton, B. E. (1987). Paramagnetic complexes of manganese(II), iron(III), and gadolinium(III) as contrast agents for magnetic resonance imaging: the influence of stability constants on the biodistribution of radioactive aminopolycarboxylate complexes. *Invest. Radiol.* 22, 322–327. doi: 10.1097/00004424-198704000-00008

Foster, M. L., Rao, D. B., Francher, T., Traver, S., and Dorman, D. C. (2018). Olfactory toxicity in rats following manganese chloride nasal instillation: a pilot study. *Neurotoxicology* 64, 284–290. doi: 10.1016/j.neuro.2017.09.004

Fredstrom, S., Rogosheske, J., Gupta, P., and Burns, L. J. (1995). Extrapyramidal symptoms in a BMT recipient with hyperintense basal ganglia and elevated manganese. *Bone Marrow Transplant.* 15, 989–992.

Gallagher, J. J., Zhang, X., Ziomek, G. J., Jacobs, R. E., and Bearer, E. L. (2012). Deficits in axonal transport in hippocampal-based circuitry and the visual pathway in APP knock-out animals witnessed by manganese enhanced MRI. *Neuroimage* 60, 1856–1866. doi: 10.1016/j.neuroimage.2012.01.132

Galosi, R., Szalay, C., Aradi, M., Perlaki, G., Pal, J., Steier, R., et al. (2017). Identifying non-toxic doses of manganese for manganese-enhanced magnetic resonance imaging to map brain areas activated by operant behavior in trained rats. *Magn. Reson. Imaging* 37, 122–133. doi: 10.1016/j.mri.2016.11.017

Gerber, G. B., Léonard, A., and Hantson, P. H. (2002). Carcinogenicity, mutagenicity and teratogenicity of manganese compounds. *Crit. Rev. Oncol. Hematol.* 42, 25–34. doi: 10.1016/s1040-8428(01)00178-0

Giordano, C. R., Roberts, R., Krentz, K. A., Bissig, D., Talreja, D., Kumar, A., et al. (2015). Catalase therapy corrects oxidative stress-induced pathophysiology in incipient diabetic retinopathy. *Invest. Ophthalmol. Vis. Sci.* 56, 3095–3102. doi: 10.1167/iovs.14-16194

Gobbo, O. L., Petit, F., Gurden, H., and Dhenain, M. (2012). *In vivo* detection of excitotoxicity by manganese-enhanced MRI: comparison with physiological stimulation. *Magn. Reson. Med.* 68, 234–240. doi: 10.1002/mrm.23210

Goesling, J., Lin, L. A., and Clauw, D. J. (2018). Psychiatry and pain management: at the intersection of chronic pain and mental health. *Curr. Psychiatry Rep.* 20:12. doi: 10.1007/s11920-018-0872-4

Goldman, M. R., Brady, T. J., Pykett, I. L., Burt, C. T., Buonanno, F. S., Kistler, J. P., et al. (1982). Quantification of experimental myocardial infarction using nuclear magnetic resonance imaging and paramagnetic ion contrast enhancement in excised canine hearts. *Circulation* 66, 1012–1016. doi: 10.1161/01.cir.66.5.1012

Grant, D., Blazak, W. F., and Brown, G. L. (1997a). The reproductive toxicology of intravenously administered MnDPDP in the rat and rabbit. *Acta Radiol.* 38, 759–769. doi: 10.3109/02841859709172409

Grant, D., Toft, K. G., Martinsen, I., and Atzpodien, E. (1997b). Tissue distribution and general safety of MnDPDP in male beagle dogs, with or without total common bile duct obstruction. *Acta Radiol.* 38, 732–739. doi: 10.3109/02841859709172406

Grillon, E., Provent, P., Montigon, O., Segebarth, C., Rémy, C., and Barbier, E. L. (2008). Blood-brain barrier permeability to manganese and to Gd-DOTA in a rat model of transient cerebral ischaemia. *NMR Biomed.* 21, 427–436. doi: 10.1002/nbm.1206

Gröschel, M., Götze, R., Müller, S., Ernst, A., and Basta, D. (2016). Central nervous activity upon systemic salicylate application in animals with kanamycin-induced hearing loss—a manganese-enhanced MRI (MEMRI) study. *PLoS One* 11:e0153386. doi: 10.1371/journal.pone.0153386

Gröschel, M., Hubert, N., Müller, S., Ernst, A., and Basta, D. (2014). Age-dependent changes of calcium related activity in the central auditory pathway. *Exp. Gerontol.* 58, 235–243. doi: 10.1016/j.exger.2014.08.014

Gröschel, M., Müller, S., Götze, R., Ernst, A., and Basta, D. (2011). The possible impact of noise-induced Ca^{2+}-dependent activity in the central auditory pathway: a manganese-enhanced MRI study. *Neuroimage* 57, 190–197. doi: 10.1016/j.neuroimage.2011.04.022

Grünecker, B., Kaltwasser, S. F., Peterse, Y., Samann, P. G., Schmidt, M. V., Wotjak, C. T., et al. (2010). Fractionated manganese injections: effects on MRI contrast enhancement and physiological measures in C57BL/6 mice. *NMR Biomed.* 23, 913–921. doi: 10.1002/nbm.1508

Gutman, D. A., Magnuson, M., Majeed, W., Keifer, O. P. Jr., Davis, M., Ressler, K. J., et al. (2013). Mapping of the mouse olfactory system with manganese-enhanced magnetic resonance imaging and diffusion tensor imaging. *Brain Struct. Funct.* 218, 527–537. doi: 10.1007/s00429-012-0413-6

Haenold, R., Herrmann, K. H., Schmidt, S., Reichenbach, J. R., Schmidt, K. F., Löwel, S., et al. (2012). Magnetic resonance imaging of the mouse visual pathway for *in vivo* studies of degeneration and regeneration in the CNS. *Neuroimage* 59, 363–376. doi: 10.1016/j.neuroimage.2011.07.069

Hamm, B., Vogl, T. J., Branding, G., Schnell, B., Taupitz, M., Wolf, K. J., et al. (1992). Focal liver lesions: MR imaging with Mn-DPDP—initial clinical results in 40 patients. *Radiology* 182, 167–174. doi: 10.1148/radiology.182.1.1309218

Hankir, M. K., Parkinson, J. R., Bloom, S. R., and Bell, J. D. (2012). The effects of glutamate receptor agonists and antagonists on mouse hypothalamic and hippocampal neuronal activity shown through manganese enhanced MRI. *Neuroimage* 59, 968–978. doi: 10.1016/j.neuroimage.2011.08.063

Hauser, R. A., Zesiewicz, T. A., Rosemurgy, A. S., Martinez, C., and Olanow, C. W. (1994). Manganese intoxication and chronic liver failure. *Ann. Neurol.* 36, 871–875. doi: 10.1002/ana.410360611

Holt, A. G., Bissig, D., Mirza, N., Rajah, G., and Berkowitz, B. (2010). Evidence of key tinnitus-related brain regions documented by a unique combination of manganese-enhanced MRI and acoustic startle reflex testing. *PLoS One* 5:e14260. doi: 10.1371/journal.pone.0014260

Howles, G. P., Qi, Y., Rosenzweig, S. J., Nightingale, K. R., and Johnson, G. A. (2012). Functional neuroimaging using ultrasonic blood-brain barrier disruption and manganese-enhanced MRI. *J. Vis. Exp.* 65:e4055. doi: 10.3791/4055

Hsu, Y. H., Lee, W. T., and Chang, C. (2007). Multiparametric MRI evaluation of kainic acid-induced neuronal activation in rat hippocampus. *Brain* 130, 3124–3134. doi: 10.1093/brain/awm207

Hubbard, J. I., Jones, S. F., and Landau, E. M. (1968). On the mechanism by which calcium and magnesium affect the release of transmitter by nerve impulses. *J. Physiol.* 196, 75–86. doi: 10.1113/jphysiol.1968.sp008495

Hughes, A. J., Daniel, S. E., Kilford, L., and Lees, A. J. (1992). Accuracy of clinical diagnosis of idiopathic Parkinson's disease: a clinico-pathological study of 100 cases. *J. Neurol. Neurosurg. Psychiatry* 55, 181–184. doi: 10.1136/jnnp.55.3.181

Hunter, D. R., Komai, H., Haworth, R. A., Jackson, M. D., and Berkoff, H. A. (1980). Comparison of Ca^{2+}, Sr^{2+} and Mn^{2+} fluxes in mitochondria of the perfused rat heart. *Circ. Res.* 47, 721–727. doi: 10.1161/01.res.47.5.721

Ikeda, S., Sera, Y., Yoshida, M., Ohshiro, H., Uchino, S., Oka, Y., et al. (2000). Manganese deposits in patients with biliary atresia after hepatic porto-enterostomy. *J. Pediatr. Surg.* 35, 450–453. doi: 10.1016/s0022-3468(00)90212-4

Immonen, R. J., Kharatishvili, I., Sierra, A., Einula, C., Pitkänen, A., and Gröhn, O. H. (2008). Manganese enhanced MRI detects mossy fiber sprouting rather than neurodegeneration, gliosis or seizure-activity in the epileptic rat hippocampus. *Neuroimage* 40, 1718–1730. doi: 10.1016/j.neuroimage.2008.01.042

Itoh, K., Sakata, M., Watanabe, M., Aikawa, Y., and Fujii, H. (2008). The entry of manganese ions into the brain is accelerated by the activation of *N*-methyl-D-aspartate receptors. *Neuroscience* 154, 732–740. doi: 10.1016/j.neuroscience.2008.03.080

Ivanova, E., Roberts, R., Bissig, D., Pan, Z. H., and Berkowitz, B. A. (2010). Retinal channelrhodopsin-2-mediated activity *in vivo* evaluated with manganese-enhanced magnetic resonance imaging. *Mol. Vis.* 16, 1059–1067.

Jackson, G. D., Kuzniecky, R. I., and Pell, G. S. (2005). "Principles of magnetic resonance imaging," in *Magnetic Resonance in Epilepsy*, eds R. I. Kuzniecky and G. D. Jackson, (San Diego, CA: Academic Press), 17–28.

Jacobs, K. E., Behera, D., Rosenberg, J., Gold, G., Moseley, M., Yeomans, D., et al. (2012). Oral manganese as an MRI contrast agent for the detection of nociceptive activity. *NMR Biomed.* 25, 563–569. doi: 10.1002/nbm.1773

Jeong, K. Y., and Kang, J. H. (2018). Investigation of spinal nerve ligation-mediated functional activation of the rat brain using manganese-enhanced MRI. *Exp. Anim.* 67, 23–29. doi: 10.1538/expanim.17-0033

Jeong, K. Y., Kim, H. M., and Kang, J. H. (2016). Investigation of the functional difference between the pathological itching and neuropathic pain-induced rat brain using manganese-enhanced MRI. *Acta Radiol.* 57, 861–868. doi: 10.1177/0284185115604514

Jin, S. U., Lee, J. J., Hong, K. S., Han, M., Park, J. W., Lee, H. J., et al. (2013). Intratympanic manganese administration revealed sound intensity and frequency dependent functional activity in rat auditory pathway. *Magn. Reson. Imaging* 31, 1143–1149. doi: 10.1016/j.mri.2013.03.003

Johnson, J. Jr., Pajarillo, E. A. B., Taka, E., Reams, R., Son, D. S., Aschner, M., et al. (2018). Valproate and sodium butyrate attenuate manganese-decreased locomotor activity and astrocytic glutamate transporters expression in mice. *Neurotoxicology* 64, 230–239. doi: 10.1016/j.neuro.2017.06.007

Jouroukhin, Y., Ostritsky, R., Assaf, Y., Pelled, G., Giladi, E., and Gozes, I. (2013). NAP (davunetide) modifies disease progression in a mouse model of severe neurodegeneration: protection against impairments in axonal transport. *Neurobiol. Dis.* 56, 79–94. doi: 10.1016/j.nbd.2013.04.012

Jung, D. J., Han, M., Jin, S.-U., Lee, S. H., Park, I., Cho, H.-J., et al. (2014). Functional mapping of the auditory tract in rodent tinnitus model using manganese-enhanced magnetic resonance imaging. *Neuroimage* 100, 642–649. doi: 10.1016/j.neuroimage.2014.06.055

Jynge, P., Brurok, H., Asplund, A., Towart, R., Refsum, H., and Karlsson, J. O. G. (1997). Cardiovascular safety of MnDPDP and $MnCl_2$. *Acta Radiol.* 38, 740–749. doi: 10.3109/02841859709172407

Karlsson, J. E., El-Saadi, W., Ali, M., Puskar, W., Skogvard, P., Engvall, J. E., et al. (2015). Mangafodipir as a cardioprotective adjunct to reperfusion therapy: a feasibility study in patients with ST-segment elevation myocardial infarction. *Eur. Heart J. Cardiovasc. Pharmacother.* 1, 39–45. doi: 10.1093/ehjcvp/pvu021

Karlsson, J. O. G., Andersson, R. G., and Jynge, P. (2017). Mangafodipir a selective cytoprotectant—with special reference to oxaliplatin and its association to chemotherapy-induced peripheral neuropathy (CIPN). *Transl. Oncol.* 10, 641–649. doi: 10.1016/j.tranon.2017.04.012

Karlsson, J. O. G., Adolfsson, K., Thelin, B., Jynge, P., Andersson, R. G. G., and Falkmer, U. G. (2012a). First clinical experience with the magnetic resonance imaging contrast agent and superoxide dismutase mimetic mangafodipir as an adjunct in cancer chemotherapy—a translational study. *Transl. Oncol.* 5, 32–38. doi: 10.1593/tlo.11277

Karlsson, J. O. G., Kurz, T., Flechsig, S., Näsström, J., and Andersson, R. G. G. (2012b). Superior therapeutic index of calmangafodipir in comparison to mangafodipir as a chemotherapy adjunct. *Transl. Oncol.* 5, 492–502. doi: 10.1593/tlo.12238

Kettritz, U., Schlund, J. F., Wilbur, K., Eisenberg, L. B., and Semelka, R. C. (1996). Comparison of gadolinium chelates with manganese-DPDP for liver lesion detection and characterization: preliminary results. *Magn. Reson. Imaging* 14, 1185–1190. doi: 10.1016/s0730-725x(96)00142-7

Kita, H., Narita, K., and Van der Kloot, W. (1981). Tetanic stimulation increases the frequency of miniature end-plate potentials at the frog neuromuscular junction in Mn^{2+}-, CO^{2+}- and Ni^{2+}-saline solutions. *Brain Res.* 205, 111–121. doi: 10.1016/0006-8993(81)90723-x

Kivity, S., Tsarfaty, G., Agmon-Levin, N., Blank, M., Manor, D., Konen, E., et al. (2010). Abnormal olfactory function demonstrated by manganese-enhanced MRI in mice with experimental neuropsychiatric lupus. *Ann. N Y Acad. Sci.* 1193, 70–77. doi: 10.1111/j.1749-6632.2009.05302.x

Kneynsberg, A., Combs, B., Christensen, K., Morfini, G., and Kanaan, N. M. (2017). Axonal degeneration in tauopathies: disease relevance and underlying mechanisms. *Front. Neurosci.* 11:572. doi: 10.3389/fnins.2017.00572

Knosche, T. R., Anwander, A., Liptrot, M., and Dyrby, T. B. (2015). Validation of tractography: comparison with manganese tracing. *Hum. Brain Mapp.* 36, 4116–4134. doi: 10.1002/hbm.22902

Kommajosyula, S. P., Randall, M. E., Brozoski, T. J., Odintsov, B. M., and Faingold, C. L. (2017). Specific subcortical structures are activated during seizure-induced death in a model of sudden unexpected death in epilepsy (SUDEP): a manganese-enhanced magnetic resonance imaging study. *Epilepsy Res.* 135, 87–94. doi: 10.1016/j.eplepsyres.2017.05.011

Kuo, Y. T., Herlihy, A. H., So, P. W., and Bell, J. D. (2006). Manganese-enhanced magnetic resonance imaging (MEMRI) without compromise of the blood-brain barrier detects hypothalamic neuronal activity *in vivo*. *NMR Biomed.* 19, 1028–1034. doi: 10.1002/nbm.1070

Lanciego, J. L., Luquin, N., and Obeso, J. A. (2012). Functional neuroanatomy of the basal ganglia. *Cold Spring Harb. Perspect. Med.* 2:a009621. doi: 10.1101/cshperspect.a009621

Lao, Y., Dion, L. A., Gilbert, G., Bouchard, M. F., Rocha, G., Wang, Y., et al. (2017). Mapping the basal ganglia alterations in children chronically exposed to manganese. *Sci. Rep.* 7:41804. doi: 10.1038/srep41804

Larsen, L. E., and Grant, D. (1997). General toxicology of MnDPDP. *Acta Radiol.* 38, 770–779. doi: 10.3109/02841859709172410

Lauterbur, P. C. (1973). Image formation by induced local interactions: examples employing nuclear magnetic resonance. *Nature* 242, 190–191. doi: 10.1038/242190a0

Lauterbur, P. C., Dias, M. M. H., and Rudin, A. M. (1980). "Augmentation of tissue water proton spin-lattice relaxation rates by *in vivo* addition of paramagnetic ions," in *Frontiers of Biological Energetics*, eds P. O. Dulton, J. Leigh and A. Scarpa (New York, NY: Academic Press), 752–759.

Leander, P., Golman, K., Månsson, S., and Höglund, P. (2010). Orally administered manganese with and without ascorbic acid as a liver-specific contrast agent and bowel marker for magnetic resonance imaging: phase I clinical trial assessing efficacy and safety. *Invest. Radiol.* 45, 559–564. doi: 10.1097/rli.0b013e3181e960ab

Lee, J. H., Silva, A. C., Merkle, H., and Koretsky, A. P. (2005). Manganese-enhanced magnetic resonance imaging of mouse brain after systemic administration of $MnCl_2$: dose-dependent and temporal evolution of T1 contrast. *Magn. Reson. Med.* 53, 640–648. doi: 10.1002/mrm.20368

Lee, R., Wong, T. Y., and Sabanayagam, C. (2015). Epidemiology of diabetic retinopathy, diabetic macular edema and related vision loss. *Eye Vis.* 2:17. doi: 10.1186/s40662-015-0026-2

Lee, H. J., Yoo, S.-J., Lee, S., Song, H.-J., Huh, M.-I., Jin, S.-U., et al. (2012). Functional activity mapping of rat auditory pathway after intratympanic manganese administration. *Neuroimage* 60, 1046–1054. doi: 10.1016/j.neuroimage.2012.01.065

Lehallier, B., Andrey, P., Maurin, Y., and Bonny, J. M. (2011). Iterative algorithm for spatial and intensity normalization of MEMRI images. Application to tract-tracing of rat olfactory pathways. *Magn. Reson. Imaging* 29, 1304–1316. doi: 10.1016/j.mri.2011.07.014

Lehallier, B., Coureaud, G., Maurin, Y., and Bonny, J. M. (2012a). Effects of manganese injected into rat nostrils: implications for *in vivo* functional study of olfaction using MEMRI. *Magn. Reson. Imaging* 30, 62–69. doi: 10.1016/j.mri.2011.08.009

Lehallier, B., Rampin, O., Saint-Albin, A., Jerôme, N., Ouali, C., Maurin, Y., et al. (2012b). Brain processing of biologically relevant odors in the awake rat, as revealed by manganese-enhanced MRI. *PLoS One* 7:e48491. doi: 10.1371/journal.pone.0048491

Lei, B. H., Chen, J. H., and Yin, H. S. (2014). Repeated amphetamine treatment alters spinal magnetic resonance signals and pain sensitivity in mice. *Neurosci. Lett.* 583, 70–75. doi: 10.1016/j.neulet.2014.09.031

Lewis, C. M., Graves, S. A., Hernandez, R., Valdovinos, H. F., Barnhart, T. E., Cai, W., et al. (2015). ^{52}Mn production for PET/MRI tracking of human stem cells expressing divalent metal transporter 1 (DMT1). *Theranostics* 5, 227–239. doi: 10.7150/thno.10185

Liang, S., Liang, M., Zhu, Y., Cheng, J., and Yang, Z. (2015). The distribution of Mn^{2+} in rabbit eyes after topical administration for manganese-enhanced MRI. *Int. J. Clin. Exp. Pathol.* 8, 836–841.

Lim, K. O., Stark, D. D., Leese, P. T., Pfefferbaum, A., Rocklage, S. M., and Quay, S. C. (1991). Hepatobiliary MR imaging: first human experience with MnDPDP. *Radiology* 178, 79–82. doi: 10.1148/radiology.178.1.1898539

Lin, Y.-J., and Koretsky, A. P. (1997). Manganese ion enhances T1-weighted MRI during brain activation: an approach to direct imaging of brain function. *Magn. Reson. Med.* 38, 378–388. doi: 10.1002/mrm.1910380305

Lin, C. P., Tseng, W. Y., Cheng, H. C., and Chen, J. H. (2001). Validation of diffusion tensor magnetic resonance axonal fiber imaging with registered manganese-enhanced optic tracts. *Neuroimage* 14, 1035–1047. doi: 10.1006/nimg.2001.0882

Lindsey, J. D., Grob, S. R., Scadeng, M., Duong-Polk, K., and Weinreb, R. N. (2013). Ocular integrity following manganese labeling of the visual system for MRI. *Magn. Reson. Imaging* 31, 865–874. doi: 10.1016/j.mri.2012.11.012

Liu, C. H., D'Arceuil, H. E., and de Crespigny, A. J. (2004). Direct CSF injection of $MnCl_2$ for dynamic manganese-enhanced MRI. *Magn. Reson. Med.* 51, 978–987. doi: 10.1002/mrm.20047

Lu, H., Demny, S., Zuo, Y., Rea, W., Wang, L., Chefer, S. I., et al. (2010). Temporary disruption of the rat blood-brain barrier with a monoclonal antibody: a novel method for dynamic manganese-enhanced MRI. *Neuroimage* 50, 7–14. doi: 10.1016/j.neuroimage.2009.12.053

Lu, H., Xi, Z. X., Gitajn, L., Rea, W., Yang, Y., and Stein, E. A. (2007). Cocaine-induced brain activation detected by dynamic manganese-enhanced magnetic resonance imaging (MEMRI). *Proc. Natl. Acad. Sci. U S A* 104, 2489–2494. doi: 10.1073/pnas.0606983104

Magen, I., and Gozes, I. (2013). Microtubule-stabilizing peptides and small molecules protecting axonal transport and brain function: focus on davunetide (NAP). *Neuropeptides* 47, 489–495. doi: 10.1016/j.npep.2013.10.011

Majid, T., Ali, Y. O., Venkitaramani, D. V., Jang, M. K., Lu, H. C., and Pautler, R. G. (2014). *In vivo* axonal transport deficits in a mouse model of fronto-temporal dementia. *Neuroimage Clin.* 4, 711–717. doi: 10.1016/j.nicl.2014.02.005

Majid, T., Griffin, D., Criss, Z. II., Jarpe, M., and Pautler, R. G. (2015). Pharmocologic treatment with histone deacetylase 6 inhibitor (ACY-738) recovers Alzheimer's disease phenotype in amyloid precursor protein/presenilin 1 (APP/PS1) mice. *Alzheimers Dement.* 1, 170–181. doi: 10.1016/j.trci.2015.08.001

Malheiros, J. M., Persike, D. S., Castro, L. U., Sanches, T. R., Andrade Lda, C., Tannus, A., et al. (2014). Reduced hippocampal manganese-enhanced MRI (MEMRI) signal during pilocarpine-induced status epilepticus: edema or apoptosis? *Epilepsy Res.* 108, 644–652. doi: 10.1016/j.eplepsyres.2014.02.007

Malheiros, J. M., Polli, R. S., Paiva, F. F., Longo, B. M., Mello, L. E., Silva, A. C., et al. (2012). Manganese-enhanced magnetic resonance imaging detects mossy fiber sprouting in the pilocarpine model of epilepsy. *Epilepsia* 53, 1225–1232. doi: 10.1111/j.1528-1167.2012.03521.x

Mantovani, S., Smith, S. S., Gordon, R., and O'Sullivan, J. D. (2018). An overview of sleep and circadian dysfunction in Parkinson's disease. *J. Sleep Res.* 27:e12673. doi: 10.1111/jsr.12673

Marques, A., Durif, F., and Fernagut, P. O. (2018). Impulse control disorders in Parkinson's disease. *J. Neural Transm.* 125, 1299–1312. doi: 10.1007/s00702-018-1870-8

Marugami, N., Takewa, M., Iwaki, Y., Hazeyama, Y., Iwato, K., Takahama, J., et al. (2013). MR signal changes on hepatobiliary imaging after oral ingestion of manganese chloride tetrahydrate: preliminary examination. *Jpn. J. Radiol.* 31, 713–723. doi: 10.1007/s11604-013-0241-5

Massaad, C. A., Amin, S. K., Hu, L., Mei, Y., Klann, E., and Pautler, R. G. (2010). Mitochondrial superoxide contributes to blood flow and axonal transport deficits in the Tg2576 mouse model of Alzheimer's disease. *PLoS One* 5:e10561. doi: 10.1371/journal.pone.0010561

Mathern, G. W., Pretorius, J. K., and Babb, T. L. (1995). Influence of the type of initial precipitating injury and at what age it occurs on course and outcome in patients with temporal lobe seizures. *J. Neurosurg.* 82, 220–227. doi: 10.3171/jns.1995.82.2.0220

Mayer, M. L., and Westbrook, G. L. (1987). Permeation and block of N-methyl-D-aspartic acid receptor channels by divalent cations in mouse cultured central neurones. *J. Physiol.* 394, 501–527. doi: 10.1113/jphysiol.1987.sp016883

Mendonça-Dias, M. H., Gaggelli, E., and Lauterbur, P. C. (1983). Paramagnetic contrast agents in nuclear magnetic resonance medical imaging. *Semin. Nucl. Med.* 13, 364–376. doi: 10.1016/s0001-2998(83)80048-8

Michaely, H. J., Metzger, L., Haneder, S., Hansmann, J., Schoenberg, S. O., and Attenberger, U. I. (2012). Renal BOLD-MRI does not reflect renal function in chronic kidney disease. *Kidney Int.* 81, 684–689. doi: 10.1038/ki.2011.455

Morad, A., Farrokh, S., and Papangelou, A. (2018). Pain management in neurocritical care; an update. *Curr. Opin. Crit. Care* 24, 72–79. doi: 10.1097/MCC.0000000000000480

Muca, A., Standafer, E., Apawu, A. K., Ahmad, F., Ghoddoussi, F., Hali, M., et al. (2018). Tinnitus and temporary hearing loss result in differential noise-induced spatial reorganization of brain activity. *Brain Struct. Funct.* 223, 2343–2360. doi: 10.1007/s00429-018-1635-z

Mueller, S. G., Bateman, L. M., and Laxer, K. D. (2014). Evidence for brainstem network disruption in temporal lobe epilepsy and sudden unexplained death in epilepsy. *Neuroimage Clin.* 5, 208–216. doi: 10.1016/j.nicl.2014.06.010

Muir, E. R., Chandra, S. B., De La Garza, B. H., Velagapudi, C., Abboud, H. E., and Duong, T. Q. (2015). Layer-specific manganese-enhanced MRI of the diabetic rat retina in light and dark adaptation at 11.7 tesla. *Invest. Ophthalmol. Vis. Sci.* 56, 4006–4012. doi: 10.1167/iovs.14-16128

Nagatomo, S., Umehara, F., Hanada, K., Nobuhara, Y., Takenaga, S., Arimura, K., et al. (1999). Manganese intoxication during total parenteral nutrition: report of two cases and review of the literature. *J. Neurol. Sci.* 162, 102–105. doi: 10.1016/s0022-510x(98)00289-5

Nair, G., Pardue, M. T., Kim, M., and Duong, T. Q. (2011). Manganese-enhanced MRI reveals multiple cellular and vascular layers in normal and degenerated retinas. *J. Magn. Reson. Imaging* 34, 1422–1429. doi: 10.1002/jmri.22719

Nairismägi, J., Pitkänen, A., Narkilahti, S., Huttunen, J., Kauppinen, R. A., and Gröhn, O. H. (2006). Manganese-enhanced magnetic resonance imaging of mossy fiber plasticity *in vivo*. *Neuroimage* 30, 130–135. doi: 10.1016/j.neuroimage.2005.09.007

Narita, K., Kawasaki, F., and Kita, H. (1990). Mn and Mg influxes through Ca channels of motor nerve terminals are prevented by verapamil in frogs. *Brain Res.* 510, 289–295. doi: 10.1016/0006-8993(90)91379-u

Nelson, K., Golnick, J., Korn, T., and Angle, C. (1993). Manganese encephalopathy: utility of early magnetic resonance imaging. *Br. J. Ind. Med.* 50, 510–513. doi: 10.1136/oem.50.6.510

Ni, Y., Petré, C., Bosmans, H., Miao, Y., Grant, D., Baert, A. L., et al. (1997). Comparison of manganese biodistribution and MR contrast enhancement in rats after intravenous injection of MnDPDP and $MnCl_2$. *Acta Radiol.* 38, 700–707. doi: 10.3109/02841859709172402

Nischwitz, V., Berthele, A., and Michalke, B. (2008). Speciation analysis of selected metals and determination of their total contents in paired serum and cerebrospinal fluid samples: an approach to investigate the permeability of the human blood-cerebrospinal fluid-barrier. *Anal. Chim. Acta* 627, 258–269. doi: 10.1016/j.aca.2008.08.018

Ogan, M. D., Revel, D., and Brasch, R. C. (1987). Metalloporphyrin contrast enhancement of tumors in magnetic resonance imaging. A study of human carcinoma, lymphoma, and fibrosarcoma in mice. *Invest. Radiol.* 22, 822–828. doi: 10.1097/00004424-198710000-00009

Ogawa, S., Lee, T. M., Kay, A. R., and Tank, D. W. (1990). Brain magnetic resonance imaging with contrast dependent on blood oxygenation. *Proc. Natl. Acad. Sci. U S A* 87, 9868–9872. doi: 10.1073/pnas.87.24.9868

Okada, M. A., Neto, F. F., Noso, C. H., Voigt, C. L., Campos, S. X., and Alberto de Oliveira Ribeiro, C. (2016). Brain effects of manganese exposure in mice pups during prenatal and breastfeeding periods. *Neurochem. Int.* 97, 109–116. doi: 10.1016/j.neuint.2016.03.009

Olanow, C. W. (2004). Manganese-induced parkinsonism and Parkinson's disease. *Ann. N Y Acad. Sci.* 1012, 209–223. doi: 10.1196/annals.1306.018

Olson, K. E., Bade, A. N., Schutt, C. R., Dong, J., Shandler, S. J., Boska, M. D., et al. (2016). Manganese-enhanced magnetic resonance imaging for detection of vasoactive intestinal peptide receptor 2 agonist therapy in a model of Parkinson's disease. *Neurotherapeutics* 13, 635–646. doi: 10.1007/s13311-016-0449-z

Oudkerk, M., Torres, C. G., Song, B., König, M., Grimm, J., Fernandez-Cuadrado, J., et al. (2002). Characterization of liver lesions with mangafodipir trisodium-enhanced MR imaging: multicenter study comparing MR and dual-phase spiral CT. *Radiology* 223, 517–524. doi: 10.1148/radiol.2232010318

Palmer, A. M., Marion, D. W., Botscheller, M. L., Swedlow, P. E., Styren, S. D., and DeKosky, S. T. (1993). Traumatic brain injury-induced excitotoxicity assessed in a controlled cortical impact model. *J. Neurochem.* 61, 2015–2024. doi: 10.1111/j.1471-4159.1993.tb07437.x

Pautler, R. G., and Koretsky, A. P. (2002). Tracing odor-induced activation in the olfactory bulbs of mice using manganese-enhanced magnetic resonance imaging. *Neuroimage* 16, 441–448. doi: 10.1006/nimg.2002.1075

Pautler, R. G., Silva, A. C., and Koretsky, A. P. (1998). *In vivo* neuronal tract tracing using manganese enhanced magnetic resonance imaging. *Magn. Reson. Med.* 40, 740–748. doi: 10.1002/mrm.1910400515

Payet, M. D., Schanne, O. F., and Ruiz-Ceretti, E. (1980). Competition for slow channel of Ca^{2+}, Mn^{2+}, Verapamil and D-600 in rat ventricular muscle? *J. Mol. Cell. Cardiol.* 12, 635–638. doi: 10.1016/0022-2828(80)90020-6

Pelled, G., Bergman, H., Ben-Hur, T., and Goelman, G. (2007). Manganese-enhanced MRI in a rat model of Parkinson's disease. *J. Magn. Reson. Imaging* 26, 863–870. doi: 10.1002/jmri.21051

Peters, O. M., and Brown, R. H. Jr. (2015). "Amyotrophic lateral sclerosis," in *Neurobiology of Brain Disorders: Biological Basis of Neurological and Psychiatric Disorders*, eds M. J. Zigmond, J. T. Coyle and L. P. Rowland (San Diego, CA: Academic Press), 262–280. doi: 10.1016/b978-0-12-398270-4.00018-5

Pomeroy, O. H., Wendland, M., Wagner, S., Derugin, N., Holt, W. W., Rocklage, S. M., et al. (1989). Magnetic resonance imaging of acute myocardial ischemia using a manganese chelate, Mn-DPDP. *Invest. Radiol.* 24, 531–536. doi: 10.1097/00004424-198907000-00004

Poole, D. S., Doorenweerd, N., Plomp, J. J., Mahfouz, A., Reinders, M. J. T., and van der Weerd, L. (2017). Continuous infusion of manganese improves contrast and reduces side effects in manganese-enhanced magnetic resonance imaging studies. *Neuroimage* 147, 1–9. doi: 10.1016/j.neuroimage.2016.09.030

Ribalet, B., and Beigelman, P. M. (1980). Calcium action potentials and potassium permeability activation in pancreatic β-cells. *Am. J. Physiol.* 239, C124–C133. doi: 10.1152/ajpcell.1980.239.3.c124

Rieber, A., Tomczak, R., Nüssle, K., Klaus, H., and Brambs, H. J. (2000). MRI with mangafodipir trisodium in the detection of pancreatic tumours: comparison with helical CT. *Br. J. Radiol.* 73, 1165–1169. doi: 10.1259/bjr.73.875.11144793

Rocklage, S. M., Cacheris, W. P., Quay, S. C., Hahn, F. E., and Raymond, K. N. (1989). Manganese(II) N,N′-dipyridoxylethylenediamine-N,N′-diacetate 5,5′-bis(phosphate). Synthesis and characterization of a paramagnetic chelate for magnetic resonance imaging enhancement. *Inorg. Chem.* 28, 477–485. doi: 10.1002/chin.198921266

Rodriguez, O., Schaefer, M. L., Wester, B., Lee, Y. C., Boggs, N., Conner, H. A., et al. (2016). Manganese-enhanced magnetic resonance imaging as a diagnostic and dispositional tool after mild-moderate blast traumatic brain injury. *J. Neurotrauma* 33, 662–671. doi: 10.1089/neu.2015.4002

Rofsky, N. M., and Weinreb, J. C. (1992). Manganese (II) N,N'-dipyridoxylethylenediamine-N,N'-diacetate 5,5'-bis(phosphate): clinical experience with a new contrast agent. *Magn. Reson. Q.* 8, 156–168.

Rofsky, N. M., Weinreb, J. C., Bernardino, M. E., Young, S. W., Lee, J. K., and Noz, M. E. (1993). Hepatocellular tumors: characterization with Mn-DPDP-enhanced MR imaging. *Radiology* 188, 53–59. doi: 10.1148/radiology.188.1.8390072

Romijn, M. G., Stoker, J., van Eijck, C. H. J., van Muiswinkel, J. M., Torres, C. G., and Laméris, J. S. (2000). MRI with mangafodipir trisodium in the detection and staging of pancreatic cancer. *J. Magn. Reson. Imaging* 12, 261–268. doi: 10.1002/1522-2586(200008)12:2<261::aid-jmri8>3.0.co;2-r

Roth, T. L., Nayak, D., Atanasijevic, T., Koretsky, A. P., Latour, L. L., and McGavern, D. B. (2014). Transcranial amelioration of inflammation and cell death after brain injury. *Nature* 505, 223–228. doi: 10.1038/nature12808

Rüber, T., David, B., and Elger, C. E. (2018). MRI in epilepsy: clinical standard and evolution. *Curr. Opin. Neurol.* 31, 223–231. doi: 10.1097/wco.0000000000000539

Rummeny, E. J., Ehrenheim, C., Gehl, H. B., Hamm, B., Laniado, M., Lodemann, K. P., et al. (1991). Manganese-DPDP as a hepatobiliary contrast agent in the magnetic resonance imaging of liver tumors: results of clinical phase II trails in Germany including 141 patients. *Invest. Radiol.* 26, S142–S145. doi: 10.1097/00004424-199111001-00048

Rummeny, E. J., Torres, C. G., Kurdziel, J. C., Nilsen, G., Op de Beeck, B., and Lundby, B. (1997). MnDPDP for MR imaging of the liver. Results of an independent image evaluation of the European phase III studies. *Acta Radiol.* 38, 638–642. doi: 10.1080/02841859709172394

Runge, V. M., Clanton, J. A., Foster, M. A., Smith, F. W., Lukehart, C. M., Jones, M. M., et al. (1984). Paramagnetic NMR contrast agents: development and evaluation. *Invest. Radiol.* 19, 408–415. doi: 10.1097/00004424-198409000-00013

Ruppel, R. A., Kochanek, P. M., Adelson, P. D., Rose, M. E., Wisniewski, S. R., Bell, M. J., et al. (2001). Excitatory amino acid concentrations in ventricular cerebrospinal fluid after severe traumatic brain injury in infants and children: the role of child abuse. *J. Pediatr.* 138, 18–25. doi: 10.1067/mpd.2001.110979

Ryu, S., Brown, S. L., Kolozsvary, A., Ewing, J. R., and Kim, J. H. (2002). Noninvasive detection of radiation-induced optic neuropathy by manganese-enhanced MRI. *Radiat. Res.* 157, 500–505. doi: 10.1667/0033-7587(2002)157[0500:ndorio]2.0.co;2

Saar, G., Cheng, N., Belluscio, L., and Koretsky, A. P. (2015). Laminar specific detection of APP induced neurodegeneration and recovery using MEMRI in an olfactory based Alzheimer's disease mouse model. *Neuroimage* 118, 183–192. doi: 10.1016/j.neuroimage.2015.05.045

Saeed, M., Wagner, S., Wendland, M. F., Derugin, N., Finkbeiner, W. E., and Higgins, C. B. (1989). Occlusive and reperfused myocardial infarcts: differentiation with Mn-DPDP—enhanced MR imaging. *Radiology* 172, 59–64. doi: 10.1148/radiology.172.1.2500678

Sandvig, A., Sandvig, I., Berry, M., Olsen, O., Pedersen, T. B., Brekken, C., et al. (2011). Axonal tracing of the normal and regenerating visual pathway of mouse, rat, frog and fish using manganese-enhanced MRI (MEMRI). *J. Magn. Reson. Imaging* 34, 670–675. doi: 10.1002/jmri.22631

Sandvig, I., Thuen, M., Hoang, L., Olsen, O., Sardella, T. C., Brekken, C., et al. (2012). *In vivo* MRI of olfactory ensheathing cell grafts and regenerating axons in transplant mediated repair of the adult rat optic nerve. *NMR Biomed.* 25, 620–631. doi: 10.1002/nbm.1778

Scharfman, H. E., Sollas, A. L., Berger, R. E., and Goodman, J. H. (2003). Electrophysiological evidence of monosynaptic excitatory transmission between granule cells after seizure-induced mossy fiber sprouting. *J. Neurophysiol.* 90, 2536–2547. doi: 10.1152/jn.00251.2003

Schima, W., Petersein, J., Hahn, P. F., Harisinghani, M., Halpern, E., and Saini, S. (1997). Contrast-enhanced MR imaging of the liver: comparison between Gd-BOPTA and mangafodipir. *J. Magn. Reson. Imaging* 7, 130–135. doi: 10.1002/jmri.1880070118

Schuh, M. J. (2016). Possible Parkinson's disease induced by chronic manganese supplement ingestion. *Consult. Pharm.* 31, 698–703. doi: 10.4140/tcp.n.2016.698

Schur, R. M., Sheng, L., Sahu, B., Yu, G., Gao, S., Yu, X., et al. (2015). Manganese-enhanced MRI for preclinical evaluation of retinal degeneration treatments. *Invest. Ophthalmol. Vis. Sci.* 56, 4936–4942. doi: 10.1167/iovs.15-16522

Sepúlveda, M. R., Dresselaers, T., Vangheluwe, P., Everaerts, W., Himmelreich, U., Mata, A. M., et al. (2012). Evaluation of manganese uptake and toxicity in mouse brain during continuous $MnCl_2$ administration using osmotic pumps. *Contrast Media Mol. Imaging* 7, 426–434. doi: 10.1002/cmmi.1469

Serrano, F., Deshazer, M., Smith, K. D., Ananta, J. S., Wilson, L. J., and Pautler, R. G. (2008). Assessing transneuronal dysfunction utilizing manganese-enhanced MRI (MEMRI). *Magn. Reson. Med.* 60, 169–175. doi: 10.1002/mrm.21648

Sharma, R., Buras, E., Terashima, T., Serrano, F., Massaad, C. A., Hu, L., et al. (2010). Hyperglycemia induces oxidative stress and impairs axonal transport rates in mice. *PLoS One* 5:e13463. doi: 10.1371/journal.pone.0013463

Shetty, A. K., Zaman, V., and Shetty, G. A. (2003). Hippocampal neurotrophin levels in a kainate model of temporal lobe epilepsy: a lack of correlation between brain-derived neurotrophic factor content and progression of aberrant dentate mossy fiber sprouting. *J. Neurochem.* 87, 147–159. doi: 10.1046/j.1471-4159.2003.01979.x

Shirakuni, T., Nagashima, T., Tamaki, N., and Matsumoto, S. (1985). Magnetic resonance imaging of experimental brain edema in cats. *Neurosurgery* 17, 557–563. doi: 10.1227/00006123-198510000-00004

Silva, A. C., Lee, J. H., Aoki, I., and Koretsky, A. P. (2004). Manganese-enhanced magnetic resonance imaging (MEMRI): methodological and practical considerations. *NMR Biomed.* 17, 532–543. doi: 10.1002/nbm.945

Sloot, W. N., and Gramsbergen, J.-B. P. (1994). Axonal transport of manganese and its relevance to selective neurotoxicity in the rat basal ganglia. *Brain Res.* 657, 124–132. doi: 10.1016/0006-8993(94)90959-8

Smith, B. N., and Dudek, F. E. (2001). Short- and long-term changes in CA1 network excitability after kainate treatment in rats. *J. Neurophysiol.* 85, 1–9. doi: 10.1152/jn.2001.85.1.1

Smith, K. D., Kallhoff, V., Zheng, H., and Pautler, R. G. (2007). *In vivo* axonal transport rates decrease in a mouse model of Alzheimer's disease. *Neuroimage* 35, 1401–1408. doi: 10.1016/j.neuroimage.2007.01.046

Smith, K. D., Paylor, R., and Pautler, R. G. (2011). R-flurbiprofen improves axonal transport in the Tg2576 mouse model of Alzheimer's disease as determined by MEMRI. *Magn. Reson. Med.* 65, 1423–1429. doi: 10.1002/mrm.22733

Smith, K. D., Peethumnongsin, E., Lin, H., Zheng, H., and Pautler, R. G. (2010). Increased human wildtype tau attenuates axonal transport deficits caused by loss of APP in mouse models. *Magn. Reson. Insights* 4, 11–18. doi: 10.4137/mri.s5237

Soria, G., Aguilar, E., Tudela, R., Mullol, J., Planas, A. M., and Marin, C. (2011). *In vivo* magnetic resonance imaging characterization of bilateral structural changes in experimental Parkinson's disease: a T2 relaxometry study combined with longitudinal diffusion tensor imaging and manganese-enhanced magnetic resonance imaging in the 6-hydroxydopamine rat model. *Eur. J. Neurosci.* 33, 1551–1560. doi: 10.1111/j.1460-9568.2011.07639.x

Southon, T. E., Grant, D., Bjørnerud, A., Moen, O. M., Spilling, B., Martinsen, I., et al. (2016). NMR relaxation studies with MnDPDP. *Acta Radiol.* 38, 708–716. doi: 10.3109/02841859709172403

Sperry, M. M., Kandel, B. M., Wehrli, S., Bass, K. N., Das, S. R., Dhillon, P. S., et al. (2017). Mapping of pain circuitry in early post-natal development using manganese-enhanced MRI in rats. *Neuroscience* 352, 180–189. doi: 10.1016/j.neuroscience.2017.03.052

Sun, S. W., Campbell, B., Lunderville, C., Won, E., and Liang, H. F. (2011). Noninvasive topical loading for manganese-enhanced MRI of the mouse visual system. *Invest. Ophthalmol. Vis. Sci.* 52, 3914–3920. doi: 10.1167/iovs.10-6363

Sun, S. W., Thiel, T., and Liang, H. F. (2012). Impact of repeated topical-loaded manganese-enhanced MRI on the mouse visual system. *Invest. Ophthalmol. Vis. Sci.* 53, 4699–4709. doi: 10.1167/iovs.12-9715

Svehla, P., Bedecarrats, A., Jahn, C., Nargeot, R., and Ciobanu, L. (2018). Intracellular manganese enhanced MRI signals reflect the frequency of action potentials in Aplysia neurons. *J. Neurosci. Methods* 295, 121–128. doi: 10.1016/j.jneumeth.2017.12.008

Takács, S., Szabo, A., Oszlanczi, G., Paulik, E., and Papp, A. (2012). A pilot study with simultaneous recording of changes in motility and cortical electrical activity of rats during four weeks of oral manganese exposure. *Int. J. Environ. Health Res.* 22, 331–339. doi: 10.1080/09603123.2011.643228

Takeda, A., Kodama, Y., Ishiwatari, S., and Okada, S. (1998). Manganese transport in the neural circuit of rat CNS. *Brain Res. Bull.* 45, 149–152. doi: 10.1016/s0361-9230(97)00330-4

Talley Watts, L., Shen, Q., Deng, S., Chemello, J., and Duong, T. Q. (2015). Manganese-enhanced magnetic resonance imaging of traumatic brain injury. *J. Neurotrauma* 32, 1001–1010. doi: 10.1089/neu.2014.3737

Tang, Y., Chen, Q., Yu, X., Xia, W., Luo, C., Huang, X., et al. (2014). A resting-state functional connectivity study in patients at high risk for sudden unexpected death in epilepsy. *Epilepsy Behav.* 41, 33–38. doi: 10.1016/j.yebeh.2014.08.140

Tang, H. L., Sun, H. P., Wu, X., Sha, H. Y., Feng, X. Y., and Zhu, J. H. (2011). Detection of neural stem cells function in rats with traumatic brain injury by manganese-enhanced magnetic resonance imaging. *Chin. Med. J.* 124, 1848–1853.

Tang, Z., Wang, J., Xiao, Z., Sun, X., Feng, X., Tang, W., et al. (2017a). Manganese-enhanced magnetic resonance imaging combined with electrophysiology in the evaluation of visual pathway in experimental rat models with monocular blindness. *Brain Behav.* 7:e00731. doi: 10.1002/brb3.731

Tang, Z., Wu, L., Xiao, Z., Sun, X., Feng, X., Chen, Q., et al. (2017b). Manganese-enhanced MR imaging (MEMRI) combined with electrophysiology in the study of cross-modal plasticity in binocularly blind rats. *Int. J. Dev. Neurosci.* 61, 12–20. doi: 10.1016/j.ijdevneu.2017.05.002

Taylor, J. M., Zhu, X. H., Zhang, Y., and Chen, W. (2015). Dynamic correlations between hemodynamic, metabolic and neuronal responses to acute whole-brain ischemia. *NMR Biomed.* 28, 1357–1365. doi: 10.1002/nbm.3408

Tham, Y.-C., Li, X., Wong, T. Y., Quigley, H. A., Aung, T., and Cheng, C.-Y. (2014). Global prevalence of glaucoma and projections of glaucoma burden through 2040: a systematic review and meta-analysis. *Ophthalmology* 121, 2081–2090. doi: 10.1016/j.ophtha.2014.05.013

Thuen, M., Berry, M., Pedersen, T. B., Goa, P. E., Summerfield, M., Haraldseth, O., et al. (2008). Manganese-enhanced MRI of the rat visual pathway: acute neural toxicity, contrast enhancement, axon resolution, axonal transport, and clearance of Mn^{2+}. *J. Magn. Reson. Imaging* 28, 855–865. doi: 10.1002/jmri.21504

Thuen, M., Olsen, O., Berry, M., Pedersen, T. B., Kristoffersen, A., Haraldseth, O., et al. (2009). Combination of Mn^{2+}-enhanced and diffusion tensor MR imaging gives complementary information about injury and regeneration in the adult rat optic nerve. *J. Magn. Reson. Imaging* 29, 39–51. doi: 10.1002/jmri.21606

Thuen, M., Singstad, T. E., Pedersen, T. B., Haraldseth, O., Berry, M., Sandvig, A., et al. (2005). Manganese-enhanced MRI of the optic visual pathway and optic nerve injury in adult rats. *J. Magn. Reson. Imaging* 22, 492–500. doi: 10.1002/jmri.20400

Tindemans, I., Boumans, T., Verhoye, M., and Van der Linden, A. (2006). IR-SE and IR-MEMRI allow *in vivo* visualization of oscine neuroarchitecture including the main forebrain regions of the song control system. *NMR Biomed.* 19, 18–29. doi: 10.1002/nbm.989

Tindemans, I., Verhoye, M., Balthazart, J., and Van der Linden, A. (2003). *In vivo* dynamic ME-MRI reveals differential functional responses of RA- and area X-projecting neurons in the HVC of canaries exposed to conspecific song. *Eur. J. Neurosci.* 18, 3352–3360. doi: 10.1111/j.1460-9568.2003.03056.x

Tjälve, H., Henriksson, J., Tallkvist, J., Larsson, B. S., and Gunnar Lindquist, N. (1996). Uptake of manganese and cadmium from the nasal mucosa into the central nervous system via olfactory pathways in rats. *Pharmacol. Toxicol.* 79, 347–356. doi: 10.1111/j.1600-0773.1996.tb00021.x

Tjälve, H., Mejàre, C., and Borg-Neczak, K. (1995). Uptake and transport of manganese in primary and secondary olfactory neurones in pike. *Pharmacol. Toxicol.* 77, 23–31. doi: 10.1111/j.1600-0773.1995.tb01909.x

Toft, K. G., Hustvedt, S. O., Grant, D., Friisk, G. A., and Skotland, T. (1997a). Metabolism of mangafodipir trisodium (MnDPDP), a new contrast medium for magnetic resonance imaging, in beagle dogs. *Eur. J. Drug Metab. Pharmacokinet.* 22, 65–72. doi: 10.1007/bf03189786

Toft, K. G., Hustvedt, S. O., Grant, D., Martinsen, I., Gordon, P. B., Friisk, G. A., et al. (1997b). Metabolism and pharmacokinetics of MnDPDP in man. *Acta Radiol.* 38, 677–689. doi: 10.3109/02841859709172400

Tofts, P. S., Porchia, A., Jin, Y., Roberts, R., and Berkowitz, B. A. (2010). Toward clinical application of manganese-enhanced MRI of retinal function. *Brain Res. Bull.* 81, 333–338. doi: 10.1016/j.brainresbull.2009.06.002

Tomson, T., Surges, R., Delamont, R., Haywood, S., and Hesdorffer, D. C. (2016). Who to target in sudden unexpected death in epilepsy prevention and how? Risk factors, biomarkers and intervention study designs. *Epilepsia* 57, 4–16. doi: 10.1111/epi.13234

Trump, B. F., and Berezesky, I. K. (1995). Calcium-mediated cell injury and cell death. *FASEB J.* 9, 219–228. doi: 10.1096/fasebj.9.2.7781924

Van der Linden, A., Van Meir, V., Tindemans, I., Verhoye, M., and Balthazart, J. (2004). Applications of manganese-enhanced magnetic resonance imaging (MEMRI) to image brain plasticity in song birds. *NMR Biomed.* 17, 602–612. doi: 10.1002/nbm.936

Van der Linden, A., Verhoye, M., Van Meir, V., Tindemans, I., Eens, M., Absil, P., et al. (2002). *In vivo* manganese-enhanced magnetic resonance imaging reveals connections and functional properties of the songbird vocal control system. *Neuroscience* 112, 467–474. doi: 10.1016/s0306-4522(02)00070-2

Van Meir, V., Verhoye, M., Absil, P., Eens, M., Balthazart, J., and Van der Linden, A. (2004). Differential effects of testosterone on neuronal populations and their connections in a sensorimotor brain nucleus controlling song production in songbirds: a manganese enhanced-magnetic resonance imaging study. *Neuroimage* 21, 914–923. doi: 10.1016/j.neuroimage.2003.10.007

Vazana, U., Veksler, R., Pell, G. S., Prager, O., Fassler, M., Chassidim, Y., et al. (2016). Glutamate-mediated blood-brain barrier opening: implications for neuroprotection and drug delivery. *J. Neurosci.* 36, 7727–7739. doi: 10.1523/JNEUROSCI.0587-16.2016

Viswanath, K., and McGavin, D. D. (2003). Diabetic retinopathy: clinical findings and management. *Community Eye Health* 16, 21–24.

Vogl, T. J., Hamm, B., Schnell, B., McMahon, C., Branding, G., Lissner, J., et al. (1993). Mn-DPDP enhancement patterns of hepatocellular lesions on MR images. *J. Magn. Reson. Imaging* 3, 51–58. doi: 10.1002/jmri.1880030110

Vousden, D. A., Cox, E., Allemang-Grand, R., Laliberte, C., Qiu, L. R., Lindenmaier, Z., et al. (2018). Continuous manganese delivery via osmotic pumps for manganese-enhanced mouse MRI does not impair spatial learning but leads to skin ulceration. *Neuroimage* 173, 411–420. doi: 10.1016/j.neuroimage.2018.02.046

Wan, X., Fu, T.-C., Smith, P. H., Brainard, J. R., and London, R. E. (1991). Magnetic resonance imaging study of the rat cerebral ventricular system utilizing intracerebrally administered contrast agents. *Magn. Reson. Med.* 21, 97–106. doi: 10.1002/mrm.1910210112

Wandschneider, B., Koepp, M., Scott, C., Micallef, C., Balestrini, S., Sisodiya, S. M., et al. (2015). Structural imaging biomarkers of sudden unexpected death in epilepsy. *Brain* 138, 2907–2919. doi: 10.1093/brain/awv233

Wang, C., Ahlström, H., Ekholm, S., Fagertun, H., Hellström, M., Hemmingsson, A., et al. (1997a). Diagnostic efficacy of MnDPDP in MR imaging of the liver. A phase III multicentre study. *Acta Radiol.* 38, 643–649. doi: 10.1080/02841859709172395

Wang, C., Gordon, P. B., Hustvedt, S. O., Grant, D., Tufte Sterud, A., Martinsen, I., et al. (1997b). MR imaging properties and pharmacokinetics of MnDPDP in healthy volunteers. *Acta Radiol.* 38, 665–676. doi: 10.1080/02841859709172399

Wang, F. H., Appelkvist, P., Klason, T., Gissberg, O., Bogstedt, A., Eliason, K., et al. (2012). Decreased axonal transport rates in the Tg2576 APP transgenic mouse: improvement with the γ-secretase inhibitor MRK-560 as detected by manganese-enhanced MRI. *Eur. J. Neurosci.* 36, 3165–3172. doi: 10.1111/j.1460-9568.2012.08258.x

Wang, Y., Wang, X., Chen, W., Gupta, K., and Zhu, X. H. (2017). Functional MRI BOLD response in sickle mice with hyperalgesia. *Blood Cells Mol. Dis.* 65, 81–85. doi: 10.1016/j.bcmd.2017.03.005

Watanabe, T., Michaelis, T., and Frahm, J. (2001). Mapping of retinal projections in the living rat using high-resolution 3D gradient-echo MRI with Mn^{2+}-induced contrast. *Magn. Reson. Med.* 46, 424–429. doi: 10.1002/mrm.1209

Watanabe, T., Natt, O., Boretius, S., Frahm, J., and Michaelis, T. (2002). *In vivo* 3D MRI staining of mouse brain after subcutaneous application of $MnCl_2$. *Magn. Reson. Med.* 48, 852–859. doi: 10.1002/mrm.10276

Weil, R. S., Costantini, A. A., and Schrag, A. E. (2018). Mild cognitive impairment in Parkinson's disease-what is it? *Curr. Neurol. Neurosci. Rep.* 18:17. doi: 10.1007/s11910-018-0823-9

Weintraub, D., Troster, A. I., Marras, C., and Stebbins, G. (2018). Initial cognitive changes in Parkinson's disease. *Mov. Disord.* 33, 511–519. doi: 10.1002/mds.27330

Weng, J.-C., Tikhonova, M. A., Chen, J.-H., Shen, M.-S., Meng, W.-Y., Chang, Y.-T., et al. (2016). Ceftriaxone prevents the neurodegeneration and decreased neurogenesis seen in a Parkinson's disease rat model: an immunohistochemical and MRI study. *Behav. Brain Res.* 305, 126–139. doi: 10.1016/j.bbr.2016.02.034

Yamamoto, T., Rossi, S., Stiefel, M., Doppenberg, E., Zauner, A., Bullock, R., et al. (1999). CSF and ECF glutamate concentrations in head injured patients. *Neuromonit. Brain Inj.* 75, 17–19. doi: 10.1007/978-3-7091-6415-0_4

Yang, P.-F., Chen, D.-Y., Hu, J. W., Chen, J.-H., and Yen, C.-T. (2011). Functional tracing of medial nociceptive pathways using activity-dependent manganese-enhanced MRI. *Pain* 152, 194–203. doi: 10.1016/j.pain.2010.10.027

Yang, J., Li, Q., Wang, M., Cao, X., Ding, Y., Wang, G., et al. (2016). Semiquantitative assessment of optic nerve injury using manganese-enhanced MRI. *Jpn. J. Radiol.* 34, 356–365. doi: 10.1007/s11604-016-0533-7

Young, W. (1992). Role of calcium in central nervous system injuries. *J. Neurotrauma* 9, S9–S25.

Yri, O. E., Vig, J., Hegstad, E., Hovde, O., Pignon, I., and Jynge, P. (2009). Mangafodipir as a cytoprotective adjunct to chemotherapy—a case report. *Acta Oncol.* 48, 633–635. doi: 10.1080/02841860802680427

Yu, X., Sanes, D. H., Aristizabal, O., Wadghiri, Y. Z., and Turnbull, D. H. (2007). Large-scale reorganization of the tonotopic map in mouse auditory midbrain revealed by MRI. *Proc. Natl. Acad. Sci. U S A* 104, 12193–12198. doi: 10.1073/pnas.0700960104

Yu, X., Zou, J., Babb, J. S., Johnson, G., Sanes, D. H., and Turnbull, D. H. (2008). Statistical mapping of sound-evoked activity in the mouse auditory midbrain using Mn-enhanced MRI. *Neuroimage* 39, 223–230. doi: 10.1016/j.neuroimage.2007.08.029

Yu, X., Wadghiri, Y. Z., Sanes, D. H., and Turnbull, D. H. (2005). *in vivo* auditory brain mapping in mice with Mn-enhanced MRI. *Nat. Neurosci.* 8, 961–968. doi: 10.1038/nn1477

Zaca, D., Agarwal, S., Gujar, S. K., Sair, H. I., and Pillai, J. J. (2014). Special considerations/technical limitations of blood-oxygen-level-dependent functional magnetic resonance imaging. *Neuroimaging Clin. N. Am.* 24, 705–715. doi: 10.1016/j.nic.2014.07.006

Zoni, S., and Lucchini, R. G. (2013). Manganese exposure: cognitive, motor and behavioral effects on children: a review of recent findings. *Curr. Opin. Pediatr.* 25, 255–260. doi: 10.1097/mop.0b013e32835e906b

18

In vivo X-Nuclear MRS Imaging Methods for Quantitative Assessment of Neuroenergetic Biomarkers in Studying Brain Function and Aging

*Xiao-Hong Zhu * and Wei Chen **

Center for Magnetic Resonance Research (CMRR), Department of Radiology, School of Medicine, University of Minnesota, Minneapolis, MN, United States

***Correspondence:**
Xiao-Hong Zhu
zhu@cmrr.umn.edu
Wei Chen
wei@cmrr.umn.edu

Brain relies on glucose and oxygen metabolisms to generate biochemical energy in the form of adenosine triphosphate (ATP) for supporting electrophysiological activities and neural signaling under resting or working state. Aging is associated with declined mitochondrial functionality and decreased cerebral energy metabolism, and thus, is a major risk factor in developing neurodegenerative diseases including Alzheimer's disease (AD). However, there is an unmet need in the development of novel neuroimaging tools and sensitive biomarkers for detecting abnormal energy metabolism and impaired mitochondrial function, especially in an early stage of the neurodegenerative diseases. Recent advancements in developing multimodal high-field *in vivo* X-nuclear (e.g., ^{2}H, ^{17}O and ^{31}P) MRS imaging techniques have shown promise for quantitative and noninvasive measurement of fundamental cerebral metabolic rates of glucose and oxygen consumption, ATP production as well as nicotinamide adenine dinucleotide (NAD) redox state in preclinical animal and human brains. These metabolic neuroimaging measurements could provide new insights and quantitative bioenergetic markers associated with aging processing and neurodegeneration and can therefore be employed to monitor disease progression and/or determine effectiveness of therapeutic intervention.

Keywords: *in vivo* X-nuclear MRS imaging, brain energy metabolism, neuroenergetics, mitochondrial function, ultra-high magnetic field (UHF), aging, neurodegeneration

MITOCHONDRIAL DYSFUNCTION AND NEUROENERGETIC DEFICIENCY AS HALLMARKS OF AGING AND NEURODEGENERATION

Aging is an inevitable process of life. With the rapid growth of the elderly population, brain diseases associated with functional decline and neurodegeneration, such as cognitive impairment (CI), Alzheimer's disease (AD) and Parkinson's disease (PD), not only have a huge impact on people's quality of life, but also greatly increase the social and economic burdens. As a complex biological process, aging (defined as an age-progressive decline in intrinsic physiological function) can be influenced by many factors other than the actual age, such as heredity, lifestyle, income and living environment.

Mitochondria are organelles found in the cells of complex organism and they produce >90% of the adenosine triphosphate (ATP) energy molecules in the brain via the oxidative phosphorylation of adenosine diphosphate (ADP). In addition to supporting unceasing neuronal activity, neurotransmission, cellular signaling and other functions under different brain states, approximately one-quarter of total ATP energy expenditure in the human brain is used for biosynthesis and "housekeeping" functions to maintain cellular integrity (Siesjo, 1978; Erecińska and Silver, 1989; Barinaga, 1997; Rolfe and Brown, 1997; Boyer, 1999; Attwell and Laughlin, 2001; Shulman et al., 2004; Hyder et al., 2006; Du et al., 2008; Zhu et al., 2015a). A coupling relationship between the neuronal activity and ATP energy consumption of the brain tissue holds for a wide range of physiological conditions and brain relies on an effective metabolic regulation to balance the ATP supply and demand through key biochemical reactions associated with energy metabolism (Du et al., 2008; Zhu et al., 2012, 2018). Under normal circumstances, the mitochondrial ATP production rate in the brain is indirectly but closely coupled with the cerebral metabolic rates of glucose (CMR_{Glc}) and oxygen ($CMRO_2$) and tightly regulated by the nicotinamide adenine dinucleotide (NAD) redox state, which can be determined by the intracellular concentration ratio of the oxidized (NAD^+) and reduced (NADH) NAD molecules (i.e., NAD redox ratio: RX_{NAD}).

As depicted in **Figure 1**, the circulating blood flow constantly supplies oxygen and glucose to the brain tissue, where the glucose is transported into the brain cells and converted to pyruvate via glycolysis and produces two ATP and two NADH molecules from each glucose molecule consumed in the cytosol. Most pyruvate molecules enter the mitochondria to form acetyl Co-A, its oxidation via the tricarboxylic acid (TCA) cycle produces eight NADH molecules that can be converted to NAD^+ molecules through oxygen metabolism (Stryer, 1988). The electron transport chain reactions extrude H^+ ions from mitochondria to generate an electrochemical potential gradient across the mitochondrial inner membrane, which is the driving force for the mitochondrial F_1F_0-ATP_{ase} mediated enzyme reaction that synthesizes ATP from ADP and inorganic phosphate (Pi; producing >30 ATPs per consumed glucose under physiological condition) and transports the H^+ ions back into mitochondria (Siesjo, 1978; Hyder et al., 2006). The ATP utilization occurs in the cytosol via the ATP hydrolysis reaction. The majority of the ATP energy are used to maintain the Na^+/K^+ ion gradients across the cell membrane for supporting action potential propagation, neuronal firing and neurotransmitter cycling (Siesjo, 1978; Stryer, 1988; Shulman et al., 1999). The rapid ATP turnover requires efficient transportation of the ATP molecules between the cytosolic and mitochondrial compartments to maintain the intracellular ATP homeostasis. This is accomplished partly by a creatine kinase (CK) catalyzed near-equilibrium chemical exchange between ATP + Creatine (Cr) and phosphocreatine (PCr) + ADP (Kemp, 2000; Du et al., 2008).

Although it only accounts for 2% of the total body weight, the human brain has enormous energy needs. The resting adult brain receives approximately 15% of the cardiac output and uses most (~20%) of systemic oxygen and glucose consumptions (Raichle, 1987; Shulman et al., 2004; Hyder et al., 2006). It is worth noting that the intracellular ATP concentration in the brain is very low (~3 mM); the entire human brain only contains approximately 2 g of ATP (assuming an average adult brain weight of 1.4 kg). In contrast, the rate of ATP synthesis by the F_1F_0-ATP_{ase} reaction is very high (8–9 µmole/g/min) in the human brain (Lei et al., 2003a; Du et al., 2007; Zhu et al., 2012), indicating that a human brain produces 7–8 kg of ATP molecules (about 5–6 times of the human brain weight) in 1 day. The extreme high turnover between the ATP production and utilization is critical in fulfilling the high energy demand of the neuronal cells and maintaining the intracellular ATP homeostasis.

The conversion between NAD^+ and NADH through the NAD redox reaction determines the intracellular NAD redox state, which controls the balance of cytosolic glycolysis and mitochondrial oxidative phosphorylation to produce adequate ATP molecules (Chance et al., 1962; Lu et al., 2014b; Zhu et al., 2015b). Mitochondrial dysfunction and energy deficiency are the key cellular hallmarks of aging and neurodegeneration, suggesting that mitochondria can serve as therapeutic targets for various neurodegenerative diseases or for monitoring the aging processes (Creasey and Rapoport, 1985; Rapoport, 1999; Balaban et al., 2005; Guarente, 2008; Yap et al., 2009; Reddy and Reddy, 2011; Nunnari and Suomalainen, 2012; López-Otín et al., 2013; Pathak et al., 2013; Lin et al., 2014; Yin et al., 2014). Therefore, the development of quantitative, reliable and sensitive neuroimaging tools or biomarkers capable of assessing mitochondrial function and cerebral energy metabolism is essential for studying the underlying mechanisms of human brain aging and monitoring the progression of aging-related brain disorders. Furthermore, biomarkers with improved specificity and sensitivity can be potentially used to distinguish normal aging from neurodegeneration, provide early diagnoses, identify therapeutic targets and evaluate treatment efficacy.

DEVELOPMENT OF NEUROIMAGING BIOMARKERS FOR STUDYING AGING AND UNDERLYING MECHANISM IN HUMAN BRAIN

Modern neuroimaging techniques have played important roles in study of human brain aging and diagnosis of neurodegenerative diseases; in particular, Positron Emission Tomography (PET) has been well established to evaluate regional brain glucose and oxygen utilization, neurochemical and neurotransmitter changes, and inflammation in AD and PD brains (Borghammer et al., 2010; Brooks and Pavese, 2011; Niccolini et al., 2014; Varley et al., 2015). For instance, the PET imaging based on radioactive fludeoxyglucose (^{18}FDG) is used to measure the glucose uptake rate that thought to reflect CMR_{Glc}. The ^{18}FDG-PET has been extensively employed to study human brain aging; however, contradictory findings with either negative (Duara et al., 1983, 1984) or positive (Pantano et al., 1984;

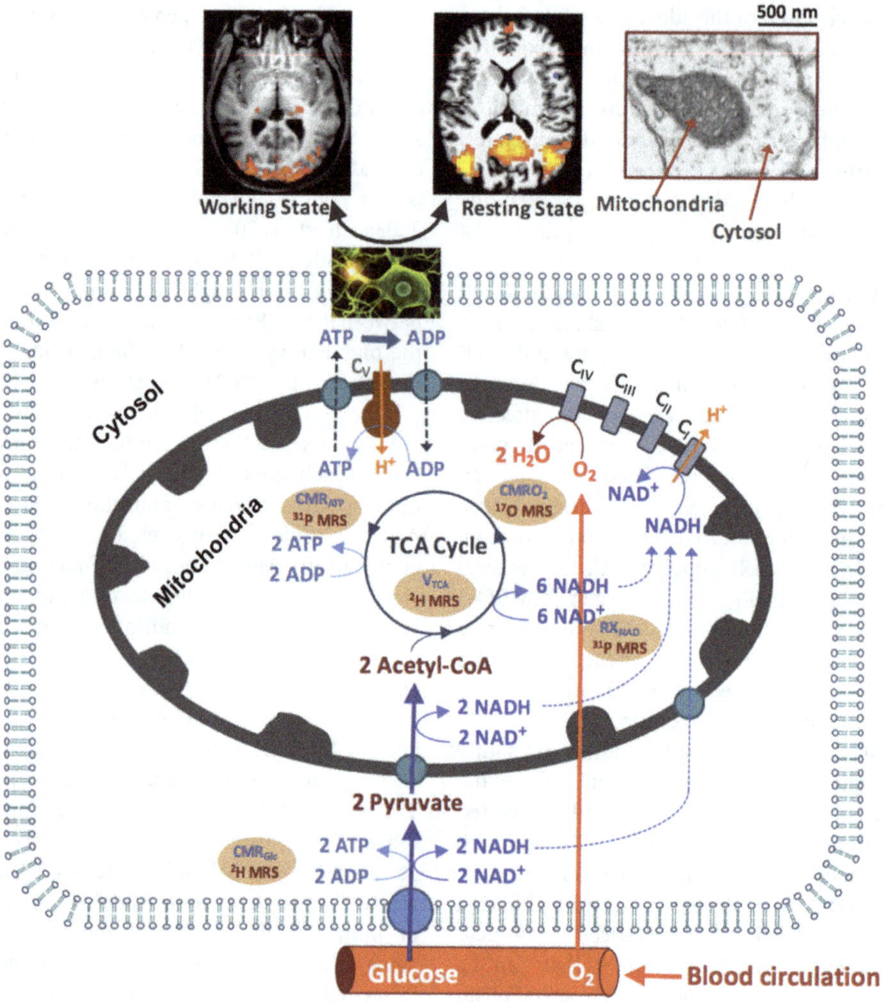

FIGURE 1 | Schematic illustration of major brain hemodynamic and metabolic processes occur in capillary, cytosol and mitochondrial sub-cellular compartments. The feeding arteries supply oxygen and glucose to the cell; glucose is converted to pyruvate, which enters mitochondrial tricarboxylic acid (TCA) cycle and oxidative metabolism pathways. The oxygen utilization is generally coupled with the adenosine triphosphate (ATP) production via the oxidative phosphorylation of adenosine diphosphate (ADP). The ATP is utilized in cytosol to support electrophysiological activities and brain functions at resting and/or working state. The NAD redox reactions are essential in regulating the ATP energy production. The cerebral metabolic rates of glucose (CMR_{Glc}), oxygen ($CMRO_2$) and ATP production (CMR_{ATP}), TCA cycle rate (V_{TAC}) and nicotinamide adenine dinucleotide (NAD) redox ratio (RX_{NAD}) representing the metabolic activities of the brain tissue can be noninvasively measured or imaged using the advanced *in vivo* X-nuclear ^2H, ^{17}O and ^{31}P MRS approaches as depicted in the shadowed texts with orange background. C_I-C_V represent five enzyme complexes involving in the cellular respiration chain reactions.

Yamaguchi et al., 1986; Leenders et al., 1990; Marchal et al., 1992; De Santi et al., 1995; Goyal et al., 2017) correlation between actual age and CMR_{Glc} in healthy human have been reported. Note that ^{18}FDG-PET based CMR_{Glc} image reflects the total glucose metabolism through both mitochondrial oxidative phosphorylation and aerobic glycolysis pathways including the conversion of pyruvates (products of glycolysis) into lactates; therefore, it does not directly represent the actual mitochondrial neuroenergetics, which can be determined by $CMRO_2$. Significant $CMRO_2$ reductions in elderly people have been reported, indicating a tight correlation between the mitochondrial energy metabolism and aging (Yamaguchi et al., 1986; Leenders et al., 1990). The $CMRO_2$ decline is consistent with significant decreases in respiratory enzyme (Complexes I–V) activities observed in aging mice brain (Ferrándiz et al., 1994; Navarro and Boveris, 2007), and is in line with a human brain study showing an approximately 30% reduction in both neuronal oxidative glucose metabolism and neurotransmission cycling rates in elderly people (Boumezbeur et al., 2010).

However, there is a lack of sophisticated neuroimaging methods that can quantitatively and noninvasively assess brain mitochondrial enzymatic activities and ATP bioenergetics, even though they play a central role in human aging and neurodegeneration. Most predictive biomarkers offered by neuroimaging are neither sufficiently nor proximal to sub-cellular mechanisms of aging to link mitochondrial and ATP bioenergetic functions. In this article, we will provide a brief review of several advanced metabolic neuroimaging methods that are based on *in vivo* X-nuclear magnetic resonance (MR) spectroscopic (MRS) imaging (MRSI) at ultra-high magnetic field (UHF) for noninvasive imaging and quantitative assessment of human brain mitochondrial functions and associated bioenergetic biomarkers, which could be highly sensitive to aging without using radioactive tracers. Three *in vivo* X-nuclear MRS methods for imaging cerebral energy metabolisms following specific metabolic pathways are discussed:

1. *In vivo* deuterium-2 (^2H) MRSI method for simultaneously measuring CMR_{Glc} and the TCA cycle rate (V_{TCA}),
2. *In vivo* oxygen-17 (^{17}O) MRSI method for quantitatively imaging three physiological parameters: $CMRO_2$, cerebral blood flow (CBF) and oxygen extraction fraction (OEF),
3. *In vivo* phosphorus-31 (^{31}P) MRSI method for simultaneous measurement of cerebral metabolic rates of ATP synthesis via the ATP_{ase} reaction (CMR_{ATP}) and CK reaction (CMR_{CK}), as well as for measuring intracellular NAD^+ and NADH, thus, the NAD redox ratio (RX_{NAD}).

These X-nuclear MRSI methods provide complementary measurements of brain energy metabolisms and ATP bioenergetics following the metabolic roadmap as shown in **Figure 1**.

In vivo carbon-13 (^{13}C) MRS is another X-nuclear MRS method that has been used to study energy metabolism and neurotransmission in animal and human brains. By combining dynamic ^{13}C MRS with ^{13}C-labeled substrates administration and compartmentalized quantification model, the metabolic fluxes of various pathways involving glucose metabolism and neuronal-astrocyte compartmental exchange can be assessed via monitoring the ^{13}C-label incorporation to the major metabolites along these pathways. The strength and limitations of the ^{13}C MRS technique and its applications have been extensively reviewed (e.g., Rothman et al., 2011 #1543; Rodrigues et al., 2013 #1544; Sonnay et al., 2017 #1542), and thus, is covered in this article.

LIMITATIONS OF *IN VIVO* X-NUCLEAR MRSI AND ADVANTAGES OF ULTRA-HIGH FIELD

To apply the *in vivo* X-nuclear MRS or MRSI in biomedical research, we face many challenges, in particular, owing to the very low concentration of detectable metabolites (in the range of few or sub-millimolar (mM)) that is several to tens of thousands of times lower than the tissue water content detected by ^1H MRI. Additionally, since the gyromagnetic ratios of the X-nuclei (e.g., ^2H, ^{13}C, ^{17}O and ^{31}P) are several times lower than that of ^1H, the intrinsic detection sensitivity and signal-to-noise ratio (SNR) of the X-nuclear MRS are further reduced, thus, extensive signal averaging is required to achieve reasonable SNR and spatial resolution. These factors have limited the reliability, applicability and spatiotemporal resolution of the *in vivo* MRSI measurements. To address these limitations, it has been shown that UHF scanners can provide a significant SNR gain and improve spectral and spatial resolutions. The advantages of the UHF for *in vivo* ^{31}P and ^{17}O MRS brain applications are described below.

The ^{31}P nuclide has been studied extensively since the inception of *in vivo* MRS (Shulman et al., 1979; Ackerman et al., 1980; Shoubridge et al., 1982). Besides high energy phosphate compounds (ATP and PCr) and Pi, other phosphorus metabolites such as NAD^+ and NADH that are actively involved in the NAD redox reaction, glycerophosphoethanolamine (GPE), glycerophosphocholine (GPC), phosphoethanolamine (PE) and phosphocholine (PC) which are essential to membrane phospholipid metabolism could also be detected by *in vivo* ^{31}P MRS. The reduced resonance linewidths (in the ppm unit) at higher field will significantly improve the ^{31}P spectral resolution, which makes it possible to resolve adjacent or overlapped phosphate resonances, determine the redox ratio of NAD (Lu et al., 2014b, 2016a; Zhu et al., 2015b), and distinguish intracellular and extracellular Pi *in vivo*. Interestingly, the T_1 values of most phosphorus metabolites decrease at higher fields, presumably the chemical shift anisotropy (CSA) dominates the longitudinal relaxation mechanism at UHF. The shortened T_1 allows more signal averaging per unit sampling time, thus, further improves the SNR and leads to a super linear dependence of the ^{31}P MRS sensitivity on the magnetic field strength (B_0) after considering the B_0 dependences of T_1 and resonance linewidth (Qiao et al., 2006; Lu et al., 2014a).

^{17}O is a stable and NMR detectable isotope of oxygen; it has a very low natural abundance (0.037%) and one-seventh gyromagnetic ratio of the ^1H. The ^{17}O isotope with a quantum number of 5/2 obeys the quadrupolar relaxation mechanism, thus, the ^{17}O nuclide in water ($H_2{}^{17}O$) has very short longitudinal (T_1) and transverse (T_2, or apparent T_2: T_2^*) relaxation times (<7 ms) that are insensitive to the B_0 inhomogeneity (Zhu et al., 2001, 2005; Lu et al., 2013). The SNR of the ^{17}O brain water signal has an approximate quadratic field dependence on the static magnetic field strength (i.e., SNR $\propto B_0^2$; Zhu et al., 2001; Lu et al., 2013), while the ^1H MRI has an approximate linear field dependence (Vaughan et al., 2001). The field dependence of the brain $H_2{}^{17}O$ signal across a wide range of B_0 indicates an over 120 times SNR gain at 16.4T as compared to a 1.5T clinical MRI scanner. Therefore, it is possible to obtain three-dimensional (3D) ^{17}O MRSI of the animal or human brain with adequate SNR and reasonable spatiotemporal resolution at ultrahigh fields. Furthermore, the sensitivity gain at UHF is essential for the development of the *in vivo* ^{17}O MR-based neuroimaging methodology in assessing cerebral oxygen metabolism and perfusion. The UHF advantages are also expected in *in vivo* ^2H MRSI applications owing to a similar quadrupolar relaxation mechanism.

SIMULTANEOUS ASSESSMENT OF CMR_{Glc} and V_{TCA} USING *IN VIVO* ^2H MRS TECHNIQUE

CMR_{Glc} and V_{TCA} are key parameters presenting the rates of glucose metabolism in brain tissue. Ability to quantify their values *in vivo* is crucial for assessing the metabolic and energetic states of the brain. As shown in **Figure 1**, the stoichiometric ratio of the CMR_{Glc} and V_{TCA} in normal brain is approximately two to one since one glucose can produce two pyruvates in cytosol before entering the mitochondrial TCA cycle; such coupling relationship can change under pathological condition, e.g., in brain tumor or stroke. Even though it is challenging, quantitative and simultaneous imaging of both CMR_{Glc} and V_{TCA} is desired for studying the complex glucose metabolic pathways and their contributions to the ATP production under normal and diseased states. Recently, we have developed an *in vivo* ^2H MRS technique for simultaneous CMR_{Glc} and V_{TCA} measurement; this technique has been validated at 16.4T using a preclinical rat model (Lu et al., 2017).

^2H nuclide is a stable isotope of hydrogen with a quantum number of 1 and has an extremely low natural abundance (0.0156%). Like ^{17}O nuclide, molecules containing ^2H obey quadrupolar relaxation mechanism and have short T_1 and T_2 values that enables rapid signal averaging for gaining the SNR. Thus, the *in vivo* ^2H MRS or MRSI becomes attractive at UHF when combining with ^2H-isotope (deuterium) labeled glucose infusion (Mateescu et al., 2011; Lu et al., 2017). After infusion, several deuterium labeled compounds, including the glycolysis and TCA cycle intermediates of the brain tissue, e.g., glutamate/glutamine (Glx), lactate (Lac) and water, can be detected using the UHF ^2H MRS with excellent sensitivity and temporal resolution and identified based on their well-resolved ^2H resonances and chemical shifts. The robust ^2H MRS signal detection, spectral analysis and kinetic modeling eventually allow for quantification of CMR_{Glc} and V_{TCA} in live brains.

Figure 2A displays the ^2H-isotope labeling scheme, labeled metabolites and associated metabolic pathways following an intravenous D-Glucose-6,6-d_2 (d66) infusion (Mateescu et al., 2011; Lu et al., 2017), where d66 glucose and non-labeled glucose are transported together into the brain and metabolized via glycolysis and oxidative phosphorylation. Along the metabolic pathways, the deuterium label on d66 can incorporate into the Lac, Glx and water pools, which can then be monitored through dynamic ^2H MRS acquisitions. Excellent spectral quality and spectral fittings can be obtained not only from d66 phantom solution (with water resonance set at 4.8 ppm as a chemical shift reference) but also from living rat brain; for instance, well-resolved deuterated resonances of glucose (3.8 ppm), Glx (2.4 ppm) and lactate (1.4 ppm) were detected following a brief (2 min) d66 infusion (**Figure 2B**). Their dynamic signal changes (15 s temporal resolution) were used to determine the CMR_{Glc} and V_{TCA} values based on a simplified kinetic model (Lu et al., 2017). The *in vivo* ^2H MRS approach has been applied to rat brains under isoflurane anesthesia and morphine analgesic condition; significant reduction of CMR_{Glc} and V_{TCA} in rat brains under 2% isoflurane (CMR_{Glc} = 0.28 ± 0.13 and V_{TCA} = 0.6 ± 0.2 μmol/g/min) as compared to that of morphine (CMR_{Glc} = 0.46 ± 0.06 and V_{TCA} = 0.96 ± 0.4 μmol/g/min) were found (Lu et al., 2017), suggesting that the *in vivo* ^2H MRS technique is highly sensitive in detecting the cerebral metabolic rate changes.

Compared with the *in vivo* ^{13}C MRS (Gruetter et al., 2003), several merits of the *in vivo* ^2H MRS technology are worth mentioning: (i) the short T_1 relaxation time of the quadrupolar ^2H nuclide (e.g., ~50 ms for d66 in rat brain at 16.4T; Lu et al., 2017) enables rapid sampling to significantly increase the SNR for *in vivo* ^2H MRS or MRSI application (see an example in **Figure 2B**); (ii) the chemical shift assignments (in ppm) and spectral patterns of the deuterated metabolites are almost identical to that of *in vivo* ^1H MRS, while the chemical shift range (in Hz) of the ^2H spectrum is ~7 times narrower than that of ^1H MRS due to a much lower ^2H gyromagnetic ratio (6.5 MHz/T for ^2H vs. 42.6 MHz/T for ^1H), thus, the chemical shift displacement artifacts should be significantly reduced for ^2H MRS localization, especially at UHF (Chen and Zhu, 2005; Lu et al., 2017); on the other hand, it is challenging to study the neurotransmission cycling between neuron and glia cells using the ^2H MRS method due to the inability of resolving ^2H-labeled glutamate from glutamine (Sibson et al., 2001; Hyder et al., 2006); (iii) in an *in vivo* ^2H MRS spectrum, the natural abundant water signal of the brain tissue can serve as an internal reference for quantifying cerebral metabolites labeled with deuterium, which makes metabolites quantification easier and more reliable; and (iv) there is no background contamination in the ^2H spectrum of living brain because no natural abundance metabolite signal other than water is detectable *in vivo*, therefore, technique commonly applied in ^{13}C and ^1H MRS to suppress intense water or lipid signal is no longer needed.

The *in vivo* ^2H MRS approach could be highly valuable for studying the decoupled relationship between glycolysis and oxidative metabolism and image the Warburg effect in brain tumor. This can be achieved through directly measuring the metabolic rates of CMR_{Glc} and V_{TCA} using the ^2H MRSI approach or by simply mapping the Glx/Lac ratio (ideally measured when Glx and Lac signals reaching a plateau after the introduction of d66), which could provide a sensitive index of the Warburg effect in brain tumor (Lu et al., 2016b). To establish a completely noninvasive metabolic imaging based on the *in vivo* ^2H MRSI measurement, the intravenous infusion of the d66 tracer can be replaced by an oral delivery of d66. The feasibility of introducing d66 via oral intake for CMR_{Glc} and V_{TCA} measurement has been recently demonstrated (Lu et al., 2018), which paves the way for translational application.

NON-INVASIVE IMAGING OF $CMRO_2$, CBF AND OEF USING *IN VIVO* ^{17}O MR TECHNIQUE

The motivation of developing *in vivo* ^{17}O MR imaging techniques is to measure $CMRO_2$ via monitoring the dynamic change of the $H_2{}^{17}O$ water that is metabolized from ^{17}O-labeled O_2 gas (Mateescu et al., 1989; Pekar et al., 1991; Fiat and Kang, 1992, 1993; Reddy et al., 1996; Arai et al., 1998; Ronen et al., 1998; Zhu et al., 2002; Zhang et al., 2004; Atkinson and Thulborn, 2010; Kurzhunov et al., 2017; Niesporek et al., 2018). Generally, *in vivo* ^{17}O-MR imaging method shares a similar principle as the well-established ^{15}O-PET technique (Lenzi et al., 1981;

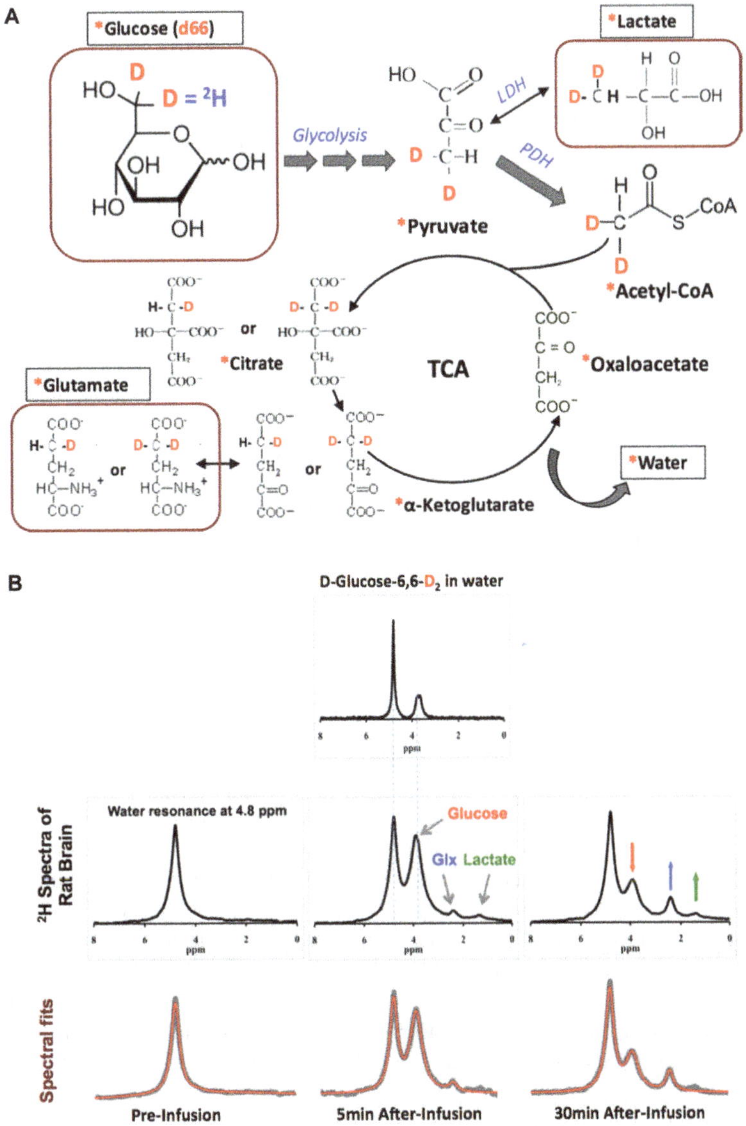

FIGURE 2 | (A) The ^{2}H-labeling scheme following the metabolic pathways of isotope-labeled glucose D-Glucose-6,6-d$_2$ (d66). The ^{2}H-labeled glucose first incorporates into pyruvate pool through glycolysis to form [3,3-d$_2$] pyruvate, some of which can be converted to [3,3-d$_2$] lactate by lactate dehydrogenase (LDH). [3,3-d$_2$] Pyruvate can also be transported into the mitochondria to form [2,2-d$_2$] Acetyl-CoA catalyzed by pyruvate dehydrogenase (PDH). After entering the TCA cycle, intermediates (4-d) or [4,4-d$_2$] citrate and (4-d) or [4,4-d$_2$] α-ketoglutarate could exchange with glutamate to generate (4-d) or [4,4-d$_2$] glutamate. In this process, the ^{2}H-labels may exchange with the proton(s) in water molecule to form deuterated water and depart from the cycle. "*": Pools labeled with ^{2}H; square boxes: highlighting the metabolites detectable by *in vivo* ^{2}H MRS. **(B)** Representative original (upper rows black traces and bottom row gray traces) and fitted (red traces in bottom row) ^{2}H spectra obtained from deuterated glucose (d66) phantom solution (top panel), and in rat brain pre- (left column) and 5 or 30 min post-deuterated glucose (d66) infusion. ^{2}H resonance assignments: water at 4.8 ppm (use as a chemical shift reference); glucose at 3.8 ppm; mixed glutamate and glutamine (Glx) at 2.4 ppm; and lactate at 1.4 ppm. Figure adapted from Lu et al. (2017).

Mintun et al., 1984) for imaging CMRO$_2$. Both modalities apply isotope-labeled oxygen gas inhalation in the measurement: $^{17}O_2$ for ^{17}O-MR and $^{15}O_2$ for ^{15}O-PET. After the inhalation, the isotope-labeled O$_2$ molecules bind to hemoglobin during the gas exchange in the lung and are subsequently delivered to the brain cells through blood circulation, perfusion and diffusion, and reduced by the cytochrome oxidase in the mitochondria to form the isotope-labeled water. One labeled oxygen molecule produces two labeled water molecules in the mitochondria, which can be washed out from the brain cells, enter the venous system and back to the heart via blood circulation.

Despite the common principle, there are fundamental differences between the ^{17}O-MR and ^{15}O-PET techniques in imaging CMRO$_2$. ^{15}O-PET cannot distinguish the radioactive signals attributed from the metabolic substrate ($^{15}O_2$) and the metabolic product ($H_2{}^{15}O$). Therefore, a standard PET-based CMRO$_2$ imaging method requires a complicate CMRO$_2$ quantification model plus multiple measurement procedures with: (i) inhalation of $^{15}O_2$ gas; (ii) injection of $H_2{}^{15}O$ tracer; and (iii) inhalation of $C^{15}O$ gas (Mintun et al., 1984), which substantially increase the total scanning time, radioactive dose and the measurement cost. The *in vivo* ^{17}O MR imaging method, on the other hand, only detects the metabolically generated and isotope-labeled $H_2{}^{17}O$. $^{17}O_2$ molecules, either freely dissolved or bound to hemoglobin are "invisible" to the *in vivo* ^{17}O detection (**Figure 3**) owing to the extremely broad ^{17}O resonance linewidth (Zhu et al., 2005; Zhu and Chen, 2011). This feature greatly simplifies the ^{17}O-MR based $CMRO_2$ imaging measurement that uses a non-radioactive and stable isotope, and thus, is more safer for human application (Zhang et al., 2004; Zhu et al., 2005; Atkinson and Thulborn, 2010).

The dynamics of the ^{17}O MR signal from the brain tissue $H_2{}^{17}O$ measured during and after an $^{17}O_2$ inhalation reflects an interplay of three physiological processes: (i) oxygen consumption to produce labeled $H_2{}^{17}O$ in the mitochondria, (ii) washout of labeled $H_2{}^{17}O$ from the brain cells via blood circulation, and (iii) "recirculation" of labeled $H_2{}^{17}O$ generated in the body re-entering the brain. The mass balance equation accounted the contributions from all three processes can be used for $CMRO_2$ quantification (Pekar et al., 1991; Zhu et al., 2002, 2005; Zhang et al., 2004; Atkinson and Thulborn, 2010):

$$\frac{dC_b(t)}{dt} = 2 \cdot \alpha(t)\, CMRO_2 + CBF \cdot \left[C_a(t) - \frac{C_b(t)}{\lambda}\right] \quad (1)$$

where $C_a(t)$, and $C_b(t)$ are the time-dependent and ^{17}O-isotope labeled $H_2{}^{17}O$ concentration in the arterial blood and brain tissue, respectively; $\alpha(t)$ is the ^{17}O enrichment fraction of the blood-contained $^{17}O_2$; λ is the brain/blood partition coefficient; the factor of 2 in Equation 1 accounts for the production of two $H_2{}^{17}O$ molecules from one $^{17}O_2$ molecule (Zhu et al., 2002; Zhang et al., 2004).

As demonstrated in **Figure 3**, there are three distinct phases in the brain $H_2{}^{17}O$ time course covering the baseline, inhalation and post-inhalation periods (Zhu et al., 2002). The signals in the first phase representing the natural abundance $H_2{}^{17}O$ in the brain tissue can serve as an internal reference for quantifying the brain $H_2{}^{17}O$ concentration and its change during the second and third phases. Equation 1 can be employed to calculate the $CMRO_2$ and CBF values, and estimate OEF (detailed quantification modeling and simplified approaches can be found in the literature (Zhu et al., 2002, 2013a,b).

One attractive feature of the ^{17}O-MR based $CMRO_2$ imaging approach is it enables repeated $CMRO_2$ measurements since the metabolized $H_2{}^{17}O$ signal in the brain can reach a new steady-state within a short time (e.g., <10 min in rodents, see **Figure 3**) at the end of the $^{17}O_2$ inhalation, so subsequent $CMRO_2$ measurements can be performed in the same subject within the same imaging session (Zhu et al., 2007). This capability is important for studying $CMRO_2$, CBF and OEF and their changes due to physiopathological perturbations where multiple measurements under different conditions are required.

For example, **Figure 4A** illustrates a functional study of blood oxygenation level dependent (BOLD) contrast and $CMRO_2$ changes in cat brain during visual stimulation (Zhu et al., 2009). Two 3D ^{17}O $CMRO_2$ imaging measurements, with and without visual stimulation, were performed on each animal. A significant increase in $CMRO_2$ (~30%) was detected in the activated visual cortical regions (**Figures 4A,B**); and interestingly, a strong inverse relation between the baseline $CMRO_2$ level and stimuli-induced $CMRO_2$ relative change across different subjects (**Figure 4C**) was observed (Zhu et al., 2009). **Figure 4D** demonstrates a preclinical application of the quantitative ^{17}O-MR imaging methodology for simultaneous and completely noninvasive mapping of $CMRO_2$, CBF and OEF in mouse brain using a brief $^{17}O_2$ inhalation (2–3 min), showing impaired $CMRO_2$ and CBF and elevated OEF in the ischemic brain region as compared to the intact brain tissue in the contralateral hemisphere (Zhu et al., 2013a).

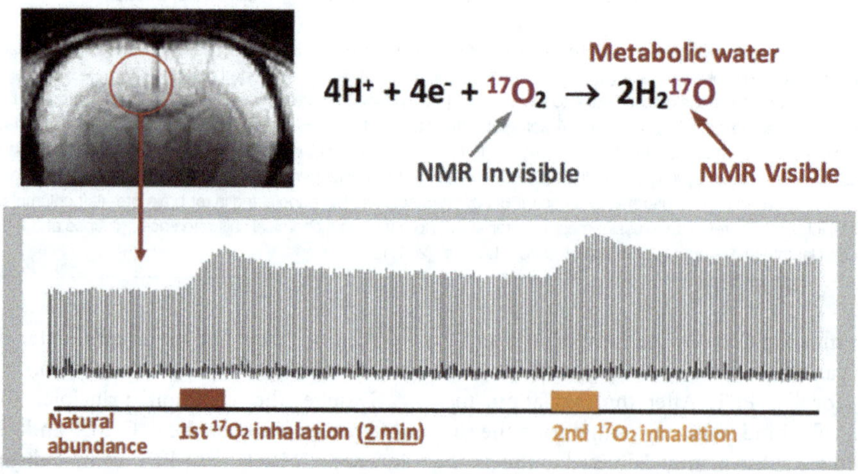

FIGURE 3 | Stack plots of rat brain tissue $H_2{}^{17}O$ spectra obtained from a single voxel selected from the 3D ^{17}O MRSI datasets with two consecutive $^{17}O_2$ inhalations (~2 min each) for repeated $CMRO_2$ and cerebral blood flow (CBF) imaging measurements. $^{17}O_2$ in either blood or brain tissue is NMR invisible. Figure adapted from Zhu et al. (2007).

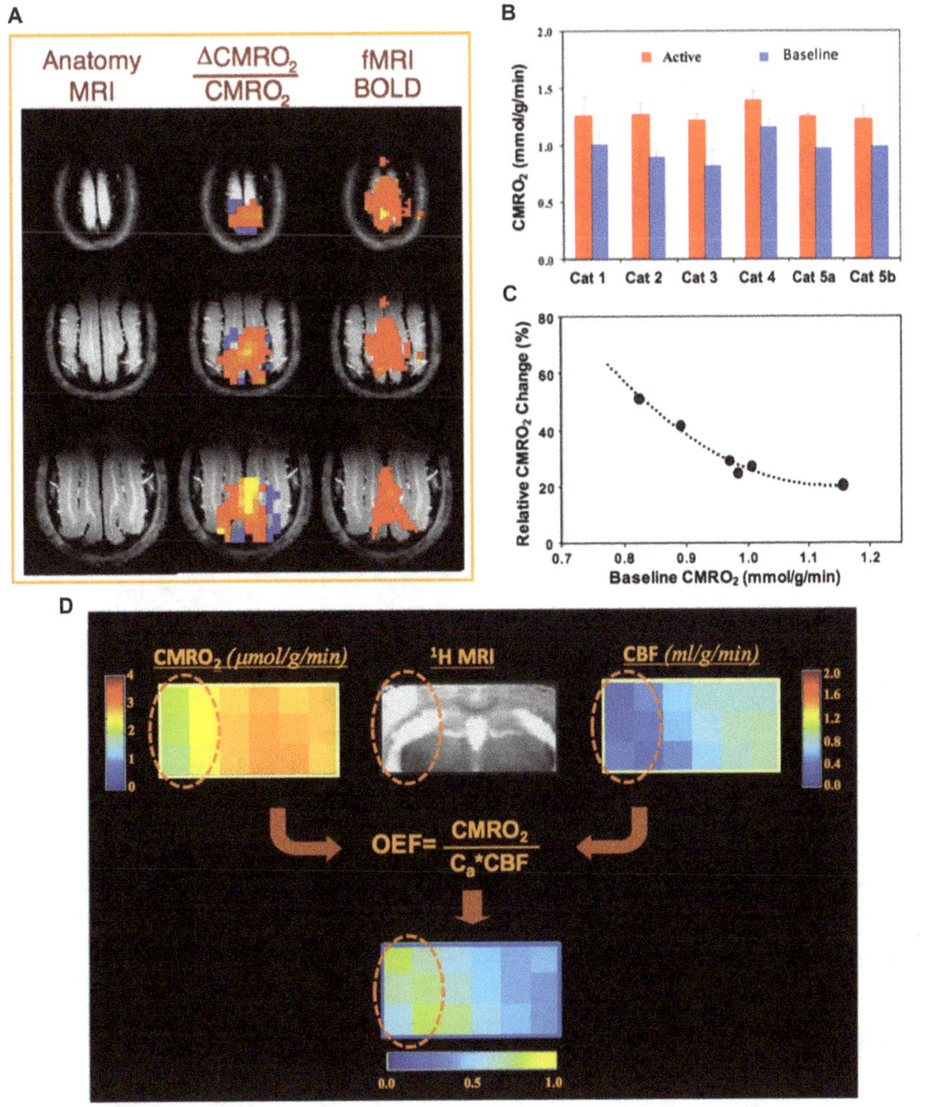

FIGURE 4 | (A) Anatomic brain images (left), fMRI blood oxygenation level dependent (BOLD) maps (right) and corresponding 3D functional $CMRO_2$ activation maps (middle) obtained from three representative image slices in a cat visual cortex, showing a significant $CMRO_2$ increase during visual stimulation. **(B)** Individual $CMRO_2$ values measured from the activated cat visual cortex region during visual stimulation as well as at control condition (baseline). Two functional studies conducted at different days in Cat 5, showing excellent $CMRO_2$ imaging reproducibility. **(C)** A strong correlation of baseline $CMRO_2$ level and activated $CMRO_2$ change among individual animals. Figure adapted from Zhu et al. (2009). **(D)** *In vivo* ^{17}O MRS imaging from a representative image slice in a mouse with middle cerebral artery occlusion (MCAO) preparation, showing significant reductions of $CMRO_2$ and CBF, and an elevated oxygen extraction fraction (OEF) in the ischemic brain region (cycled) affected by MCAO as compared to the intact tissue in the contralateral hemisphere. Figure adapted from Zhu et al. (2013a) with permission of Elsevier Inc.

For human brain application, due to the large body size, slow blood circulation and exchange of ^{17}O labeled and non-labeled oxygen gas in human lung, it is more challenging to reliably quantify $CMRO_2$, and a more sophisticated $CMRO_2$ quantification model is required (Atkinson and Thulborn, 2010; Zhu et al., 2014). Recently, we have demonstrated the feasibility for noninvasively imaging all three parameters of $CMRO_2$, CBF and OEF using a brief (2–3 min) $^{17}O_2$ inhalation in human visual cortex under resting condition and their changes in response to visual stimulation (Zhu et al., 2014).

STUDYING CEREBRAL ATP ENERGY METABOLISM AND NAD REDOX USING *IN VIVO* ^{31}P MRS TECHNIQUE

In vivo ^{31}P MRS is a powerful tool for studying cerebral phosphorus metabolism and neuroenergetics without the need for any isotopically labeled substrate. It not only detects various phosphorus metabolites, but also determines intracellular pH and free Mg^{2+} concentration of the brain tissue (Ackerman et al., 1980; Hetherington et al., 2002; Lei et al., 2003b; Du et al.,

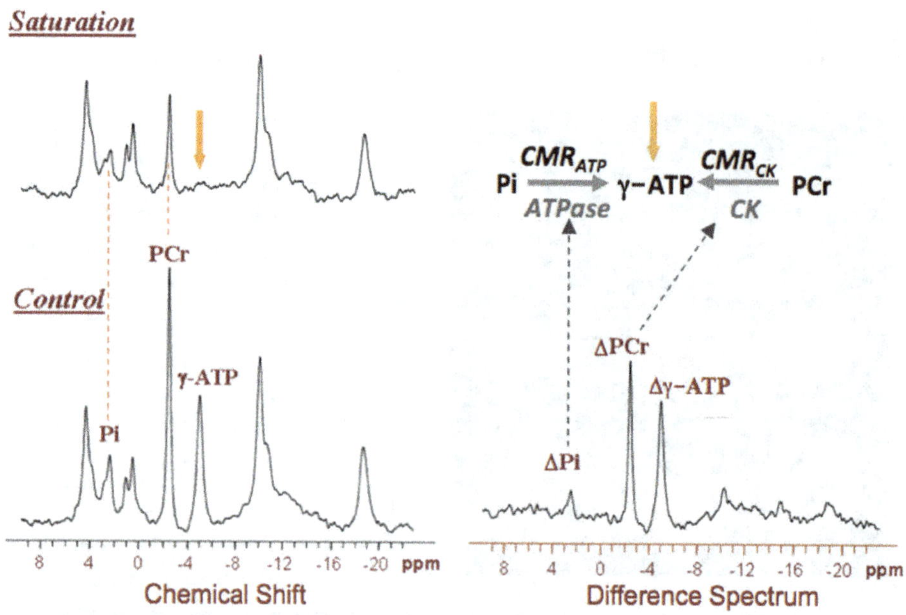

FIGURE 5 | *In vivo* ^{31}P spectra obtained from a representative healthy human brain in the absence (control) and presence of γ-ATP resonance saturation at 7T, and their difference spectrum. The signal reductions in the Pi and Phosphocreatine (PCr) resonances can be used to calculate the values of CMR_{ATP} and CMR_{CK}, respectively. Figure adapted from Lei et al. (2003a).

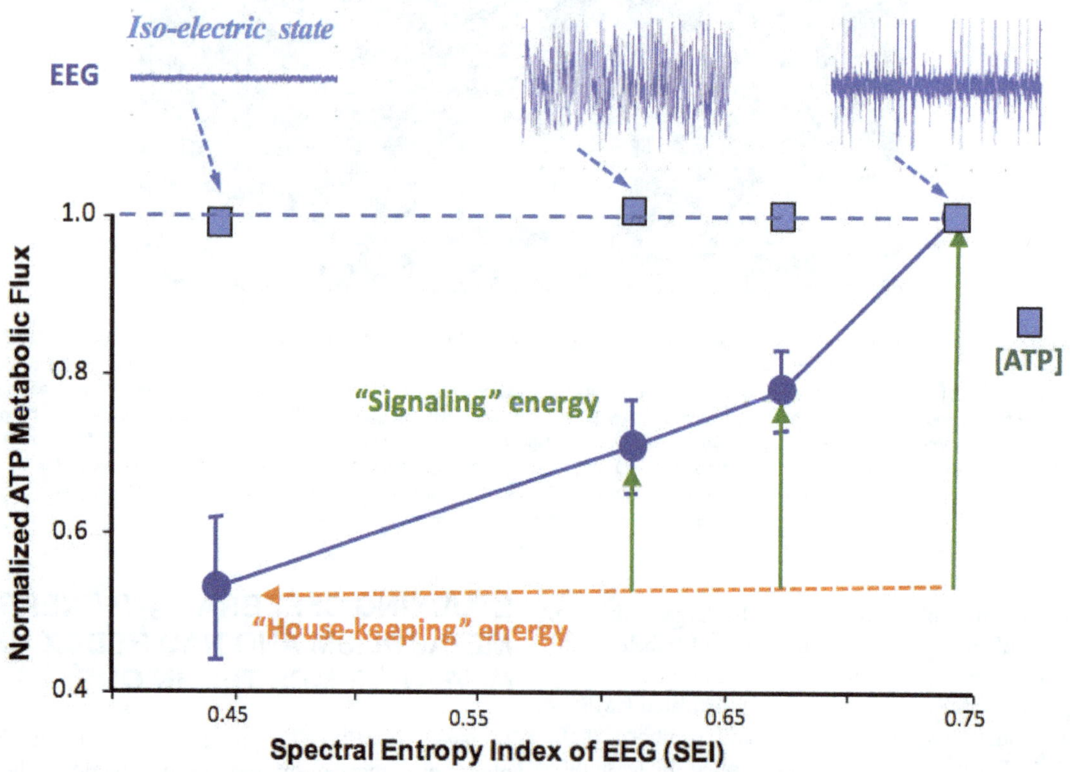

FIGURE 6 | Relationship of the rat brain electroencephalogram (EEG) activity level (top tracers) and normalized CMR_{ATP} or cerebral ATP concentration determined under different brain states. The EEG signal was quantified by the spectral entropy index (SEI). The CMR_{ATP} value correlates strongly with SEI, while intracellular ATP concentration remains constant even at the iso-electric state. Figure adapted from Du et al. (2008).

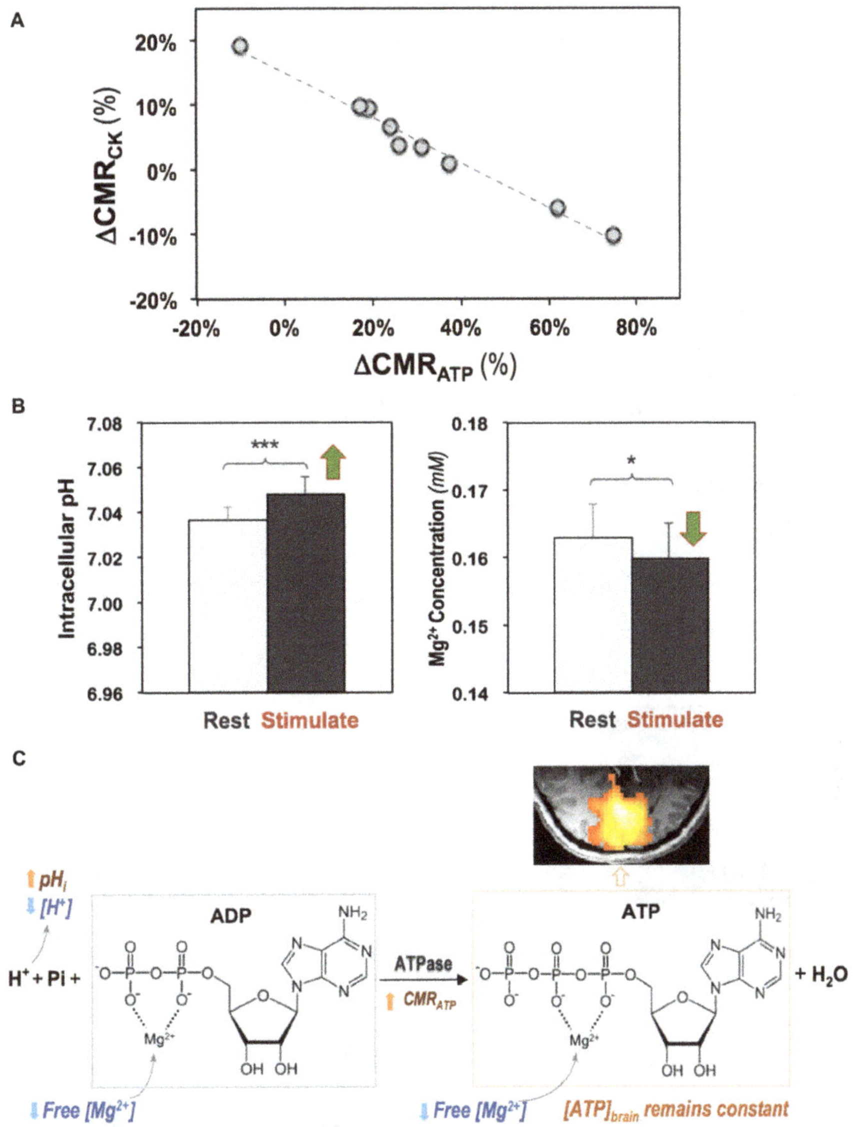

FIGURE 7 | (A) A strong and negative correlation between the stimulus-evoked CMR_{CK} and CMR_{ATP} changes among individual subjects; and **(B)** increased intracellular pH and decreased intracellular free Mg^{2+} level in human visual cortex during visual stimulation. **(C)** Schematic illustration of complex and coherent changes in ATPase activity, ATP production rate (CMR_{ATP}), intracellular pH and free (Mg^{2+}) in response to brain stimulation (Zhu et al., 2018). Two-tailed paired *t*-test indicating significant differences detected comparing the two conditions with $^{*}p < 0.05$ and $^{***}p < 0.001$.

2007, 2008; Zhu et al., 2012). Furthermore, when it combines with the magnetization transfer (MT) preparation (^{31}P MRS-MT), the enzyme activities and metabolic fluxes via the F_1F_0-ATPase and CK reactions can be measured and quantified (Frosén and Hoffman, 1963; Shoubridge et al., 1982; Uğurbil, 1985; Lei et al., 2003a; Du et al., 2007; Ren et al., 2017). Therefore, the *in vivo* ^{31}P MRS-MT technique can be used to noninvasively study abnormal mitochondrial function associated with energetic impairment in neurodegenerative diseases such as AD (Schägger and Ohm, 1995). **Figure 5** displays a typical ^{31}P MRS-MT dataset obtained in human brain at 7T. The signal reductions of the PCr and Pi resonances in the presence of γ-ATP saturation as compared to that of control can be used to calculate the "forward" metabolic fluxes for the CK reaction (i.e., PCr→ATP) and ATPase reaction (i.e., Pi→ATP), i.e., CMR_{CK} and CMR_{ATP}, respectively (Lei et al., 2003a; Du et al., 2007).

As shown in **Figure 6**, the *in vivo* ^{31}P MRS-MT method can be used to investigate the relation between the neuronal activity level and the ATP production rates at different brain states (Du et al., 2008). In this study, a strong positive correlation between the spontaneous brain electroencephalogram (EEG) activity and CMR_{ATP} was reported (Du et al., 2008); it was also found that when all electrophysiological signals are stopped (i.e., in an isoelectric state), the brain still consumes a significant portion of ATP energy for "house-keeping"

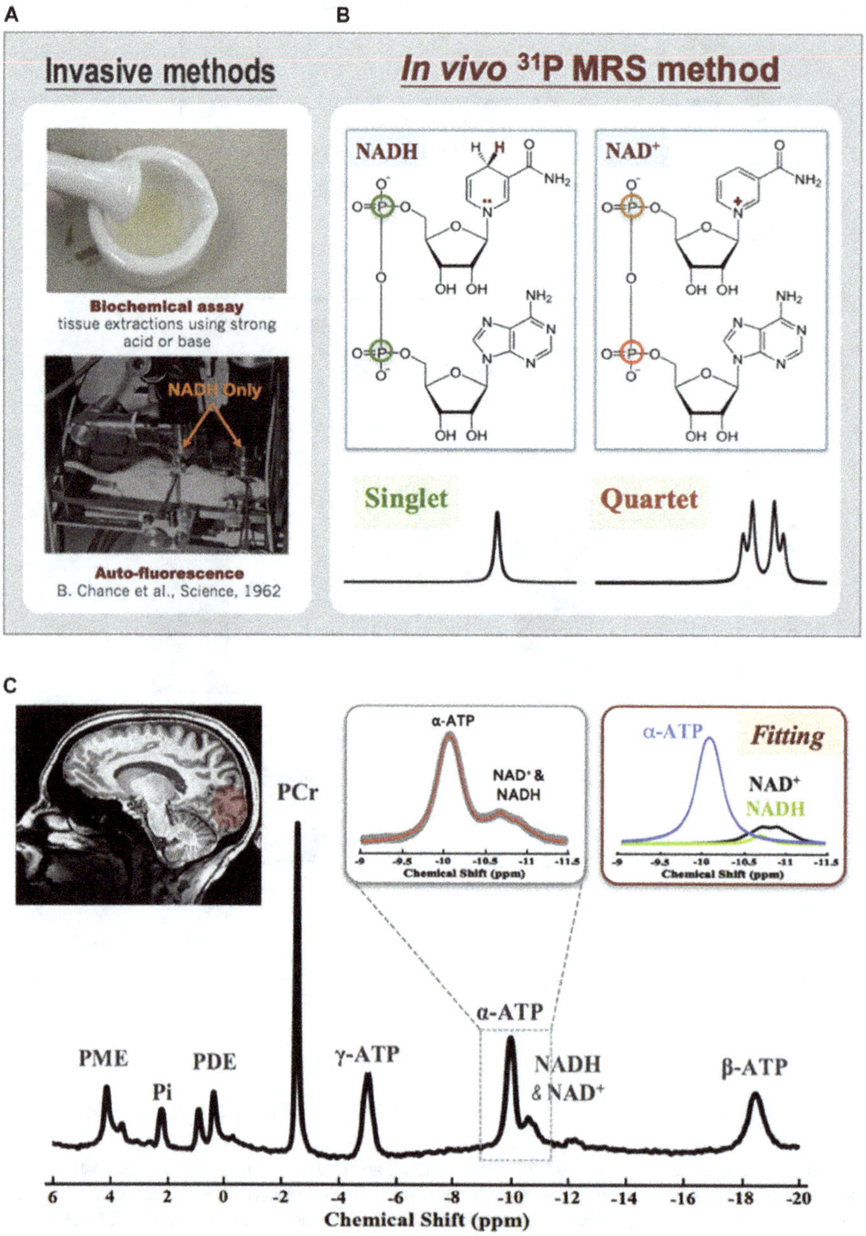

FIGURE 8 | (A) Two invasive methods are available for assessing intracellular NAD contents based on biochemical assay (top) or auto-fluorescence technique. **(B)** Molecular structures of NAD^+ and NADH and their distinct ^{31}P spectral patterns (singlet for NADH and quartet for NAD^+). **(C)** A representative ^{31}P spectrum obtained from the occipital lobe of a healthy subject at 7T. The expanded spectra in the inserts display a chemical shift range of −9.0 to −11.5 ppm with original ^{31}P signal (gray trace) and model fitted spectrum (red trace) of α-ATP and NAD. The individual fitting components of γ-ATP (blue), NAD^+ (black) and NADH (green) are also showed in the top-right panel. Figure adapted from Zhu et al. (2015b).

and maintaining the cellular integrity; and the brain ATP concentration remains constant while CMR_{ATP} could vary ~50% over a wide range of neuronal activity levels (see **Figure 6**). These findings suggest that under physiological conditions, the cerebral energy metabolism is effectively regulated to maintain the intracellular ATP homeostasis; and the metabolic rate of CMR_{ATP} should be a better biomarker for assessing energetic state of healthy brains (Du et al., 2008).

With improved sensitivity and spectral resolution at ultrahigh field of 7T and advancement in developing UHF radiofrequency (RF) coils, *in vivo* ^{31}P MRS-MT approach can be combined with 3D chemical shift imaging (CSI) to map the ATP metabolic rates in human brain with whole-head coverage. This makes it possible to differentiate CMR_{ATP} and CMR_{CK} between the human brain gray matter (GM) and white matter (WM), which led to the finding of three times higher CMR_{ATP} and CMR_{CK} in GM than WM. Also, it has been found that on average, a single neuron

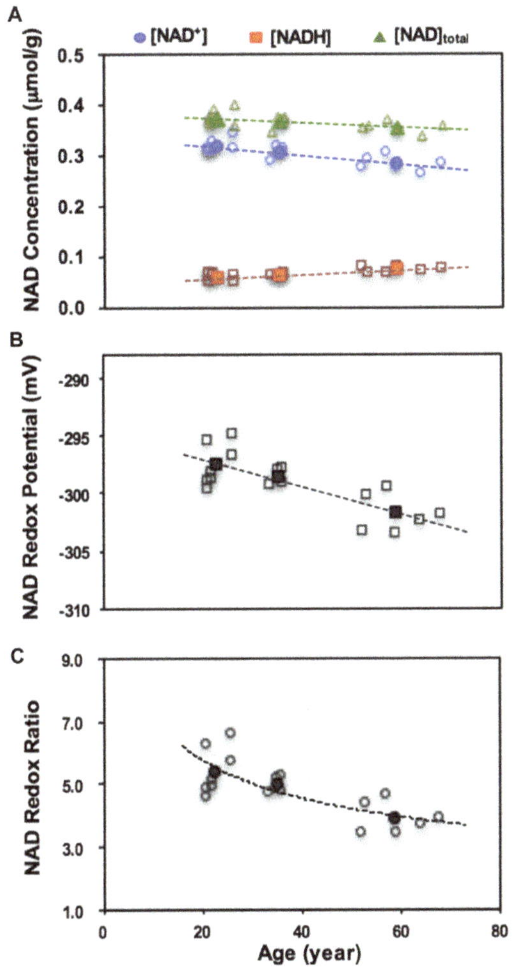

FIGURE 9 | Age dependences of intracellular NAD^+, NADH, total NAD concentrations **(A)**, the NAD redox potential **(B)** or redox ratio **(C)** observed in healthy human brains. The open symbols represent data of individual subjects and the filled symbols are the average data from three age groups of young (21–26 year, $n = 7$), middle (33–36 year, $n = 4$) and old (59–68 year, $n = 6$) subjects. Figure adapted from Zhu et al. (2015b).

consumes ~4.7 billion ATP molecules per second in human cortex at resting condition based on the direct CMR_{ATP} imaging measurement (Zhu et al., 2012).

Given the high ATP expenditure in a resting human brain, how a brain at working-state fulfills its energetic requirement is an important question for understanding the fundamental role of cerebral energetics in brain function and health. By applying the 3D ^{31}P CSI-MT imaging technique in human visual cortex at 7T, the regional CMR_{ATP} and CMR_{CK} at rest and during visual stimulation were directly measured; and a significant stimulus-induced and highly correlated neuroenergetic changes was detected, indicating that the ATPase and CK reactions play distinctive and complementary roles in supporting evoked neuronal activity and maintaining the intracellular ATP homeostasis (Zhu et al., 2018). **Figure 7** summarizes the results of this study showing a strong and negative correlation between the task-evoked CMR_{ATP} and CMR_{CK} changes in the activated human visual cortex among individual subjects (**Figure 7A**), and a significant increase in the intracellular pH accompanied by a reduction in the intracellular free $[Mg^{2+}]$ during the visual stimulation (**Figure 7B**). The findings of this original study provide interesting new insights into the mechanism of brain ATP energy metabolism and regulation in supporting evoked neuronal activity (**Figure 7C**), and demonstrate that the *in vivo* ^{31}P-MT imaging technique is a sensitive and highly valuable neuroimaging tool for quantitatively studying energy metabolism in human brain.

Brain energy metabolism and regulation are controlled by the metabolic coenzyme NAD and its redox state presented by the parameter of RX_{NAD} (= $[NAD^+]/[NADH]$). Extensive biological and cellular studies indicate that NAD^+ also functions as a co-substrate for several important enzymes including Sirtuins, poly-ADP-ribose polymerases (PARPs) and CD38/157 that play critical roles in cellular signaling, cell death, aging and longevity. Intracellular NAD^+ depletion has emerged as an indicator of aging and neurodegeneration, and thus, it is considered as a new therapeutic target for aging-related disorders and neurodegenerative diseases (Ying, 2007; Mouchiroud et al., 2013; Imai and Guarente, 2014; Verdin, 2015; Guarente, 2016; Mills et al., 2016; Schultz and Sinclair, 2016; Fang et al., 2017).

Despite the crucial roles of NAD in cellular energy metabolism and signaling, determining intracellular NAD contents and redox state is difficult, especially in live brains. Only two invasive methods are available: one is the biochemical assay (Zhang et al., 2006; Yang et al., 2007; Xie et al., 2009) and the other relies on the auto-fluorescence signal of the NADH but not NAD^+ (Chance et al., 1962; see **Figure 8A**). Few years ago, an *in vivo* ^{31}P MRS-based NAD assay was developed in our laboratory that enables noninvasive assessment of NAD^+ and NADH contents and RX_{NAD} in animal and human brains (Lu et al., 2014b, 2016a; Zhu et al., 2015b). This new method utilizes a theoretical NMR spectral model to describe the ^{31}P resonances of NAD^+ and NADH and their spectral patterns at a given magnetic field strength. As shown in **Figure 8B**, the molecular structure of NAD^+ only differs from NADH by one H^+ and two electrons. This subtle structural difference makes the shielding environment of the phosphorus spins in the NAD^+ molecule (two different ^{31}P spins) substantially different from that of NADH (two identical ^{31}P spins). Based on the NMR theory, the second-order coupling effect applies to the two-spin system of NAD^+, leading to a well-defined quartet of resonances with the signal intensity ratios and chemical shifts varying with the field strength; conversely, the NADH displays a single resonance with doubled intensity. The spectral patterns of NAD^+ quartet and NADH singlet, therefore, can be precisely predicted at any given field strength using a quantification model that describes all ^{31}P signals of NAD^+, NADH and α-ATP. After least-square fitting of the *in vivo* ^{31}P spectrum, the values of $[NAD^+]$, [NADH] and RX_{NAD} can be calculated using the α-ATP signal as an internal concentration reference (Lu et al., 2014b). The newly developed *in vivo* NAD assay has been applied to the healthy human at 7T. Excellent SNR and spectral quality as shown in **Figure 8C** ensures the reliable fitting of NAD^+, NADH and α-ATP resonances and the quantification of $[NAD^+]$ (≈0.30 ± 0.02 mM), [NADH]

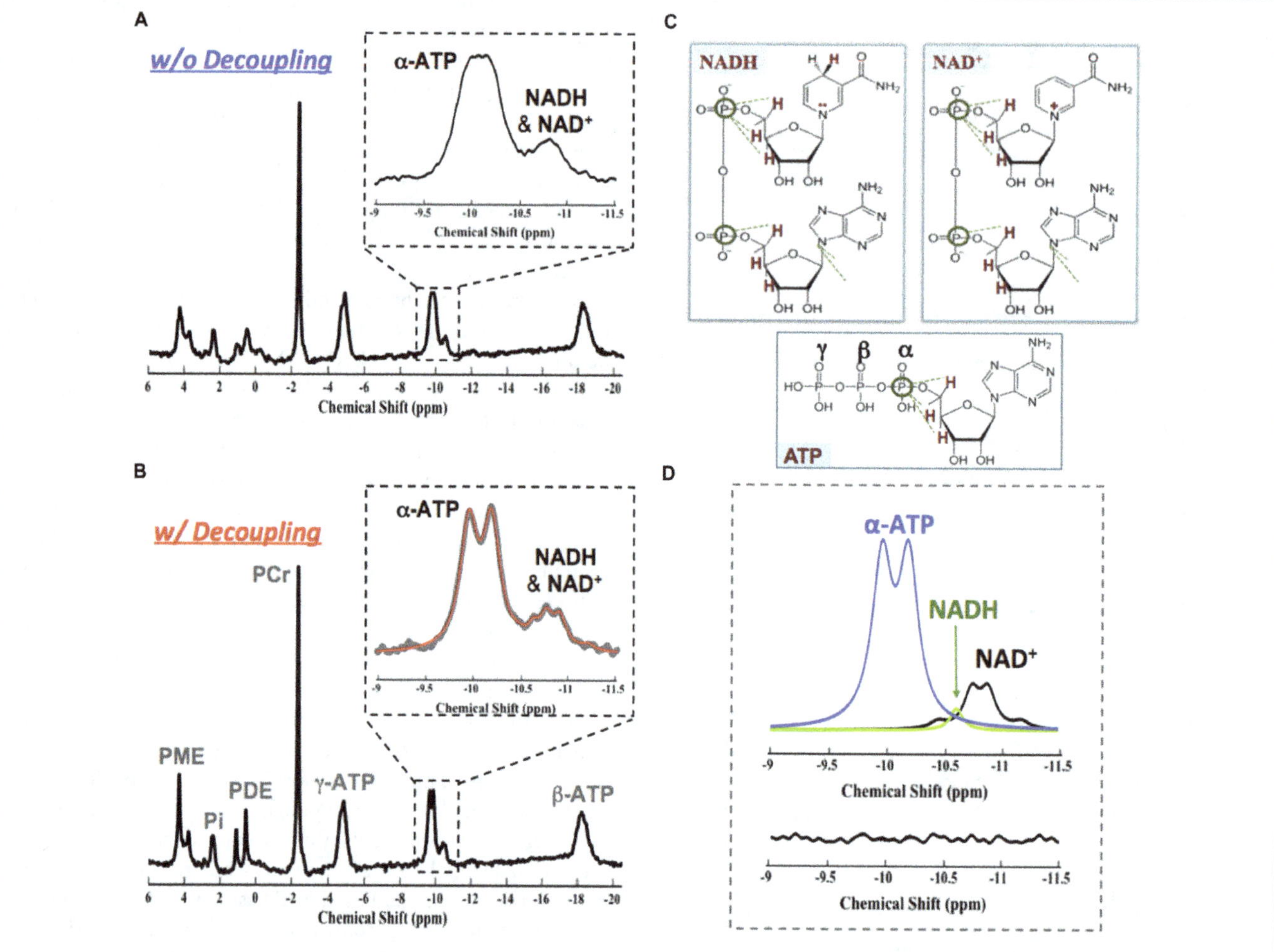

FIGURE 10 | *In vivo* ^{31}P brain spectrum collected in the absence **(A)** and presence **(B)** of ^{1}H decoupling on the water resonance from a representative healthy subject at 4T. The ^{1}H decoupling significantly reduces the linewidth of γ-ATP, NAD^{+} and NADH resonances owing to the close proximity between their phosphorus spins to the protons as shown in **(C)**. **(D)** Fitting results showing individual components of γ-ATP (blue), NAD^{+} (black) and NADH (green) signals and a small residue. Figure adapted from Lu et al. (2016a).

(≈0.06 ± 0.01 mM) and RX_{NAD} (= 4.8 ± 0.9) in the healthy human brain (Zhu et al., 2015b).

A growing number of evidence suggests a close link between the abnormal brain NAD^{+} and amyloid beta-peptide in AD (Wu et al., 2014), and therapies that aim to restore intracellular NAD^{+} level have shown promise for repairing the DNA damage or protecting against age-related cellular damage (Braidy et al., 2008, 2011). The ^{31}P MRS-based *in vivo* NAD assay provides an ideal tool to monitor the NAD changes in the human brain. **Figure 9** shows an application of the NAD assay in healthy subjects, which detected strong age-dependent changes in [NAD^{+}], [NADH], $[NAD]_{total}$ (=[NAD^{+}]+[NADH]) and RX_{NAD} (Zhu et al., 2015b). A decrease in the NAD^{+}/NADH redox ratio in normal human brain indicates that the glucose-oxygen metabolic balance is shifted toward a slower mitochondrial oxidative phosphorylation, leading to a lack of ATP production capacity in the aging brain.

Interestingly, we have reported that the *in vivo* ^{31}P MRS NAD assay could also be employed at relatively lower field. Similar performance at 7T can be achieved at 4T with incorporation of ^{1}H decoupling into the ^{31}P NAD assay (Zhu et al., 2015b; Lu et al., 2016a). The advanced NAD assay approach at 4T significantly improves the spectral resolution and the SNR of the NAD^{+}, NADH and α-ATP (**Figures 10A,B**) owing to the proximity of the nearby protons (**Figure 10C**); excellent model fittings (**Figure 10D**) and identical RX_{NAD} value (5.3 ± 0.4, $N = 7$, age: 23 ± 4 years) as that of 7T (5.4 ± 0.8, $N = 7$, age 23 ± 2 years) were obtained (Zhu et al., 2015b; Lu et al., 2016a). This result confirms the potential of *in vivo* NAD assay for translational applications at the field strength of clinical scanners, for instance, at 3T.

In summary, the advanced *in vivo* X-nuclear MRS imaging techniques as reviewed in this article can provide quantitative measures of key physiological parameters representing metabolite contents, tissue properties and metabolic rates involving major energetic pathways in live brains. The multi-nuclear MRS imaging measurements can benefit substantially from the high/ultrahigh magnetic field for improving sensitivity and reliability, and thus, these valuable metabolic imaging tools can be used to noninvasively assess the brain energetic changes in aging and neurodegenerative diseases. Although the neuroenergetic measurements and the quantitative markers described herein have shown feasibility and great potential in early detection of abnormal cerebral metabolism related to aging and neurodegeneration, their use in clinical practice still requires time and more efforts; nevertheless, the FDA approval of the 7T human scanner for clinical diagnosis of brain diseases will speed up the process. The same imaging methods are also suitable for studying the physiological functions and aging dependence of other organs such as the heart and skeletal muscle.

AUTHOR CONTRIBUTIONS

X-HZ and WC made equal contribution for writing and editing this review article.

FUNDING

The work reviewed in this article was partly supported by National Institutes of Health (NIH) grants of R01 NS041262, NS057560, NS070839 and MH111413, R24 MH106049, P41 EB015894, P30 NS5076408; the W.M. Keck Foundation.

ACKNOWLEDGMENTS

The authors thank Drs. Ming Lu, Byeong-Yeul Lee, Fei Du, Nanyin Zhang, Xiaoliang Zhang, Hao Lei, Gregor Adriany, Kamil Uğurbil, Yi Zhang and Mr. Hannes Wiesner, for their support, technical assistance and contribution to the development of the *in vivo* MRS imaging technologies as described in this review article. This article is also to commemorate Dr. Ming Lu for his seminal contributions to science and technology development.

REFERENCES

Ackerman, J. J. H., Grove, T. H., Wong, G. G., Gadian, D. G., and Radda, G. K. (1980). Mapping of metabolites in whole animals by ^{31}P NMR using surface coils. *Nature* 283, 167–170. doi: 10.1038/283167a0

Arai, T., Nakao, S., Morikawa, S., Inubushi, T., Yokoi, T., Shimizu, K., et al. (1998). Measurement of local cerebral blood flow by magnetic resonance imaging: *in vivo* autoradiographic strategy using ^{17}O-labeled water. *Brain Res. Bull.* 45, 451–456. doi: 10.1016/s0361-9230(97)00369-9

Atkinson, I. C., and Thulborn, K. R. (2010). Feasibility of mapping the tissue mass corrected bioscale of cerebral metabolic rate of oxygen consumption using 17-oxygen and 23-sodium MR imaging in a human brain at 9.4 T. *Neuroimage* 51, 723–733. doi: 10.1016/j.neuroimage.2010.02.056

Attwell, D., and Laughlin, S. B. (2001). An energy budget for signaling in the grey matter of the brain. *J. Cereb. Blood Flow Metab.* 21, 1133–1145. doi: 10.1097/00004647-200110000-00001

Balaban, R. S., Nemoto, S., and Finkel, T. (2005). Mitochondria, oxidants, and aging. *Cell* 120, 483–495. doi: 10.1016/j.cell.2005.02.001

Barinaga, M. (1997). What makes brain neurons run. *Science* 276, 196–198. doi: 10.1126/science.276.5310.196

Borghammer, P., Chakravarty, M., Jonsdottir, K. Y., Sato, N., Matsuda, H., Ito, K., et al. (2010). Cortical hypometabolism and hypoperfusion in Parkinson's disease is extensive: probably even at early disease stages. *Brain Struct. Funct.* 214, 303–317. doi: 10.1007/s00429-010-0246-0

Boumezbeur, F., Mason, G. F., de Graaf, R. A., Behar, K. L., Cline, G. W., Shulman, G. I., et al. (2010). Altered brain mitochondrial metabolism in healthy aging as assessed by *in vivo* magnetic resonance spectroscopy. *J. Cereb. Blood Flow Metab.* 30, 211–221. doi: 10.1038/jcbfm.2009.197

Boyer, P. D. (1999). What makes ATP synthase spin? *Nature* 402, 247–249. doi: 10.1038/46193

Braidy, N., Guillemin, G., and Grant, R. (2008). Promotion of cellular NAD^+ anabolism: therapeutic potential for oxidative stress in ageing and Alzheimer's disease. *Neurotox. Res.* 13, 173–184. doi: 10.1007/bf03033501

Braidy, N., Guillemin, G. J., Mansour, H., Chan-Ling, T., Poljak, A., and Grant, R. (2011). Age related changes in NAD^+ metabolism oxidative stress and Sirt1 activity in wistar rats. *PLoS One* 6:e19194. doi: 10.1371/journal.pone.0019194

Brooks, D. J., and Pavese, N. (2011). Imaging biomarkers in Parkinson's disease. *Prog. Neurobiol.* 95, 614–628. doi: 10.1016/j.pneurobio.2011.08.009

Chance, B., Cohen, P., Jobsis, F., and Schoener, B. (1962). Intracellular oxidation-reduction states *in vivo*: the microfluorometry of pyridine nucleotide gives a continuous measurement of the oxidation state. *Science* 137, 499–508. doi: 10.1126/science.137.3529.499

Chen, W., and Zhu, X. H. (2005). Dynamic study of cerebral bioenergetics and brain function using *in vivo* multinuclear MRS approaches. *Concepts Magn. Reson.* 27, 84–121. doi: 10.1002/cmr.a.20046

Creasey, H., and Rapoport, S. I. (1985). The aging human brain. *Ann. Neurol.* 17, 2–10. doi: 10.1002/ana.410170103

De Santi, S., de Leon, M. J., Convit, A., Tarshish, C., Rusinek, H., Tsui, W. H., et al. (1995). Age-related changes in brain: II. Positron emission tomography of frontal and temporal lobe glucose metabolism in normal subjects. *Psychiatr. Q.* 66, 357–370. doi: 10.1007/bf02238755

Du, F., Zhu, X. H., Qiao, H., Zhang, X., and Chen, W. (2007). Efficient *in vivo* ^{31}P magnetization transfer approach for noninvasively determining multiple kinetic parameters and metabolic fluxes of ATP metabolism in the human brain. *Magn. Reson. Med.* 57, 103–114. doi: 10.1002/mrm.21107

Du, F., Zhu, X. H., Zhang, Y., Friedman, M., Zhang, N., Uğurbil, K., et al. (2008). Tightly coupled brain activity and cerebral ATP metabolic rate. *Proc. Natl. Acad. Sci. U S A* 105, 6409–6414. doi: 10.1073/pnas.0710766105

Duara, R., Grady, C., Haxby, J., Ingvar, D., Sokoloff, L., Margolin, R. A., et al. (1984). Human brain glucose utilization and cognitive function in relation to age. *Ann. Neurol.* 16, 703–713. doi: 10.1002/ana.410160613

Duara, R., Margolin, R. A., Robertson-Tchabo, E. A., London, E. D., Schwartz, M., Renfrew, J. W., et al. (1983). Cerebral glucose utilization, as measured with positron emission tomography in 21 resting healthy men between the ages of 21 and 83 years. *Brain* 106, 761–775. doi: 10.1093/brain/106.3.761

Erecińska, M., and Silver, I. A. (1989). ATP and brain function. *J. Cereb. Blood Flow Metab.* 9, 2–19. doi: 10.1038/jcbfm.1989.2

Fang, E. F., Lautrup, S., Hou, Y., Demarest, T. G., Croteau, D. L., Mattson, M. P., et al. (2017). NAD^+ in aging: molecular mechanisms and translational implications. *Trends Mol. Med.* 23, 899–916. doi: 10.1016/j.molmed.2017.08.001

Ferrándiz, M. L., Martínez, M., De Juan, E., Díez, A., Bustos, G., and Miquel, J. (1994). Impairment of mitochondrial oxidative phosphorylation in the brain of aged mice. *Brain Res.* 644, 335–338. doi: 10.1016/0006-8993(94)91699-3

Fiat, D., and Kang, S. (1992). Determination of the rate of cerebral oxygen consumption and regional cerebral blood flow by non-invasive ^{17}O *in vivo* NMR spectroscopy and magnetic resonance imaging: Part 1. Theory and data analysis methods. *Neurol. Res.* 14, 303–311. doi: 10.1080/01616412.1992.11740074

Fiat, D., and Kang, S. (1993). Determination of the rate of cerebral oxygen consumption and regional cerebral blood flow by non-invasive ^{17}O *in vivo* NMR spectroscopy and magnetic resonance imaging. Part 2. Determination of $CMRO_2$ for the rat by ^{17}O NMR and $CMRO_2$, rCBF and the partition coefficient for the cat by ^{17}O MRI. *Neurol. Res.* 15, 7–22. doi: 10.1080/01616412.1993.11740100

Frosén, S., and Hoffman, R. A. (1963). Study of moderately rapid chemical exchange by means of nuclear magnetic double resonance. *J. Chem. Phys.* 39, 2892–2901. doi: 10.1063/1.1734121

Goyal, M. S., Vlassenko, A. G., Blazey, T. M., Su, Y., Couture, L. E., Durbin, T. J., et al. (2017). Loss of brain aerobic glycolysis in normal human aging. *Cell Metab.* 26, 353.e3–360.e3. doi: 10.1016/j.cmet.2017.07.010

Gruetter, R., Adriany, G., Choi, I. Y., Henry, P. G., Lei, H. X., and Oz, G. L. (2003). Localized *in vivo* C-13 NMR spectroscopy of the brain. *NMR Biomed.* 16, 313–338. doi: 10.1002/nbm.841

Guarente, L. (2008). Mitochondria—a nexus for aging, calorie restriction, and sirtuins? *Cell* 132, 171–176. doi: 10.1016/j.cell.2008.01.007

Guarente, L. (2016). CELL METABOLISM. The resurgence of NAD^+. *Science* 352, 1396–1397. doi: 10.1126/science.aag1718

Hetherington, H. P., Pan, J. W., and Spencer, D. D. (2002). ^1H and ^{31}P spectroscopy and bioenergetics in the lateralization of seizures in temporal lobe epilepsy. *J. Magn. Reson. Imaging* 16, 477–483. doi: 10.1002/jmri.10177

Hyder, F., Patel, A. B., Gjedde, A., Rothman, D. L., Behar, K. L., and Shulman, R. G. (2006). Neuronal-glial glucose oxidation and glutamatergic-GABAergic function. *J. Cereb. Blood Flow Metab.* 26, 865–877. doi: 10.1038/sj.jcbfm.9600263

Imai, S., and Guarente, L. (2014). NAD^+ and sirtuins in aging and disease. *Trends Cell Biol.* 24, 464–471. doi: 10.1016/j.tcb.2014.04.002

Kemp, G. J. (2000). Non-invasive methods for studying brain energy metabolism: what they show and what it means. *Dev. Neurosci.* 22, 418–428. doi: 10.1159/000017471

Kurzhunov, D., Borowiak, R., Reisert, M., Joachim Krafft, A., Caglar Özen, A., and Bock, M. (2017). 3D $CMRO_2$ mapping in human brain with direct ^{17}O MRI: comparison of conventional and proton-constrained reconstructions. *Neuroimage* 155, 612–624. doi: 10.1016/j.neuroimage.2017.05.029

Leenders, K. L., Perani, D., Lammertsma, A. A., Heather, J. D., Buckingham, P., Healy, M. J., et al. (1990). Cerebral blood flow, blood volume and oxygen utilization. Normal values and effect of age. *Brain* 113, 27–47. doi: 10.1093/brain/113.1.27

Lei, H., Uğurbil, K., and Chen, W. (2003a). Measurement of unidirectional Pi to ATP flux in human visual cortex at 7 Tesla using *in vivo* ^{31}P magnetic resonance spectroscopy. *Proc. Natl. Acad. Sci. U S A* 100, 14409–14414. doi: 10.1073/pnas.2332656100

Lei, H., Zhu, X. H., Zhang, X. L., Uğurbil, K., and Chen, W. (2003b). *In vivo* ^{31}P magnetic resonance spectroscopy of human brain at 7 T: an initial experience. *Magn. Reson. Med.* 49, 199–205. doi: 10.1002/mrm.10379

Lenzi, G. L., Jones, T., and Frackowiak, R. S. (1981). Positron emission tomography: state of the art in neurology. *Prog. Nucl. Med.* 7, 118–137.

Lin, A. L., Coman, D., Jiang, L., Rothman, D. L., and Hyder, F. (2014). Caloric restriction impedes age-related decline of mitochondrial function and neuronal activity. *J. Cereb. Blood Flow Metab.* 34, 1440–1443. doi: 10.1038/jcbfm.2014.114

López-Otín, C., Blasco, M. A., Partridge, L., Serrano, M., and Kroemer, G. (2013). The hallmarks of aging. *Cell* 153, 1194–1217. doi: 10.1016/j.cell.2013.05.039

Lu, M., Chen, W., and Zhu, X. H. (2014a). Field dependence study of *in vivo* brain ^{31}P MRS up to 16.4 T. *NMR Biomed.* 27, 1135–1141. doi: 10.1002/nbm.3167

Lu, M., Zhu, X. H., Zhang, Y., and Chen, W. (2014b). Intracellular redox state revealed by *in vivo* ^{31}P MRS measurement of NAD^+ and NADH contents in brains. *Magn. Reson. Med.* 71, 1959–1972. doi: 10.1002/mrm.24859

Lu, M., Zhang, Y., Uğurbil, K., Chen, W., and Zhu, X. H. (2013). *In vitro* and *in vivo* studies of ^{17}O NMR sensitivity at 9.4 and 16.4 T. *Magn. Reson. Med.* 69, 1523–1527. doi: 10.1002/mrm.24386

Lu, M., Zhu, X. H., and Chen, W. (2016a). *In vivo* ^{31}P MRS assessment of intracellular NAD metabolites and NAD^+/NADH redox state in human brain at 4 T. *NMR Biomed.* 29, 1010–1017. doi: 10.1002/nbm.3559

Lu, M., Zhu, X. H., Zhang, Y., Low, W., and Chen, W. (2016b). "Simultaneous assessment of abnormal glycolysis and oxidative metabolisms in brain tumor using *in vivo* deuterium (^2H) MRS imaging," in *Proceedings of the International Society for Magnetic Resonance in Medicine* (Singapore), 3962.

Lu, M., Zhu, X. H., Zhang, Y., and Chen, W. (2018). "A pilot study for *in vivo* measurement and quantification of brain glucose metabolic rates using oral uptake of deuterated glucose," in *Proceedings of the International Society for Magnetic Resonance in Medicine* (Paris, France), 907.

Lu, M., Zhu, X. H., Zhang, Y., Mateescu, G., and Chen, W. (2017). Quantitative assessment of brain glucose metabolic rates using *in vivo* deuterium magnetic resonance spectroscopy. *J. Cereb. Blood Flow Metab.* 37, 3518–3530. doi: 10.1177/0271678x17706444

Marchal, G., Rioux, P., Petit-Taboué, M. C., Sette, G., Travère, J. M., Le Poec, C., et al. (1992). Regional cerebral oxygen consumption, blood flow, and blood volume in healthy human aging. *Arch. Neurol.* 49, 1013–1020. doi: 10.1001/archneur.1992.00530340029014

Mateescu, G. D., Ye, A., Flask, C. A., Erokwu, B., and Duerk, J. L. (2011). *In vivo* assessment of oxygen consumption via deuterium magnetic resonance. *Adv. Exp. Med. Biol.* 701, 193–199. doi: 10.1007/978-1-4419-7756-4_26

Mateescu, G. D., Yvars, G., Pazara, D. I., Alldridge, N. A., Lamanna, J. C., Lust, D. W., et al. (1989). "^{17}O-^1H magnetic resonance imaging in plants, animals, and materials," in *Synthesis and Application of Isotopically Labeled Compounds*, eds T. A. Baillie and J. R. Jones (Amsterdam: Elsevier), 499–508.

Mills, K. F., Yoshida, S., Stein, L. R., Grozio, A., Kubota, S., Sasaki, Y., et al. (2016). Long-term administration of nicotinamide mononucleotide mitigates age-associated physiological decline in mice. *Cell Metab.* 24, 795–806. doi: 10.1016/j.cmet.2016.09.013

Mintun, M. A., Raichle, M. E., Martin, W. R., and Herscovitch, P. (1984). Brain oxygen utilization measured with O-15 radiotracers and positron emission tomography. *J. Nucl. Med.* 25, 177–187.

Mouchiroud, L., Houtkooper, R. H., and Auwerx, J. (2013). NAD^+ metabolism: a therapeutic target for age-related metabolic disease. *Crit. Rev. Biochem. Mol. Biol.* 48, 397–408. doi: 10.3109/10409238.2013

Navarro, A., and Boveris, A. (2007). The mitochondrial energy transduction system and the aging process. *Am. J. Physiol. Cell Physiol.* 292, C670–C686. doi: 10.1152/ajpcell.00213.2006

Niccolini, F., Su, P., and Politis, M. (2014). Dopamine receptor mapping with PET imaging in Parkinson's disease. *J. Neurol.* 261, 2251–2263. doi: 10.1007/s00415-014-7302-2

Niesporek, S. C., Umathum, R., Lommen, J. M., Behl, N. G. R., Paech, D., Bachert, P., et al. (2018). Reproducibility of $CMRO_2$ determination using dynamic ^{17}O MRI. *Magn. Reson. Med.* 79, 2923–2934. doi: 10.1002/mrm.26952

Nunnari, J., and Suomalainen, A. (2012). Mitochondria: in sickness and in health. *Cell* 148, 1145–1159. doi: 10.1016/j.cell.2012.02.035

Pantano, P., Baron, J. C., Lebrun-Grandie, P., Duquesnoy, N., Bousser, M. G., and Comar, D. (1984). Regional cerebral blood flow and oxygen consumption in human aging. *Stroke* 15, 635–641. doi: 10.1161/01.STR.15.4.635

Pathak, D., Berthet, A., and Nakamura, K. (2013). Energy failure: does it contribute to neurodegeneration? *Ann. Neurol.* 74, 506–516. doi: 10.1002/ana.24014

Pekar, J., Ligeti, L., Ruttner, Z., Lyon, R. C., Sinnwell, T. M., van Gelderen, P., et al. (1991). *In vivo* measurement of cerebral oxygen consumption and blood flow using ^{17}O magnetic resonance imaging. *Magn. Reson. Med.* 21, 313–319. doi: 10.1002/mrm.1910210217

Qiao, H., Zhang, X., Zhu, X. H., Du, F., and Chen, W. (2006). *In vivo* ^{31}P MRS of human brain at high/ultrahigh fields: a quantitative comparison of NMR detection sensitivity and spectral resolution between 4 T and 7 T. *Magn. Reson. Imaging* 24, 1281–1286. doi: 10.1016/j.mri.2006.08.002

Raichle, M. E. (1987). "Circulatory and metabolic correlates of brain function in normal humans," in *Handbook of Physiology—The Nervous System*, eds V. B. Mountcastle, F. Plum and S. R. Geiger (Bethesda, MD: American Physiological Society), 643–674.

Rapoport, S. I. (1999). Functional brain imaging in the resting state and during activation in Alzheimer's disease. Implications for disease mechanisms involving oxidative phosphorylation. *Ann. N Y Acad. Sci.* 893, 138–153. doi: 10.1111/j.1749-6632.1999.tb07823.x

Reddy, P. H., and Reddy, T. P. (2011). Mitochondria as a therapeutic target for aging and neurodegenerative diseases. *Curr. Alzheimer Res.* 8, 393–409. doi: 10.2174/156720511795745401

Reddy, R., Stolpen, A. H., Charagundla, S. R., Insko, E. K., and Leigh, J. S. (1996). ^{17}O-decoupled 1H detection using a double-tuned coil. *Magn. Reson. Imaging* 14, 1073–1078. doi: 10.1016/s0730-725x(96)00227-5

Ren, J., Sherry, A. D., and Malloy, C. R. (2017). Efficient ^{31}P band inversion transfer approach for measuring creatine kinase activity, ATP synthesis, and molecular dynamics in the human brain at 7 T. *Magn. Reson. Med.* 78, 1657–1666. doi: 10.1002/mrm.26560

Rodrigues, T. B., Valette, J., and Bouzier-Sore, A.-K. (2013). 13_C NMR spectroscopy applications to brain energy metabolism. *Front. Neuroenergetics* 5:9. doi: 10.3389/fnene.2013.00009

Rolfe, D. F., and Brown, G. C. (1997). Cellular energy utilization and molecular origin of standard metabolic rate in mammals. *Physiol. Rev.* 77, 731–758. doi: 10.1152/physrev.1997.77.3.731

Ronen, I., Merkle, H., Uğurbil, K., and Navon, G. (1998). Imaging of $H_2{}^{17}O$ distribution in the brain of a live rat by using proton-detected ^{17}O MRI. *Proc. Natl. Acad. Sci. U S A* 95, 12934–12939. doi: 10.1073/pnas.95.22.12934

Rothman, D. L., De Feyter, H. M., de Graaf, R. A., Mason, G. F., and Behar, K. L. (2011). 13_C MRS studies of neuroenergetics and neurotransmitter cycling in humans. *NMR Biomed.* 24, 943–957. doi: 10.1002/nbm.1772

Schägger, H., and Ohm, T. G. (1995). Human diseases with defects in oxidative phosphorylation. 2. F_1F_0 ATP-synthase defects in Alzheimer disease revealed by blue native polyacrylamide gel electrophoresis. *Eur. J. Biochem.* 227, 916–921. doi: 10.1111/j.1432-1033.1995.tb20219.x

Schultz, M. B., and Sinclair, D. A. (2016). Why NAD^+ declines during aging: it's destroyed. *Cell Metab.* 23, 965–966. doi: 10.1016/j.cmet.2016.05.022

Shoubridge, E. A., Briggs, R. W., and Radda, G. K. (1982). ^{31}P NMR saturation transfer measurements of the steady state rates of creatine kinase and ATP synthetase in the rat brain. *FEBS Lett.* 140, 288–292. doi: 10.1016/0014-5793(82)80916-2

Shulman, R. G., Brown, T. R., Uğurbil, K., Ogawa, S., Cohen, S. M., and Den Hollander, J. A. (1979). Cellular applications of ^{31}P and ^{13}C nuclear magnetic resonance. *Science* 205, 160–166. doi: 10.1126/science.36664

Shulman, R. G., Rothman, D. L., Behar, K. L., and Hyder, F. (2004). Energetic basis of brain activity: implications for neuroimaging. *Trends Neurosci.* 27, 489–495. doi: 10.1016/j.tins.2004.06.005

Shulman, R. G., Rothman, D. L., and Hyder, F. (1999). Stimulated changes in localized cerebral energy consumption under anesthesia. *Proc. Natl. Acad. Sci. U S A* 96, 3245–3250. doi: 10.1073/pnas.96.6.3245

Sibson, N. R., Mason, G. F., Shen, J., Cline, G. W., Herskovits, A. Z., Wall, J. E., et al. (2001). *In vivo* ^{13}C NMR measurement of neurotransmitter glutamate cycling, anaplerosis and TCA cycle flux in rat brain during. *J. Neurochem.* 76, 975–989. doi: 10.1046/j.1471-4159.2001.00074.x

Siesjo, B. K. (1978). *Brain Energy Metabolism.* New York, NY: Wiley.

Sonnay, S., Gruetter, R., and Duarte, J. M. N. (2017). How energy metabolism supports cerebral function: insights from 13_C magnetic resonance studies *In vivo*. *Front. Neurosci.* 11:288. doi: 10.3389/fnins.2017.00288

Stryer, L. (1988). *Biochemistry.* New York, NY: W.H. Freeman & Company.

Uğurbil, K. (1985). Magnetization transfer measurements of individual rate constants in the presence of multiple reactions. *J. Magn. Reson.* 64, 207–219. doi: 10.1016/0022-2364(85)90345-2

Varley, J., Brooks, D. J., and Edison, P. (2015). Imaging neuroinflammation in Alzheimer's and other dementias: recent advances and future directions. *Alzheimers Dement.* 11, 1110–1120. doi: 10.1016/j.jalz.2014.08.105

Vaughan, J. T., Garwood, M., Collins, C. M., Liu, W., Delabarre, L., Adriany, G., et al. (2001). 7T vs. 4T: RF power, homogeneity, and signal-to-noise comparison in head images. *Magn. Reson. Med.* 46, 24–30. doi: 10.1002/mrm.1156

Verdin, E. (2015). NAD^+ in aging, metabolism, and neurodegeneration. *Science* 350, 1208–1213. doi: 10.1126/science.aac4854

Wu, M. F., Yin, J. H., Hwang, C. S., Tang, C. M., and Yang, D. I. (2014). NAD attenuates oxidative DNA damages induced by amyloid β-peptide in primary rat cortical neurons. *Free Radic. Res.* 48, 794–805. doi: 10.3109/10715762.2014.907889

Xie, W. J., Xu, A. S., and Yeung, E. S. (2009). Determination of NAD^+ and NADH in a single cell under hydrogen peroxide stress by capillary electrophoresis. *Anal. Chem.* 81, 1280–1284. doi: 10.1021/ac802249m

Yamaguchi, T., Kanno, I., Uemura, K., Shishido, F., Inugami, A., Ogawa, T., et al. (1986). Reduction in regional cerebral metabolic rate of oxygen during human aging. *Stroke* 17, 1220–1228. doi: 10.1161/01.str.17.6.1220

Yang, H. Y., Yang, T., Baur, J. A., Perez, E., Matsui, T., Carmona, J. J., et al. (2007). Nutrient-sensitive mitochondrial NAD^+ levels dictate cell survival. *Cell* 130, 1095–1107. doi: 10.1016/j.cell.2007.07.035

Yap, L. P., Garcia, J. V., Han, D., and Cadenas, E. (2009). The energy-redox axis in aging and age-related neurodegeneration. *Adv. Drug Deliv. Rev.* 61, 1283–1298. doi: 10.1016/j.addr.2009.07.015

Yin, F., Boveris, A., and Cadenas, E. (2014). Mitochondrial energy metabolism and redox signaling in brain aging and neurodegeneration. *Antioxid. Redox Signal.* 20, 353–371. doi: 10.1089/ars.2012.4774

Ying, W. H. (2007). NAD^+ and NADH in brain functions, brain diseases and brain aging. *Front. Biosci.* 12, 1863–1888. doi: 10.2741/2194

Zhang, Q. H., Wang, S. Y., Nottke, A. C., Rocheleau, J. V., Piston, D. W., and Goodman, R. H. (2006). Redox sensor CtBP mediates hypoxia-induced tumor cell migration. *Proc. Natl. Acad. Sci. U S A* 103, 9029–9033. doi: 10.1073/pnas.0603269103

Zhang, N., Zhu, X. H., Lei, H., Uğurbil, K., and Chen, W. (2004). Simplified methods for calculating cerebral metabolic rate of oxygen based on ^{17}O magnetic resonance spectroscopic imaging measurement during a short $^{17}O_2$ inhalation. *J. Cereb. Blood Flow Metab.* 24, 840–848. doi: 10.1097/01.WCB.0000125885.54676.82

Zhu, X. H., and Chen, W. (2011). *In vivo* oxygen-17 NMR for imaging brain oxygen metabolism at high field. *Prog. Nucl. Magn Reson. Spectrosc.* 59, 319–335. doi: 10.1016/j.pnmrs.2011.04.002

Zhu, X. H., Chen, J. M., Tu, T. W., Chen, W., and Song, S. K. (2013a). Simultaneous and noninvasive imaging of cerebral oxygen metabolic rate, blood flow and oxygen extraction fraction in stroke mice. *Neuroimage* 64, 437–447. doi: 10.1016/j.neuroimage.2012.09.028

Zhu, X. H., Zhang, Y., Wiesner, H. M., Uğurbil, K., and Chen, W. (2013b). *In vivo* measurement of CBF using ^{17}O NMR signal of metabolically produced $H_2{}^{17}O$ as a perfusion tracer. *Magn. Reson. Med.* 70, 309–314. doi: 10.1002/mrm.24469

Zhu, X. H., Du, F., Zhang, N., Lu, M., Zhang, Y., Liu, X., et al. (2015a). *Study of Brain Bioenergetics and Function Using In Vivo MRS.* New York, NY: Springer.

Zhu, X. H., Lu, M., Lee, B. Y., Uğurbil, K., and Chen, W. (2015b). *In Vivo* NAD assay reveals the intracellular NAD contents and redox state in healthy human brain and their age dependences. *Proc. Natl. Acad. Sci. U S A* 112, 2876–2881. doi: 10.1073/pnas.1417921112

Zhu, X. H., Lee, B. Y., and Chen, W. (2018). Functional energetic responses and individual variance of the human brain revealed by quantitative imaging of adenosine triphosphate production rates. *J. Cereb. Blood Flow Metab.* 38, 959–972. doi: 10.1177/0271678x18769039

Zhu, X. H., Liu, X., Lu, M., Wiesner, H. M., Uğurbil, K., and Chen, W. (2014). "*In vivo* ^{17}O MR imaging and quantification of $CMRO_2$, CBF and OEF in human visual cortex at rest and during activation," in *Proceedings of the International Society for Magnetic Resonance in Medicine* (Milan, Italy), 3763.

Zhu, X. H., Merkle, H., Kwag, J. H., Uğurbil, K., and Chen, W. (2001). ^{17}O relaxation time and NMR sensitivity of cerebral water and their field dependence. *Magn. Reson. Med.* 45, 543–549. doi: 10.1002/mrm.1073

Zhu, X. H., Qiao, H., Du, F., Xiong, Q., Liu, X., Zhang, X., et al. (2012). Quantitative imaging of energy expenditure in human brain. *Neuroimage* 60, 2107–2117. doi: 10.1016/j.neuroimage.2012.02.013

Zhu, X. H., Zhang, Y., Tian, R. X., Lei, H., Zhang, N., Zhang, X., et al. (2002). Development of ^{17}O NMR approach for fast imaging of cerebral metabolic rate of oxygen in rat brain at high field. *Proc. Natl. Acad. Sci. U S A* 99, 13194–13199. doi: 10.1073/pnas.202471399

Zhu, X. H., Zhang, Y., Zhang, N., Uğurbil, K., and Chen, W. (2007). Noninvasive and three-dimensional imaging of $CMRO_2$ in rats at 9.4 T: reproducibility test and normothermia/hypothermia comparison study. *J. Cereb. Blood Flow Metab.* 27, 1225–1234. doi: 10.1038/sj.jcbfm.9600421

Zhu, X. H., Zhang, N., Zhang, Y., Uğurbil, K., and Chen, W. (2009). New insights into central roles of cerebral oxygen metabolism in the resting and stimulus-evoked brain. *J. Cereb. Blood Flow Metab.* 29, 10–18. doi: 10.1038/jcbfm.2008.97

Zhu, X. H., Zhang, N., Zhang, Y., Zhang, X., Uğurbil, K., and Chen, W. (2005). *In vivo* ^{17}O NMR approaches for brain study at high field. *NMR Biomed.* 18, 83–103. doi: 10.1002/nbm.930

19

Neuroimaging Biomarkers of mTOR Inhibition on Vascular and Metabolic Functions in Aging Brain and Alzheimer's Disease

*Jennifer Lee[1], Lucille M. Yanckello[1,2], David Ma[1], Jared D. Hoffman[1,2], Ishita Parikh[1], Scott Thalman[3], Bjoern Bauer[4], Anika M. S. Hartz[1,2], Fahmeed Hyder[5] and Ai-Ling Lin[1,2,3]**

[1] Sanders-Brown Center on Aging, University of Kentucky, Lexington, KY, United States, [2] Department of Pharmacology and Nutritional Science, University of Kentucky, Lexington, KY, United States, [3] F. Joseph Halcomb III, M.D. Department of Biomedical Engineering, University of Kentucky, Lexington, KY, United States, [4] Department of Pharmaceutical Sciences, University of Kentucky, Lexington, KY, United States, [5] Departments of Radiology and Biomedical Engineering, Magnetic Resonance Research Center, Yale University, New Haven, CT, United States

***Correspondence:**
Ai-Ling Lin
ailing.lin@uky.edu

The mechanistic target of rapamycin (mTOR) is a nutrient sensor of eukaryotic cells. Inhibition of mechanistic mTOR signaling can increase life and health span in various species via interventions that include rapamycin and caloric restriction (CR). In the central nervous system, mTOR inhibition demonstrates neuroprotective patterns in aging and Alzheimer's disease (AD) by preserving mitochondrial function and reducing amyloid beta retention. However, the effects of mTOR inhibition for *in vivo* brain physiology remain largely unknown. Here, we review recent findings of *in vivo* metabolic and vascular measures using non-invasive, multimodal neuroimaging methods in rodent models for brain aging and AD. Specifically, we focus on pharmacological treatment (e.g., rapamycin) for restoring brain functions in animals modeling human AD; nutritional interventions (e.g., CR and ketogenic diet) for enhancing brain vascular and metabolic functions in rodents at young age (5–6 months of age) and preserving those functions in aging (18–20 months of age). Various magnetic resonance (MR) methods [i.e., imaging (MRI), angiography (MRA), and spectroscopy (MRS)], confocal microscopic imaging, and positron emission tomography (PET) provided *in vivo* metabolic and vascular measures. We also discuss the translational potential of mTOR interventions. Since PET and various MR neuroimaging methods, as well as the different interventions (e.g., rapamycin, CR, and ketogenic diet) are also available for humans, these findings may have tremendous implications in future clinical trials of neurological disorders in aging populations.

Keywords: mechanistic target of rapamycin (mTOR), rapamycin, caloric restriction, ketogentic diet, MRI, PET, Aging, Alzheimer's disease

INTRODUCTION

The mechanistic target of rapamycin (mTOR) is a nutrient sensor that mediates the responses to energy status and growth factor in eukaryotic cells (Laplante and Sabatini, 2009). Discovered by three groups in 1994, mTOR is a particular protein bound by rapamycin (Brown et al., 1994; Cafferkey et al., 1994; Sabatini et al., 1994). mTOR activity can be inhibited by both rapamycin and nutritional signaling, such as caloric restriction (CR) (Perluigi et al., 2015). Inhibition of mTOR can switch cellular response from reproduction/growth to somatic maintenance, with decreased protein synthesis and cell growth, and increased autophagy in animal models (Harrison et al., 2009; Stanfel et al., 2009). As such, mTOR inhibition has shown to increase resistance to stresses resulting in lifespan extension in various mammalian species, and being considered central to the regulation of both aging and age-related diseases (Johnson et al., 2013).

In the central nervous system, mTOR inhibition has been shown to prevent neurodegeneration and protect brain functions in aging. Notably, rapamycin reduces amyloid-beta (Aβ) plaques and neurofibrillary tau tangles and improves cognitive functions in mice that model human Alzheimer's disease (AD) (Spilman et al., 2010; Majumder et al., 2011). Similarly, CR (without malnutrition) is able to alleviate AD-like pathology (Lee et al., 2000, 2002; Thrasivoulou et al., 2006). In addition, CR protects mitochondrial function (the powerhouse in the cells), maintains glucose homeostasis, and reduces oxidative stress – all phenotypes of aging (Park et al., 2005; Duan and Ross, 2010; Perluigi et al., 2015). Thus, CR (reduced caloric and glucose intake) shifts metabolism toward ketone body utilization (Guo et al., 2015; Lin et al., 2015). Elevated ketone body metabolism or the administration of the ketogenic diet (KD) is also evident to be neuroprotective against AD, aging, epilepsy, brain injury, and neurodegeneration (Van der Auwera et al., 2005; Yang et al., 2017). However, biochemical and molecular experiments may limit mTOR-related research to *in vitro* or *ex vivo* cell culture or animal models. Such findings may be incapable of being completely translated and applied to humans.

Powerful brain imaging tools have been refined to visualize changes in brain function *in vivo* over time (Lavina, 2016; Hyder and Rothman, 2017). In particular, functional imaging can be used to determine changes in physiology before AD-like pathology appears and before the onset of cognitive impairment. Brain vascular and metabolic dysfunction plays a critical role in driving neurodegeneration and dementia (Reiman et al., 2001, 2004, 2005; Thambisetty et al., 2010; Fleisher et al., 2013). We have recently demonstrated that early detection of these physiological changes and identification of effective interventions using imaging would be critical to potentially slow down brain aging and prevent AD. **Table 1** summarizes the imaging techniques used in the studies we review, ranging from various magnetic resonance imaging (MRI) and spectroscopy (MRS) methods to positron emission tomography (PET) to confocal microscopic imaging, where the last method is primarily for preclinical research. To assess vascular functions, we used MRI-based arterial spin labeling (ASL), which measures quantitative cerebral blood flow (CBF) values by utilizing arterial blood water as an endogenous tracer. We also determined vascular density with magnetic resonance angiography (MRA) and blood-brain barrier (BBB) P-glycoprotein transport activity with live-cell imaging confocal microscopy. To assess metabolic functions, we used well-established PET protocols and proton magnetic resonance spectroscopy (^{1}H-MRS) to quantify glucose uptake and brain metabolites, respectively (Lin et al., 2012; Lin and Rothman, 2014). We have also included the novel MRS techniques of ^{1}H[^{13}C] proton-observed-carbon-edited (POCE) to determine neurotransmission rate and mitochondrial oxidative metabolism in the aging brain.

In this review, we will discuss our neuroimaging findings on mTOR inhibition in the aging and AD brain. First, we will address the effectiveness of rapamycin in reducing AD-like pathology by restoring cerebrovascular functions in mice. Second, we will address our recent findings on CR and KD in enhancing brain vascular functions and shifting metabolism in young healthy mice. Third, we will provide evidence that CR preserves brain metabolic and vascular functions in aging in both mice and rats. Finally, we will discuss the translational potential of mTOR-related interventions in future human studies.

RAPAMYCIN RESTORES BRAIN VASCULAR AND METABOLIC FUNCTIONS IN MICE MODELING HUMAN ALZHEIMER'S DISEASE

Rapamycin was discovered in 1970s from soil samples in Easter Island Rapa Nui (Sehgal et al., 1975); thus, the compound was named rapamycin (also known as sirolimus) after its place of origin (Johnson et al., 2013). It was discovered in 1988 that rapamycin contained immunosuppressive properties (Camardo, 2003). This finding led to the FDA's approval of rapamycin in 1999 as an immunosuppressant preventative of the rejection in organs transplant patients (Camardo, 2003). Over the past two decades, rapamycin or its analogs have been widely used in the clinic and their toxicity profiles have been well characterized (Soefje et al., 2011).

Preclinical studies have been conducted to analyze the potential effectiveness of rapamycin to treat AD (Caccamo et al., 2010; Spilman et al., 2010; Majumder et al., 2011). In a recent study (Lin et al., 2017a), we focused on the effects of rapamycin in presymptomatic mice carrying the human apolipoprotein ε4 (APOE4) allele, given that APOE4 is the most significant genetic risk factor for AD (Liu et al., 2013). Neuroimaging studies in humans have shown that cognitively normal APOE4 carriers develop vascular and metabolic deficits decades before the aggregation of Aβ and tau tangles (Reiman et al., 2001, 2004, 2005; Thambisetty et al., 2010; Fleisher et al., 2013). In particular, researchers conducting PET studies found that cognitively normal carriers of the APOE4 allele have abnormally low cerebral metabolic rates of glucose (CMRglc) in similar brain regions as patients diagnosed with AD (Reiman et al., 2001, 2004, 2005; Thambisetty et al., 2010; Fleisher et al., 2013). This metabolic abnormality was observed both in late-middle-aged (40–60 years of age) and young (20–39 years of age) carriers, who have normal memory and cognitive ability and are without Aβ or tau pathology. These PET findings suggest that APOE4 carriers develop functional brain abnormalities several decades prior to the potential onset of dementia. Longitudinal research using MRI has displayed

TABLE 1 | List of discussed neuroimaging methods.

Modality	Methods	Measurements	Applications
Magnetic resonance imaging (MRI) and spectroscopy (MRS)	ASL	Cerebral blood flow	Humans and animals
	MRA	Vascular density	
	^{1}H-MRS	A variety of essential brain metabolites	
	POCE	Mitochondrial function; Neurotransmission rate; neuronal and glial activities	
Positron emission tomography (PET)	^{18}FDG	Cerebral glucose metabolism	
Confocal Microscopy	Live-cell imaging	Blood brain barrier P-gp transport activity	Mainly in animals

ASL, arterial spin labeling; MRA, magnetic resonance angiography; ^{1}H-MRS, proton magnetic resonance spectroscopy; POCE, ^{1}H[^{13}C] proton-observed-carbon-edited MRS; ^{18}FDG, fluorine-18 (^{18}F)-labeled 2-fluoro-2-deoxy-d-glucose.

that CBF is reduced in an accelerated manner in similar brain regions (e.g., frontal, parietal, and temporal cortices) in cognitively healthy APOE4 carriers (Thambisetty et al., 2010). The APOE4-related neurovascular risk is strongly correlated with an accelerated decline in verbal memory, language capability, attention, and visual/spatial abilities in midlife (Bangen et al., 2013).

A similar situation is seen in transgenic mice that express the human APOE4 isoform that is driven by the human glial fibrillary acidic protein promoter. Young, presymptomatic APOE4 mice have significantly lower CMRglc and CBF, as well as increased BBB leakage compared to the wild-type (WT) non-APOE4 mice (Bell et al., 2012; Lin et al., 2017a). Treating asymptomatic female APOE4 mice with rapamycin for 1 month resulted in a significant increase in CBF compared to the non-treated littermates. After 6 months of treatment, we found that rapamycin-treated APOE4 mice had normal CBF that was comparable to that of the sex- and age-matched WT mice. Similarly, rapamycin-treated mice also had lower BBB leakage. Furthermore, we found that BBB leakage could potentially be blocked by inhibiting cyclophilin A-dependent proinflammatory pathways with rapamycin (Bell et al., 2012). In addition, CMRglc was also restored to WT level as observed in the rapamycin-treated APOE4 mice (Lin et al., 2017a).

In another study with hAPP(J20) mice (a mouse model of human AD) that already developed significant Aβ pathology and cognitive decline, we found that rapamycin was also effective in restoring neurovascular function. Symptomatic hAPP(J20) 11 month old mice treated with rapamycin for 16 weeks had restored CBF to the level of WT mice (Lin et al., 2013). In addition, rapamycin restored vascular density, determined by MR angiography, in the brains of hAPP(J20) mice. The restored vascular integrity was highly correlated with reduced Aβ, cerebral amyloid angiopathy (CAA), and microhemorrhages in treated hAPP(J20) mice. These findings were consistent with the literature showing that rapamycin can reduce Aβ (Liu et al., 2017). In this study, we also identified that mTOR inhibition activates endothelial nitric oxide synthase (eNOS), and thus, released nitric oxide (NO), a vasodilator (Cheng et al., 2008; Lin et al., 2013). Therefore, rapamycin activating eNOS may be critical for restoring CBF in hAPP(J20) mice. In addition to restored cerebrovascular function and reduced AD-like pathology, hAPP(J20) mice also had improved memory and learning performance after 16 weeks of rapamycin treatment (Lin et al., 2013). Collectively, data generated from the two imaging studies show that rapamycin can potentially prevent AD phenotypes in APOE4 mice and reverse the effects of AD in hAPP(J20) transgenic mice (Richardson et al., 2015).

CALORIC RESTRICTION AND KETOGENIC DIET ENHANCE BRAIN VASCULAR FUNCTIONS AND SHIFT METABOLISM IN YOUNG MICE

In the early 1930s, Clive McCay demonstrated that restricting calorie intake without malnutrition can prolong both the mean and maximal lifespan in rats when compared to animals on *ad libitum* diet (AL; free eating) (McCay et al., 1989; Park, 2010). Since then, CR is perhaps the most studied anti-aging manipulation within a broad range of species (Colman et al., 2009; Choi et al., 2011; Rahat et al., 2011). This is further supported by other studies that display lower incidences of age-related neurodegenerative disorders found in animals treated with CR (Park et al., 2005; Duan and Ross, 2010).

Recently, our efforts have been focused on understanding how CR impacts brain function in the early stage. In particular, we would like to know how brain vascular and metabolic functions might be impacted with CR in young mice. We imaged mice at 5–6 months of age, either on 40% CR diet or AL, and found that CR significantly enhanced CBF (>20%) both globally and in the hippocampus, compared to their AL littermates (Parikh et al., 2016). The increase in CBF was associated with reduced mTOR and increased eNOS levels that were similar to what we observed with rapamycin. In addition, CR-fed mice had significantly increased P-glycoprotein (P-gp) transport activity levels at the BBB, which facilitates clearance of Aβ out of the brain. These findings are consistent with literature showing that CR reduces AD-like pathology and the onset of cognitive impairment (Mouton et al., 2009; Schafer et al., 2015).

We used ^{1}H-MRS to determine energy metabolites in the hippocampus (Guo et al., 2015). We observed that CR mice displayed significantly increased levels of total creatine (tCr), a high-energy substrate, in comparison to AL mice. Given that tCr is the sum of creatine and phosphocreatine, we posited that CR increases adenosine triphosphate (ATP) production in young CR mice since phosphocreatine acts in a central role as an intracellular buffer during ATP production in mitochondria. This finding is consistent with literature that CR enhances ATP production by activating AMP-activated protein kinase (AMPK) and sirtuins pathways, which in turn suppresses the mTOR pathway (Blagosklonny, 2010). It has been found that the level of glucose regulates the AMPK pathway. With low levels of glucose and metabolic stress that accompany CR, there is a depletion of energy (low ATP: AMP ratio), which in turn activates AMPK (Salt et al., 1998; Hardie, 2014). AMPK, when activated, can be seen as an indicator of cellular energy status, turning on catabolic pathways that generate ATP while inhibiting cellular processes that consume ATP such as the mTOR pathway.

We also found significantly elevated levels of taurine in the CR mice when compared to the AL mice. Since taurine is correlated with neuromodulation, higher levels imply that young CR mice might have augmented excitability compared to the age-matched AL mice. Interestingly, both globally and in the hippocampus and frontal cortex (regions related to cognitive functions), CR mice displayed significantly reduced brain glucose uptake as determined by PET imaging (Guo et al., 2015). Our imaging findings are consistent with Western blot data showing that CR reduces glucose transporter 1 (GLUT-1) in brain capillaries of the mice (Parikh et al., 2016). As a result, we found a mismatch of CBF-CMRglc coupling induced by CR, opposite to tight coupling of CBF-CMRglc in a normal brain at rest (Fox et al., 1988; Lin et al., 2010).

These reduced glucose uptake results led us to hypothesize that in order to sustain essential mitochondrial activity and neuronal functions, the brain may utilize alternative fuel substrates as an energy source. As the brain would also use ketone bodies as energy source (Akram, 2013), we measured ketone body levels in the brain and blood and found that CR rodents had a significantly higher concentration of ketone bodies in comparison to AL animals (Guo et al., 2015; Lin et al., 2015). The findings indicated that CR may, at a very early stage in the brain, induce a metabolic switch from glucose to ketones.

To verify the impact of elevated ketone bodies on vascular functions, we fed young, age-matched WT mice with the KD for 16 weeks. Similar to what we observed with young CR mice, mice fed with KD also had significant increases in CBF and P-gp transport activity levels in brain capillaries compared to control mice (Ma et al., 2018). These neurovascular enhancements were also associated with reduced mTOR and increased eNOS protein expressions. The result is consistent with previous reports that ketogenesis is associated with the down-regulation of mTOR (McDaniel et al., 2011). In line with this, two other studies indicate that an acute increase in ketone body concentration (via infusion of β-hydroxyl butyrate) elevated CBF independent of overall cerebral metabolic activity. This suggests that ketone bodies can directly increase CBF via the cerebral endothelium (Hasselbalch et al., 1996; Roy et al., 2013).

CALORIC RESTRICTION PRESERVES BRAIN VASCULAR AND METABOLIC FUNCTIONS IN AGING RODENTS

Healthy aging is accompanied by CBF reduction, BBB impairment and Aβ retention (Lin et al., 2015; Parikh et al., 2016; Hoffman et al., 2017). To identify CR effects on the aging brain, we included old CR and AL mice (18–20 months of age) in the same CR experiments and compared them with young mice (5–6 months of age). We found that CR enhanced CBF in young mice; moreover, CR also reduced the CBF decline in aging (Parikh et al., 2016). As a result, when compared to young AL mice, old CR mice had comparable levels of CBF, indicating that CR preserves CBF with age. Similar results were found in rats, showing that old rats with chronic CR diet had much higher CBF compared to the age-matched animal, and had comparable CBF level compared to the young AL rats (Lin et al., 2015). These results support that CR has an early enhancement effect on CBF that is preserved with aging. In addition, the preserved CBF in the hippocampus and frontal cortex were highly associated with the preserved memory and learning, as well as the reduced anxiety (Parikh et al., 2016). Our results suggest that dietary intervention initiated at a young age (e.g., young adults) may prove beneficial in the preservation of cognitive and mental abilities in aging.

A similar trend was also observed in hippocampal tCr concentration. As mentioned above, tCr was enhanced in young CR mice. Although tCr dropped dramatically as the CR mice getting older, tCr levels remained comparable to those in young AL mice and were higher than those in old AL mice. This suggests that CR increases ATP production in young CR mice while preserving ATP production in old CR mice (Guo et al., 2015).

Using advanced MRS techniques like POCE, we were able to trace *in vivo* mitochondrial oxidative metabolisms in neurons and neurotransmitter cycling between neuronal and glial cells (Lin et al., 2014). We found that, compared with the young AL rats, old CR rats had similar levels of neuronal glucose oxidation and neurotransmitter cycling, suggesting CR preserved mitochondrial functions and neuronal activity with age. In contrast, old AL rats had much lower levels in both measures. When calculating the ATP production rates for the three groups we found that old CR and young AL animals also had comparable levels of ATP production. We also observed metabolic shifts in aging animals. When compared to age-matched AL rats, old CR rats had significantly lower glucose uptake values in the various brain regions but had significantly higher levels of ketone bodies, β-hydroxyl butyrate (BHB) in the brain (Lin et al., 2015). The metabolic shift may play a critical role in sustaining brain energetics in aging.

Taken together, using multi-modal imaging methods we demonstrated that CR enhances vascular and metabolic functions in early life stages and decelerates the decline with age. Maintaining a healthy brain homeostasis may be due to the metabolic shift from glucose to ketone bodies (Lin et al., 2017b).

TRANSLATIONAL POTENTIAL OF mTOR INTERVENTIONS IN CLINICAL TRIALS

Many mTOR inhibitors (including rapamycin, rapalogs, and Everolimus) have already been approved by the FDA and are widely used in clinics (Soefje et al., 2011). Since 1999, rapamycin, alongside other immunosuppressive agents, has been administered to transplant patients to prevent the rejection of organs (Camardo, 2003). Over the past decade, studies also showed that rapamycin or rapalogs have an anti-tumor property; for relatively long periods of time, cancer patients with rapamycin show little change in their quality of life (Mita et al., 2003). Other studies reported that Everolimus improved cognition and reduced depression in humans (Lang et al., 2009). Recent studies showed that with low doses of rapamycin (e.g., lower than half of the therapeutic dosage; 0.5 mg daily or 5 mg weekly), cognitively normal elderly had improved immune functions with minimal side effects (Mannick et al., 2014). The results of the studies support that a short-term rapamycin treatment can be used safely in otherwise healthy older person.

To date, most rapamycin and rapalog clinical studies focus on structural neuroimaging to examine changes in brain tumor mass (Tillema et al., 2012; Fukumura et al., 2015; Ma et al., 2015; Sasongko et al., 2016), metastatic cancer (Subbiah et al., 2015), or active lesions (Moraal et al., 2010). However, functional neuroimaging such as EEG has been clinically applied to assess the efficacy of rapamycin in treating epilepsy (Cambiaghi et al., 2015), and MRS was used to study metabolic implications of rapamycin (Serkova et al., 1999).

CR has also been studied in humans. A recent publication by Redman et al. shows that young, healthy individuals having achieved 15% CR experienced about 8 kg weight loss over 2 years (Redman et al., 2018). Energy expenditure (measured over 24 h of awake and sleep cycle) was reduced beyond weight loss and systemic oxidative stress was also reduced. Findings from this 2 year CR trial in healthy, non-obese humans provide new evidence of persistent systemic metabolic slowing accompanied by reduced oxidative stress, which supports the rate of living and oxidative damage theories of mammalian aging.

CR has also been observed to improve memory in older adults (Fontan-Lozano et al., 2008; Witte et al., 2009; Mattson, 2010; Valdez et al., 2010). Using functional and structural MRI measurements, Witte et al. (2014) reported that resveratrol, a CR-mimetic nutrient, enhanced word retention over a 30-min period in older adults when compared with placebo.

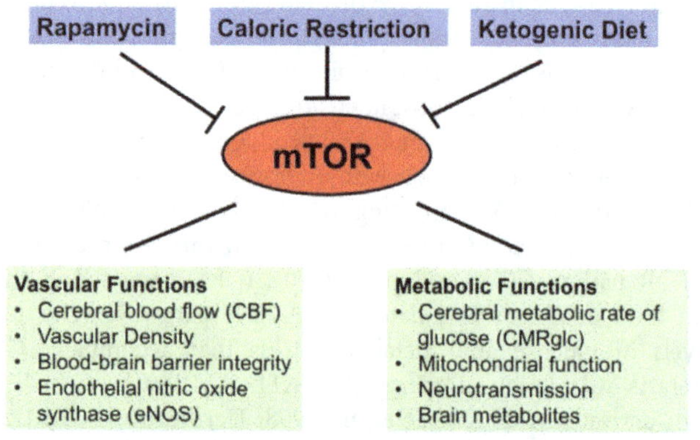

FIGURE 1 | Diagram showing vascular and metabolic changes induced by mTOR inhibition through rapamycin, caloric restriction, and ketogenic diet.

These results support that supplementary resveratrol can improve memory performance, as well as improve glucose metabolism and increase hippocampal functional connectivity in older adults. In another study, Jakobsdottir et al. (2016) reported that CR reserved abnormal brain activity in brain areas (e.g., amygdala) involved in the processing of visual food-related stimuli in postmenopausal women with obesity. It should be noted, however, there are studies that these studies have only investigated the short-term benefits of CR.

The KD has been used in the clinic to treat epilepsy (Baranano and Hartman, 2008; Walczyk and Wick, 2017), Parkinson's disease (Vanitallie et al., 2005), and autism (Evangeliou et al., 2003). The use of neuroimaging in clinical KD studies include EEG and functional MRI to define the extent of dysplasia (Guerrini et al., 2015), and ^{1}H-MRS to assess GABAergic activity (Wang et al., 2003) and glucose metabolism (Fujii et al., 2007). Recent studies also investigated the efficacy of ketone utilization in the brain. Using PET, it was found that the cerebral metabolic rate of ketones represents about 33% of the brain's energy requirements after 4 days on KD (Courchesne-Loyer et al., 2017). POCE studies in human have reported that consumption of ketones (BHB) is predominantly neuronal (Pan et al., 2002). These results support that ketone bodies are an effective alternative fuel substrate in the non-fasted adult human brain.

Collectively, rapamycin, CR, and KD have been widely applied to human studies, which indicates that our work with animal models has the potential to be translated to human studies. To date, little has been reported regarding *in vivo* vascular and metabolic measures in aging and AD with these interventions. The use of quantitative neuroimaging methods (e.g., ^{18}FDG-PET, POCE, ^{1}H-MRS, MRA, and ASL) would be vital in future use to identify the efficacy of mTOR-related interventions and treatments for protecting brain functions in aging and various AD-related neurodegeneration, including vascular dementia and Down syndrome (Lin et al., 2016).

CONCLUSION

In this review, we discussed the neuroprotective effects of mTOR inhibition in aging and AD. Specifically, rapamycin is a preventative, and possibly a treatment, for the effects of the AD phenotype observed in APOE4 and hAPP(J20) transgenic mouse models of AD; CR and KD can enhance brain vascular functions and shift metabolism in young healthy mice; and CR can preserve brain metabolic and vascular functions in aging. We summarize these findings in **Figure 1**. As the quantitative PET and MRI neuroimaging methods used in these studies in animal models can be translated into human studies, they will be greatly useful in future studies to examine the effects of these mTOR-related interventions in preventing brain function declines associated with aging and neurodegeneration in clinical trials.

AUTHOR CONTRIBUTIONS

All authors listed have made a substantial, direct and intellectual contribution to the work, and approved it for publication.

FUNDING

The studies were supported by National Institutes of Health (NIH)/National Institute on Aging (NIA) Grant K01AG040164, NIH/NIA Grant R01AG054459, NIH/CTSA Grant UL1TR000117, and American Federation for Aging Research Grant #A12474 to A-LL, NIH/NIA Grant R01AG039621 to AH, NIH/NINDS Grant R01NS079507 to BB, NIH/NIMH Grant R01MH067528 to FH, and NIH Training Grant T32DK007778 to JH, and T32AG057461 to ST.

REFERENCES

Akram, M. (2013). A focused review of the role of ketone bodies in health and disease. *J. Med. Food* 16, 965–967. doi: 10.1089/jmf.2012.2592

Bangen, K. J., Beiser, A., Delano-Wood, L., Nation, D. A., Lamar, M., Libon, D. J., et al. (2013). APOE genotype modifies the relationship between midlife vascular risk factors and later cognitive decline. *J. Stroke Cerebrovasc. Dis.* 22, 1361–1369. doi: 10.1016/j.jstrokecerebrovasdis.2013.03.013

Baranano, K. W., and Hartman, A. L. (2008). The ketogenic diet: uses in epilepsy and other neurologic illnesses. *Curr. Treat Options Neurol.* 10, 410–419. doi: 10.1007/s11940-008-0043-8

Bell, R. D., Winkler, E. A., Singh, I., Sagare, A. P., Deane, R., Wu, Z., et al. (2012). Apolipoprotein E controls cerebrovascular integrity via cyclophilin A. *Nature* 485, 512–516. doi: 10.1038/nature11087

Blagosklonny, M. V. (2010). Calorie restriction: decelerating mTOR-driven aging from cells to organisms (including humans). *Cell Cycle* 9, 683–688. doi: 10.4161/cc.9.4.10766

Brown, E. J., Albers, M. W., Shin, T. B., Ichikawa, K., Keith, C. T., Lane, W. S., et al. (1994). A mammalian protein targeted by G1-arresting rapamycin-receptor complex. *Nature* 369, 756–758. doi: 10.1038/369756a0

Caccamo, A., Majumder, S., Richardson, A., Strong, R., and Oddo, S. (2010). Molecular interplay between mammalian target of rapamycin (mTOR), amyloid-beta, and Tau: effects on cognitive impairments. *J. Biol. Chem.* 285, 13107–13120. doi: 10.1074/jbc.M110.100420

Cafferkey, R., Mclaughlin, M. M., Young, P. R., Johnson, R. K., and Livi, G. P. (1994). Yeast TOR (DRR) proteins: amino-acid sequence alignment and identification of structural motifs. *Gene* 141, 133–136. doi: 10.1016/0378-1119(94)90141-4

Camardo, J. (2003). The Rapamune era of immunosuppression 2003: the journey from the laboratory to clinical transplantation. *Transplant. Proc.* 35(Suppl. 3), 18S–24S. doi: 10.1016/S0041-1345(03)00356-7

Cambiaghi, M., Magri, L., and Cursi, M. (2015). Importance of EEG in validating the chronic effects of drugs: suggestions from animal models of epilepsy treated with rapamycin. *Seizure* 27, 30–39. doi: 10.1016/j.seizure.2015.02.015

Cheng, C., Tempel, D., Oostlander, A., Helderman, F., Gijsen, F., Wentzel, J., et al. (2008). Rapamycin modulates the eNOS vs. shear stress relationship. *Cardiovasc. Res.* 78, 123–129. doi: 10.1093/cvr/cvm103

Choi, J. S., Choi, K. M., and Lee, C. K. (2011). Caloric restriction improves efficiency and capacity of the mitochondrial electron transport chain in *Saccharomyces cerevisiae*. *Biochem. Biophys. Res. Commun.* 409, 308–314. doi: 10.1016/j.bbrc.2011.05.008

Colman, R. J., Anderson, R. M., Johnson, S. C., Kastman, E. K., Kosmatka, K. J., Beasley, T. M., et al. (2009). Caloric restriction delays disease onset and mortality in rhesus monkeys. *Science* 325, 201–204. doi: 10.1126/science.1173635

Courchesne-Loyer, A., Croteau, E., Castellano, C. A., St-Pierre, V., Hennebelle, M., and Cunnane, S. C. (2017). Inverse relationship between brain glucose and ketone metabolism in adults during short-term moderate dietary ketosis: a dual tracer quantitative positron emission tomography study. *J. Cereb. Blood Flow Metab.* 37, 2485–2493. doi: 10.1177/0271678X16669366

Duan, W., and Ross, C. A. (2010). Potential therapeutic targets for neurodegenerative diseases: lessons learned from calorie restriction. *Curr. Drug Targets* 11, 1281–1292. doi: 10.2174/1389450111007011281

Evangeliou, A., Vlachonikolis, I., Mihailidou, H., Spilioti, M., Skarpalezou, A., Makaronas, N., et al. (2003). Application of a ketogenic diet in children with autistic behavior: pilot study. *J. Child Neurol.* 18, 113–118. doi: 10.1177/08830738030180020501

Fleisher, A. S., Chen, K., Liu, X., Ayutyanont, N., Roontiva, A., Thiyyagura, P., et al. (2013). Apolipoprotein E epsilon4 and age effects on florbetapir positron emission tomography in healthy aging and Alzheimer disease. *Neurobiol. Aging* 34, 1–12. doi: 10.1016/j.neurobiolaging.2012.04.017

Fontan-Lozano, A., Lopez-Lluch, G., Delgado-Garcia, J. M., Navas, P., and Carrion, A. M. (2008). Molecular bases of caloric restriction regulation of neuronal synaptic plasticity. *Mol. Neurobiol.* 38, 167–177. doi: 10.1007/s12035-008-8040-1

Fox, P. T., Raichle, M. E., Mintun, M. A., and Dence, C. (1988). Nonoxidative glucose consumption during focal physiologic neural activity. *Science* 241, 462–464. doi: 10.1126/science.3260686

Fujii, T., Ho, Y. Y., Wang, D., De Vivo, D. C., Miyajima, T., Wong, H. Y., et al. (2007). Three Japanese patients with glucose transporter type 1 deficiency syndrome. *Brain Dev.* 29, 92–97. doi: 10.1016/j.braindev.2006.07.007

Fukumura, S., Watanabe, T., Takayama, R., Minagawa, K., and Tsutsumi, H. (2015). Everolimus treatment for an early infantile subependymal giant cell astrocytoma with tuberous sclerosis complex. *J. Child Neurol.* 30, 1192–1195. doi: 10.1177/0883073814544703

Guerrini, R., Duchowny, M., Jayakar, P., Krsek, P., Kahane, P., Tassi, L., et al. (2015). Diagnostic methods and treatment options for focal cortical dysplasia. *Epilepsia* 56, 1669–1686. doi: 10.1111/epi.13200

Guo, J., Bakshi, V., and Lin, A. L. (2015). Early shifts of brain metabolism by caloric restriction preserve white matter integrity and long-term memory in aging mice. *Front. Aging Neurosci.* 7:213. doi: 10.3389/fnagi.2015.00213

Hardie, D. G. (2014). AMP-activated protein kinase: maintaining energy homeostasis at the cellular and whole-body levels. *Annu. Rev. Nutr.* 34, 31–55. doi: 10.1146/annurev-nutr-071812-161148

Harrison, D. E., Strong, R., Sharp, Z. D., Nelson, J. F., Astle, C. M., Flurkey, K., et al. (2009). Rapamycin fed late in life extends lifespan in genetically heterogeneous mice. *Nature* 460, 392–395. doi: 10.1038/nature08221

Hasselbalch, S. G., Madsen, P. L., Hageman, L. P., Olsen, K. S., Justesen, N., Holm, S., et al. (1996). Changes in cerebral blood flow and carbohydrate metabolism during acute hyperketonemia. *Am. J. Physiol.* 270, E746–E751. doi: 10.1152/ajpendo.1996.270.5.E746

Hoffman, J. D., Parikh, I., Green, S. J., Chlipala, G., Mohney, R. P., Keaton, M., et al. (2017). Age drives distortion of brainmetabolic, vascular and cognitive functions, and the gut microbiome. *Front. Aging Neurosci.* 9:298. doi: 10.3389/fnagi.2017.00298

Hyder, F., and Rothman, D. L. (2017). Advances in imaging brain metabolism. *Annu. Rev. Biomed. Eng.* 19, 485–515. doi: 10.1146/annurev-bioeng-071516-044450

Jakobsdottir, S., Van Nieuwpoort, I. C., Van Bunderen, C. C., De Ruiter, M. B., Twisk, J. W., Deijen, J. B., et al. (2016). Acute and short-term effects of caloric restriction on metabolic profile and brain activation in obese, postmenopausal women. *Int. J. Obes.* 40, 1671–1678. doi: 10.1038/ijo.2016.103

Johnson, S. C., Rabinovitch, P. S., and Kaeberlein, M. (2013). mTOR is a key modulator of ageing and age-related disease. *Nature* 493, 338–345. doi: 10.1038/nature11861

Lang, U. E., Heger, J., Willbring, M., Domula, M., Matschke, K., and Tugtekin, S. M. (2009). Immunosuppression using the mammalian target of rapamycin (mTOR) inhibitor everolimus: pilot study shows significant cognitive and affective improvement. *Transplant. Proc.* 41, 4285–4288. doi: 10.1016/j.transproceed.2009.08.050

Laplante, M., and Sabatini, D. M. (2009). mTOR signaling at a glance. *J. Cell Sci.* 122, 3589–3594. doi: 10.1242/jcs.051011

Lavina, B. (2016). Brain vascular imaging techniques. *Int. J. Mol. Sci.* 18:E70. doi: 10.3390/ijms18010070

Lee, J., Duan, W., Long, J. M., Ingram, D. K., and Mattson, M. P. (2000). Dietary restriction increases the number of newly generated neural cells, and induces BDNF expression, in the dentate gyrus of rats. *J. Mol. Neurosci.* 15, 99–108. doi: 10.1385/JMN:15:2:99

Lee, J., Seroogy, K. B., and Mattson, M. P. (2002). Dietary restriction enhances neurotrophin expression and neurogenesis in the hippocampus of adult mice. *J. Neurochem.* 80, 539–547. doi: 10.1046/j.0022-3042.2001.00747.x

Lin, A. L., Coman, D., Jiang, L., Rothman, D. L., and Hyder, F. (2014). Caloric restriction impedes age-related decline of mitochondrial function and neuronal activity. *J. Cereb. Blood Flow Metab.* 34, 1440–1443. doi: 10.1038/jcbfm.2014.114

Lin, A. L., Gao, J. H., Duong, T. Q., and Fox, P. T. (2010). Functional neuroimaging: a physiological perspective. *Front. Neuroenergetics* 2:17. doi: 10.3389/fnene.2010.00017

Lin, A. L., Jahrling, J. B., Zhang, W., Derosa, N., Bakshi, V., Romero, P., et al. (2017a). Rapamycin rescues vascular, metabolic and learning deficits in apolipoprotein E4 transgenic mice with pre-symptomatic Alzheimer's disease. *J. Cereb. Blood Flow Metab.* 37, 217–226.

Lin, A. L., Laird, A. R., Fox, P. T., and Gao, J. H. (2012). Multimodal MRI neuroimaging biomarkers for cognitive normal adults, amnestic mild cognitive impairment, and Alzheimer's disease. *Neurol. Res. Int.* 2012:907409. doi: 10.1155/2012/907409

Lin, A. L., Parikh, I., Hoffman, J. D., and Ma, D. (2017b). Neuroimaging biomarkers of caloric restriction on brain metabolic and vascular functions. *Curr. Nutr. Rep.* 6, 41–48. doi: 10.1007/s13668-017-0187-9

Lin, A. L., Powell, D., Caban-Holt, A., Jicha, G., Robertson, W., Gold, B. T., et al. (2016). ^{1}H-MRS metabolites in adults with down syndrome: effects of dementia. *Neuroimage Clin.* 11, 728–735. doi: 10.1016/j.nicl.2016.06.001

Lin, A. L., and Rothman, D. L. (2014). What have novel imaging techniques revealed about metabolism in the aging brain? *Future Neurol.* 9, 341–354. doi: 10.2217/fnl.14.13

Lin, A. L., Zhang, W., Gao, X., and Watts, L. (2015). Caloric restriction increases ketone bodies metabolism and preserves blood flow in aging brain. *Neurobiol. Aging* 36, 2296–2303. doi: 10.1016/j.neurobiolaging.2015.03.012

Lin, A. L., Zheng, W., Halloran, J. J., Burbank, R. R., Hussong, S. A., Hart, M. J., et al. (2013). Chronic rapamycin restores brain vascular integrity and function through NO synthase activation and improves memory in symptomatic mice modeling Alzheimer's disease. *J. Cereb. Blood Flow Metab.* 33, 1412–1421. doi: 10.1038/jcbfm.2013.82

Liu, C. C., Kanekiyo, T., Xu, H., and Bu, G. (2013). Apolipoprotein E and Alzheimer disease: risk, mechanisms and therapy. *Nat. Rev. Neurol.* 9, 106–118. doi: 10.1038/nrneurol.2012.263

Liu, Y. C., Gao, X. X., Chen, L., and You, X. Q. (2017). Rapamycin suppresses Abeta25-35- or LPS-induced neuronal inflammation via modulation of NF-kappaB signaling. *Neuroscience* 355, 188–199. doi: 10.1016/j.neuroscience.2017.05.005

Ma, D., Wang, A., Parikh, I., Green, S. J., Hoffman, J. D., Chlipala, G., et al. (2018). Ketogenic diet enhances neurovascular function with altered gut microbiome in young healthy mice. *Sci. Rep.* 8:6670. doi: 10.1038/s41598-018-25190-5

Ma, D. J., Galanis, E., Anderson, S. K., Schiff, D., Kaufmann, T. J., Peller, P. J., et al. (2015). A phase II trial of everolimus, temozolomide, and radiotherapy in patients with newly diagnosed glioblastoma: NCCTG N057K. *Neuro Oncol.* 17, 1261–1269. doi: 10.1093/neuonc/nou328

Majumder, S., Richardson, A., Strong, R., and Oddo, S. (2011). Inducing autophagy by rapamycin before, but not after, the formation of plaques and tangles ameliorates cognitive deficits. *PLoS One* 6:e25416. doi: 10.1371/journal.pone.0025416

Mannick, J. B., Del Giudice, G., Lattanzi, M., Valiante, N. M., Praestgaard, J., Huang, B., et al. (2014). mTOR inhibition improves immune function in the elderly. *Sci. Transl. Med.* 6:268ra179. doi: 10.1126/scitranslmed.3009892

Mattson, M. P. (2010). The impact of dietary energy intake on cognitive aging. *Front. Aging Neurosci.* 2:5. doi: 10.3389/neuro.24.005.2010

McCay, C. M., Crowell, M. F., and Maynard, L. A. (1989). The effect of retarded growth upon the length of life span and upon the ultimate body size. 1935. *Nutrition* 5, 155–171; discussion 172.

McDaniel, S. S., Rensing, N. R., Thio, L. L., Yamada, K. A., and Wong, M. (2011). The ketogenic diet inhibits the mammalian target of rapamycin (mTOR) pathway. *Epilepsia* 52, e7–e11. doi: 10.1111/j.1528-1167.2011.02981.x

Mita, M. M., Mita, A., and Rowinsky, E. K. (2003). The molecular target of rapamycin (mTOR) as a therapeutic target against cancer. *Cancer Biol. Ther.* 2, S169–S177. doi: 10.4161/cbt.365

Moraal, B., Van Den Elskamp, I. J., Knol, D. L., Uitdehaag, B. M., Geurts, J. J., Vrenken, H., et al. (2010). Long-interval T2-weighted subtraction magnetic resonance imaging: a powerful new outcome measure in multiple sclerosis trials. *Ann. Neurol.* 67, 667–675. doi: 10.1002/ana.21958

Mouton, P. R., Chachich, M. E., Quigley, C., Spangler, E., and Ingram, D. K. (2009). Caloric restriction attenuates amyloid deposition in middle-aged dtg APP/PS1 mice. *Neurosci. Lett.* 464, 184–187. doi: 10.1016/j.neulet.2009.08.038

Pan, J. W., De Graaf, R. A., Petersen, K. F., Shulman, G. I., Hetherington, H. P., and Rothman, D. L. (2002). [2,4-^{13} C_2]-beta-Hydroxybutyrate metabolism in human brain. *J. Cereb. Blood Flow Metab.* 22, 890–898. doi: 10.1097/00004647-200207000-00014

Parikh, I., Guo, J., Chuang, K. H., Zhong, Y., Rempe, R. G., Hoffman, J. D., et al. (2016). Caloric restriction preserves memory and reduces anxiety of aging mice with early enhancement of neurovascular functions. *Aging* 8, 2814–2826. doi: 10.18632/aging.101094

Park, H. W. (2010). Longevity, aging, and caloric restriction: Clive Maine McCay and the construction of a multidisciplinary research program. *Hist. Stud. Nat. Sci.* 40, 79–124. doi: 10.1525/hsns.2010.40.1.79

Park, S. Y., Choi, G. H., Choi, H. I., Ryu, J., Jung, C. Y., and Lee, W. (2005). Calorie restriction improves whole-body glucose disposal and insulin resistance in association with the increased adipocyte-specific GLUT4 expression in Otsuka Long-Evans Tokushima fatty rats. *Arch. Biochem. Biophys.* 436, 276–284. doi: 10.1016/j.abb.2005.01.010

Perluigi, M., Di Domenico, F., and Butterfield, D. A. (2015). mTOR signaling in aging and neurodegeneration: at the crossroad between metabolism dysfunction and impairment of autophagy. *Neurobiol. Dis.* 84, 39–49. doi: 10.1016/j.nbd.2015.03.014

Rahat, O., Maoz, N., and Cohen, H. Y. (2011). Multiple pathways regulating the calorie restriction response in yeast. *J. Gerontol. A Biol. Sci. Med. Sci.* 66, 163–169. doi: 10.1093/gerona/glq165

Redman, L. M., Smith, S. R., Burton, J. H., Martin, C. K., Il'yasova, D., and Ravussin, E. (2018). Metabolic slowing and reduced oxidative damage with sustained caloric restriction support the rate of living and oxidative damage theories of aging. *Cell Metab.* 27, 805.e4–815.e4. doi: 10.1016/j.cmet.2018.02.019

Reiman, E. M., Caselli, R. J., Chen, K., Alexander, G. E., Bandy, D., and Frost, J. (2001). Declining brain activity in cognitively normal apolipoprotein E epsilon 4 heterozygotes: a foundation for using positron emission tomography to efficiently test treatments to prevent Alzheimer's disease. *Proc. Natl. Acad. Sci. U.S.A.* 98, 3334–3339. doi: 10.1073/pnas.061509598

Reiman, E. M., Chen, K., Alexander, G. E., Caselli, R. J., Bandy, D., Osborne, D., et al. (2004). Functional brain abnormalities in young adults at genetic risk for late-onset Alzheimer's dementia. *Proc. Natl. Acad. Sci. U.S.A.* 101, 284–289. doi: 10.1073/pnas.2635903100

Reiman, E. M., Chen, K., Alexander, G. E., Caselli, R. J., Bandy, D., Osborne, D., et al. (2005). Correlations between apolipoprotein E epsilon4 gene dose and brain-imaging measurements of regional hypometabolism. *Proc. Natl. Acad. Sci. U.S.A.* 102, 8299–8302. doi: 10.1073/pnas.0500579102

Richardson, A., Galvan, V., Lin, A. L., and Oddo, S. (2015). How longevity research can lead to therapies for Alzheimer's disease: the rapamycin story. *Exp. Gerontol.* 68, 51–58. doi: 10.1016/j.exger.2014.12.002

Roy, M., Hennebelle, M., St-Pierre, V., Courchesne-Loyer, A., Fortier, M., Bouzier-Sore, A. K., et al. (2013). Long-term calorie restriction has minimal impact on brain metabolite and fatty acid profiles in aged rats on a Western-style diet. *Neurochem. Int.* 63, 450–457. doi: 10.1016/j.neuint.2013.08.006

Sabatini, D. M., Erdjument-Bromage, H., Lui, M., Tempst, P., and Snyder, S. H. (1994). RAFT1: a mammalian protein that binds to FKBP12 in a rapamycin-dependent fashion and is homologous to yeast TORs. *Cell* 78, 35–43. doi: 10.1016/0092-8674(94)90570-3

Salt, I. P., Johnson, G., Ashcroft, S. J., and Hardie, D. G. (1998). AMP-activated protein kinase is activated by low glucose in cell lines derived from pancreatic beta cells, and may regulate insulin release. *Biochem. J.* 335(Pt 3), 533–539. doi: 10.1042/bj3350533

Sasongko, T. H., Ismail, N. F., and Zabidi-Hussin, Z. (2016). Rapamycin and rapalogs for tuberous sclerosis complex. *Cochrane Database Syst. Rev.* 7:CD011272. doi: 10.1002/14651858.CD011272.pub2

Schafer, M. J., Alldred, M. J., Lee, S. H., Calhoun, M. E., Petkova, E., Mathews, P. M., et al. (2015). Reduction of beta-amyloid and gamma-secretase by calorie restriction in female Tg2576 mice. *Neurobiol. Aging* 36, 1293–1302. doi: 10.1016/j.neurobiolaging.2014.10.043

Sehgal, S. N., Baker, H., and Vezina, C. (1975). Rapamycin (AY-22,989), a new antifungal antibiotic. II. Fermentation, isolation and characterization. *J. Antibiot.* 28, 727–732. doi: 10.7164/antibiotics.28.727

Serkova, N., Litt, L., James, T. L., Sadee, W., Leibfritz, D., Benet, L. Z., et al. (1999). Evaluation of individual and combined neurotoxicity of the immunosuppressants cyclosporine and sirolimus by in vitro multinuclear NMR spectroscopy. *J. Pharmacol. Exp. Ther.* 289, 800–806.

Soefje, S. A., Karnad, A., and Brenner, A. J. (2011). Common toxicities of mammalian target of rapamycin inhibitors. *Target Oncol.* 6, 125–129. doi: 10.1007/s11523-011-0174-9

Spilman, P., Podlutskaya, N., Hart, M. J., Debnath, J., Gorostiza, O., Bredesen, D., et al. (2010). Inhibition of mTOR by rapamycin abolishes cognitive deficits and reduces amyloid-beta levels in a mouse model of Alzheimer's disease. *PLoS One* 5:e9979. doi: 10.1371/journal.pone.0009979

Stanfel, M. N., Shamieh, L. S., Kaeberlein, M., and Kennedy, B. K. (2009). The TOR pathway comes of age. *Biochim. Biophys. Acta* 1790, 1067–1074. doi: 10.1016/j.bbagen.2009.06.007

Subbiah, V., Berry, J., Roxas, M., Guha-Thakurta, N., Subbiah, I. M., Ali, S. M., et al. (2015). Systemic and CNS activity of the RET inhibitor vandetanib combined with the mTOR inhibitor everolimus in KIF5B-RET re-arranged non-small cell lung cancer with brain metastases. *Lung Cancer* 89, 76–79. doi: 10.1016/j.lungcan.2015.04.004

Thambisetty, M., Beason-Held, L., An, Y., Kraut, M. A., and Resnick, S. M. (2010). APOE epsilon4 genotype and longitudinal changes in cerebral blood flow in normal aging. *Arch. Neurol.* 67, 93–98. doi: 10.1001/archneurol.2009.913

Thrasivoulou, C., Soubeyre, V., Ridha, H., Giuliani, D., Giaroni, C., Michael, G. J., et al. (2006). Reactive oxygen species, dietary restriction and neurotrophic factors in age-related loss of myenteric neurons. *Aging Cell* 5, 247–257. doi: 10.1111/j.1474-9726.2006.00214.x

Tillema, J. M., Leach, J. L., Krueger, D. A., and Franz, D. N. (2012). Everolimus alters white matter diffusion in tuberous sclerosis complex. *Neurology* 78, 526–531. doi: 10.1212/WNL.0b013e318247ca8d

Valdez, G., Tapia, J. C., Kang, H., Clemenson, G. D. Jr., Gage, F. H., Lichtman, J. W., et al. (2010). Attenuation of age-related changes in mouse neuromuscular synapses by caloric restriction and exercise. *Proc. Natl. Acad. Sci. U.S.A.* 107, 14863–14868. doi: 10.1073/pnas.1002220107

Van der Auwera, I., Wera, S., Van Leuven, F., and Henderson, S. T. (2005). A ketogenic diet reduces amyloid beta 40 and 42 in a mouse model of Alzheimer's disease. *Nutr. Metab.* 2:28.

Vanitallie, T. B., Nonas, C., Di Rocco, A., Boyar, K., Hyams, K., and Heymsfield, S. B. (2005). Treatment of Parkinson disease with diet-induced hyperketonemia: a feasibility study. *Neurology* 64, 728–730. doi: 10.1212/01.WNL.0000152046.11390.45

Walczyk, T., and Wick, J. Y. (2017). The ketogenic diet: making a comeback. *Consult. Pharm.* 32, 388–396. doi: 10.4140/TCP.n.2017.388

Wang, Z. J., Bergqvist, C., Hunter, J. V., Jin, D., Wang, D. J., Wehrli, S., et al. (2003). In vivo measurement of brain metabolites using two-dimensional double-quantum MR spectroscopy–exploration of GABA levels in a ketogenic diet. *Magn. Reson. Med.* 49, 615–619. doi: 10.1002/mrm.10429

Witte, A. V., Fobker, M., Gellner, R., Knecht, S., and Floel, A. (2009). Caloric restriction improves memory in elderly humans. *Proc. Natl. Acad. Sci. U.S.A.* 106, 1255–1260. doi: 10.1073/pnas.0808587106

Witte, A. V., Kerti, L., Margulies, D. S., and Floel, A. (2014). Effects of resveratrol on memory performance, hippocampal functional connectivity, and glucose metabolism in healthy older adults. *J. Neurosci.* 34, 7862–7870. doi: 10.1523/JNEUROSCI.0385-14.2014

Yang, Q., Guo, M., Wang, X., Zhao, Y., Zhao, Q., Ding, H., et al. (2017). Ischemic preconditioning with a ketogenic diet improves brain ischemic tolerance through increased extracellular adenosine levels and hypoxia-inducible factors. *Brain Res.* 1667, 11–18. doi: 10.1016/j.brainres.2017.04.010

Permissions

All chapters in this book were first published by Frontiers; hereby published with permission under the Creative Commons Attribution License or equivalent. Every chapter published in this book has been scrutinized by our experts. Their significance has been extensively debated. The topics covered herein carry significant findings which will fuel the growth of the discipline. They may even be implemented as practical applications or may be referred to as a beginning point for another development.

The contributors of this book come from diverse backgrounds, making this book a truly international effort. This book will bring forth new frontiers with its revolutionizing research information and detailed analysis of the nascent developments around the world.

We would like to thank all the contributing authors for lending their expertise to make the book truly unique. They have played a crucial role in the development of this book. Without their invaluable contributions this book wouldn't have been possible. They have made vital efforts to compile up to date information on the varied aspects of this subject to make this book a valuable addition to the collection of many professionals and students.

This book was conceptualized with the vision of imparting up-to-date information and advanced data in this field. To ensure the same, a matchless editorial board was set up. Every individual on the board went through rigorous rounds of assessment to prove their worth. After which they invested a large part of their time researching and compiling the most relevant data for our readers.

The editorial board has been involved in producing this book since its inception. They have spent rigorous hours researching and exploring the diverse topics which have resulted in the successful publishing of this book. They have passed on their knowledge of decades through this book. To expedite this challenging task, the publisher supported the team at every step. A small team of assistant editors was also appointed to further simplify the editing procedure and attain best results for the readers.

Apart from the editorial board, the designing team has also invested a significant amount of their time in understanding the subject and creating the most relevant covers. They scrutinized every image to scout for the most suitable representation of the subject and create an appropriate cover for the book.

The publishing team has been an ardent support to the editorial, designing and production team. Their endless efforts to recruit the best for this project, has resulted in the accomplishment of this book. They are a veteran in the field of academics and their pool of knowledge is as vast as their experience in printing. Their expertise and guidance has proved useful at every step. Their uncompromising quality standards have made this book an exceptional effort. Their encouragement from time to time has been an inspiration for everyone.

The publisher and the editorial board hope that this book will prove to be a valuable piece of knowledge for researchers, students, practitioners and scholars across the globe.

List of Contributors

Kang Ko
Department of Neuropsychiatry, Seoul National University Hospital, Seoul, South Korea
Department of Psychiatry, Yonsei University College of Medicine, Seoul, South Korea

Min Soo Byun and Dahyun Yi
Institute of Human Behavioral Medicine, Medical Research Center, Seoul National University, Seoul, South Korea

Jun Ho Lee
Department of Neuropsychiatry, Seoul National University Hospital, Seoul, South Korea
Department of Psychiatry, Seoul National University College of Medicine, Seoul, South Korea

Chan Hyung Kim
Department of Psychiatry, Yonsei University College of Medicine, Seoul, South Korea
Institute of Behavioral Science in Medicine, Yonsei University College of Medicine, Seoul, South Korea

Dong Young Lee
Department of Neuropsychiatry, Seoul National University Hospital, Seoul, South Korea
Institute of Human Behavioral Medicine, Medical Research Center, Seoul National University, Seoul, South Korea
Department of Psychiatry, Seoul National University College of Medicine, Seoul, South Korea

J. J. Chen
Rotman Research Institute, Baycrest, Toronto, ON, Canada
Department of Medical Biophysics, University of Toronto, Toronto, ON, Canada

Elizabeth Head
Department of Pharmacology & Nutritional Sciences, Sanders Brown Center on Aging, University of Kentucky, Lexington, KY, United States

David K. Powell
Magnetic Resonance Imaging and Spectroscopy Center, Sanders Brown Center on Aging, University of Kentucky, Lexington, KY, United States

Frederick A. Schmitt
Department of Neurology, Sanders Brown Center on Aging, University of Kentucky, Lexington, KY, United States

Ruta Nylander, Håkan Ahlström and Elna-Marie Larsson
Department of Surgical Sciences, Radiology, Uppsala University, Uppsala, Sweden

Lena Kilander
Department of Public Health and Caring Sciences, Geriatrics, Uppsala University, Uppsala, Sweden

Lars Lind
Department of Medical Sciences, Uppsala University, Uppsala, Sweden

Bin Wang
College of Computer Science and Technology, Taiyuan University of Technology, Taiyuan, China
Department of Radiology, First Hospital of Shanxi Medical University, Taiyuan, China

Yan Niu, Liwen Miao, Rui Cao, Pengfei Yan, Hao Guo, Dandan Li, Yuxiang Guo and Jie Xiang
College of Computer Science and Technology, Taiyuan University of Technology, Taiyuan, China

Tianyi Yan
School of Life Science, Beijing Institute of Technology, Beijing, China
Key Laboratory of Convergence Medical Engineering System and Healthcare Technology, Ministry of Industry and Information Technology, Beijing Institute of Technology, Beijing, China

Jinglong Wu
Key Laboratory of Biomimetic Robots and Systems, Ministry of Education, Beijing Institute of Technology, Beijing, China
Graduate School of Natural Science and Technology, Okayama University, Okayama, Japan

Hui Zhang
Department of Radiology, First Hospital of Shanxi Medical University, Taiyuan, China

Francesco Cerritelli
Department of Neuroscience, Imaging and Clinical Sciences, Università degli Studi G. d'Annunzio Chieti e Pescara, Chieti, Italy
Institute for Advanced Biomedical Technologies (ITAB), Università degli Studi G. d'Annunzio Chieti e Pescara, Chieti, Italy
Clinical-Based Human Research Department—C.O.M.E. Collaboration ONLUS, Pescara, Italy

Piero Chiacchiaretta, Giovanna Bubbico, Mauro Gianni Perrucci and Antonio Ferretti
Department of Neuroscience, Imaging and Clinical Sciences, Università degli Studi G. d'Annunzio Chieti e Pescara, Chieti, Italy
Institute for Advanced Biomedical Technologies (ITAB), Università degli Studi G. d'Annunzio Chieti e Pescara, Chieti, Italy

Bryan J. Neth and Suzanne Craft
Department of Internal Medicine, Section on Gerontology and Geriatric Medicine, Wake Forest School of Medicine, Winston-Salem, NC, United States

Jason A. Brandon, Brandon C. Farmer, Holden C. Williams and Lance A. Johnson
Department of Physiology, University of Kentucky, Lexington, KY, United States

Scott W. Thalman
F. Joseph Halcomb III, Department of Biomedical Engineering, University of Kentucky, Lexington, KY, United States
Sanders-Brown Center on Aging, University of Kentucky, Lexington, KY, United States

David K. Powell
F. Joseph Halcomb III, Department of Biomedical Engineering, University of Kentucky, Lexington, KY, United States
Magnetic Resonance Imaging and Spectroscopy Center, University of Kentucky, Lexington, KY, United States

Margo Ubele
Sanders-Brown Center on Aging, University of Kentucky, Lexington, KY, United States

Christopher M. Norris
Sanders-Brown Center on Aging, University of Kentucky, Lexington, KY, United States
Department of Pharmacology and Nutritional Sciences, University of Kentucky, Lexington, KY, United States

Elizabeth Head
Department of Pathology and Laboratory Medicine, University of California, Irvine, Irvine, CA, United States
University of California Irvine Institute for Memory Impairments and Neurological Disorders (UCI MIND), University of California, Irvine, Irvine, CA, United States

Katherine J. Bangen, Alexandra J. Weigand and Emily C. Edmonds
Research Service, VA San Diego Healthcare System, San Diego, CA, United States
Department of Psychiatry, University of California, San Diego, San Diego, CA, United States

Ai-Ling Lin
F. Joseph Halcomb III, Department of Biomedical Engineering, University of Kentucky, Lexington, KY, United States
Sanders-Brown Center on Aging, University of Kentucky, Lexington, KY, United States
Department of Pharmacology and Nutritional Sciences, University of Kentucky, Lexington, KY, United States
Department of Neuroscience, University of Kentucky, Lexington, KY, United States

David J. Braun
Sanders-Brown Center on Aging, University of Kentucky, Lexington, KY, United States

Linda J. Van Eldik
Sanders-Brown Center on Aging, University of Kentucky, Lexington, KY, United States
Spinal Cord and Brain Injury Research Center, University of Kentucky, Lexington, KY, United States
Department of Neuroscience, University of Kentucky, Lexington, KY, United States

Madeleine L. Werhane and Alexandra L. Clark
Department of Psychiatry, University of California, San Diego, San Diego, CA, United States
Department of Psychology, San Diego State University, San Diego, CA, United States

Lisa Delano-Wood, Kelsey R. Thomas and Mark W. Bondi
Department of Psychiatry, University of California, San Diego, San Diego, CA, United States
Psychology Service, VA San Diego Healthcare System, San Diego, CA, United States

Daniel A. Nation
Department of Psychology, University of Southern California, Los Angeles, CA, United States

Nicole D. Evangelista
Research Service, VA San Diego Healthcare System, San Diego, CA, United States

Thomas T. Liu
Department of Radiology and Bioengineering, University of California, San Diego, San Diego, CA, United States

Anika M. S. Hartz
Sanders-Brown Center on Aging, University of Kentucky, Lexington, KY, United States
Department of Pharmacology and Nutritional Sciences, University of Kentucky, Lexington, KY, United States

Yu Zhong, Andrew N. Shen and Erin L. Abner
Sanders-Brown Center on Aging, University of Kentucky, Lexington, KY, United States

Björn Bauer
Department of Pharmaceutical Sciences, College of Pharmacy, University of Kentucky, Lexington, KY, United States

Brittani R. Price, Donna M. Wilcock and Erica M. Weekman
Department of Physiology, Sanders-Brown Center on Aging, University of Kentucky, Lexington, KY, United States

Scott W. Thalman
F. Joseph Halcomb III, MD Department of Biomedical Engineering, University of Kentucky, Lexington, KY, United States
Sanders-Brown Center on Aging, University of Kentucky, Lexington, KY, United States

David K. Powell
F. Joseph Halcomb III, MD Department of Biomedical Engineering, University of Kentucky, Lexington, KY, United States
Magnetic Resonance Imaging and Spectroscopy Center, University of Kentucky, Lexington, KY, United States

Ai-Ling Lin
F. Joseph Halcomb III, MD Department of Biomedical Engineering, University of Kentucky, Lexington, KY, United States
Magnetic Resonance Imaging and Spectroscopy Center, University of Kentucky, Lexington, KY, United States
Department of Pharmacology and Nutritional Sciences, University of Kentucky, Lexington, KY, United States
Department of Neuroscience, University of Kentucky, Lexington, KY, United States

Andrée-Anne Berthiaume, David A. Hartmann and Narayan R. Bhat
Department of Neuroscience, Medical University of South Carolina, Charleston, SC, United States

Mark W. Majesky
Center for Developmental Biology and Regenerative Medicine, Seattle Children's Research Institute, Seattle, WA, United States
Departments of Pediatrics and Pathology, University of Washington, Seattle, WA, United States

Andy Y. Shih
Department of Neuroscience, Medical University of South Carolina, Charleston, SC, United States
Center for Developmental Biology and Regenerative Medicine, Seattle Children's Research Institute, Seattle, WA, United States
Center for Biomedical Imaging, Medical University of South Carolina, Charleston, SC, United States

Helene Benveniste and Hedok Lee
Department of Anesthesiology, Yale School of Medicine, Yale University, New Haven, CT, United States

Gerald Dienel
Department of Neurology, University of Arkansas for Medical Sciences, Little Rock, AR, United States
Department of Cell Biology and Physiology, University of New Mexico, Albuquerque, NM, United States

Zvi Jacob and Rany Makaryus
Department of Anesthesiology, Stony Brook University, Stony Brook, NY, United States

Albert Gjedde
Department of Translational Neurobiology, University of Southern Denmark, Odense, Denmark

Fahmeed Hyder and Douglas L. Rothman
Department of Biomedical Engineering & Radiology and Biomedical Imaging, Yale School of Medicine, Yale University, New Haven, CT, United States

Ryan A. Cloyd
Department of Physiology, University of Kentucky, Lexington, KY, United States
College of Medicine, University of Kentucky, Lexington, KY, United States
Sanders-Brown Center on Aging, University of Kentucky, Lexington, KY, United States

Shon A. Koren
Department of Physiology, University of Kentucky, Lexington, KY, United States
Sanders-Brown Center on Aging, University of Kentucky, Lexington, KY, United States
Department of Neuroscience & Center for Translational Research in Neurodegenerative Disease University of Florida, Gainesville, FL, United States

Jose F. Abisambra
Department of Physiology, University of Kentucky, Lexington, KY, United States
Sanders-Brown Center on Aging, University of Kentucky, Lexington, KY, United States
Department of Neuroscience & Center for Translational Research in Neurodegenerative Disease, University of Florida, Gainesville, FL, United States
Spinal Cord and Brain Injury Research Center, University of Kentucky, Lexington, KY, United States

Xiao-Hong Zhu and Wei Chen
Center for Magnetic Resonance Research (CMRR), Department of Radiology, School of Medicine, University of Minnesota, Minneapolis, MN, United States

Jennifer Lee, David Ma and Ishita Parikh
Sanders-Brown Center on Aging, University of Kentucky, Lexington, KY, United States

Lucille M. Yanckello, Jared D. Hoffman and Anika M. S. Hartz
Sanders-Brown Center on Aging, University of Kentucky, Lexington, KY, United States
Department of Pharmacology and Nutritional Science, University of Kentucky, Lexington, KY, United States

Scott Thalman
F. Joseph Halcomb III, M.D. Department of Biomedical Engineering, University of Kentucky, Lexington, KY, United States

Bjoern Bauer
Department of Pharmaceutical Sciences, University of Kentucky, Lexington, KY, United States

Fahmeed Hyder
Departments of Radiology and Biomedical Engineering, Magnetic Resonance Research Center, Yale University, New Haven, CT, United States

Ai-Ling Lin
Sanders-Brown Center on Aging, University of Kentucky, Lexington, KY, United States
Department of Pharmacology and Nutritional Science, University of Kentucky, Lexington, KY, United States
F. Joseph Halcomb III, M.D. Department of Biomedical Engineering, University of Kentucky, Lexington, KY, United States

Index

www.ingramcontent.com/pod-product-compliance
Lightning Source LLC
LaVergne TN
LVHW060517210926
848485LV00005B/1094
9781639279425